TO A REAL
PROFESSIONAL
AND
GOOD FRIEND
Alan M. Markham
7/29/93

Accidental Injury

Biomechanics and Prevention

Alan M. Nahum   John W. Melvin

Editors

Accidental Injury

Biomechanics and Prevention

With 288 Figures

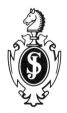

Springer-Verlag

New York Berlin Heidelberg London Paris
Tokyo Hong Kong Barcelona Budapest

Alan M. Nahum
University of California at San Diego
    School of Medicine
La Jolla, CA 92093, USA

John W. Melvin
Biomedical Science Department
General Motors Research Laboratories
Warren, MI 48090, USA

Library of Congress Cataloging-in-Publication Data
Accidental injury : biomechanics and prevention / Alan Nahum, John
   Melvin (editors).
          p.   cm.
   Includes bibliographical references and index.
   ISBN 0-387-97881-X. — ISBN 3-540-97881-X
   1. Crash injuries—Physiological aspects. 2. Wounds and injuries.
3. Human mechanics. I. Nahum, Alan M., 1931–   . II. Melvin,
John.
   [DNLM: 1. Biomechanics. 2. Wounds and Injuries—prevention &
control.   WO 700 A1714]
RD96.6.A23 1993
617.1′028—dc20
DNLM/DLC
for Library of Congress   92-2381

Printed on acid-free paper.

Production managed by Terry Kornak. Manufacturing supervised by Jacqui Ashri.
Typeset by Best-set, Chaiwan, Hong Kong.
Printed and bound by Edwards Brothers Inc., Ann Arbor, MI.
Printed in the United States of America.

9 8 7 6 5 4 3 2 1

ISBN 0-387-97881-X Springer-Verlag New York Berlin Heidelberg
ISBN 3-540-97881-X Springer-Verlag Berlin Heidelberg New York

To Julie, David, Bob, and Victoria, whose love and support make all things possible.

Preface

Writing on accidental injury often seems to occur from one of two perspectives. One perspective is that of those involved in aspects of injury diagnosis and treatment and the other is that of those in the engineering and biologic sciences who discuss mechanical principles and simulations.

From our point of view, significant information problems exist at the interface: Persons in the business of diagnosis and treatment do not know how to access, use, and evaluate theoretical information that does not have obvious practical applications; persons on the theoretical side do not have enough real-life field data with which to identify problems or to evaluate solutions.

The ideal system provides a constant two-way flow of data that permits continuous problem identification and course correction.

This book attempts to provide a state-of-the-art look at the applied biomechanics of accidental-injury causation and prevention. The authors are recognized authorities in their specialized fields.

It is hoped that this book will stimulate more applied research in the field of accidental-injury causation and prevention.

Alan M. Nahum
John W. Melvin

Contents

Contributors

Douglas "L" Allsop, Collision Safety Engineering, Inc., Orem, UT 84058, USA

John M. Cavanaugh, Bioengineering Center, Wayne State University, Detroit, MI, 48202 USA

Richard F. Chandler, Protection and Survival Research, FAA Civil Aeromedical Institute, Oklahoma City, OK, USA

C. C. Chou, Alpha Simultaneous Engineering, Ford Motor Co., Detroit, MI, USA

Charles P. Compton, Transportation Data Center, University of Michigan Transportation Research Institute, Ann Arbor, MI 48109-2150, USA

Jeffrey C. Elias, Transportation Research, Inc., East Liberty, OH 43319, USA

Rolf Eppinger, Biomechanics Division, NHTSA, Washington, DC 20590, USA

Elizabeth Frankenburg, Orthopaedic Surgery Department University of Michigan Medical School, Ann Arbor, MI 48109, USA

Y. C. Fung, Professor Emeritus of Bioengineering, University of California, San Diego, La Jolla, CA 92037, USA

Steven Goldstein, Orthopaedic Surgery Department, University of Michigan Medical School, Ann Arbor, MI 48109, USA

Warren N. Hardy, Bioengineering Center, Wayne State University, Detroit, MI 48202, USA

Roger C. Haut, College of Osteopathic Medicine, Michigan State University, East Lansing, MI 48824, USA

Albert I. King, Bioengineering Center, Wayne State University, Detroit, MI 48202, USA

Janet Kuhn, Orthopaedic Surgery Department, University of Michigan Medical School, Ann Arbor, MI 48109, USA

Robert Levine, Division of Orthopedics, Wayne State University, Bloomfield Hills, MI 48013, USA

James W. Lighthall, Biomedical Sciences Department, General Motors Research Laboratory, Warren, MI 48202, USA

Thomas F. MacLaughlin, S.E.A. Inc. 7349 Worthington-Galena Rd., Columbus, OH 43085, USA

James H. McElhaney, Biomedical Engineering Department, Duke University, Durham, NC 27706, USA

John W. Melvin, Biomedical Science Department, General Motors Research Laboratories, Warren, MI 48202, USA

Harold J. Mertz, Injury Assessment Technology, Safety and Crashworthiness Systems, General Motors Corporation, Warren, MI 48202, USA

Barry S. Myers, Division of Orthopaedics, Duke University Medical Center, Durham, NC 27706, USA

James A. Newman, Biokinetics & Associates Ltd., Ottawa, Canada

Mini N. Pathria, Department of Radiology, University of California at San Diego Medical Center, San Diego, CA 92110 USA

Priya Prasad, Advanced Vehicle Engineering and Technology, Ford Motor Co., Detroit, MI, USA

Donald Resnick, Department of Radiology, Veterans Administration Medical Center, San Diego, CA 92110

Stephen W. Rouhana, General Motors Research Labs, Warren, MI 48202, USA

C. Brian Tanner, Transportation Research, Inc., East Liberty, OH 43319, USA

Lawrence E. Thibault, Department of Bioengineering, University of Pennsylvania, Philadelphia, PA 19104, USA

Kazunari Ueno, Biomedical Science Department, General Motors Research Laboratories, Warren, MI 48202, USA

Kathleen Weber, Child Passenger Protection, University of Michigan Medical School, Bloomfield Hills, MI 48109, USA

David S. Zuby, Transportation Research, Inc., East Liberty, OH 43319, USA

1
The Application of Biomechanics to the Understanding of Injury and Healing

Y.C. Fung

Introduction

In this chapter, I will first consider the mechanics of organ and tissue injury and then go on to discuss the mechanics of tissue growth and resorption. The former is relevant to understanding accidents and to engineering designs to avoid accidental injury; the latter is relevant to treatment, healing, repair, recovery, and rehabilitation. Tissue injury, repair, and growth are all related to physical stress; that is why mechanics is important. The body's response to physical stress is biology. The computation involved in learning how large the stress is mechanics. The design of vehicles or equipment to impose proper stress or to avoid excessive stress is engineering. Mechanics connects engineering to medical arts. The more we know mechanics, the better the job we can do at both ends.

Stress Is the Main Parameter to Consider in Trying to Understand Trauma

Since not all the readers of this book are engineers, and since the lawyer's, psychologist's or physician's concept of stress and strain may be quite different from that of the engineer's, I will begin this chapter with an explanation of terminology.

Trauma to a person is equivalent to the failure of a machine or a structure. Genera-

tions of engineers have studied the failure of machines and structures, and they have come to the conclusion that everything depends on stress. Every material has a critical value of stress below which it is "safe," and above which it "fails." An external load causes stress everywhere in a structure. The safety of the structure is judged by the stress at every point relative to the strength of the material. The safety of the structure is determined by the weakest link. If the critical stress is exceeded at the weakest spot, then the whole structure may be considered failed, seriously or otherwise. Engineers can design structures against failure. A person has to live with the structure he has. So a person has to understand the stress in one's body under traumatic circumstances.

Stress as a Quantity Needs Six Numbers to Specify It

Consider a little cube of material in one's body, as shown in Fig. 1.1A. The cube has six faces. On face No. 1, which is perpendicular to the X_1 coordinate axis, three forces act: one is perpendicular to the surface and acts in the X_1-axis direction. Another one is parallel to the surface and acts in the direction of the X_2 axis. The third one is also parallel to the surface but acts in the direction of the X_3 axis. Dividing these forces by the area of the surface, we obtain three numbers, T_{11}, T_{12}, T_{13}. T_{11} is called a *normal stress*. T_{12} and T_{13} are called

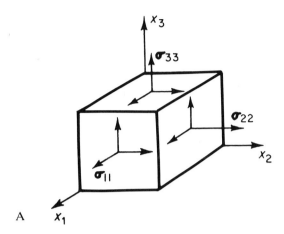

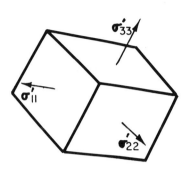

FIGURE 1.1. (A) Stress is force per unit area acting on a surface. The component perpendicular to the surface is normal stress. The components tangential to the surface is shear stress. On a small cube, each face has three stresses acting on it. (B) At any point in a body, one can find a set of principal axes. If we imagine isolating a little cube oriented in the principal direction, then on each face there acts only one stress: the normal, principal stress.

shear stresses. T_{11}, T_{12}, and T_{13} have the units of force per unit area. In the English system we measure stresses in *pounds per square inch*. In the *International System of Units* (SI Units) stresses are expressed in *Newtons per square meter*. One pound per square inch is equal to 6,894 Newtons per square meter. One Newton per square meter is also said to be one *Pascal*. It is so named internationally in honor of Louis Pascal.

Similarly, on surface No. 2, which is perpendicular to the X_2 axis, there act three stresses, T_{21}, T_{22}, and T_{33}, as shown in Fig. 1.1. On surface No. 3, which is perpendicular to the X_3 axis, there are three stresses, T_{31}, T_{32}, and T_{33}. On the other three surfaces, perpendicular to the negative X_1 axis, negative X_2 axis, negative X_3 axis, the stresses are respectively the same as those acting on the surfaces perpendicular to the positive X_1, X_2, and X_3 axes. Thus, the stresses acting in the little cube can be listed in a matrix, as below:

	Components of stresses		
	1	2	3
Surface normal to X_1	T_{11}	T_{12}	T_{13}
Surface normal to X_2	T_{21}	T_{22}	T_{23}
Surface normal to X_3	T_{31}	T_{32}	T_{33}

The whole table specifies the state of stress in the little cube. Hence at every point in a body, where such a cube can be drawn, there are nine components of stresses. Fortunately, it can be shown that the three pairs of shear stresses are always equal:

$$T_{12} = T_{21}, \quad T_{23} = T_{32}, \quad T_{31} = T_{13}$$

Therefore, at every point, there are six independent components of stresses. Thus stress is a quantity that needs six numbers (components) to describe it at every point.

It can be shown that at any given point in a body, one can find a certain orientation of the cube on whose surfaces all the shear stresses are zero. (See Fig. 1.1B.) In such a so-called *principal orientation*, the stress components listed as a matrix appear as

	Principal stresses		
	1	2	3
Surface ⊥ principal direction 1	T_{11}	0	0
Surface ⊥ principal direction 2	0	T_{22}	0
Surface ⊥ principal direction 3	0	0	T_{33}

Then the components of stresses T_{11}, T_{22}, and T_{33} are called *principal stresses*. To describe the state of stress at any point in a body by the principal stresses, one must specify also the principal directions. Hence one still need six numbers to describe the stress.

Conclusion: Stress is a quantity that needs six numbers to specify it. The six numbers can be the six components of the stress, or the three principal stresses together with three angles that describe the orientation of the principal axes.

When a Load Hits a Person, the Stress in the Person Depends on how Fast the Body Material Moves

The impact load that may cause injury to a person frequently comes as a moving mass (e.g., a bullet, a flying object, a car), or as an obstruction to a moving person (e.g., falling to the ground, running into a tree). The impact causes the material of the human body in con-

tact with the load to move relative to the rest of the body. The initial velocity induced in the body material particles that come into contact with the load has a decisive influence on the stress distribution in the body following the impact. This velocity can be supersonic, transonic, subsonic, or so slow as to be almost static. The body reacts differently to these speeds. This is of central importance to the understanding of trauma, and is explained below.

If a load comes like a bullet from a gun, it sets up a shock wave. The shock wave will move in a person's body with a speed faster than the speed of sound in the body. At supersonic speed, the shock wave carries energy that is concentrated at the shock-wave front. Thus in a thin layer in the body, a great concentration of strain energy exists, which has a high potential for injury. This is analogous to the sonic boom coming from a supersonic airplane. People are familiar with the window-

TABLE 1.1. Velocity of sound in various tissues, air, and water.

Tissue	Density (g/cm³)	TPP[a] (kPa)	Sound speed mean ± S.D. (m/sec)	Reference
Muscle	1		1,580	Ludwig (1950), Frucht (1953),von Gierke (1964)
Fat	1		1,450	Ludwig (1950), Frucht (1953)
Bone	2.0		3,500	Clemedson and Jönsson (1962)
Collapsed lung	0.4		650 (ultrasound)	Dunn and Fry (1961)
Collapsed lung pneumonitis	0.8		320 (ultrasound)	Dunn and Fry (1961)
Lung, horse	0.6		25	Rice (1983)
Lung, horse	0.125		70	Rice (1983)
Lung, calf			24–30	Clemedson and Jönsson (1962)
Lung, goat		0	31.4 ± 0.4	Yen et al. (1986)
		0.5	33.9 ± 2.3	
		1.0	36.1 ± 1.9	
		1.5	46.8 ± 1.8	
		2.0	64.7 ± 3.9	
Lung, rabbit		0	16.5 ± 2.4	Yen et al. (1986)
		0.4	28.9 ± 3.3	
		0.8	31.3 ± 0.9	
		1.2	35.3 ± 0.8	
		1.6	36.9 ± 1.7	
Air			340	Dunn and Fry (1961)
Water, distilled, 0°C			1,407	Kaye and Labby (1960)
Air bubbles (45% by vol) in glycerol and H₂O			20	Campbell and Pitcher (1958)

[a] TPP = Transpulmonary pressure = airway pressure − pleural pressure; $1 kPa = 10^3 N/m^2 \sim 10.2 cm$ H_2O

shaking, roof-shattering thunder of the sonic booms. In these booms the shock energy of the airplane is transmitted down to the house. Similarly, the shock wave created by a load that hits at a supersonic load can cause damage to a human body. A fast-moving blunt load that does not penetrate can nevertheless cause shock-wave damage.

If the body material moves at a transonic or subsonic velocity, stress waves will move in the body at sonic speed. These stress waves can focus themselves into a small area and cause concentrated damage in that area. They can also be reflected at the border of organs and cause greater damage in the reflection process.

The complex phenomena of shock- and elastic-wave reflection, refraction, interference, and focusing are made more complex in the human body by the fact that different organs have different sound speed, as listed in Table 1.1 (from Fung,[1] 1990, in which original references are listed). It is seen from this table that the cortical bone has a sound speed of 3,500 m/sec. This may be compared with the sound speed of 4,800 m/sec in steel, aluminum, copper, etc. The speed of elastic waves in the lung is of the order of 30–45 m/sec.[2] This is much lower than the sound speed in the air, almost ten times slower. The lung has such a low sound speed is because it has a gas-filled, foamy structure. Roughly speaking, the lung tissue has the elasticity of the gas and mass of the tissue. Sound speed being proportional to the square root of elastic modulus divided by the mass density, the lowering of sound speed by the tissue mass is understandable. The lung structure is so complex that several types of stress waves can exist. Table 1.1 lists several sound speeds in the lung. The speeds given by Yen et al.[2] (1986) were measured from the lungs of man, cat, and rabbit under impact pressures and wall velocities comparable with those induced by shock waves of an air blast (e.g., due to a bomb explosion, or a gun fired not too far away, or a gasoline tank explosion). The wave speeds found by Yen et al. depend on the transpulmonary pressure of the lung (i.e., on how large the lung is inflated) and the animal species. The sound speed given by Rice[3] (1983) was measured by a microphone

picking up to a sound made by an electric spark. The speed given by Dunn and Fry[4] (1961) was measured by ultrasound waves, which appear to be quite different from the waves measured by Yen et al. and Rice.

At an impact speed like that of an automobile in city driving, vibrations can be induced in the external or internal organs of the passenger or driver, resulting in a dynamic stress higher than the stress that would have existed if the load were applied statically.

Finally, a force may be applied very slowly, as if it were in a steady-state or static condition. Material at every point in the body responds to the static load with a static stress.

In general, for the same force, the stress induced in the body is the smallest if it is applied very slowly. The stress will generally be larger when the rate at which the load is applied is increased. As the rate increases, first the induced vibration may cause additional stress. Then the elastic waves may cause stress concentration. The spatial distribution of stress is different in static, vibratory, and elastic wave regimes.

In the following section we shall discuss the strength of the materials, i.e., the maximum stress a material can bear without failure. It will be seen that the strength depends on the rate of change of strain. Therefore, the effects of the speed of loading are twofold: the strain rate influences the maximum stress induced by the impact, and it influences the strength of the material. Thus the limit of safety, defined by having the maximum stress staying below the critical limit of strength, depends on the rate of loading.

The Strength of A Tissue or Organ Is Expressed by a Tolerable Stress, Which May Vary with the Condition with Which the Load Is Applied

We spoke in the preceding section about the stresses induced in the tissues and organs due to an external load. Now let us consider the

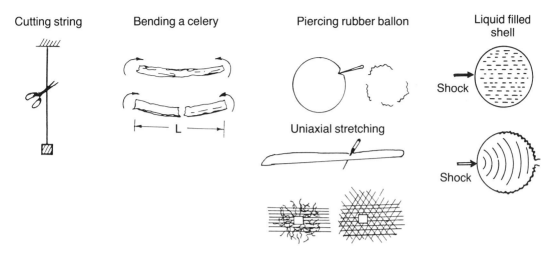

FIGURE 1.2. Several experiments demonstrating that the meaning of the term "strength" depends on the type of stress, whether it is uniaxial, biaxial, or triaxial. Strength also depends on the fluid content of a tissue, or whether a body contains fluid or not, and or whether elastic and shock waves cause concentration of stress, or propagating kinetic energy away by elastic waves. The rate of change of strain affects the critical stress at which rupture occurs. From Fung.[1] Reproduced by permission.

strength of the tissues and organs in greater detail. We have to define strength and tolerance very carefully, because they depend on what we mean by failure. Careful experiments and definitions of injury will be described in the remainder of this book, organ by organ, and tissue by tissue. In this chapter I will discuss only the general concepts.

To discuss strength, failure, and tolerance, let us consider first the simple experiments shown in Fig. 1.2:

1. A piece of twine is to be cut by a pair of dull scissors. I have difficulty cutting it when the twine is relaxed. But if I pull it tight and then cut it, it breaks easily. Why?
2. A stalk of fresh celery breaks very easily in bending. An old, dehydrated one does not. Practice on carrots, also!
3. A balloon is inflated. Another is not inflated but is stretched to a great length. Prick them with a needle. One explodes. The other does not. Why?
4. A thin-walled metal tube is filled with a liquid. Strike it on one side. Sometimes the shell fails on the other side. This is known as *contre coup*. How can this happen?
5. Take a small nylon ball, or a pearl, or a ball

bearing, and throw it onto a hard surface. It bounces. Throw it onto a thin metal plate such as that used in the kitchen for baking, and it won't bounce.

We can explain the first example by computing the maximum principal stress in the string due to the action of shear and the pulling. Pulling the string taut increases the maximum principal stresses. When a limit is exceeded, the string breaks.

In the second example, the specimen fails by bending. The bending stress in the fibers of the celery is higher in the fresh and plump celery, lower in the dehydrated specimen.

To explain the phenomenon shown in the third example, we have to think of the long-chain molecules of the rubber membrane. These molecules or fibers are bent and twisted randomly in every direction. When the balloon is inflated, fibers in every direction are stretched taut. A prick of the pin breaks fibers in every direction passing through the hole, and the membrane breaks with an explosion. On the other hand, when the rubber membrane is stretched uniaxially, only the fibers in the direction of the stretching are pulled taut.

Those in other directions are still relaxed. The pin prick breaks only the fibers in one direction; those in other directions remain intact. Hence no explosion.

The fourth example shows what focusing of stress waves can do. The compression wave in the fluid initiated by the impact moves to the right. The flexural wave of the metal shell also moves to the right along the curved surface of the tube wall. If the flexural wave and the compression wave arrive at the other side simultaneously, a concentration of stress may occur that may exceed the ultimate stress of the materials and cause fracture on the far side. This may occur in head injury.

There are many biological analogs of these examples. Altogether they tell us that in answering questions of strength and tolerance, we must consider the magnitude of the maximum principal stress, the rate at which the stress varies with time in a material, the molecular configuration of the material, which depends on the nature of the stress, whether it is uniaxial, biaxial, or triaxial; and the stress waves around the point of concern in the material. The fourth example shows that the stress concentration due to the elastic waves may result in a weakness. In all cases, however, for safety, the focus of attention is on stress.

In summary, we have explained that the stress in the body in response to external force depends on the speed at which the force is applied onto the human body. In making a stress analysis, we first obtain the static stress distribution in the body under the external load (e.g., the inertia force due to deceleration of a car), then determine the dynamic amplification due to vibrations, then assess the stress concentration due to elastic waves and shock waves.

We see that the strength of an organ or a tissue in our body depends not only on the magnitude of the stress, static or dynamic, but also on the type of the stress: whether it is uniaxial, biaxial, or triaxial.

In sections following, we consider in greater detail the meaning of the strength of material relative to *injury*, *repair*, *growth*, and *resorption*.

Injury of Organs and Tissues

In human society, the concept of injury is largely subjective. To bring some order into this subjective world, objective clinical observations and tests are desirable, but not necessarily easy. For example, consider head injury. The brain can be injured by fracture, impingement, excessively high localized pressure or tensile stress, high localized shear stress and strain, and cavitation in high-tension regions. The regions where the maximum normal stress occurs are usually different from where the maximum shear stress occurs; and they are affected significantly by the flow through foramen magnum (opening at the base of the skull) during impact. The brain tissue can be contused and blood vessels may be ruptured.

A well-known trauma is brain *concussion*, which is defined as a clinical syndrome characterized by immediate transient impairment of neural function, such as loss of consciousness, and disturbances of vision and equilibrium due to mechanical forces. Normally, concussion does not cause permanent damage. It is the first functional impairment of the brain to occur as the severity of head impact increases. It is reproducible in experimental animals. It has been studied with respect to rotational acceleration and flexion-extension of the upper cervical cord during motion of the head-neck junction.

Logically, one could correlate lesions, immunochemical changes, and neurological observations with the stress in the brain. But today, a thorough correlation still does not exist. There are a number of difficulties. First of all, the evaluation of stress distribution in the brain is difficult. Not only is the computation of stress distribution in a specific boundary-value problem difficult, but the identification of the boundary conditions in known automobile collisions or aircraft accidents is nearly impossible today. And the neurological data that must be correlated with the stress distribution have not yet been collected in controlled experiments. Obviously the situation calls for an extensive basic-research program. Without true understanding headway cannot be made. This has been the situation for three decades. Researchers know how to proceed but support has not been forthcoming.

Brain injury is perhaps the most difficult problem in trauma research, and the most important because of its prevalence. Injury to other organs, e.g., fracture of bone, sprain of a tendon, bursting of an aneurysm of aorta, etc., is more tractable. Each organ has its own characteristics. Subsequent chapters of this book will deal with various organs. In understanding these chapters, the two concepts discussed in the preceding sections, namely, the rate of application of the load (static, subsonic, or supersonic), and the type of the critical stress, (uniaxial, biaxial, or triaxial) are important. They play roles in the mechanism of injury.

A recent publication edited by Woo and Buckwalter[5] presents a detailed discussion of injury and repair of the musculoskeletal soft tissues, including tendon, ligament, bone-tendon and myotendinous junctions, skeletal muscle, peripheral nerve, peripheral blood vessel, articular cartilage, and meniscus. A detailed mechanical analysis of vibration and amplification and elastic waves is presented in the author's book.[1] The trauma of the lung due to impact load and the cause of subsequent edema are examined in detail in Fung.[1] Existing data on the tolerance of organs to impact loads are quite extensive. See References at end of chapter 12, ref. 1. The book edited by Nahum and Melvin,[6] a predecessor of the present volume, presents an extensive current view on this subject.

Biomechanical Analysis

In assessing human tolerance of impact loads and in designing vehicles for crashworthiness, it is necessary to calculate the stress and strain at specific points in various organs, and this is best done by mathematical modeling. Through mathematical modeling, one can connect pieces of information on anatomy, physiology, and clinical observations with people, vehicle,

and accident. A validated model can then become a foundation of engineering.

Biomechanical modeling is being developed vigorously. A selected bibliography is given in Fung.[1]

Healing and Rehabilitation Are Helped by Proper Stress

Living organisms are endowed with a certain ability to heal when damaged. Orthopedic surgeons were the first to pay attention to the role played by biomechanics in the healing of bone fracture. In 1866, G.H. Meyer[7] presented a paper on the structure of cancellous bone and demonstrated that "the spongiosa showed a well-motivated architecture which is closely connected with the statics of bone." A mathematician, C. Culmann,[8] was in the audience. In 1867, Culmann presented Meyer a drawing of the principal stress trajectories on a curved beam similar to a human femur. The similarity between the principal stress trajectories and the trabecular lines of the cancellous bone is remarkable. In 1869, J. Wolff[9] claimed that there is a perfect mathematical correspondence between the structure of cancellous bone in the proximal end of the femur and the trajectories in Culmann's crane. In 1880, W. Roux[10] introduced the idea of "functional adaptation." A strong line of research followed Roux. Pauwels,[11,12] beginning in his paper in 1935 and culminating in his book of 1965, which was translated into English in 1980, turned these thoughts to precise and practical arts of surgery. Vigorous development continues. In the 1980s, Carter[13] and his associates have published a hypothesis about the relationship between stress and calcification of the cartilage into bone. Cowin[14] and his associates have developed a mathematical theory of Wolff's law. Fukada,[15] Yasuda,[16] Bassett,[17] Salzstein and Pollack,[18] and others have studied piezoelectricity of bone and developed the use of electromagnetic waves to assist healing of bone fracture. E.J. Lund,[19] R. Becker,[20] S.D. Smith,[21] and others have studied the effect of electric field on the growth of cells and on the growth of amputated limb of frog. Recently, the biology of bone cells is advancing rapidly, and molecular biological transformation of muscle into bone has been announced.

Thus both the motivation and the knowledge and art of providing a suitable stress to the bone and cartilage to promote healing and rehabilitation are clear and advancing rapidly.

Remodeling of Soft Tissues in Response to Stress Changes

The best-known example of soft-tissue re-modeling due to change of stress is the hyper-trophy of the heart caused by a rise in blood pressure. Another famous example was given by Cowan and Crystal,[22] who showed that when one lung of a rabbit was excised, the remaining lung expanded to fill the thoracic cavity, and it grew until it weighed approxi-mately the initial weight of both lungs.

On the other hand, animals exposed to the weightless condition of space flight have demonstrated skeletal muscle atrophy.[1] Leg volumes of astronauts are diminished in flight.[1] In-flight vigorous daily exercise is necessary to keep astronauts in good physical fitness over a longer period of time.[1]

Immobilization of muscle causes atrophy. But there is a marked difference between stretched immobilized muscle vs. muscle immobilized in the resting or shortened posi-tion. Fundamentally, growth is a cell-biological phenomenon at molecular level. Stress and strain keep the cells in a certain specific con-figuration. Since growth depends on cell con-figuration, it depends on stress and strain.

How fast do soft tissues remodel when stress is changed? To find out, Dr. S.Q. Liu and I did an experiment.[23] We created high blood pressure in rat's lung by putting rats in a low-oxygen chamber. The chamber's oxygen con-centration is about the same as that at the Continental Divide of the Rocky Mountains in Colorado, about 12,000 ft. Nitrogen is added so that the total pressure is the same as the atmospheric pressure at sea level. When a rat enters such a chamber, its systolic blood pressure in the lung will shoot up from the normal 15 mm Hg to 22 mm Hg within minutes, and maintain in the elevated pressure of 22 mm Hg for a week, then gradually rise to 30 mm Hg in a month. (The systemic blood pressure remains essentially unchanged in the mean-time.) Under such a step rise in blood pressure in the lung, the pulmonary blood vessel remodels. To examine the change, a rat is taken out of the chamber at a scheduled time. It was anesthetized immediately by an intra-peritoneal injection of pentobarbital sodium according to a procedure and dosage approved by the University, NIH, and Department of Agriculture, and then dissected according to an approved protocol. The specimens were fixed first in glutaraldehyde, then in osmium tetraoxide, embedded in Medcast resin, stained with toluidine blue O, and examined by light microscopy.

Figure 1.3 shows how fast the remodeling proceeds. In this figure, the photographs in each row refers to a segment of the pulmonary artery as indicated by the leader line. The first photograph of the top row shows the cross section of the arterial wall of the normal 3-month-old rats. The specimen was fixed at the no-load condition. In the figure, the endo-thelium is facing upward. The vessel lumen is on top. The endothelium is very thin, of the order of a few microns. The scale of 100 μm is shown at the bottom of the figure. The dark lines are elastin layers. The upper, darker half of the vessel wall is the media. The lower, lighter half of the vessel wall is the adventitia. The second photo in the first row shows the cross section of the main pulmonary artery 2 hours after exposure to lower oxygen pressure. There is evidence of small fluid vesicles and some accumulation of fluid in the endothelium and media. There is a biochemical change of elastin staining in vessel wall at this time. The third photograph shows the wall structure 12 hours later. It is seen that the media is greatly thickened, while the adventitia has not changed very much. At 96 hours of exposure to hypoxia, the photograph in the fourth column shows that the adventitia has thickened to about the same thickness as the media. The next two photos show the pulmonary arterial

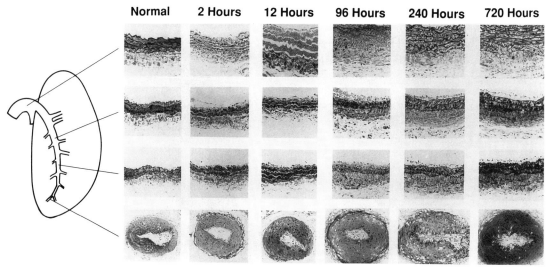

| Normal | 2 Hours | 12 Hours | 96 Hours | 240 Hours | 720 Hours |

100 μm

FIGURE 1.3. Photographs of histological slides from four regions of main pulmonary artery of a normal rat and hypertensive rats with different periods of hypoxia. Specimens were fixed at no-load condition. See text for details. From Fung and Liu.[23] Reproduced by permission.

wall structure when the rat lung is subjected to 10 and 30 days of lowered oxygen concentration. The major change in these later periods is the continued thickening of the adventitia.

The photographs of the second row show the progressive changes in the wall of a smaller pulmonary artery. The third and fourth rows are photographs of arteries of even smaller diameter. The inner diameter of the arteries in the fourth row is of the order of 100 μm, approaching the range of sizes of the arterioles. The remodeling of the vessel wall is evident in pulmonary arteries of all sizes.

Thus we see that the active remodeling of blood-vessel wall proceeds quite fast. Histological changes can be identified within hours. The maximum rate of change occurs within a day or 2.

Morphometric changes are not the only changes occurring in blood vessel wall when the blood pressure changes as a step function. The zero-stress state of the vessel and the mechanical properties of the vessel wall also change gradually as the remodeling proceeds. This is expected because the mechanical properties follow material composition and structure, so the properties will change when the composition and structure changes. Data on zero-stress state changes during tissue remodeling in pulmonary and system arteries and veins are given in papers by Fung and Liu[23,24] and Liu and Fung.[25] Data on changes in mechanical properties due to tissue remodeling in arteries are presented in Liu and Fung.[26]

A corresponding program of research on the hypertrophy of the heart leads also to many new findings. Increased stress in the heart also leads to hypertrophy, and morphometric, structural, and mechanical properties change.

What these experiments reveal is that other things being equal, tissue growth is related to stress. The growth-stress relationship plays a role in the healing of the tissues and in rehabilitation to normal life.

Tissue Engineering

Looming large in the future is tissue engineering, which can be defined as engineering the improvement of natural tissues of man, or creating living artificial tissue substitutes with human cells. One example is the skin substitute made with a patient's own cells cultured in a biodegradable scaffold. Another example is the blood-vessel substitute seeded with the patient's own endothelial cells. Work on cartilage, bone, and other organs is in progress. These new techniques became possible because major advances were made in the art of tissue culture in recent years as a consequence of the discovery of growth factors and various culture media. These discoveries make tissue engineering thinkable. With the feasibility established, we can now think of practical applications of the stress-growth laws to engineering living tissues. Success in this area will have great impact on healing and rehabilitation of injuries.

Conclusion

Biomechanics is a key factor in understanding accidental injury and healing. This chapter presents an overview and an introduction to some terminology and basic concepts. The substantive details follow in the rest of the book.

Accidental injury is a national problem. It is a special problem for American society. Violence fills our TV. Drug using is out of control. Thus a large factor in accident prevention is not biomechanics, not medicine, not surgery, not rehabilitation, not law. It is culture. It is good for the professional people to think of the big picture, too. However, the professional side must not be minimized. The injured persons need care. The society needs injury prevention. At the level of emergency care, medical and surgical treatment, physical rehabilitation, designing of a safer vehicle, providing better protection of man, and establishing a better public policy, we need the best of scientific knowledge. A thorough understanding of the fundamental topics discussed in this article will help.

References

1. Fung YC. *Biomechanics: motion, flow, stress, and growth.* Springer-Verlag, New York, 1990.

2. Yen RT, Fung YC, Ho HH, Butterman G (1986) Speed of stress wave propagation in the lung. J Appl Physiol 61(2):701–705.
3. Rice DA (1983) Sound speed in pulmonary parenchyma. J Appl Physiol 54(1):304–308.
4. Dunn F, Fry WJ (1961) Ultrasonic absorption and reflection of lung tissue. Phys Med Biol 5:401–410.
5. Woo SLY, Buckwalter JA (eds) *Injury and repair of the musculoskeletal soft tissues.* American Academy of Orthopedic Surgeons, Park Ridge, IL, 1988.
6. Nahum AM, Melvin J (eds) *The biomechanics of trauma.* Appleton-Century-Crofts, Norwalk, CT, 1985.
7. Meyer GH (1867) Die Architektur der spongiosa. Archiv fur Anatomië, Physiologie, und wissenschaftliche Medizin (Reichert und wissenschafliche Medizin, Reichert und Du Bois-Reymonds Archiv) 34:615–625.
8. Culmann C. *Die graphische Statik.* Meyer und Zeller, Zurich, 1866.
9. Wolff J (1869) Über die bedeutung der Architektur der spondiösen Substanz. *Zentralblatt für die medizinische Wissenschaft.* 6:223–234.
10. Roux W *Gesammelte Abhandlungen über die entwicklungs mechanik der Organismen.* W Engelmann, Leipzig, 1880–1895.
11. Pauwels F *Biomechanics of the locomotor apparatus*, German ed 1965. English translation by P Maqnet and R Furlong, Springer-Verlag, Berlin, New York, 1980.
12. Carter DR, Fyhrie DP, Whalen RT (1987) Trabecular bone density and loading history: regulation of connective tissue biology by mechanical energy. J Biomech 20:785–794.
13. Carter DR, Wong M (1988) Mechanical stresses and endochondral ossification in the chondroepiphysis. J Orthop Res 6:148–154.
14. Cowin SC (1986) Wolff's law of trabecular architecture at remodeling equilibrium. J Biomech Eng 108:83–88.
15. Fukada E (1974) Piezoelectric properties of biological macromolecules. Adv Biophys 6:121.
16. Yasuda I (1974) Mechanical and electrical callus. Ann NY Acad Sci 238:457–465.
17. Bassett CAL Pulsing electromagnetic fields: A new approach to surgical problems. In Buchwald H, Varco RL (eds) *Metabolic surgery.* Grune and Stratton, New York, pp 255–306, 1978.
18. Satzstein RA, Pollack SR (1987) Electromechanical potentials in cortical bone. II. Experimental analysis. J Biomech 20:271.

19. Lund EJ (1921) Experimental control of organic polarity by the electric current I. Effects of the electric current of regenerating internodes of obelia commisuralis. J Exp Zool 34:471.

20. Becker RO (1961) The bioelectric factors in amphibian limb regeneration. J Bone Joint Surg 43A:6431.

21. Smith SD (1974) Effects of electrode placement on stimulation of adult frog limb regeneration. Ann NY Acad Sci 238:500.

22. Cowan MJ, Crystal RG (1975) Lung growth after unilateral pneumonectomy: Quantitation of collagen synthesis and content. Am Rev Respir Disease 111:267–276.

23. Fung YC, Liu SQ (1989) Change of residual strains in arteries due to hypertrophy caused by aortic constriction. Circ Res 65:1340–1349.

24. Liu SQ, Fung YC (1989) Relationship between hypertension, hypertrophy, and opening angle of zero-stress state of arteries following aortic constriction. J Biomech Eng 111:325–335.

25. Liu SQ, Fung YC (1992) Influence of STZ-induced diabetes on zero-stress states of rat pulmonary and systemic arteries. Diabetes. 41:136–146.

26. Fung YC, Liu SQ (1992) Strain distribution in small blood vessels with zero-stress state taken into consideration. Am J Physiol: *Heart & Circ.* 262:H544–H552.

2
Instrumentation in Experimental Design

Warren N. Hardy

Introduction

Insightful experimental design is crucial to the success of investigative science. Application of appropriate technique and technology follows recognition of the problem to be solved. When considering the biomechanics of trauma, the task most often involves the discovery of how input energy relates to output kinematics and dynamics and how these quantities correlate with observed injury. Therein lies the key to discovering the physical nature of a subject under test and its system performance and parameters. It is in this way that responses, tolerances, and mechanisms are determined. Obtaining this information is an integral part of developing the predictive models that assist engineers, physicians, and scientists in their efforts to understand and reduce injury.

Assuming a problem has been identified and adequately characterized, it remains for the researcher to create a representative and repeatable event, measure it, and analyze it such a way that meaningful conclusions may be drawn. From an instrumentation perspective, this process encompasses selection or design of transducers, signal conditioning equipment, data acquisition and storage equipment, signal and data processing methods, and an experimental control regime.

If one wishes to measure the load a subject experiences during impact, a load cell can generally not be affixed to the subject. The size and mass of the load cell would alter the response of the test specimen. However, reac-tion loads may be measured instead. Even though the inertial properties of any mass in front of the gages in the load cell would cause erroneous measurement, acceleration of the load cell may be used for "mass correction" to obtain the proper value of force. The size and mass of an accelerometer usually produce negligible effects on the parameters to be measured. This provides a better signal-to-noise ratio as well as a direct measurement of load than if an accelerometer alone were used. It also provides a redundancy. Proper cancellation of inertial effects generates confidence in the data, while improper cancellation in-dicates the presence of error. This approach is straightforward.

If one needs to measure deflection of the chest of a human cadaver undergoing impact, a targeted rod may be driven through the chest, and its motion may be recorded photo-graphically. The drawbacks to this approach are numerous. The rod is invasive and alters the internal structure of the chest. It can very easily bend and vibrate during the test. Also, it gives an indication of deflection at only one point. Reduction of high speed film data is tedious and can be plagued with error. How-ever, a thin band with numerous full-bridge strain-gage arrays may be wrapped about the chest and used to generate planar contours from measured curvatures. Although challeng-ing to implement, this approach could generate a wealth of information. This approach is newer, and more esoteric.

This chapter concerns itself primarily with

the transformation of one type of energy to another, usually mechanical to electrical. It is this function that transducers perform. Researchers in biomechanics employ specialized measurement techniques to provide elegant solutions to intricate problems. Some of these techniques are widely accepted and almost classic in nature, and some are very new and barely off the laboratory benches. The following is a discussion of the more important transducer and signal conditioning basics and a noncritical review of some of the ways that manufacturers and researchers associated with injury-related biomechanics have solved specific measurement problems.

Transducer Fundamentals[1-12]

A transducer performs two functions in the energy transformation process: sensing of the quantity to be measured and conversion of that quantity to a proportional electrical parameter. For example, an input of force, displacement, velocity, or acceleration effects a change in resistance, capacitance, inductance, or charge. Often this is an indirect process, where it is not the quantity of interest but a related quantity that is actually measured. Consider a piezoresistive accelerometer. Conceptually, a seismic mass attached to a thin beam experiences or "senses" an acceleration, but it is the change in resistance of strain gages affixed to the beam undergoing bending that produces "output."

While transforming energy, a transducer should not alter the level of energy of the system of which it is a part. That is, transducers should measure responses of a system without changing them. An ideal transducer would be massless and without volume. It would be able to measure at a point, measure only in the direction(s) of interest, and be sensitive only to the quantities of interest. Electrically, an ideal transducer would have DC to infinite frequency response with minimal phase shift. It would be highly sensitive throughout a broad input range and have negligible output impedance. Finally, it should be linear, in both an algebraic and a systems sense. That is, a regression coefficient may be found to relate output to input with a high degree of correlation, and the frequency of the output function is identical to the frequency of the input.

Unfortunately, the ideal is never practically attainable. Every transducer has some mass and occupies some space. Therefore, every transducer has the potential to alter the performance of a system. A load cell cannot function without deforming. Force is required to stroke a linear potentiometer and move the mass within an accelerometer. The volume of a pressure sensor changes. when accelerated in a direction orthogonal to its sensitive axis, an accelerometer will produce an output. Strain-gage and load-cell output will drift with changing temperature. The change in resistance of a thermistor is logarithmic with respect to temperature. It is up to the researcher to determine the desired, or even acceptable, electromechanical qualities of a transducer and the performance characteristics of any associated signal conditioning equipment that will produce a measurement system with appropriate response capabilities.

Most transducers can be separated into two categories. Those that require electrical energy input and those that do not. Those that require input, either a constant supply or a time-variant input signal that is to be modulated, can be described as non-self-generating. Those that generate their own output, such as charge, can be described as self-generating. The following section pertains to operational theory for simple examples of the two types: Resistive strain gages and piezoelectric crystals. Transducers not employing resistive strain gages or piezoelectric crystals are left largely undiscussed in this section. This includes thermocouples and thermistors, linear variable differential transformers (LVDTs) and potentiometers, capacitive transducers, and optical encoders.

Resistive-Gage Measurement

Subjecting a system to mechanical input results in stresses within the system. Stress is defined as force per unit area. Lack of deformation within a system (infinitesimal strains) would suggest the system could withstand infinite stresses. This clearly is not the case. Therefore, with each stress there is an associated strain. Strain is defined as a change in length per unit length. Within the elastic region of a homogeneous isentropic material, stress is a linear function of strain related by the modulus of elasticity of the material. A measurement system sensitive to strain can be used to describe a number of parameters related to stress. Frequently, devices whose resistance changes with geometric changes related to strain are employed in strain measurement. A metal conductor, or resistance strain gage is such a device. A material whose electrical resistivity changes when the material is subjected to stress is often described as piezoresistive. Semiconductor strain gages are fabricated from such materials. These definitions suggest that a large collection of dissimilar substances, including electrolytic solutions (when appropriately physically constrained), could be used

as resistive elements. However, the following discussion is limited to metallic strain gages, specifically the foil-alloy type, and semiconductor strain gages.

The Metallic Strain Gage[1,5,8]

The resistance of a conductive material element varies with strain. This change is not due to intrinsic changes in the resistivity of the material but to the changes in geometry of the element. Resistance (in ohms) of a specimen with known geometry is equal to the resistivity of the material multiplied by the length and divided by the cross-sectional area.

$$R = \rho L/A \qquad (2.1)$$

Consider a length of wire. A change in the length of the wire is accompanied by a change in the cross-sectional area such that the volume of the wire remains constant. Given the new

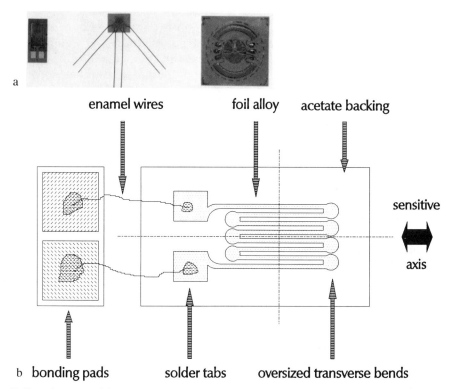

FIGURE 2.1. Foil strain gages. (a) Single axis, stacked rosette, and diaphragm types. (b) Conceptualization of an axial foil strain gage.

geometry of the wire, a new value of its resistance may be found. After some manipulation it can be shown that for small changes in length the ratio of the change in resistance to the original resistance of a wire is:

$$\Delta R/R = Gf\Delta L/L \qquad (2.2)$$

where the ratio of the change in length to the original length of the wire is strain. Therefore, the mechanical property of strain can be related to the electrical property, resistance. It can be shown that this is a linear relationship. The constant term Gf is the gage factor. The gage factor for most metals is approximately 2. A gage factor is unique to a particular gage, or batch of gages, and is provided by the manufacturer. The gage factor directly relates percentage change in resistance to applied strain.

Foil gauges (Fig. 2.1a) typically consist of an alloy such as Advance or Isoelastic (both alloys of nickel) fixed to an acetate base. The gage is sensitive in the direction of the thin metal grid. The bulges of material located at the bends of the grid (Fig. 2.1b) are designed to desensitize the gage to transmit strains. Fine enamel wire connects the gage to bonding pads, where the larger conductors of a shielded cable are soldered. The complicated technique for mounting a strain gage to a specimen is left undescribed.

The Semiconductor Strain Gage[1,2]

In the face-centered lattice of silicon, adjacent atoms share electrons, forming covalent bonds. These electron pairs in the orbital subshells are strongly bound to the nucleus, and there are no free electrons, or charge carriers. However, impurities may be added to the silicon to change its electrical properties. This is referred to as doping. Silicon atoms have four valence electrons. Atoms with three valence electrons, such as boron, are called acceptors. Adding an acceptor to silicon creates "holes," or areas or electron vacancies. These holes are considered majority charge carriers and "migrate" through the semiconductor. This migration is actually the breaking and reforming of covalent bonds. When an acceptor is added to

silicon it forms a p-type substance. When a donor such as arsenic, with five valence electrons, is added to provide surplus electrons as the majority charge carriers, an n-type substance is formed. Semiconductor strain gages typically employ doping concentrations of $10^{16}-10^{20}$ atoms/cc. Resistivity is expressed in terms electron charge (e), the number of charge carriers (N), and the mobility of the charge carriers, and is given by:

$$\rho = 1/(eN\mu) \qquad (2.3)$$

While N depends on the type and concentration of impurities, mobility depends on the level of strain and its direction with respect to the crystalline structure. The mobility is direction sensitive because a semiconductor strain gage is electrically anisotropic. Therefore, the orientation in which a gage is cut from a crystallographic structure affects its performance. The resistivity of a semiconductor strain gage is on the order of 1,000 times greater than that of a foil gage. Also the sensitivity to strain of a semiconductor gage can be greater than 100 times that of a foil gage. Therefore, highly sensitive and very small semiconductor gages can be manufactured in a variety of ranges, in simple shapes. Increasing the doping of a substance decreases its sensitivity to strain and its sensitivity to temperature. Increased doping also increases its linearity. However, because gages can be produced with negative gage factors (n-type) and used in tandem with p-type gages, much of the nonlinearity and temperature effects can be canceled, and lesser doped gages with higher sensitivities can be used. Additionally, semiconductor gages allow the fabrication of transducers with higher frequency response, greater longevity, and smaller hysteresis than foil gages.

Semiconductor gages can be manufactured as flat gages or sculptured gages. Flat gages (Fig. 2.2a) can be considered as Euler's columns with bonding stresses that are low in comparison with the stresses that are developed at the center of the gage. Sculptured gages (Fig. 2.2b) can be formed by a combination of chemical etching and a pattern of diffused doping.

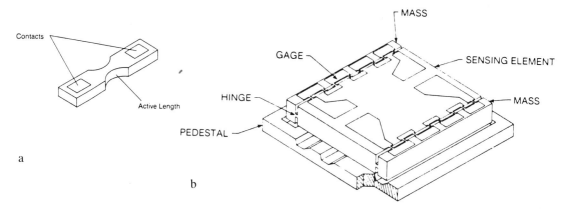

FIGURE 2.2. Piezoresistive semiconductor strain gages: (a) Flat (bulk). (b) Sculptured. (Courtesy of Endevco.)

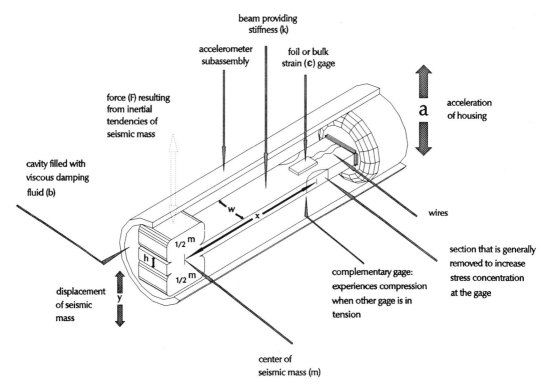

FIGURE 2.3. Conceptualization of a beam accelerometer showing seismic mass ang gage placement. (See eq. 4–7.)

Basic Strain-Gage Transducers[1,5,11]

One of the most widely employed kinematic transducers in biomechanics research is the accelerometer. Based on strain in a deflected thin beam and Newton's second law, the beam accelerometer is essentially a second-order spring, mass, and damper system. Newton's second law states that the time rate of change of momentum of a body is equal to the force required to produce said change. This is commonly written as:

$$\Sigma F = m \cdot a \qquad (2.4)$$

where F is force, m is the mass of the body, and a is acceleration (dv/dt). Strain in a deflected thin beam produced by transverse application of force may be described in terms of the resulting bending moment, the section modulus of the beam, and the modulus of elasticity of the beam material. This is known as the beam equation and is commonly written as:

$$\varepsilon = M/(E \cdot I/C) \qquad (2.5)$$

M is the bending moment (force F applied at a distance x), E is the modulus of elasticity, and I/C is the elastic section modulus. The section modulus for a thin beam is equal to the width of the beam, w, times the square of the height, h, divided by 6. Therefore, the beam equation may be rewritten as:

$$\varepsilon = F \cdot x \cdot 6/(E \cdot w \cdot h^2) \qquad (2.6)$$

A beam accelerometer (Fig. 2.3) may be conceptualized as a thin beam with a seismic mass fixed to one end of the beam, and the other end of the beam being built into the housing, or subassembly, of the accelerometer. The inertial tendencies of the seismic mass are resisted by stresses developed in the beam during acceleration of the beam. This may be represented by a reaction force at the end of the beam. Resultant strains may be measured at a distance x from this force by complementary strain gages placed on either side of the beam. These gages are typically bulk piezoresistive gages. Motion of the mass relative to the accelerometer body may be described by the second-order differential force balance:

$$m\ddot{y} + b\dot{y} + ky = F \qquad (2.7)$$

where y is linear displacement for small excursions due to application of force F. The seismic mass, m, can often simply be the mass of part of the beam itself and damping, b, is usually small and provided by silicon oil within the subassembly. Stiffness is provided by the

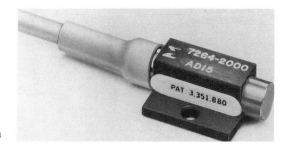

a

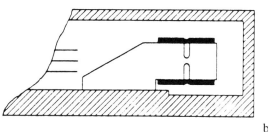

b

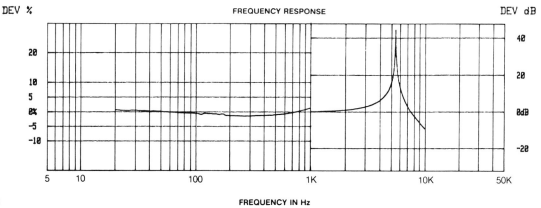

c

FIGURE 2.4. Piezoresistive accelerometer: (a) The Endevco 7264. (b) Internal conceptualization of the 7264. (c) Frequency (amplitude) response of a typical 7264. (Courtesy of Endevco.)

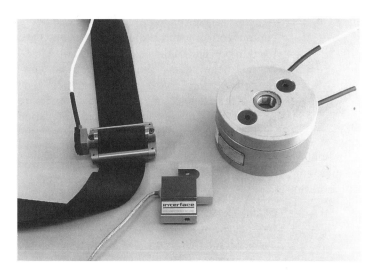

FIGURE 2.5. Example load cells: From left, Robert A. Denton, Incorporated seat-belt load cell, an Interface SM 250 shear-beam load cell, and a GSE 3182 biaxial column load cell.

beam and the gages bonded to it. The Endevco model 7264 piezoresistive accelerometer (Fig. 2.4a–c) is an example of a classic industry workhorse.

One of the most widely employed dynamic transducers in biomechanics research is the load cell. Strain-gage load cells are available in a variety of configurations including shear beam, cantilever beam, membrane, and column structures.

Stress (pressure) results from the application of a force (load) over a given area. The resulting stress and hence strain distribution in a load cell depends on the structural geometry of the load cell. A conventional tensile and compressive column load cell is sensitive to forces applied along the longitudinal axes of the internal beam structure. It is based on the linear relationship between stress and strain in the elastic region of a homogeneous isentropic

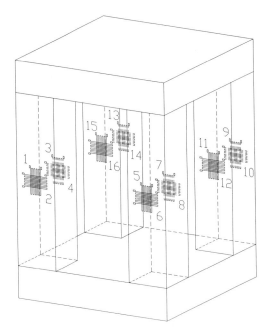

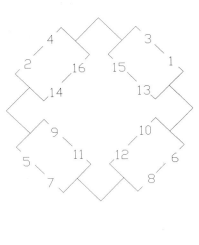

FIGURE 2.6. Column load-cell concepts. Left is a possible strain gage configuration and on the right is the corresponding bridge wiring. (Adapted from material from Denton, Inc.)

material relating axial and transverse strain to axial stress. Axial strain is related to axial stress by Young's modulus, and transverse strain is related to axial stress by Poisson's ratio.

Pictured clockwise from upper left (Fig. 2.5) is a Denton model BELT seat-belt load cell, a GSE model 3182 column load cell, and an Interface model SM-250 shear beam load cell. Structural, gage placement, and bridge con-

figurations (Fig. 2.6) for a load cell can be elaborate and vary among manufacturers.

Piezoelectric Measurement

Some naturally occurring crystals such as quartz and tourmaline, and artificially created ceramic crystals such as barium titanate, exhibit a phenomenon known as piezoelectricity. The piezoelectric effect is characterized by the

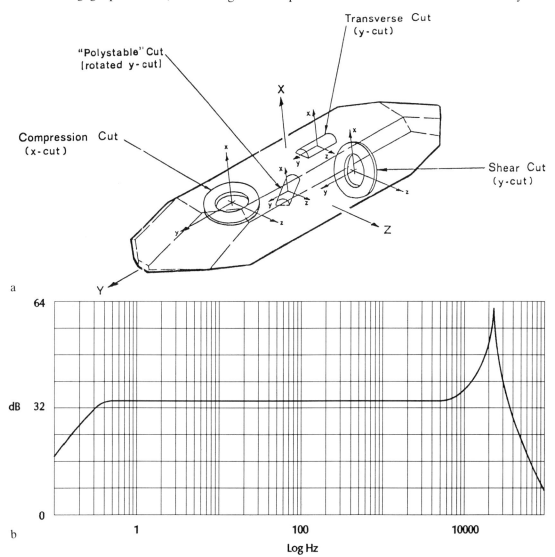

FIGURE 2.7. Piezoelectric concepts. (a) The SiO_2 crystal bar (y-grown). The orientiation of the cut corresponds to the transducer's application. Transverse and polystable cuts are used in pressure transducers. (Courtesy of Kistler Instrument Cor-

poration.) (b) Conceptual representation of a typical piezoelectric accelerometer frequency response. (Adapted from material provided by Kistler Instrument Corporation.)

development of charge, and hence a measurable potential, on opposing faces of a crystal subjected to stress. Crystals capable of this behavior possess an asymmetrical lattice structure. External stress distorts this lattice causing reorientation of internal charges. This, in turn, results in relative displacement of positive and negative internal charges. The effect of this internal reorientation extends to the surface of the crystal, where it is measurable. The transducer application determines the type of cut that is made from a crystal to form a piezoelectric element (Fig. 2.7a).

Piezoelectric Response[4,8,9]

The charge that is developed across a piezoelectric crystal will dissipate through the internal resistance of the crystal. Therefore, a piezoelectric transducer is incapable of monitoring a steady-state condition as its frequency response does not extend to DC. Static calibration is then, not possible. Very high internal resistances can produce a usable range to fractions of a hertz but also create very high output impedances, however. A very pronounced and stable resonance peak is characteristic of piezoelectric crystals as they are essentially undamped. Both of these phenomena are illustrated in the amplitude response (Fig. 2.7b) of a typical piezoelectric transducer.

Basic Piezoelectric Transducers[4, 8, 9]

Piezoelectric crystals are generally used in accelerometer or load cell applications. The Pennwalt ACH-01 accelerometer (Fig. 2.8) contains integral electronics to reduce its output impedance and its dependence on high-grade capacitance cable. The Kistler load washer (Fig. 2.9) is capable of measuring large compressive forces. Generally, if a piezoelectric load cell is to be capable of bipolar operation, the crystals of the load cell must be prestressed. Because the charge across the crystals dissipates through internal resistance, this static load does not produce an output or offset. Therefore, when the load cell experiences tension, the crystal will be slightly unloaded, and will produce a change in output. Compression further loads the transducer, and again a change in output is produced. A load washer may be preloaded by the user, and will then measure compressive and tensile loads.

Signal Conditioning Fundamentals[1–12]

Given that a transducer is capable of sensing a physical quantity and converting it to a proportional electrical quantity, it remains to use the varying electrical parameters as part of a

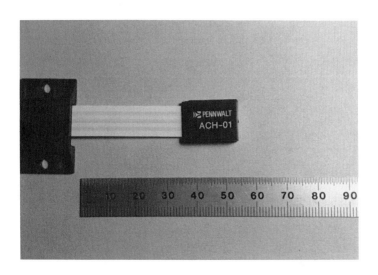

FIGURE 2.8. Piezoelectric accelerometer: An example with integral electronics: The Pennwalt ACH-01.

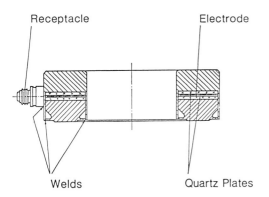

FIGURE 2.9. Conceptual representation of a Kistler load washer (Courtesy of Kistler Instrument Corporation.)

practical measurement system. Typically a transducer's varying electrical parameter is not one that is conveniently directly monitored, particularly in a dynamic situation. For example, the small rapid changes in resistance of a semiconductor strain gage in a piezoresistive accelerometer are impossible to measure directly. Proper signal conditioning techniques are required to integrate the electrical-parameter changes of a transducer into an accurate measurement system. It is necessary to use a transducer's varying resistance, inductance, capacitance, or charge to affect a change in voltage. This is just one of the functions of a signal conditioning system. A signal conditioning system is responsible for everything that occurs between the sensing and conversion process of a transducer and the actual sampling performed by a digitizer. Connectors and cabling, completion and calibration and balance circuits, isolators and amplifiers, filters and multiplexers are all considered part of a complete signal conditioning system. With this in mind, it can be said that the response of a data acquisition system is governed primarily by the performance and limitations of the signal conditioning equipment involved.

Signal conditioning systems must perform a number of functions and meet a wide range of specifications. Functionally, a system must supplement transducers with external elements, such as completion resistors or dummy gages, to create viable, linear temperature-compensated, measurement networks. It must also provide a method for connecting remote transducers and measurement networks to stationary electronics. In strain-gage bridge systems this could be multiconductor twisted pair cable with excitation and sense leads, output and calibration leads, a foil shield, and a PVC jacket. In piezoelectric systems this could be coaxial capacitive cable. A system must supply non-self-exciting networks with excitation in the form of a constant voltage or current source, or an alternating carrier frequency. With self-generating networks the system must provide a method of converting electrical changes in a measurement network to a voltage signal, such as a charge amplifier. It should provide methods to obtain quiescent balancing of the network, such as T balance or voltage-insertion circuits to remove offsets. Once a network is balanced, high gain may subsequently be applied. High gains are required in many signal conditioning systems due to the relatively small changes in many measurement networks. Amplification, and much of other signal conditioning, is often accomplished using operational amplifier (op amp) circuitry. The system must also, if necessary, supply components to linearize the relationship between the physical quantity being observed and the voltage signals. This can often be accomplished by judicious selection of passive components or by an active implementation. The final functional requirement of a signal-conditioning system is that it be able to provide a method of calibration. Depending upon the nature of the transducers being used, this may be accomplished by shunt calibration or voltage substitution, or stepped sensitivity calibration.

There are a number of specifications that components of a signal conditioning system must meet while performing the aforementioned functions. Of primary concern are input and output impedances. Input impedance of a device must be kept high enough so as not to load the output of previous stages. This is particularly important when considering the output impedance of a transducer and the input of a buffer or amplifier. If the input impedance of an amplifier is 100 times as great as the output impedance of the measurement network there will be a 1% error in measurement due to loading. Therefore, input impedances of amplifiers are generally thousands of times greater than the output impedances of the transducer networks they are designed to work with. Alternately, output impedances are generally kept as low as possible, to accommodate long lead lengths, capacitive loads, and subsequent low-input impedance devices. Also of importance are frequency bandwidth and dynamic range, differential and common mode, noise and distortion, thermal response and drift, sensitivity and gain, and linearity and hysteresis, among others.

The following is a description of representative resistive gage and piezoresistive crystal circuit applications and of cabling and calibration techniques for each, followed by a discussion of overall system performance requirements and specifications.

Resistive Measurement Applications

Given that the electrical resistance of a gage is a linear function of applied strain, it remains to use this change in resistance to change a more easily measurable electrical quantity, specifically voltage. The simplest implementation of such a circuit is a voltage divider network comprised of a regulated DC power supply and an active gage in series with a fixed resistor of the same value as the gage. This arrangement has a number of drawbacks. It is inherently nonlinear and susceptible to temperature. It also possesses a large quiescent state offset, making direct application of high gains impossible. However, other configurations help solve these problems. Additional resistors, dummy gages and active gages can be used to form bridge circuits. The most-often found circuit is the Wheatstone bridge and T balance network. The following is an introduction to single and multiple active gage resistive networks and a discussion of associated cabling and calibration concerns.

Gage Circuitry[1,4,5,8,9]

Fortunately, when confronted with a single active strain-gage measurement scheme, a number of things may be done to compensate for temperature, linearity, and offset. The response of a single gage in series with a resistor can be very linear about a point or within a small range of strains. Typically strains should be kept below 5,000 microstrains, and the resistor is of the same value as the strain-gage resistance corresponding to a midscale strain (usually 0%). Also, to assist in temperature compensation, a foil strain gage should have the same coefficient of thermal expansion as the specimen to which it is mounted. This brings the value of apparent strain much closer to the actual value. A three-wire configuration may be used for a single gage (Fig. 2.10a). This allows more equal division of voltage due to temperature induced changes in resistance of the lead wires. Where possible, a dummy gage may be employed. A dummy gage is a second identical strain gage mounted to a specimen of identical thermal characteristics as the primary gage. This gage replaces the fixed resistor in the voltage divider and is placed in the same environment (as physically close as is practical) to the active gage. In this configuration both the active and dummy gages experience the same temperature changes and the division of voltage remains constant as each resistance changes equally.

Offset voltage may be reduced by adding another series voltage divider in parallel with the first. If the two resistors in this added divider are of an equal value, the quiescent difference in voltage between the two sides is zero. This parallel configuration of two series voltage dividers is referred to as a Wheatstone bridge (Fig. 2.10b). If two complementary gages are used as one of the voltage divider networks, the bridge circuit exhibits a greater degree of linearity, temperature compensation, and sensitivity than a single active gage bridge. For example, two like gages with like orientation fixed to opposite sides of a point on a thin beam form a complementary pair of active gages. As the beam deforms, one gage experiences tension, and its resistance increases. The other gage experiences compression, and its resistance decreases, theoretically by the same amount as the first gage increases. Both gages are in the same environ-

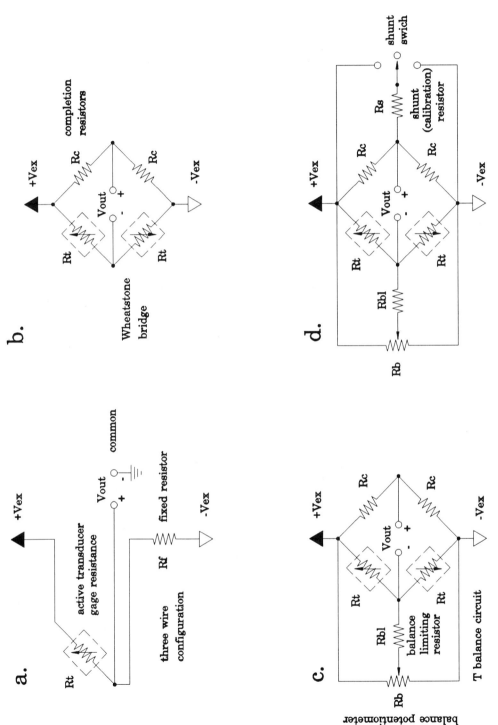

FIGURE 2.10. Bridge-circuit concepts. (a) The three-wire, single-temperature-compensated gage, voltage divider circuit. (b) The Wheatstone bridge with two active gages (or one active, one dummy gage) and two completion resistors. (c) The T balance circuit with balance-limiting resistor. (d) Bipolar shunt calibration concept. In high-gain applications the shunt resistor is generally hundreds of times the value of the transducer resistance.

ment, providing good temperature compensation. The resistance of both gages is changing equally and oppositely so the output is linear with respect to strain, and is greater (roughly twice) than it would have been when using a single gage. The fixed resistors on the opposite half of the bridge are referred to as completion resistors. Transducers employing a Wheatstone bridge configuration typically possess 1, 2, or 4 active gages with 3, 2, or no completion resistors, respectively. It is also typical that gages and resistors within each divider have similar nominal values. In general, output impedances of resistive measurement networks range between 120 and 2,000 Ω. It is not necessary, though often preferable, to have the same values in both of the dividers. Although the Wheatstone bridge approach can provide quiescent output values very close to zero, when high gain is applied a prohibitively large offset again appears. If a method were available to create perfectly equal division of voltage in each half of the bridge under a variety of initial conditions, then high gains could be used safely. Such a circuit is the T balance network. It is named so because it consists of a variable-resistance element and a fixed resistor shunted in a T configuration (Fig. 2.10c) across the Wheatstone bridge. The variable resistor is a balance potentiometer and the fixed resistor is a balance-limiting resistor. The limiting resistor is used to restrict the amount of shunting that can occur across either arm of the bridge. Using improperly low values for the balance and balance-limiting resistors can cause gage heating, bridge loading, non-linearity, and sensitivity shifts. If values are used that are too large, the range of balancing ability by this circuit would be seriously limited. Compromise values for the balance potentiometer and the limiting resistor are 20 times the bridge output impedance and 50 times the bridge output impedance, respectively.

Static Calibration[4,8]

Once a linear, temperature-compensated, balanceable measurement network has been obtained, at least two steps remain: amplification and calibration. The transducer measurement network provides a means of relating a physical parameter to voltage, and amplification increases this voltage to workable levels. Calibration provides a method for determining this relationship exactly. For example, an accelerometer used in a balanced bridge and differential amplifier configuration experiences an acceleration and an output voltage is recorded. How much acceleration, or how many gravities, does this voltage represent? To find the answer to this question the measurement system must be calibrated.

Consider that the change in resistance of a strain element is linear with respect to the strain it is experiencing, and the strain it is experiencing is linear with respect to the deflection of the thin beam to which it is mounted. Consider also that the deflection of the beam is linear with respect to acceleration experienced by a mass attached to the end of the beam. Therefore, for a given acceleration there will be a corresponding change in the resistance of the strain element. This change in resistance can be statically simulated. It can be simulated by placing a resistor in parallel with the strain element or another resistive element in a bridge circuit (Fig. 2.10d). This parallel placement is referred to as a shunt, and the resistor is termed a shunt or calibration resistor. The resulting equivalent parallel resistance represents a given physical situation or acceleration. Changing the resistance of one of the arms in a bridge network causes an unequal division of voltage and hence a measurable output voltage. This output (shunt) voltage corresponds to the physical level of acceleration represented by the change in bridge arm resistance caused by the shunting. In this way, the sensitivity of each channel may be determined through the entire measurement system:

$$\text{Sensitivity} = \frac{\text{simulated physical parameter}}{\text{shunt voltage}} \quad (2.8)$$

What remains to be found is the physical level that is simulated for a given value of shunt resistance.

If the simulated physical level is a simple strain, the calibration strain for a given shunt resistor may be found from the gage factor for the strain gage used. If the system is measuring another parameter such as acceleration or load, the transducer must initially be subjected to incremental steps of known (reference/calibration) quantities. Preferably these calibration quantities are either directly or indirectly traceable to the National Bureau of Standards. Once known values have been applied and output voltages have been measured, a linear regression between input and output may be found. Then the voltage obtained from a resistor shunt may be used to predict a physical value from the calibration curve. This physical value is then intimately associated with the transducer network being calibrated and shunt resistor being used and is independent of gain. Shunt calibration is typically a bipolar operation, with the resistor being shunted over upper and lower adjacent arms of the bridge, producing a positive and negative shunt voltage. Taking the average of the absolute values of the two shunt voltages provides a calibration voltage that is insensitive to small offsets.

There are several guidelines to follow when applying a shunt calibration technique. First, the shunt calibration voltage should be approximately 75% of the expected maximum output voltage when initially calibrating a device and when setting up for an actual test. This is to assure that calibration of the system does not rely too heavily on interpolation or extrapolation. For instance, using a calibration voltage that corresponds to a value much beyond the range of interest assumes that the slope of the linearized calibration curve out to a distant point is the same as the slope of a calibration curve found using only points within the range of interest. This is an incorrect assumption. Second, if a different physical value (PV) is required, allowing the user to design to a different range of sensitivity, a new (very closely approximated) value may be found by the reciprocal relationship:

$$\frac{R_{shunt_a}}{R_{shunt_b}} = \frac{PV_b}{PV_a} \qquad (2.9)$$

This holds true because as the value of the parallel shunt resistance increases, the change in the equivalent parallel resistance decreases, so a smaller physical quantity is being simulated. A more accurate, and typically used, formula relies on the value of the bridge arm that is being shunted as well. This is particularly necessary when considering large changes in shunt resistance, i.e., $600\,K\Omega$ to $10\,K\Omega$. Lastly, the relationship between physical value and shunt voltage may be used to maximize the output of a data-acquisition system, and hence to obtain optimal signal-to-noise ratios, while staying within the limitations of the system and avoiding clipped data. The following equation can be used to accomplish this:

$$\frac{Physical\ value}{V_{calibration}} \cdot V_{output} = engineering\ units$$

$$(2.10)$$

The above equation suggests that if a physical value is known for a given transducer measurement network and a given shunt resistor, the sensitivity through an entire chain of signal conditioning elements may be found without needing to know individual sensitivities for each element. Shunt voltages for each channel may simply be digitized prior to a test event.

However, prior to actually conducting a test, an initial calibration must be performed. Adhering to the accelerometer example, a static calibration may be performed using a device known as a rate table (Fig. 2.11). A platter is mounted to the shaft of a servomotor, and an accelerometer is mounted to the platter with its sensitive axis positioned radially at a given radius. Because centripetal acceleration at a rotating point is a function of angular velocity and distance from the center of rotation, the accelerometer experiences a steady acceleration for a given constant angular velocity of the motor. The accelerometer leads are connected to stationary electronics via slip rings. Stepping the motor through a series of known angular velocities provides a series of known accelerations and measurable outputs. It is from this information that a calibration is obtained. Because the measurements are made under steady-state conditions, this form of calibration is static in nature, as is dead-weight calibration of a load cell. (Dynamic calibration

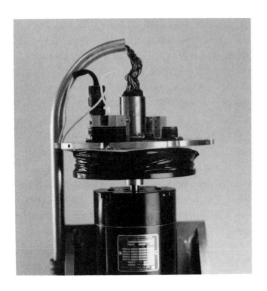

FIGURE 2.11. Rate table: A static (constant centri-petal acceleration) calibration fixture for accelero-meters. The rotating accelerometer mounting platter is driven by an AC servomotor.

is addressed with respect to piezoelectric considerations.)

Cabling[3,4]

A cabling system makes the physical connection between remote transducer networks and signal conditioning electronics. It must do this in a way that introduces minimal noise and error into the measurement system. Cables are frequently subjected to repeated abuse, such as in the case of crash-sled trailing cables, so they must be rugged. However, durable cables tend to have thick jacketing, which creates undesirable increases in weight and reduces flexibility. Low conductor resistance and shielding are desired, which also promote increased dimensions. Additionally, the optimal cabling configurations for minimizing errors in a bridge measurement circuit can require up to ten conductors per channel. Frequently, a compromise is necessary. Systems are able to perform well using only four conductors and a shield. Bundles of cables serving multiple channels may be wrapped within a sleeve made of very strong material such as Kevlar to reduce the amount of jacket required for each individual cable.

When using a great length of cable (1,000 ft) between a bridge transducer and signal-conditioning electronics, or when attempting to provide an ideal cabling environment, the conductor configuration can become complex (Fig. 2.12). Two conductors are used to supply the excitation voltage to the bridge. Because through long cables there is often a drop in potential along the length of a conductor due to its resistance, the voltage seen at the bridge is not the same as the regulated supply voltage at the amplifier. Therefore, many systems have the ability to monitor (sense) and regulate voltage at a remote point. The sense leads serve this monitoring function. Ideally, no current flows through these wires. The positive and negative output leads return the signal from the bridge to noninverting and inverting inputs of the amplifier. Separate calibration lines are provided so that there is equal shunting of all gages and/or resistors. This scheme assures that any drop in potential along the excitation lines is not involved in the shunting process, and that cable resistances have a balanced effect. It is common to combine the function of the calibration lines with the sense leads, thereby reducing the number of conductors. In some cases, especially where large conductors in short lengths (100 ft) are used, the sense leads and the calibration lines are not used.

Unwanted noise can pose a large problem, especially in large measurement systems. Cabling can contribute substantially to the level of noise within a system. Passing a conductor through an environment filled with electric and magnetic fields assures the presence of noise. Lighting and solenoids contribute heavily to the amount of noise, especially 60 Hz, in a system. Long cables and high-impedance sources pose a particular problem. Proper shielding and cabling techniques can reduce noise levels significantly. One of the most effective methods of reducing magnetic (inductive) noise is to use twisted pairs of wires for related conductors. One of the most effective means of eliminating electric (capacitive) noise is to use thin foil shields. The shielding is then either connected to a ground or common, or driven at a variable potential, accommodat-

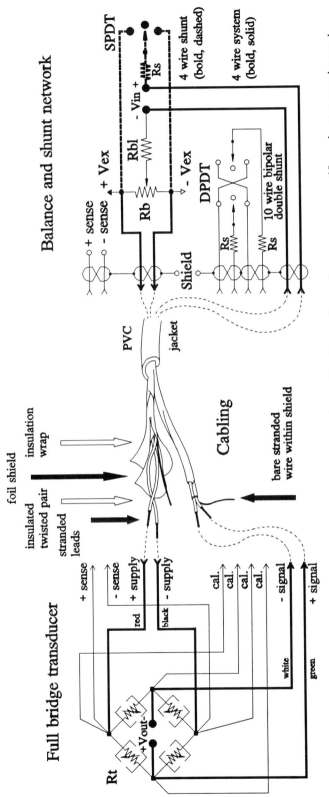

FIGURE 2.12. Resistive bridge cabling arrangement. Depending on the application, as few as four or as many as 10 conductors may be used.

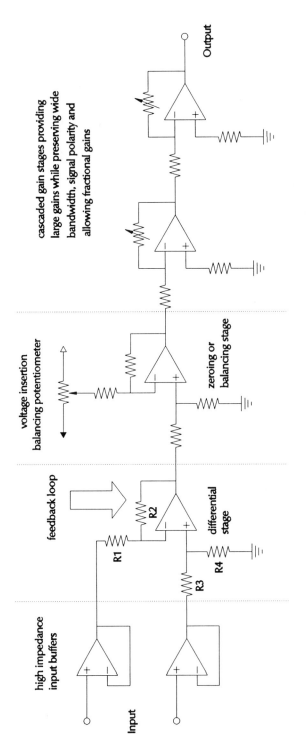

FIGURE 2.13. Fundamental amplifier concepts for resistive applications.

ing unbalanced source impedances. In each case care must be taken to avoid loops formed by the shield being tied to more than one potential. This includes different grounds that may be at different potentials, causing a current to flow through the shielding (ground). However, if it is simply possible to reduce the length of cabling used, the amount of noise will be reduced.

Amplification[2,4,5,9]

The full-scale output of excited measurement networks may be on the order of tens of millivolts or less. However, the full-scale input range of many indicating devices, such as an analog meter or analog-to-digital conversion (A/D) system, may be ± 5 V or higher. The ability of a high-level indicating system to accurately distinguish levels of a weak signal is poor. Therefore, amplification is needed to obtain maximum resolution of the measurement signal.

One of the most widely used amplification devices is the op amp. Two qualities make some op amps particularly well suited to the task of instrumentation amplification: extremely high input impedance (up to one million MΩ) and extremely large open loop gain (up to one million times). Field effect transistor (FET) input stages make ultra-high input impedances possible because of nearly infinite gate-to-channel isolation. Cascading multiple gain stages allows for large open loop gains. A typical, though not optimal, amplifier may be configured with as few as three op amps (Fig. 2.13). The op amps are represented by the triangular symbols. The output voltage is equal to the difference between the two input voltages. The input stages are high-impedance followers ($V_{out} = V_{in}$), and the second stage is a differential amplifier.

Nearly infinite input impedance and open loop gain make the solution or design of ideal op-amp circuits straightforeword. Infinite input impedance suggests that no current flows into the noninverting (+) or inverting (−) terminals. Infinite open loop gain suggests that:

$$V_{out} = \infty \left[(V+) - (V-)\right] \quad (2.11)$$

where $(V+)$ and $(V-)$ are input voltages applied to the (+) and (−) terminals, respectively. This relationship is generally difficult to satisfy. However, when using negative feedback (applying a portion of the output to the inverting terminal) this equation can be satisfied. When using negative feedback, the output of the amplifier is continually adjusting so that the (+) and (−) terminals are held at equal potential. When $(V+) = (V-)$, the quantity $(V+) - (V-) = 0$, satisfying the open loop gain condition. This describes the fundamental principles of an operational amplifier. In practical analysis of a negative-feedback op-amp circuit it is typical to apply Kirchoff's Current Law, Ohm's Law, and the $(V+) = (V-)$ concept to derive a network's transfer function.

The importance of using high input impedances to avoid output loading of measurement networks has been discussed. Another important concept that depends on the resistance values of this circuit is common mode rejection, or CMR. CMR is the rejection or blocking of like signals. The open loop condition suggests that when the signal appearing at the two input terminals is the same (common-mode), the output should be zero. Ideally, this is the case. Practically, however, there is some gain. A measure of how well an amplifier rejects like signals is the common-mode rejection ratio, or CMRR. CMRR is specified in decibels (dB), or

$$20\text{Log}_{10}(DG/CMG) \quad (2.12)$$

where DG is the differential gain and CMG is the common mode gain. This specification is generally 90 dB or greater. In differential amplifier circuits, care must be taken to preserve equal weighting or amplification of the two inputs to maintain high values of CMRR. It can be shown this occurs when R2R3 = R1R4 in the example circuit. Under these circumstances, only differing signals, not like signals, are amplified. The immediate benefit of this is that most noise, such as 60-Hz interference, can be rejected by the amplifier, providing good signal-to-noise ratios when using long cables in a noisy environment.

For instrumentation amplification applications, care must be taken to select components and design circuits that meet other requirements as well. Amplifier circuits with frequency response from DC to 100 kHz are suitable for most biomechanics applications, and accuracies of 0.1% and linearities of 0.01% are similarly within reason. Signal-to-noise ratios, usually specified at a given frequency and power level, can be 80 dB or greater. Input impedances should be on the order of 50 MΩ. It should be noted that the above specifications are for the amplification section of a data acquisition system, not the entire system.

Piezoelectric Measurement Applications

Piezoelectric transducers are characterized by small size, low cost, high linearity, and a wide frequency response. Unfortunately, they also possess high output impedance (older transducers), require specialized cabling and signal-conditioning and calibration techniques, and have zero output at steady state. it is primarily for these reasons, and the lack of static calibration ability that piezoresistive transducers have enjoyed popularity over piezoelectric transducers in impact biomechanics research.

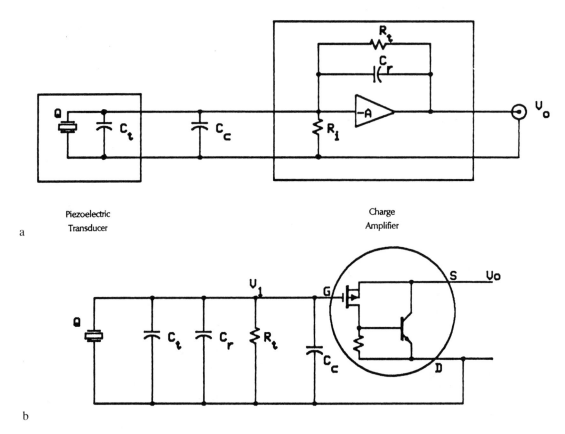

FIGURE 2.14. Piezoelectric signal-conditioning concepts. (a) A simplified charge amplifier model where Q is transducer charge, C_t is transducer capacitance, C_c is cable capacitance, R_i is insulation resistance (cable and transducer), C_r is range or feedback capacitance, and R_t is time constant or range capacitor resistance. (Courtesy of Kistler Instrument Corporation.) (b) The integral charge-to-voltage Piezotron circuit employing MOSFET input and bipolar transistor output (BIFET) conversion where Q is the piezoelectric element charge, C_t is transducer capacitance, C_r is range capacitance, R_t is time-constant resistance, and C_i is BIFET input capacitance. (Courtesy of Kistler Instrument Corporation.)

Crystal Circuits[4,8,9]

Two parameters are of extreme importance when dealing with piezoelectric transducers: charge and capacitance. The signal conditioning techniques used in piezoresistive systems do not apply. Piezoelectric transducers require charge amplifiers. The charge generated by the transducer is transferred to a capacitor in the feedback loop of the first amplification stage. The transducer is connected to the charge amp by means of capacitance (coaxial) cable. Unfortunately, the output of the transducer performance is influenced by the input resistance and capacitance of the amplifier being used (Fig. 2.14a). However, piezoelectric transducers are available with integral eletronics to eliminate many of these problems. Often, the output of the crystal is connected directly to a high-impedance buffer within the transducer (Fig. 2.14b).

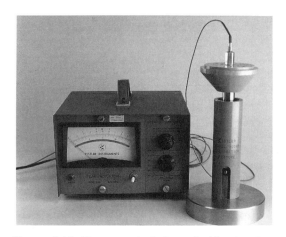

FIGURE 2.15. Drop stand: A dynamic (deceleration pulse) calibration fixture. To the left is a peak hold meter and charge amplifier. On the right is the drop stand and a Kistler piezoelectric accelerometer that serves as a reference.

Dynamic Calibration[4,8,9]

Because piezoelectric transducers do not respond to steady-state excitation, static calibration is not possible. This means that piezoelectrics cannot be calibrated using constant levels or steps of input. It also means that a calibration value cannot be simulated in a static fashion, such as shunt calibration. Therefore piezoelectric transducers must be calibrated using a transient or time variant (dynamic) physical input. A common type of calibration is drop calibration. The transducer to be calibrated, an accelerometer, for instance, is subjected to a transient pulse of acceleration, or deceleration, and its output is compared to that of a known reference accelerometer that experienced the same acceleration pulse. A drop calibration fixture (Fig. 2.15) consists of a reference accelerometer mounted upon a pedestal that can accommodate other transducers that are to be calibrated, and a reference load cell within the pedestal. After the transducer in question has been mounted to the pedestal, the pedestal is raised and dropped. The maximum acceleration experienced by the reference accelerometer is captured on a peak meter monitoring the output of the charge amplifier. This output

is compared to the peak acceleration of the transducer being calibrated. In this way the magnitude performance of a piezoelectric accelerometer may be compared to a transducer of known calibration. Dynamic calibration may also be performed with respect to phase as well as magnitude. Again comparison is made to a reference transducer, but while using sinusoidal, not pulse input. This can be achieved on a shaker. The reference transducer and the transducer to be calibrated are again mounted to a common surface, and experience identical input. However, the outputs may be compared both in terms of amplitude and phase through a range of frequencies. Both of the aforementioned calibration methods are indirect. That is, the performance of a given transducer is evaluated with respect to another transducer, which in turn has been compared to a known, direct standard. Indirect calibration may involve a number of levels, but becoming far removed from a direct calibration is unadvisable.

Because of the inability to be statically calibrated, piezoelectric systems depend upon sensitivity calibrations. As an example, sensitivity for a piezoelectric accelerometer may be expressed in terms of millivolts per volt per gravity. Not only must the sensitivities for each

of the transducers in a system be known, but
the sensitivity of each element in the signal
processing chain must also be known, i.e.,
amplifier gains, filter gains, and digitizer gains.
To determine the gains of each stage and
subsequently the sensitivity of the entire
system, known stepped voltages may be sub-
stituted for the transducer outputs at the
amplifier inputs. These signals are digitized,
and the sensitivity through each channel can
then be calculated.

System Performance

After developing a system of transducer
measurement networks, cabling, balancing and
calibration networks, and amplifier circuits, it
remains to devise a method of obtaining a
permanent record of the event to be observed.
This requires an indicating device. This can be
as simple as a voltmeter (the values to be read
and recorded by hand) in static test involving
a few channels. It could also involve chart
recorders when doing quasi-static or some
dynamic tests. If only transient maxima are
of interest, sample and peak hold indicators
(meters) may be used. However, multichannel
systems capable of dynamic measurements
typically rely on discrete sampling of continuous signals. This process is A/D conversion.

Care must be taken in the conversion of
continuous signals to discrete data points to
assure that the digital information accurately
represents the original waveform. This can be
accomplished by adhering to sampling theory
principles and applying proper filtering techniques. However, it is important that the
information obtained at one research institution be comparable to that collected at another,
and that present data can be related to future
and past data. It is also important that signal-
conditioning and data acquisition techniques
be appropriate for the nature of the parameters
being examined. To address this issue, there
exists the Society of Automotive Engineers
(SAE) J211 specification entitled Instrumentation for Impact Test. The following section is a
review of sampling techniques and theory, and
the associated filtering requirements. Also

included is a discussion of the SAE J211
specification.

Sampling[2,4,6,9]

Analog-to-digital conversion is often accomplished by using data acquisition cards that are
part of a personal computer system. Measurement systems that require greater channel
capacity and higher speed often use dedicated
digitizing systems. Each method uses A/D
converters to perform the sampling. Smaller
systems may use only one converter for several
channels and sequentially multiplex the signals
to be sampled. This requires the use of sample
and hold amplifiers so that sampling of each
channel is simultaneous. Larger, more expensive systems may dedicate a converter for each
channel. The A/D converters themselves are
available in a variety of classes, using a variety
of conversion methods. Examples include
parallel or flash conversion, dual slope or
integrating, successive approximation, and
tracking.

One of the most important concepts associated with digitizing is aliasing. Aliasing is the
misrepresentation of a waveform. The Nyquist
Criterion states that for accurate representation of a waveform, it must be sampled at
a rate at least twice that of its highest frequency content. This is a minimal requirement.
Because filters do not possess ideal cutoff
characteristics and common waveform reconstruction methods are simplistic, practical
sampling ratios are usually many times that of
the waveform's highest-frequency component.
Graphically, a 100-Hz waveform sampled
at 133.3 Hz appears to have a frequency of
33.3 Hz (Fig. 2.16a). This 33.3-Hz alias would
appear on a harmonic spectrum (Fig. 2.16b)
as having "wrapped around" the point corresponding to one-half the value of the sampling frequency.

Filtering[2,4,6,9]

The key to successfully representing a continuous waveform in sampled form is the use of
antialiasing filtering. Antialiasing filters are
low-pass filters of moderate order, an example
being a fourth-order Butterworth filter with

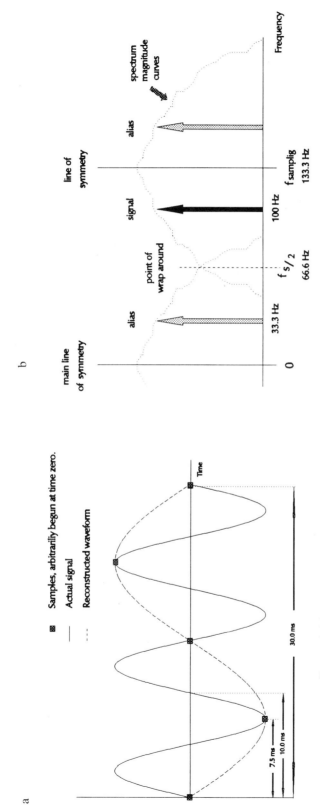

FIGURE 2.16. Representation of an aliased signal in (a) the time domain and (b) the frequency domain.

a cutoff frequency of 1,650 Hz. The cutoff frequency is specified as the -3-dB point, or the frequency at which the amplitude of the output is 0.707 of the input of the input amplitude. An ideal low-pass filter allows only frequencies below the cutoff point to pass and rejects all frequencies above this point. Butterworth filters have a unique quality—the natural frequency is always the same as the -3-dB frequency, regardless of what the natural frequency, damping factor, or attenuation rate is. The attenuation rate for a fourth-order filter is 80 dB/decade. Filtering not only affects amplitude response, but phase response as well. Filtering can be used to remove unwanted frequency components from a signal. Filters that reject a range of frequencies are termed band block. If the band is very narrow it is referred to as a notch filter. The most prevalent implementation of this is the 60-Hz notch filter.

Postprocessing of sampled data often involves digital filtering. There are recursive and nonrecursive filters, phase and phaseless filters, and finite and infinite impulse response filters. Although considered part of a data channel, these are data processing algorithms, and not actual instrumentation. Therefore they are left undiscussed.

Instrumentation for Impact Test—SAE J211[10]

The SAE J211 specification is designed to provide uniform guidelines for the conditioning, acquisition, and processing of data. This form of standardization provides a common basis

TABLE 2.1. SAE J211[10] channel class specifications. The channel class provides recommendations for data handling depending upon the nature of the source of the data.

Typical Test Measurements	Channel class#
Vehicle structural accelerations for use in:	
Total vehicle comparison	60
Collision simulation input	60
Component analysis	600
Integration for velocity or displacement	180
Barrier face force	60
Belt restraint system loads	60
Anthropomorphic Test Device	
Head accelerations (linear and angular)	1,000
Neck	
Forces	1,000
Moments	600
Thorax	
Spine accelerations	180
Rib accelerations	1,000
Sternum accelerations	1,000
Deflections	180
Lumbar	
Forces	1,000
Moments	1,000
Pelvis	
Accelerations	1,000
Forces	1,000
Moments	1,000
Femur/Knee/Tibia/Ankle	
Forces	600
Moments	600
Displacements	180
Sled acceleration	60
Steering column loads	600
Headform acceleration	1,000

(Reprinted with permission from SAE Handbook, Volume 4 © 1990 Society of Automotive Engineers, Inc.)

for comparison of past, present, and future information, and information that is generated from different sources. It is important to note that the specifications within J211 are only guidelines. A researcher may elect to step outside of the guidelines for a particular application. This is accepted practice, as long as the procedures actually used are well described when the data are presented.

Channel class specifications (Table 2.1) describe the entire channel, including the transducer, cabling, signal conditioning, multiplexing, filtering, sampling, and post-processing. A response corridor is specified for each channel class (Fig. 2.17). The J211 specification also addresses minimum sampling rates, maximum phase shifts, and allowable error limits. Additionally J211 provides

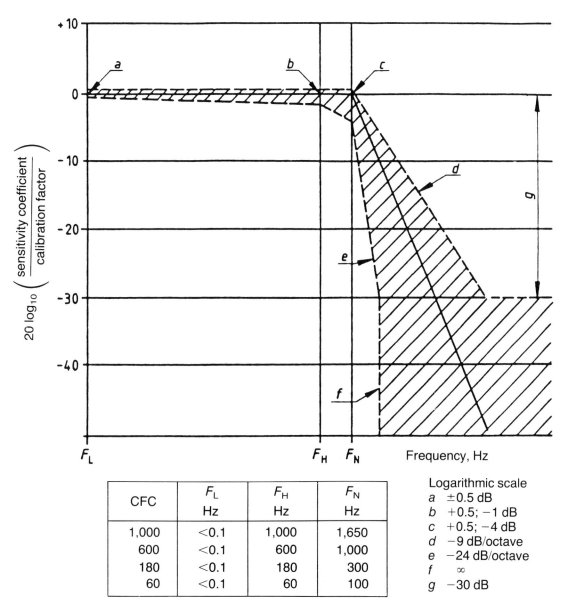

CFC	F_L Hz	F_H Hz	F_N Hz
1,000	<0.1	1,000	1,650
600	<0.1	600	1,000
180	<0.1	180	300
60	<0.1	60	100

Logarithmic scale
a ±0.5 dB
b +0.5; −1 dB
c +0.5; −4 dB
d −9 dB/octave
e −24 dB/octave
f ∞
g −30 dB

FIGURE 2.17. SAE J211[10] normalized response corridor. Amplitude response windows for channel class recommendations. (Reprinted with permission from SAE Handbook, Volume 4. © 1990 Society of Automotive Engineers, Inc.)

Hybrid III sign conventions and photographic instrumentation guidelines.

Specialized Measurement Techniques

When posed with a measurement task, a researcher may often find that readily available technology is not entirely suited for adequate solution of the problem. The researcher may then either attempt to improve upon existing technology or develop a new technology altogether. This process is not limited to those involved in research, as the transducer manufacturers contribute heavily to the development of new measurement technologies. The following is a brief discussion of some unique measurement solutions created by both researchers and industry in the areas of kinematics, displacement and deformation measurement, and pressure and force measurement.

Rigid Body Kinematics and Accelerometry[12]

A subject that has long captured the attention of researchers in impact biomechanics is the determination of generalized three-dimensional motion of a rigid body. Historically, efforts have focused upon improving the performance of preceding methods of solution. With each newly proposed solution, however, came an associated new set of considerations. These considerations were frequently in the form of conceptual theory not being physically realizable because of technical and practical limitations. Researchers have addressed and argued both the advantages and shortcomings of a collection of methods. As no single definitive method has been developed, researchers have generally employed the method that represents the most appropriate compromise for their particular application.

Conceptually, generalized three-dimensional motion of a point on a rigid body is easily described. Used in the derivation are: the fixed laboratory reference frame, a translating frame

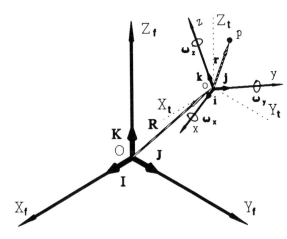

FIGURE 2.18. Rigid body kinematics coordinate systems. Equations are written to describe the motion at a point p on a rigid body with origin o.

having the same orientation as the laboratory system attached to the rigid body, and a body fixed rotational frame sharing its origin with the translating frame (Fig. 2.18). Beginning with the velocity of a point on the rigid body being expressed in terms of the time derivative of position vectors, taking appropriate derivatives and making subsequent substitutions the acceleration at point p on the rigid body may be written as:

$$\mathbf{a}_p = \ddot{\mathbf{R}} + \boldsymbol{\omega} \times (\boldsymbol{\omega} \times \mathbf{r}) + \dot{\boldsymbol{\omega}} \times \mathbf{r} \quad (2.13)$$

As point p is on a rigid body, there are no complementary (Coriolis) effects present in this equation. A component-level representation is given in eq. 2.14. Judicious selection of transducer location and orientation allow a variety of equations to be written using this relation.

$$\begin{aligned}
\mathbf{a}_p = {} & \ddot{x}\mathbf{i} + \ddot{y}\mathbf{j} + \ddot{z}\mathbf{k} \\
& + (-\omega_y^2 r_x - \omega_z^2 r_x + \omega_y \omega_x r_y + \omega_z \omega_x r_z)\mathbf{i} \\
& + (\omega_x \omega_y r_x - \omega_x^2 r_y - \omega_z^2 r_y + \omega_z \omega_y r_z)\mathbf{j} \\
& + (\omega_x \omega_z r_z + \omega_y \omega_z r_y - \omega_x^2 r_z - \omega_y^2 r_z)\mathbf{k} \\
& + (-\dot{\omega}_z^2 r_y + \dot{\omega}_y^2 r_z)\mathbf{i} \\
& + (\dot{\omega}_z^2 r_x - \dot{\omega}_x^2 r_z)\mathbf{j} \\
& + (\dot{\omega}_y^2 r_x + \dot{\omega}_x^2 r_y)\mathbf{k}
\end{aligned}$$

$$(2.14)$$

Implementation of a practical method of applying the given relationships has been a difficult task. The process of measuring rigid body

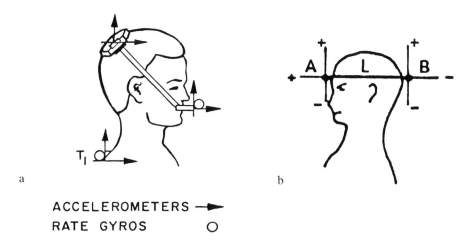

ACCELEROMETERS ➤

RATE GYROS ○

FIGURE 2.19. Early efforts to describe angular accelerations and velocity in a plane. Accelerometer placement used by (a) Ewing et al.[14] and (b) Clarke et al.[16] (Reprinted with permission from SAE 680792. © 1968 and SAE 710857. © 1971 Society of Automotive Engineers, Inc., respectively.)

motion in impact biomechanics was forwarded by Mertz.[13] Linear accelerometry was used in the determination of angular acceleration during investigation of the mechanics of whiplash. This study determined planar angular acceleration of the center of gravity (c.g.) of the head by measuring linear "tangential" accelerations at known distances from each other. Linear accelerometers were oriented with their sensitive axes perpendicular to the line that could be drawn between them in the median plane. This technique relied on measurement of tangential accelerations at a given radius from the origin of a system experiencing angular acceleration.

This concept, coupled with the use of rate gyroscopes, was furthered by Ewing et al.[14,15] Anatomical mounts were positioned over the posterior spinous process of the first thoracic vertebra (T1), over the posterior superior aspect of the head and at the mouth. Each anatomical mount was fitted with a transducer mount. Each transducer mount consisted of an orthogonal pair of linear accelerometers with their sensitive axes in the median plane (Fig. 2.19a). The T1 and mouth mounts also included miniature rate gyroscopes. The acceleration data were resolved into a pair of accelerations parallel to the line drawn between the two head transducer mounts, and a pair of accelerations perpendicular to this line. these pairs were averaged to produce

one orthogonal pair at the midpoint of this line. This procedure was designed to remove angular acceleration effects from the tangential accelerations and to remove centripetal effects from the radial accelerations. The rate gyroscopes were used to obtain planar angular velocity and integration of angular velocity produced angular displacement, or orientation.

Clarke[16] used orthogonal biaxial pairs of linear accelerometers fixed in frontal and occipital mounts to investigate linear and angular accelerations of the human head in volunteer restraint system testing, which included air bags. Again, angular components in the median plane are reduced from measured linear accelerations. The acceleration vectors resolved from the two biaxial clusters mounted at points A and B (Fig. 2.19b) were summed to produce a relative acceleration vector between points A and B. This vector was analyzed in terms of normal and tangential components. Given a fixed distance L between points A and B, the normal acceleration component was proportional to the product of the distance L and the square of angular velocity and the tangential acceleration component was proportional to the product of the distance L and angular acceleration. These relationships assume planar rotation.

The previously discussed efforts generally employed two biaxial linear accelerometer

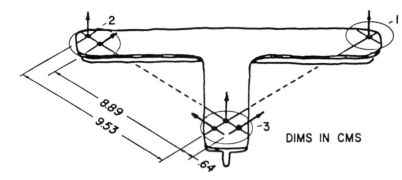

FIGURE 2.20. The 3-2-1 accelerometer array used by Becker et al.[17] to determine generalized 3D motion of a rigid body. (Reprinted with permission from SAE 751173. © 1975 Society of Automotive Engineers, Inc.)

arrays to determine planar rotational quantities. However, the determination of generalized three-dimensional rigid body motion required an increase in the number of measured accelerations. Becker et al.[17] used six accelerometers in a 3-2-1 "tee" configuration (Fig. 2.20). To avoid unnecessary weight increases, rate gyroscopes were not used. It was stated that this technique was sufficient for trajectories involving less than 90 degrees of rotation, and when the accelerometer mount was not impacted directly.

It is generally accepted that the first stable solution to the problem was presented by Padgaonkar et al.[18] This solution is the Wayne State University (WSU) nine-accelerometer mount, or the 3-2-2-2 method. A representative WSU 3-2-2-2 fixture used in cadaver testing

is shown (Fig. 2.21). A unique geometric array of linear accelerometers allows the calculation of angular acceleration, which can be integrated to find angular velocity. A cluster of three mutually orthogonal linear accelerometers are positioned at the origin, while three pairs of orthogonally mounted accelerometers are mounted at a constant distance from the origin along each of the axes. The position and orientation of each of the nine accelerometers are given (Fig. 2.22). Using this geometry, angular velocity cross terms may be eliminated, and the equations of motion are reduced to:

$$\dot{\omega}_x = \tfrac{1}{2}((a_{y_{zl}} - a_{o_z})/r_{y_{zl}} - (a_{z_{yl}} - a_{o_y})/r_{z_{yl}})$$
$$\dot{\omega}_y = \tfrac{1}{2}((a_{z_{xl}} - a_{o_x})/r_{z_{xl}} - (a_{x_{zl}} - a_{o_z})/r_{x_{zl}})$$
$$\dot{\omega}_z = \tfrac{1}{2}((a_{x_{yl}} - a_{o_y})/r_{x_{yl}} - (a_{y_{xl}} - a_{o_x})/r_{y_{xl}})$$

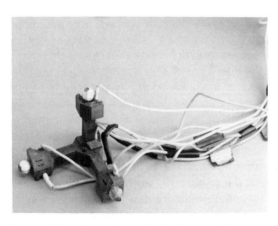

FIGURE 2.21. Wayne State 3-2-2-2 fixture. This nine-accelerometer array is used in the analysis of 3D motion in cadaver testing (specifically of the impaced the head).

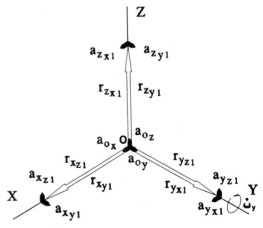

FIGURE 2.22. Conceptual illustration of the WSU 3-2-2-2 showing the linear accelerometer positions and orientations.

Therefore, angular accelerations are essentially found by averaging differences of linear accelerations measured at points at a given separation. This concept is extended by Chou et al.[19] to determine linear components of acceleration at a point on the rigid body, namely the c.g. of an impacted head, to facilitate the calculation of head injury criterion (HIC). This corresponds to substituting measured and calculated values back into the original equations to find the linear accelerations at a point with known coordinates on the rigid body. Mital et al.[20] address the problem of noncommutativity of finite rotations and developed a method based on an orientation and-noncommutative-rate-vectors approach to determine 3D angular displacements relative to an inertially fixed frame. In this way both rotations and order of rotations are accountable. Also, the matrix that transforms the position vector from its body fixed frame to an inertially fixed frame is not updated after every time-step, but after a specified threshold of rotation has been reached.

Since the inception of the 3-2-2-2 method, researchers have repeatedly struggled to develop an improved concept. Common sources of error have been cross-axis sensitivity of transducers, machining errors in the mount, mismatched transducer pairs, signal noise (and loss), mounting fixture vibrations, zero shift, and errors associated with numerical and recursive techniques. This was discussed by Johnson et al.[21] In this discussion, the use of rate gyroscopes was recommended.

Stalnaker et al.[22] employ a minimization of the least square of error in a system of equations generated from a 3-3-3 scheme, using three triaxial clusters of linear accelerometers. This method provides least-square estimate solutions for angular acceleration and angular velocity. Interest in application of linear accelerometry to the determination of angular kinematic quantities is often renewed as researchers discover better methods of measuring, or calculating the required parameters. An in-line 15-accelerometer approach is outlined by Viano et al.[23] Component sums of angular acceleration and angular velocity cross terms are obtained by linear regression, resulting in three coupled first-order differential equations. Subsequent decoupling of these equations permitted recursive solution. The primary application of this fixture (Fig. 2.23) is the

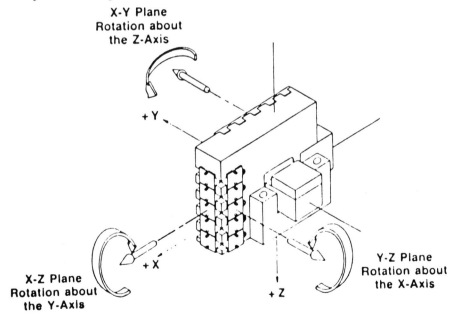

**X-Y Plane
Rotation about
the Z-Axis**

+ Y

**X-Z Plane
Rotation about
the Y-Axis**

+ X

+ Z

**Y-Z Plane
Rotation about
the X-Axis**

FIGURE 2.23. The rigid block in-line 15-accelerometer array developed for dummy use by Viano et al.[23] (Reprinted with permission from SAE 861891. © 1986 Society of Automotive Engineers, Inc.)

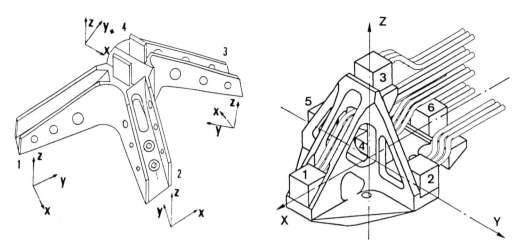

FIGURE 2.24. The (a) MS-I and (b) APR 89-III rigid body kinematics fixtures used by Bendjellal et al.[24] (Each reprinted with permission from SAE 902320. © 1990 Society of Automotive Engineers, Inc.)

determination of the generalized motion and contact forces experienced by the impacted Hybrid III head.

Bendjellal et al.[24] employ the MS-I mount (Fig. 2.24a) for cadaver testing and the 18-channel APR 89-III (Fig. 2.24b) for dummy testing. The APR 89-III consists of six triaxial clusters, and is capable of 3-2-2-2, 3-3-3, or in-line measurement techniques, and provides a means of direct comparison between these methods. Spherical geometric analysis (SGA) is applied to a noncollinear accelerometer array using centripetal accelerations (normal) to calculate angular velocity directly by Nusholtz et al.[25] (Fig. 2.25). Presently under development is the WSU RBKTA, or rigid body kinematics transducer array (not shown). It is a 24-channel device that applies a least-square approach to the calculation of angular acceleration and a centripetal approach to the calculation of angular velocity. It is thought to be suitable for both cadaver and dummy use.

Transducer manufacturers also provide methods of direct measurement, with some

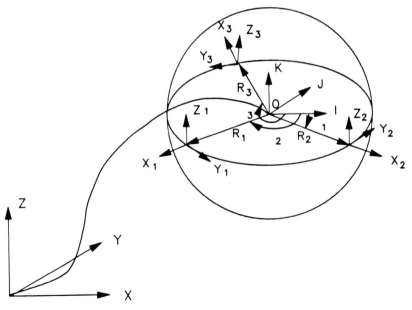

FIGURE 2.25. Illustration of the concepts behind the innovative spherical geometric analysis (SGA) used in the determination of generalized rigid body motion by Nusholtz et al.[25] (Reprinted with permission from Experimental Mechanics. © 1991 Society for Experimental Mechanics.)

success, of angular kinematic quantities. Examples include the Endevco 7302B angular accelerometer (Fig. 2.26) and the IETL-001 angular velocity sensor discussed by Laughlin[26] (Fig. 2.27). The IETL is a magneto-hydrodynamic (MHD) angular motion *sensor* that produces a voltage across a conductive fluid (mercury) annulus experiencing relative motion with respect to a magnetic field. The relative velocity between the fluid and magnetic field is induced when the sensor experiences rotation, and the inertia of the fluid resists rotation about the sensitive axis (Fig. 2.28).

ICSensors, and others, now produce integrated accelerometers (Fig. 2.29). The smaller of the two devices is an 8063-200 die, and the larger device is a 3031-500 surface-mount plastic package. The small size of these accelerometers makes them suitable for a number of applications, including transducers that are to be implanted. Such a transducer is the NDA, or neutral density cranial accelerometer, designed at Wayne State University. The NDA is designed to be implanted in cadaver brain. It is used in the investigation of brain-injury mechanisms. When used with an extracorporal rigid body array, such as the 3-2-2-2, relative kinematic quantities between the skull and brain are investigated in cadavers undergoing facial impacts. It consists of a polyurethane-foam-injected, acrylic-coated, polyester resin shell housing integrated accelerometer dies.

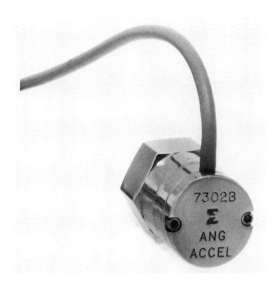

FIGURE 2.26. The 7302B angular accelerometer. (Courtesy of Endevco.)

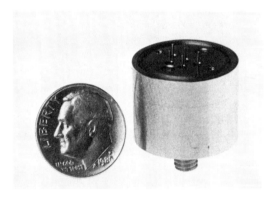

FIGURE 2.27. The IETL-001 angular veloity sensor. (Courtesy of Applied Technology Associates, Inc.)

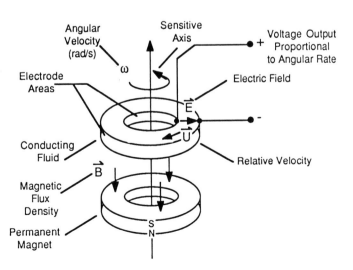

FIGURE 2.28. Illustration of the concepts behind the IETL-001. From Laughlin.[26] (Reprinted with permission from SAE 892428. © 1989 Society of Automotive Engineers, Inc.)

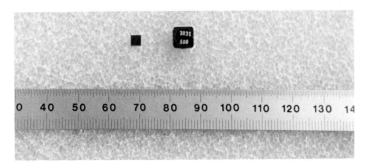

FigURE 2.29. Integrated accelerometers: To the left, the ICSensors
8063 die; on right, the ICSensors
3031 surface-mount accelerometer
package.

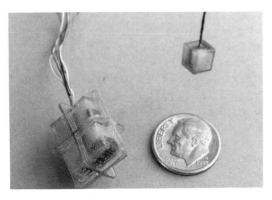

FigURE 2.30. Neutral density cranial accelerometers: The larger flanged unit is a functional biaxial
unit. The smaller device (less than 0.2 ml) is a
triaxial prototype.

Recent models include a functional biaxial
unit that uses model 3001 dies, and a smaller
triaxial prototype that uses model 8063 dies
(Fig. 2.30).

Displacement and Deformation

Deflection measurement techniques in impact
biomechanics range from the simple to the complex. From linear and rotary potentiometers,
linear variable differential transformers
(LVDTs), position resolvers and encoders, to
complex film and optical methods, researchers
labor to better describe the displacement and
deformation of objects undergoing impact.
Often the motion to be described is general,
and there exists no convenient method of
deflection measurement. For example, the
chest potentiometer in Hybrid III that measures anterior-posterior (AP) motion of the

"sternum" with respect to the "spine" provides
limited information, and thoracic compression
in cadaver testing is difficult to assess, especially
without compromising the integrity of the
specimen. Therefore, inventive ways to
measure displacement and deformation are
required.

When measuring either position or displacement the linear potentiometer (pot) is
one of the most widely used transducers.
Technological advances are improving the
dynamic capabilities of potentiometers. The
Novotechnik T 150 (Fig. 2.31) employs a conductive plastic resistive element and is rated for
$20 g$ vibration and 10 m/sec. The Space Age
Control Incorporated string pot (Fig. 2.32) uses
a cable wound about a pulley to drive a single
turn rotary potentiometer. Typically, the body
of the potentiometer is mounted to a reference
point and the cable (by means of a clamp fixed

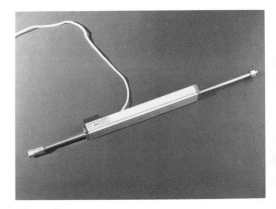

FigURE 2.31. The plastic resistive element Novotechnik T 150 (150 mm) linear potentiometer.

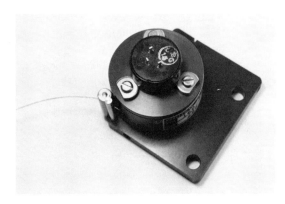

FIGURE 2.32. Space Age Control position transducer, commonly referred to as a string potentiometer.

to it) is anchored to a point on the object of interest. Tension is maintained in the cable by means of a torsional spring that resists rotation of the pulley when the cable is pulled. This spring allows the cable to retract when the distance between the potentiometer body and the object to which the cable is fastened decreases. These devices are used in Hybrid III in triangulation schemes for the determination of planar deflections of points on the rib cage, and in the side-impact dummy Biosid to measure lateral deflections of the ribs. String pots in complex gimbaled configurations, developed as part of an effort to enhance frontal dummy-impact performance, are used to measure 3D displacements of points within the dummy chest.

When it is not possible to attach a device, such as a potentiometer, to the test subject, or when the information that a potentiometer can provide is inadequate, optical methods are often employed. Such methods could include a Kodak SP2000 high-speed video system using CCD (charge-coupled device) image sensors, a Redlake Fastax 16-mm high-speed film camera using a rotary prism, or a Northern Digital Optotrak system, which tracks infrared emitting markers in 3D space (Fig. 2.33). Ogata et al.[27] describe an optical method for measuring deformation of the Hybrid III chest. This system is referred to as a 3D multipoint sternum displacement sensing system, or 3D-MUSTERDS. It employs position-sensing detector cameras to follow light-emitting diodes mounted to the sternum. There are four cameras and four diodes (Fig. 2.34). The control and computation circuitry is housed in a chassis external to the dummy.

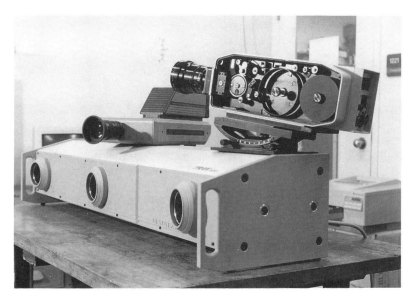

FIGURE 2.33. Optic measurement equipment. A Kodak SP2000 image-sensing camera (left), a Redlake Fastax high-speed 16-mm film camera (right), and a Northern Digital Optotrak (bottom).

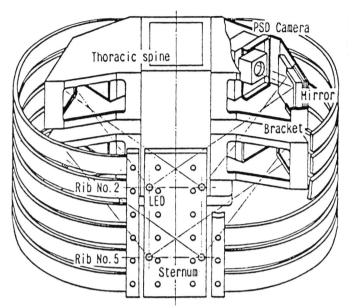

FIGURE 2.34. Concept of the 3D-MUSTERDS developed by Ogata et al.[27] (Reprinted with permission from Toyota Motor Corporation.)

Similarly, when desiring to measure strain in a ligament without modifying the performance of the ligament, Woo et al.[28] employ a video dimension analyzer, or VDA. With this system, the distance between lines stained on a ligament is determined by finding the horizontal scan time taken between the stain lines. The voltage output of the VDA is proportional to this scan time. Using the initial distance between these line as a baseline, strain in a ligament may be determined. More conventional methods of ligament analysis include the mercury strain gage, such as that described by Brown et al.[29] and buckle transducers.

As it is not always possible to mount measurement devices within a test subject, and cinemagraphic data analysis is tedious and does not always provide the needed information, an alternate method of deformation measurement is developed by Eppinger.[30] This method is

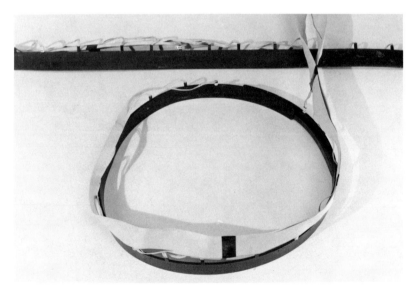

FIGURE 2.35. The EPIDM (external peripheral instrument for deformation measurement) or *chestband* developed by Eppinger.[30] Shown are 16-gage-array models. Subsequent models have up to 40 arrays.

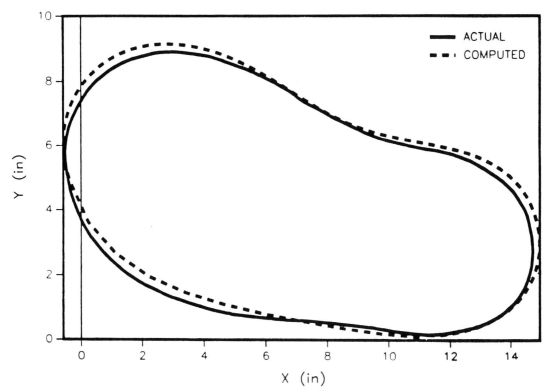

FIGURE 2.36. Comparison of actual chestband geometry to Rband pc output illustrating the contour generating ability of an early EPIDM. From Eppinger.[30] (Reprinted with permission from SAE 892426. © 1989 Society of Automotive Engineers, Inc.)

known as the external peripheral instrument for deformation measurement, or EPIDM. The EPIDM is more commonly referred to as the *chestband*. The chestband (Fig. 2.35) consists of multiple arrays of full bridge strain-gage circuits bonded to a thin steel band. The chestband is 1,422 mm (56 inches) long, and the active portion of the band is surrounded by a urethane jacket. The chestband may be used with varying numbers of gage arrays, in various configurations. The band describes the contour of an object in the plane about which it is wrapped. The concepts behind the EPIDM are straightforward. First, a point rotating about some arbitrary axis at a known radius, through a given angle, describes a length of arc. Second, curvature is the reciprocal of the radius of rotation. Third, curvature is proportional to strain. In this way, the output of the chestband relates to curvature directly.

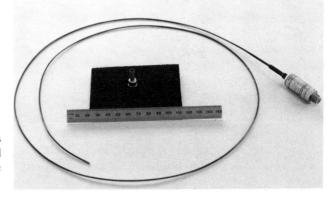

FIGURE 2.37. A Nova Sensor NPH series solid-state pressure sensor surrounded by a Millar Mikro-Tip catheter pressure transducer.

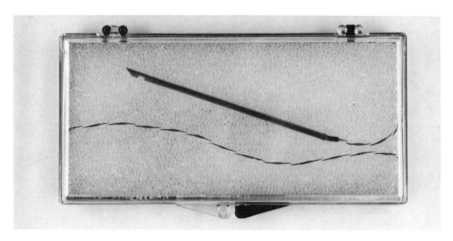

FIGURE 2.38. Needle pressure transducer designed for use in the intervertebral disk.

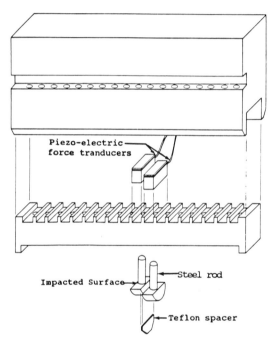

FIGURE 2.39. The load-sensing impact fixture used by Allsop et al.[31] to investigate facial bone fracture. Load is transmitted to a series of piezoelectric force transducers by an array of 18 small impactors. (Reprinted with permission from SAE 881719. © Society of Automotive Engineers, Inc.)

Knowing the distances between the gages along the band's length, a contour of the test specimen may be represented using measured curvatures. A companion to the EPIDM is the Rband_pc program, which generates planar

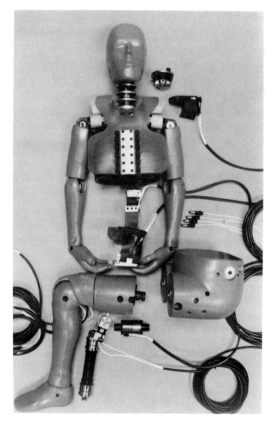

FIGURE 2.40. The various load-sensing elements available for the Hybrid III frontal crash dummy. (Courtesy of Denton, Inc.)

contour plots from the chestband data at specified time-steps. The Rband_pc program constrains the band output to form a closed contour; i.e., there must be 360 degrees through the contour. It also constrains the last point of the contour to be coincident with the first point. Additionally, the point specified as the "spine" is fixed, and an equally distributed additive factor is applied to the data to correct errors in total rotation. An example comparing Rband_pc output to the known test geometry of the chestband (Fig. 2.36) illustrates the type of information that may be obtained from the EPIDM.

Pressure and Force

Miniaturization and specialization of pressure and force transducers facilitate the measurement of quantities that would otherwise be unmeasurable. These transducers find application in both cadaver and dummy testing.

Pictured (Fig. 2.37) are a Nova Sensor NPH series solid-state low-pressure sensor and a Millar Mikro-Tip catheter pressure transducer. The catheter transducer is useful in measuring arterial pressures in repressurized cadavers during impact testing.

An intradiscal pressure transducer fabricated by Robert A. Denton Incorporated (Fig. 2.38) uses a 1.575-mm (0.062-inch) hypodermic needle and a Precision Measurement Company model 060 pressure transducer. It is used in the study of back pain and vertebral disk injury.

The study of facial impact response is furthered by Allsop et al.[31] with the use of two unique measurement techniques. The first is a linear array of 18 miniature piezoelectric force transducers used to measure force distributions, to characterize fracture, and to develop force-deflection response curves. These transducers were mounted to an aluminum block that served as a vertical impactor (Fig. 2.39). The second is the use of acoustic emissions to identify the occurrence of fracture.

One of the most specialized measurement systems is the Hybrid III frontal dummy itself. Many of the components of the Hybrid III are actually load-sensing elements (Fig. 2.40). These transducers are an integral part of the dummy's injury-assessment capabilities. Proceeding from the superior aspect of the dummy, and not including acceleration measurement provisions, the Hybrid III may be fitted with an upper-neck load cell, a lower-neck load cell, a thoracic-spine load cell, a lumbar-spine load cell, load bolt sensors, an upper-femur load cell, a femur load cell, and an instrumented lower leg consisting of upper- and lower-tibia load cells. Each of these load cells is available as a multiaxis unit, capable of measuring various combinations of forces and moments.

Conclusion

Although within this forum a comprehensive treatment of instrumentation methods is not possible, it is hoped that a number of points of interest are touched upon. For some this material may serve as an introduction to an aspect of research with which they are not familiar. For others it may serve as a review, or a compact collection of fundamental concepts. It is also hoped, irrespective of what else is or is not gained from this exercise, that those who read this text develop a greater understanding of some of the challenges confronting researchers from a purely technical aspect and of the level of patience and care that is required to achieve successful experimental results in injury-related biomechanics.

References

1. Dally JW, Riley WF. *Experimental stress analysis*. 2nd ed. McGraw-Hill, New York, 1978.
2. Millman J. *Microelectronics: digital and analog circuits and systems*. McGraw-Hill, New York, 1979.
3. Morrison R. *Grounding and shielding techniques in instrumentation*. 3rd ed. John Wiley, New York, 1986.
4. Nachtigal CL (ed) *Instrumentation and control: fundamentals and applications*. John Wiley, New York, 1990.
5. Normann RA. *Principles of bioinstrumentation*. John Wiley, New York, 1988.
6. Oppenheim AV, Willsky AS, Young IT. *Signals and systems*. Prentice-Hall, Englewood Cliffs, NJ, 1983.

7. Ribbens WB. *Fundamentals of electronic instrumentation for measurement.* Campus Publishers, Ann Arbor, MI, 1973.

8. Tse FS, Morse IE. *Measurement and instrumentation in engineering: principles and basic laboratory experiments.* Marcel Dekker, New York, 1989.

9. Webster JG (ed) *Medical instrumentation: application and design.* Houghton Mifflin, Boston, 1978.

10. SAE J211. Instrumentation for impact test (A.) In 1990 SAE Handbook, Volume 4. Society of Automotive Engineers, pp 34, 185–34, 191, Warrendale, PA, 1990.

11. Beer FP, Johnston ER. *Mechanics of materials.* McGraw-Hill, New York, 1981.

12. Beer FP, Johnston ER. *Vector mechanics for engineers: dynamics.* 2nd ed. McGraw-Hill, New York, 1972.

13. Mertz HJ. Kinematics and kinetics of whiplash. PhD Dissertation. Wayne State University, Detroit, MI, 1967.

14. Ewing CL, Thomas DJ, Beeler GW, Patrick LM, Gillis DB. Dynamic response of the head and neck of the living human to -Gx impact acceleration. Twelveth Stapp Car Crash Conference. SAE 680792, pp 424–439, 1968.

15. Ewing CL, Thomas DJ, Patrick LM, Beeler GW, Smith MJ. Living human dynamic response to -Gx impact acceleration. II. Accelerations measured on the head and neck. Thirteenth Stapp Car Crash Conference. SAE 690817, pp 400–415, 1969.

16. Clarke TD, Gragg CD, Sprouffske JF, Trout EM, Zimmerman RM, Muzzy WH. Human head linear and angular accelerations during impact. Fifteenth Stapp Car Crash Conference. SAE 710857, pp 269–286, 1971.

17. Becker E, Willems G. An experimentally validated 3-D inertial tracking package for application in biodynamic research. Nineteenth Stapp Car Crash Conference. SAE 751173, pp 899–930, 1975.

18. Padgaonkar AJ, Krieger KW, King AI (1975) Measurement of angular acceleration of a rigid body using linear accelerometers. J Appl Mechanics 42:552–556.

19. Chou CC, Sinha SC (1976) On the kinematics of the head using linear acceleration measurements. J Biomech 9:607–613.

20. Mital NK, King AI (1979) Computation of rigid-body rotation in three-dimensional space from body-fixed linear acceleration measurements. J Appl Mech 46:925–930.

21. Johnson AK, Hu AS. Review of head rotational measurements during biomechanical impact tests. National Highway Traffic Safety Administration Technical Report, DOT-HS 80925-68, 1977.

22. Stalnaker RL, Melvin JW, Nusholtz GS, Alem NM, Benson JB. Head impact response. Twenty-first Stapp Car Crash Conference. SAE 770921, pp 303–335, 1977.

23. Viano DC, Melvin JW, McLeary JC, Madeira RG, Shee TR, Horsh JD. Measurement of head dynamics and facial contact forces in the Hybrid III dummy. Thirtieth Stapp Car Crash Conference. SAE 861891, pp 269–289, 1986.

24. Bendjellal F, Oudenard L, Uriot J, Brigout C, Brun-Cassan F. Computation of Hybrid III head dynamics in various impact situations. Thirty-fourth Stapp Car Crash Conference SAE 902320, pp 207–232, 1990.

25. Nusholtz GS, Wu J, Kaiker P (1991) Passenger air-bag study using geometric analysis of rigid-body motion. Exp Mech 3:264–371.

26. Laughlin DR. A magnetohydrodynamic angular motion sensor for anthropomorphic test device instrumentation. Thirty-third Stapp Car Crash Conference SAE 892428, pp 43–77, 1989.

27. Ogata K, Chiba M, Asakura HKF. Development of a sternum displacement sensing system for Hybrid III dummy. Toyota Motor Corporation, 1991.

28. Woo SL-Y, Gomez MA, Seguchi Y, Endo CM, Akeson WH (1983) Measurement of mechanical properties of ligament substance from bone-ligament-bone preparation. J Orthop Res 1: 22–29.

29. Brown TD, Sigal L, Njus GO, Njus NM, Singerman RJ, Brand RA (1986) Dynamic performance characteristics of the liquid metal strain gage. J Biomech 19:165–173.

30. Eppinger RH. On the development of a deformation measurement system and its application toward developing mechanically based injury indices. Thirty-third Stapp Car Crash Conference SAE 892426, pp 21–28, 1989.

31. Allsop DL, Warner CY, Wille MG, Schneider DC, Nahum AM. Facial impact response—a comparison of the Hybrid III dummy and human cadaver. Thirty-second Stapp Car Crash Conference. SAE 881719, pp 139–155, 1988.

3
The Use of Public Crash Data in Biomechanical Research

Charles P. Compton

Introduction

One of the primary contributors to the injury problem is the automobile crash. Information collected about crashes has the potential to aid researchers in understanding the mechanisms of injuries and to point the way to possible solutions. Unlike the laboratory experiment, in which all variables are measured, held constant, or monitored, most variables in an automobile collision are not monitored and are changing rapidly.

The problem for the researcher is to find enough information with which to understand the mechanism of injury causation. Automobile crashes are one of the largest contributors of injuries and one of the most difficult to document. There are currently two levels of detail in publicly available computer files, police investigations, and in-depth investigations done by professional accident teams.

Police data files contain very little specific information about injuries but represent almost all injury-producing crashes. Often the investigating officer, who is at the scene, knows what specific injuries are sustained and their causes, but the data-collection forms used do not allow for entry of this information in the database.

Accident-investigation teams collect a great deal of information, usually after the crash, about injuries and their causation. This includes reviewing the police report, examining the vehicle, interviewing the occupants, and obtaining medical reports. Due to the costs of this time-consuming process the number of these types of investigation is very limited.

In this chapter we will examine the different types of databases available to the researcher and discuss the types of analysis that can be done using those databases. This review will be limited to those data sets publicly available from the United States government, state governments, and research organizations such as the University of Michigan Transportation Research Institute. Future directions in crash-data collection and linkage to other trauma data will be discussed. A bibliography of information sources relevant to crash-data collection and databases appears at the end of this chapter.

Types of Crash-Data Files

Police-Collected Data

Police data sets generally contain information on all injury-producing collisions on public roads in a given state. States differ on the reporting criteria for property-damage crashes and off-road crashes. The state of Michigan, for example, does not include off-road crashes or private-property crashes even when these collisions result in a fatality.

Information on the location, environment, vehicles, and injured occupants is recorded along with a narrative and diagram of the accident. States collect and computerize these records for many purposes: driver records, traffic engineering, selective enforcement, and problem identification, to name a few. Details of the location, environment, vehicles, and circumstances of the accident are of primary importance for these uses. Appendix A contains a case listing for a 1990 Michigan accident as an example of the type of data available from police files. Some states, such as Florida, have begun testing computers for data entry by the police. At this time there are no states computerizing either the narrative or the diagram; however, as the price of computer technology drops the opportunity to capture this information becomes more possible.

The National Safety Council has published standard coding formats for data elements (ANSI D16.1) since 1970, but changes come slowly and the value of such standardization is not always apparent to those with decision-making authority. The federal government has become more involved recently in encouraging this standardization and the Federal Highway Administration is researching methods that can be used to improve data quality.

Injuries are coded using the KABCO scale: K is fatal, A is incapacitating injury, B is nonincapacitating injury, C is minor injury, and O is not injured. The officer in the field has little time to make an injury-severity assessment, so even these rough estimates of injury severity are imprecise. For the researcher interested in the specific mechanisms of injury causation there is little detail to be found in police data files.

Vehicle damage may be indicated by an area of damage to the vehicle and, perhaps, the use of a damage scale to indicate severity of damage. Many states use the TAD scale (the name comes from the Traffic Accident Data project of the National Safety Council) to indicate the level of damage to the vehicle. This scale, a 0–7 scale of damage to the vehicle, relies on the investigating officer comparing pictures of damage to example vehicles with the damage confronting him at the scene of the crash.

Vehicle identification is a particularly dif-ficult proposition with state data sets. Some states, such as Texas, have make and model coded for a large but incomplete list of vehicles while some other states only identify the vehicle as a car or truck. Some states include the vehicle identification number while others do not. In general, the more specific the desired identification the less likely a state data set will be to contain the information. The identification of vehicles with unusual characteristics, such as modified suspensions, is impossible.

This level of detail, a lack of specific injury information, and a very general estimate of crash severity relegate the use of police data files to defining the frequency of accident types, identifying roadways and driver characteristics, and answering other general questions about the crash-involved population.

In addition to a dearth of specific information, some of the data items collected are suspect. In a state with mandatory seat-belt laws, when the officer arrives on the scene and asks the driver if he was using his restraints the answer is frequently yes. In fact, if one were to believe the state crash files, persons in accidents are more likely to be using the available restraints than those randomly observed in the driving population.

Police officers seldom witness the accident they are investigating. They have limited time to collect data and limited training in accident reconstruction. There are many fine investigators in police work but the researcher analyzing a mass accident file has no knowledge of the proportion of good information nor any means of identifying the bad information.

The most thoroughly investigated crashes are fatal crashes, and thus the information collected on those crashes is more complete. The National Highway Traffic Safety Administration (NHTSA) has, since 1975, sponsored the centralized collection of fatal crash data in the Fatal Accident Reporting System (FARS). Analysts in each state, trained by NHTSA, transcribe all fatal crashes in their state onto a common and more-complete report that is stored in Washington. A listing of a sample case is contained in appendix B. This file is publicly available from NHTSA.

In-Depth Investigations

The second type of accident data file is that which collects in-depth investigations done by trained investigators. This data collection may be sponsored by insurance companies, automobile manufacturers, or government agencies. The data collected by commercially sponsored investigation programs are generally not publicly available while government-sponsored investigations generally are available to the researcher for analysis.

In-depth investigations may or may not involve on-scene investigation, but working from the police report the investigator will evaluate the vehicle and obtain occupant-injury information, including hospital reports and autopsies. Data-collection forms tend to be much more specific than police reports and usually contain detailed measurements of vehicle damage as well as a method for coding specific occupant injuries. Because the investigator has multiple sources of information and the training to reconstruct the collision dynamics, in-depth investigation computer data files are much more specific and useful to the researcher.

Unfortunately, because of the time, and therefore money, it takes to collect these additional data, relatively few in-depth investigations are done each year. The current NHTSA in-depth investigation program, the National Accident Sampling System (NASS) Crashworthiness Data System (CDS), contains just 4,648 accidents in the 1989 file. A sample case listing from this file may be found in appendix C.

While police files are a census of all crashes, the in-depth files are a very small sample. Early investigation efforts tended to collect data on specific accident types—rollover, fires, or fatals—in an attempt to determine causes and identify means of prevention of the accident type or to mitigate injury causation. This required an identification of some characteristics of the crash in advance and assumed the chosen characteristics were the most important. The NASS system, operating since 1979, randomly selects cases in randomly selected areas of the country. The hope is that this small sample will statistically represent all crashes in the United States.

The information contained in the NASS file is quite specific in some areas and lacking in others. In 1988 the program became the Crashworthiness Data System (CDS) and has focused on the crashworthiness of the vehicle under investigation. A parallel data-collection program, the General Estimates System (GES), collects police reports from the same sampling area for comparative purposes.

In the CDS system detailed information is available on items such as crash damage, door and window integrity, intrusions into the passenger compartment, and identification for the vehicle along with the VIN. Crash severity is determined as DELTA V (the change in velocity due to impact) by the CRASH3 computer program. Injuries and the specific contacts that caused them are listed in detail when known. Also information on the occupant, such as height, weight, seating position, and details of restraint use, are available. In all, several hundred data items are collected or derived for each vehicle.

Access to Data Files

Many state data files are available to the public. Some states, such as Texas, sell the data on magnetic tapes, while others, such as Michigan, provide it free. Some states have guarded their data closely and have not released it unless forced to by court action (North Carolina), while others are only too happy to share their information for the public good. Federal data files, the NASS CDS and GES databases and FARS, are publicly available from NHTSA.

In addition to acquiring the actual data sets there are also computer systems to which access can be obtained. Contractors with the federal government may be allowed access to government computers. The University of Michigan Transportation Research Institute Transportation Data Center sets up computer accounts on the U of M mainframe computer system, accessible through Sprintnet from anywhere in the world. Databases residing on the system include Michigan, Washington, Texas, FARS, NASS, and many other data files. Other public research facilities such as the Texas Transportation Institute or the Highway Safety Research Center in North Carolina also may have access to such files. Some private engineering and consulting firms also maintain their own copies of crash databases.

The NHTSA, as well as some states such as New York, will do computer runs on their data for the researcher. There is often a fee for such work. As personnel and policy change rapidly in government organizations, no list of contact people or even state organizations would remain correct for long. Statewide crash data is usually processed by a central agency assigned the task; in Michigan it recently became the Office of Highway Safety Planning, while in Texas it is the Department of Public Safety. It is recommended that the potential user contact the organization of interest well in advance of any expected need for such information, as the one thing all states and the federal government have in common is their speed.

Problem Identification Using Crash Data

The identification of specific problems in the crash data sets we have been discussing is not always straightforward. Details of injury

mechanisms, crash forces, and occupant kinematics are limited at best. No one crash file can define the scope of a given problem because no one crash file has both the large numbers of cases required to identify rare events such as serious injury or fatality and the specific details to fully understand the mechanisms of injury that occur in such events.

Police files represent most accidents but contain little information on injuries, while in-depth investigations identify in detail the injuries to a very small sample of the crash population. The researcher must construct a picture of the injury type of interest by analyzing the large crash files to define the population of all crashes and analyzing the more detailed in-depth files to identify specific injury circumstances.

An example of the type of analysis that can be done on state accident databases might be the distribution of occupant age and injury severity. Changing demographics in the United States make the older occupant a topic of considerable interest. Figure 3.1 shows occupant age by occupant injury severity from the 1989 Michigan data for occupants of passenger cars. Besides seating position, restraint use, and perhaps some information on the vehicle in which the injured person was an occupant, there is little other specific information available from a state accident data file.

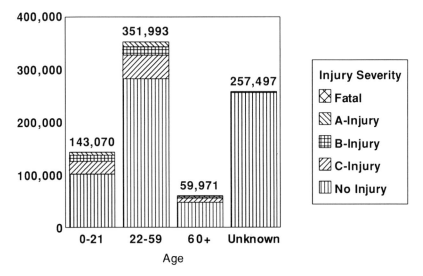

FIGURE 3.1. Injury severity by age, 1989 Michigan passenger car occupants.

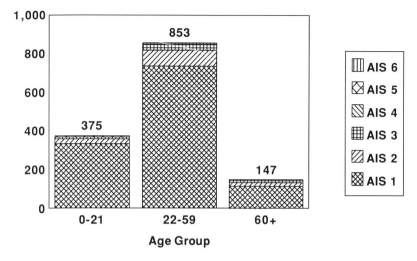

Unweighted

FIGURE 3.2. Neck injury severity by age, 1989 NASS passenger car occupants.

Figure 3.1 shows the distribution of age and injury severity in Michigan, but it may not reflect the national picture. The FARS file could be used to find the age and injury severity of occupants in fatal accidents nationwide while the NASS GES file could be used to look at a statistical sample of occupants in all severities of crashes.

Analysis of in-depth data can be much more specific. Using neck injury as an example, one might speculate that neck injuries would occur more often in older occupants. Figure 3.2 shows age and injury severities for all neck injuries in 1989 NASS CDS for persons in passenger cars. The injury severity is rated according to the Abbreviated Injury Scale, and the body region is from the Occupant Injury Classification (OIC).

Figure 3.2 would suggest that neck injury does indeed occur more frequently to older

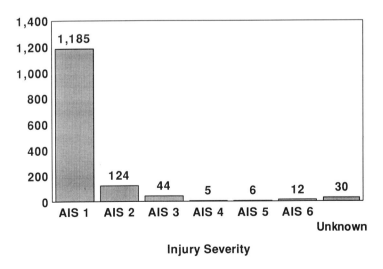

Unweighted

FIGURE 3.3. Neck injuries, 1989 NASS passenger car occupants.

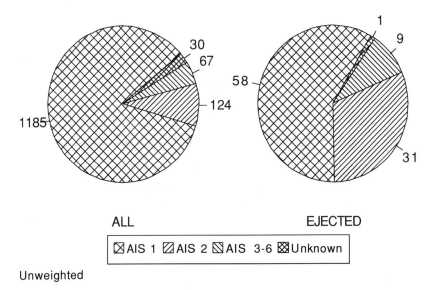

ALL   EJECTED

☒AIS 1 ☐AIS 2 ☐AIS 3-6 ☒Unknown

Unweighted

FIGURE 3.4. Ejection and neck injuries, NASS 1989 passenger car occupants.

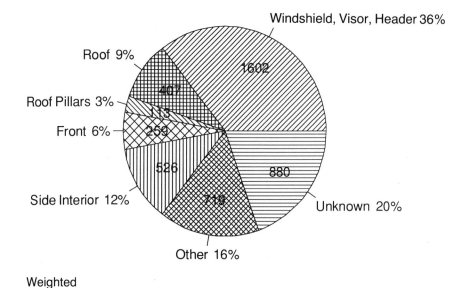

Weighted

FIGURE 3.5. AIS 3–6 neck injury and contacts, NASS 1989 passenger car occupants.

occupants than to younger ones. Far more extensive computer analysis could be done using the NASS CDS files, filtering occupant information such as injury contacts or height of the occupant. Vehicle-specific information such as crash severity and types and location of occupant compartment intrusions could also be taken into account. Figures 3.3–3.8 contain more sample charts of neck-injury severity distributions for some variables available in the CDS. The researcher must take into account factors such as ejection, rollover, belt use, and age, as they all play a significant part of the injury picture.

The NASS CDS file contains a weighting variable to estimate how many cases might be represented nationally from CDS analysis. To get a feeling for how accurate this weighting

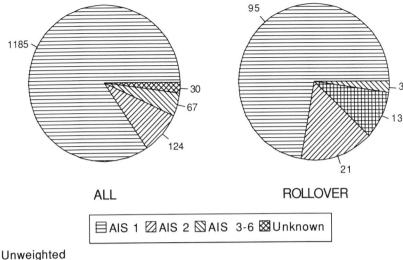

ALL   ROLLOVER

⊟ AIS 1 ⧄ AIS 2 ◩ AIS 3-6 ⊠ Unknown

Unweighted

FIGURE 3.6. Rollover and neck injury, NASS 1989 passenger car occupants.

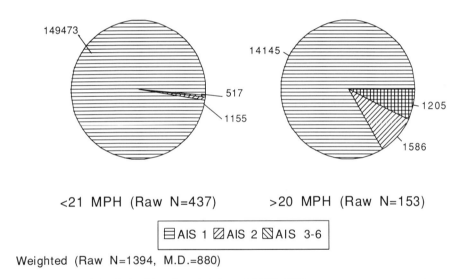

<21 MPH (Raw N=437)   >20 MPH (Raw N=153)

⊟ AIS 1 ⧄ AIS 2 ◩ AIS 3-6

Weighted (Raw N=1394, M.D.=880)

FIGURE 3.7. Delta V and neck injury, NASS 1989 passenger car occupants.

is, consider the GES weighting system. The GES system collects 5–10 times the number of cases the CDS system collects (although the sampling system is different) and the NHTSA has reported that an estimate of 1,000 from the 1989 GES has a standard error of 50%. The error decreases as the estimated number increases; at an estimate of 100,000 the reported standard error is less than 10%. This suggests that most weighted estimates derived from

CDS data, a much smaller sampling system, have a very large standard error.

Changes in Crash-Data Collection

It has long been recognized that the standardization of crash data collection and computerization would facilitate comparisons of

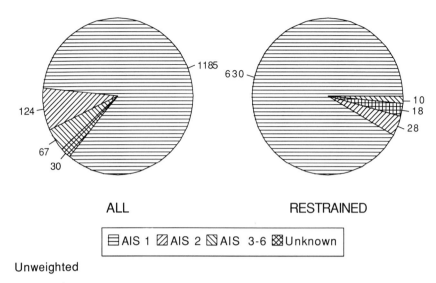

FIGURE 3.8. Belt use and neck injury, NASS 1989 passenger car occupants.

different states' data for problem identification in safety, roadway engineering, and a host of other areas. The National Safety Council has recommended standard coding practices and recently the NHTSA has recommended a core set of data elements, the Critical Automated Data Reporting Elements (CADRE), for all states to collect. As the NHTSA states in the *Federal Register* (May 1990), "if States would collect these data elements on Police Traffic Accident Reports and include them on automated databases, the usefulness of these files in support of highway safety analysis would increase dramatically." The adoption of these recommendations and the sharing of the data would represent a major advancement in the overall field of highway safety.

Another area that will potentially provide detailed information for research is the trauma registry, or database of hospital information on trauma victims. Hospitals have computerized their records for years, and many researchers have linked patient data with accident data, but only in studies of limited scope. There are many difficulties to overcome, not the least of which are the legal ramifications of allowing access to patient data, but if large-scale linking of accident and trauma data does occur it will provide very detailed information about the injuries and costs of automobile crashes.

Bibliography of Crash Data Files and Related Documentation[1]

American Association of Motor Vehicle Administrators, American National Standards Institute, and National Highway Traffic Safety Administration, Data Element Dictionary for Traffic Records Systems. Report No. ANSI D20.1-1979/ DOT-HS-805-226. American National Standards Institute, New York, March 1980.

Association for the Advancement of Automotive Medicine. *The abbreviated injury scale*, 1985 Revision, AAAM, Des Plaines, IL, 1985.

Collision deformation classification. SAE J224a, Society of Automotive Engineers.

CRASH3 User's guide and technical manual. DOT-HS-805-732, January 1981.

Critical automated data reporting elements. National Highway Traffic Safety Administration, Fed Reg 55(84):18220, May 1, 1990.

Evans L. *Traffic safety and the driver*. Van Nostrand Reinhold Co, New York, 1991.

Fatal accident reporting system coding and validation manual. National Highway Traffic Safety Administration, National Center for Statistics and Analysis, 1991.

Hight PV, et al. Barrier equivalent velocity, delta-V, and crash 3 stiffness in automobile collisions.

[1] Contact For NHTSA data files: Marjorie Saccoccio, DTS-44, DOT/Transportation Systems Center, Kendall Square, Cambridge, MA 02142.

In *Field accidents: data collection, analysis, methodologies, and crash injury reconstructions*, Society of Automotive Engineers, Warrendale, PA, 1985.

National Accident Sampling System, *General estimates system, analytical user's manual*. National Highway Traffic Safety Administration, National Center for Statistics and Analysis, 1989 File.

National Accident Sampling System, General Estimates System. *A review of information on police-reported Traffic crashes in the United States*. National Highway Traffic Safety Administration, National Center for Statistics and Analysis, 1989.

National Accident Sampling System, *Crashworthiness data subsystem, analytical user's manual*. National Highway Traffic Safety Administration, National Center for Statistics and Analysis, 1989 File.

National Accident Sampling System, *Crashworthiness data subsystem, Data collection, coding, and editing manual*. National Highway Traffic Safety Administration, National Center for Statistics and Analysis, 1989 File.

National accident sampling system, injury coding manual. National Highway Traffic Safety Administration, National Center for Statistics and Analysis, 1988 File.

Manual on classification of motor vehicle traffic accidents, ANSI D16.1 National Safety Council, 1990.

O'Day, James, Waissi, Gary R Worldwide Accident Data Standardization. The UMTRI Research Review, 17(6) May–June 1987.

Trauma Registry Users' Manual. Centers For Disease Control, Atlanta, Georgia, July 1990.

Appendix A: Sample Police File Data, MICHIGAN 1990, UMTRI File Listing

V1:CASE SEQUENCE NUMBER = 999997
V2:ACCIDENT MONTH = January
V3:ACCIDENT DAY = 3
V4:ACCIDENT YEAR = 90
V5:TIME OF DAY = 9 am–10 am
V8:DAY OF WEEK = Wednesday
V10:HIGHWAY DEPT DISTRICT = 3rd district
V11:STATE POLICE POST = Cadillac

V12:COUNTY = Wexford
V13:CITY OR TOWNSHIP = 12
V17:HIGHWAY AREA TYPE = Intersection
V18:HIGHWAY AREA CODE = In intersection
V19:ACCIDENT LOCATION = On regular road
V20:HIGHWAY CLASS = M route
V21:HIGHWAY CLASS SUBSCRIPT = Nonlim acc M rt
V22:ROAD ALIGNMENT = Straight
V23:ROAD SURFACE = Wet
V24:ROAD DEFECT = None
V25:TRAFFIC CONTROL = Stop sign
V26:CONSTRUCTION ZONE = Non const zone
V27:WEATHER = Clear/cloudy
V28:LIGHT = Daylight
V29:POPULATION = Township
C30:ACCIDENT TYPE = Col w other veh
V31:ACC ANALYSIS—WHERE = Angle - at int
V32:ACC ANALYSIS—HOW = 1 (based on value of V30)
V33:ACC ANALYSIS SUBSCRIPT = 1
V34:SPECIAL ACCIDENT TAG = None of above
V35:ACCIDENT TYPE SUBSCRIPT = Col w veh-no med
V36:NSC ACC CIRCUMSTANCE = Failed to yield
V37:TWO VEH ACC SUBSCRIPT = Angle
V38:ACCIDENT CONFIGURATION = 2 veh -angle
V39:TRAFFIC UNIT MIX = Car-truck
V40:DRINKING IN ACCIDENT = No drinking
V41:PED INVOL VED IN ACCIDENT = Ped/cycl uninvld
V42:ACCIDENT INVESTIGATED BY = County sheriff
V43:INVESTIGATED AT SCENE = Investigated
V44:ENFORCEMENT IN ACCIDENT = No violation
V45:SEVERITY OF ACCIDENT = Fatal
V46:TOTAL TRAFFIC UNITS = 2
V47:TOTAL MOVING VEHICLES = 2
V48:WORST INJURY IN ACC = Fatal
V49:TOTAL KILLED IN ACC = 1

V50:TOTAL A INJURED IN ACC = 0
V51:TOTAL B INJURED IN ACC = 0
V52:TOTAL C INJURED IN ACC = 0
V53:TOTAL INJURED IN ACC = 0
V54:TOTAL CASUALTIES IN ACC = 1
V55:TOTAL UNINJURED IN ACC = 1
V101:TRAFFIC UNIT NUMBER = 1
V102:TRAFFIC UNIT TYPE = Passenger car
V103:VEHICLE MAKE = Chevrolet
V104:VEHICLE TYPE = Car -1500-2499lb
V105:NSC VEHICLE TYPE = Passenger car
V106:YEAR MANUFACTURED = 87
V107:VEHICLE CONDITION = No defect
V108:VEHICLE   DRIVEN/TOWED   =
  Towed away
V109:TRAILER TYPE = No trailer
V110:TRUCK CARGO TYPE = Not a truck
V111:TRUCK CARGO SPILLAGE = Not a
  truck
V112:DRIVER INTENT = Going straight
V113:PEDESTRIAN   INTENT   =   MD/
  non ped/cycl
V114:DIRECTION OF TRAVEL = West
V115:OBJECT HIT = No object hit
V116:SITUATION = None above/non v
V117:IMPACT CODE = Left side
V118:VEHICLE DAMAGE SEVERITY = 8
V119:FUEL LEAK OR FIRE = No leak or
  fire
V120:HIT AND RUN DRIVER = Driver
  known
V121:DRINKING OR DRUG USE = No
  alcohol/drugs
V122:DRINKING TEST RESULT = Not
  tested
V123:VISUAL   OBSTRUCTION   =   No
  obstruction
V124:CONTRIBUTNG   CIRCUMSTANCE
  = Other/unknown -(by combining the codes
  ("other" with "unknown" the analytic value
  of the variable is diminished)
V125:HAZARDOUS ACTION = Failed to
  yield
V126:POLICE ACTION = No citation
V127:TU TOTAL OCCUPANTS = 1
V128:LF RESTRAINT USAGE = Belt used
V134:TOTAL OCC UNRESTRAINED = 0
V135:TOTAL OCC RESTRAINED = 1
V136:TOTAL OCC W UNK RES USE = 0
V137:DRIVER HELMET USE = Helmet not
  used

V138:PASSENGER HELMET USE = Info
  not coded
V139:TU WORST INJURY = Fatal
V140:TU TOTAL KILLED = 1
V141:TU TOTAL A INJURED = 0
V142:TU TOTAL B INJURED = 0
V143:TU TOTAL C INJURED = 0
V144:TU TOTAL INJURED = 0
V145:TU TOTAL CASUALTIES = 1
V146:TU TOTAL UNINJURED = 0
V147:DRIVER/PED AGE = 53
V150:DRIVER/PED SEX = Female
V151:DRIVER/PED   RESIDENCE   =
  Michigan
V201:OCCUPANT NUMBER = 1
V202:OCCUPANT   LOCATION   =   Driver
  (1988)
V203:OCCUPANT POSITION = Driver/ped/
  cyclst
V204:OCCUPANT   RESTRAINT   USE   =
  Belt used
V205:OCCUPANT HELMET USE = Helmet
  not used
V206:OCCUPANT AGE = 53
V209:OCCUPANT SEX = Female
V210:OCCUPANT INJURY SEVERITY =
  Fatal

Appendix B: Fatal Accident Reporting System 1990, UMTRI File Listing

V1:CASE STATE = Alabama
V2:CASE NUMBER = 1
V3:SEQUENCE NUMBER = 0
V4:VEHICLE NUMBER = No veh number
V5:RECORD TYPE = Accident Record
V6:PERSON NUMBER = No person number
V7:CITY = 0
V8:COUNTY = 117
V9:ACCIDENT DATE—MONTH = January
V10:ACCIDENT DATE—DAY = 7
V11:ACCIDENT DATE—YEAR = 90
V12:ACCIDENT TIME—HOUR = 6:00 am–
  6:59 am
V13:ACCIDENT TIME—MINUTE = 45
V14:NUMBER OF VEHICLE FORMS = 1
V15:NUMBER OF PERSON FORMS = 1
V16:FEDERAL-AID SYSTEM = Interstate

V17:ROADWAY FUNCTION CLASS = Rur interstate

V18:ROUTE SIGNING = Interstate

V19:TRAFFICWAY IDENTIFIER = 165

V20:MILEPOINT = 2350

V21:SPECIAL JURISDICTION = None

V22:FIRST HARMFUL EVENT = Tree

V23:MANNER OF COLLISION = Not transp coll

V24:RELATION TO JUNCTION = Nonjunction

V25:RELATION TO ROADWAY = Median

V26:TRAFFICWAY FLOW = Dv hwy, med, n/bar

V27:NUMBER OF TRAVEL LANES = 2 lanes

V28:SPEED LIMIT = 65 mph

V29:ROADWAY ALIGNMENT = Straight

V30:ROADWAY PROFILE = Grade

V31:ROADWAY SURFACE TYPE = Blacktp/btuminus

V32:ROADWY SURFACE CONDITION = Wet

V33:TRAFFIC CONTROL DEVICE = No controls

V34:TRAFFIC CONT FUNCTIONING = No controls

V35:HIT AND RUN = No hit and run

V36:LIGHT CONDITION = Daylight

V37:ATMOSPHERIC CONDITIONS = Rain

V38:CONSTRUCTION/MAINT ZONE = None

V39:EMS NOTIFIED—HOUR = 8

V40:EMS NOTIFIED—MINUTE = 11

V41:EMS ARRIVAL—HOUR = 8

V42:EMS ARRIVAL—MINUTE = 12

V43:EMS HOSPITAL—HOUR = 0

V44:EMS HOSPITAL—MINUTE = 0

V45:SCHOOL BUS RELATED = No

V46:ACCIDENT RELATED FACTORS = 000000 (3,2-digit codes, 00 = none)

V47:RAIL GRADE CROSSING ID = 0000000

V48:NUMBER FATALITIES IN ACC = 1

V49:DAY OF WEEK = Sunday

V50:NUMBER DRINKING DRIVERS = 1

V51:ACCIDENT DATE-JULIAN = 32820

V52:NUMBER UNINJURED IN ACC = 0

V53:NUMBER C-INJURED IN ACC = 0

V54:NUMBER B-INJURED IN ACC = 0

V55:NUMBER A-INJURED IN ACC = 0

V56:NUMBER K-INJURED IN ACC = 1

V57:NUM UNK INJURED IN ACC = 0

V104:VEHICLE NUMBER = 1

V105:RECORD TYPE = Vehicle record

V106:PERSON NUMBER = No person number

V107:VEHICLE MAKE = Pontiac

V108:VEHICLE MAKE-MODEL = Firebrd/ Trans Am

V109:BODY TYPE = 2dr sdn, hdtp, cpe

V110:MODEL YEAR = 84

V111:VIN = 1G2AW87G4E

V112:VIN—LETTER #1 = 1

V113:VIN—LETTER #2 = G

V114:VIN—LETTER #3 = 2

V115:VIN—LETTER #4 = A

V116:VIN—LETTER #5 = W

V117:VIN—LETTER #6 = 8

V118:VIN—LETTER #7 = 7

V119:VIN—LETTER #8 = G

V120:VIN—LETTER #9 = 4

V121:VIN—LETTER #10 = E

V122:REGISTRATION STATE = Alabama

V123:ROLLOVER = No rollover

V124:JACKKNIFE = N/articulatd veh

V125:TRAVEL SPEED = 70

V126:HAZARDOUS CARGO = No

V127:VEHICLE TRAILERING = No

V128:SPECIAL USE = No special use

V129:EMERGENCY USE = No

V130:IMPACT POINT—INITIAL = 7 o'clock

V131:IMPACT POINT—PRINCIPAL = 7 o'clock

V132:EXTENT OF DEFORMATION = Disabling (sev)

V133:VEHICLE ROLE = Striking

V134:MANNER OF LEAVING SCENE = Towed away

V135:FIRE OCCURRENCE = No fire

V136:NUMBER OF OCCUPANTS = 1

V137:NUMBER OF DEATHS IN VEH = 1

V138:VEHICLE RELATED FACTORS = 0100

V139:VEHICLE MANEUVER = Going straight

V140:MOST HARMFUL EVENT = Tree

V141:VIN AUTO MODEL = FAM

V142:VIN BODY TYPE = 2H

V143:VIN AUTO WEIGHT = 3189

V144:VIN AUTO WHEELBASE SHORT = 1010

V145:VIN AUTO WHEELBASE LONG = 0

V146:VIN TRUCK FUEL CODE = Not available

V147:VIN TRUCK WEIGHT CODE = Not coded

V148:VIN TRUCK SERIES = ***

V149:VIN MOTORCYCLE DSPLACMNT = 9999

V150:LENGTH OF VIN = 17

V151:NUMBER UNINJURED IN VEH = 0

V152:NUMBER C-INJURED IN VEH = 0

V153:NUMBER B-INJURED IN VEH = 0

V154:NUMBER A-INJURED IN VEH = 0

V155:NUMBER K-INJURED IN VEH = 1

V156:NUM UNK INJURED IN VEH = 0

V205:RECORD TYPE = Driver record

V206:PERSON NUMBER = No person number

V207:DRIVER PRESENCE = Drvr operatd veh

V208:DRIVER DRINKING = Drinking reportd

V209:LICENSE STATE = Georgia

V210:LICENSE STATUS = Single class

V211:LICENSE CLASS COMPLIANCE = Valid license

V212:LICENSE RESTRICTIONS MET = Not restrictions

V213:VIOLATIONS CHARGED = None

V214:NUMBER OF PREV ACCIDENTS = 0

V215:NUMBER PREV SUSPENSIONS = 0

V216:NUMBER OF PREV DWI CONV = 0

V217:NUM PREV SPEEDING CONV = 0

V218:NUM PREV OTHER MV CONV = 0

V219:LAST ACCIDENT—MONTH = No record

V220:LAST ACCIDENT—YEAR = 0

V221:FIRST ACCIDENT—MONTH = No record

V222:FIRST ACCIDENT—YEAR = 0

V223:DRIVER ZIP CODE = 35214

V224:DRIVER RELATED FACTORS = 442800

V305:RECORD TYPE = Occupant record

V306:OCCUPANT NUMBER = 1

V307:FILLER O1 = 0

V308:OCCUPANT AGE = 25

V309:OCCUPANT SEX = Male

V310:OCCUPANT TYPE = Drv m.v. in tran

V311:OCC SEATING POSITION = Ft st-lt side

V312:RESTRAINT SYSTEM USE = None used/NA

V313:AIR BAG AVAIL/FUNCTION = Unknown/NA

V314:FILLER O2 = 0

V315:OCCUPANT EJECTION = Not ejected/NA

V316:OCCUPANT EXTRICATION = None/NA

V317:OCC METH ALC DETERMINAT = Not reported

V318:OCC ALCOHOL INVOLVEMENT = Alcohol involved

V319:OCC ALCOHOL TEST RESULT = 0.15

V320:OCC DRUG TOXICOLOGY = No drugs reportd

V321:OCCUPANT INJURY SEVERITY = K fatal injury

V322:OCC TAKEN TO HOSPITAL = No

V323:OCC DEATH DATE—MONTH = January

V324:OCC DEATH DATE—DAY = 7

V325:OCC DEATH DATE—YEAR = 90

V326:OCC DEATH TIME—HOURS = 6:00 am–6.59 am

V327:OCC DEATH TIME—MINUTES = 45

V328:LAG TIME ACC/DEATH—HRS = 0

V329:LAG TIME ACC/DEATH—MIN = 0

V330:OCCUPANT RELATED FACTORS = 000000

V331:OCC DEATH CERTIFICATE = ************

V332:OCC FATAL INJURY AT WORK = No

Appendix C: National Accident Sampling System, Crashworthiness Data System 1989, UMTRI File Listing

V101:PSU NUMBER = 1

V102:CASE NUMBER = 001E

V103:RECORD NUMBER = Accident record

V104:VERSION NUMBER = Version 2

V105:NUM GEN VEH FORMS SUBMIT = 2

V106:ACCIDENT MONTH = January

V107:ACCIDENT YEAR = 1989

V108:ACCIDENT DAY OF WEEK = Thursday

V109:ACCIDENT TIME = 806

V110:ANTI-LACERATIVE WINDSHLD = No

V111:NUM EVENTS RECORDED = 2

V112:MAXIMUM TREATMENT = Hospitalization

V113:MAXIMUM KNOWN AIS = Moderate injury

V114:NUM SERIOUSLY INJ OCC = None

V115:NUM INJURED OCCUPANTS = 2

V116:ALCOHOL/DRUG INVOL VEMENT = No

V117:PSU INFLATION FACTOR = 8.900

V118:NAT INFLATION FACTOR = 711.199

V205:EVENT SEQUENCE NUMBER = 1st event

V206:VEHICLE NUMBER (1) = Vehicle #1

V207:CLASS OF VEHICLE (1) = Intermediate (wh

V208:GEN AREA OF DAMAGE (1) = (R)Right Side

V209:VEH NUM (2)/OBJ CONTACT = Vehicle num 2

V210:CLASS OF VEHICLE (2) = Intermediate (wh

V211:GEN AREA OF DAMAGE (2) = (F)Front

V303:RECORD NUMBER = General Vehicle

V304:VERSION NUMBER = Version 2

V305:VEHICLE NUMBER = Vehicle #1

V306:MODEL YEAR = 1980

V307:VEHICLE MAKE = Pontiac

V308:MAKE/MODEL = Pont LeMans/Temp

V309:BODY TYPE = 4-door sedan, ha

V310:VIN = 2D19KAB100

V311:VIN—CHARACTER #1 = 2

V312:VIN—CHARACTER #2 = D

V313:VIN—CHARACTER #3 = 1

V314:VIN—CHARACTER #4 = 9

V315:VIN—CHARACTER #5 = K

V316:VIN—CHARACTER #6 = A

V317:VIN—CHARACTER #7 = B

V318:VIN—CHARACTER #8 = 1

V319:VIN—CHARACTER #9 = 0

V320:VIN—CHARACTER #10 = 0

V321:VEHICLE DISPOSITION = Towed due to dam

V322:TRAVEL SPEED = Unknown

V323:ALCOHOL/DRUG PRESENCE = N/alcohol n/drug

V324:ALCOHOL TEST RESULT = None given

V325:SPEED LIMIT = 45

V326:ATTEMPTED AVOID MANEUVER = Braking (lockup)

V327:ACCIDENT TYPE = 64

V328:DRIVER PRESENCE = Driver present

V329:NUMBER OF OCCUPANTS = 1

V330:NUMBER OCCUPANT FORMS = 1

V331:CURB WEIGHT = 31

V332:CARGO WEIGHT = <50 lbs

V333:TOWED TRAILING UNIT = No towed unit

V334:TRAJECTORY DATA DOC = No

V335:POST COLL TREE/POLE COND = N/coll w/tree

V336:ROLLOVER = No rollover

V337:FRONT OVERRIDE/UNDERRIDE = No over/underide

V338:REAR OVERRIDE/UNDERRIDE = No over/underide

V339:HEADING ANGLE—THIS VEH = 30

V340:HEADING ANGLE—OTH VEH = 278

V341:BASIS FOR TOTAL DELTA-V = CRASH dam only

V342:TOTAL DELTA-V = 22

V343:LONG COMPONENT DELTA-V = 0

V344:LAT COMPONENT DELTA-V = -22

V345:ENERGY ABSORPTION = 435

V346:RECONSTRUCT CONFIDENCE = results reasonab

V347:TYPE OF VEH INSPECTION = Complete inspect

V348:MAXIMUM TREATMENT = Hospitalization

V349:MAXIMUM KNOWN AIS = Moderate injury

V350:NUM SERIOUSLY INJURED = None

V351:NUMBER INJURED = 1

V352:FRONT/REAR WHEEL DRIVE = Rear wheel drive

V353:VIN LENGTH = 13

V354:WEIGHT—OTHER VEHICLE = 32

V355:BODY TYPE—OTHER VEH = 2-door sedan, cp

V356:AOPS VEHICLE = Unk if Equipped

V403:RECORD NUMBER = Exterior Damage
V404:VERSION NUMBER = Version 2
V405:VEHICLE NUMBER = Vehicle #1
V406:ACCIDENT SEQUENCE (1) = 1
V407:OBJECT CONTACTED (1) = Vehicle num 2
V408:DIRECTION OF FORCE (1) = 3 o'clock
V409:DEFORMATION LOCATION (1) = R
V410:LONG/LAT LOCATION (1) = Y
V411:VERT/LAT LOCATION (1) = A
V412:TYPE OF DISTRIB (1) = W
V413:DEFORMATION EXTENT (1) = Extent zone 3
V414:ACCIDENT SEQUENCE (2) = 2
V415:OBJECT CONTACTED (2) = Vehicle num 2
V416:DIRECTION OF FORCE (2) = 3 o'clock
V417:DEFORMATION LOCATION (2) = R
V418:LONG/LAT LOCATION (2) = B
V419:VERT/LAT LOCATION (2) = E
V420:TYPE OF DISTRIB (2) = W
V421:DEFORMATION EXTENT (2) = Extent zone 1
V422:HIGHEST DELTA-V—"L" = 101
V423:HIGHEST DELTA-V—"C1" = 1
V424:HIGHEST DELTA-V—"C2" = 14
V425:HIGHEST DELTA-V—"C3" = 14
V426:HIGHEST DELTA-V—"C4" = 14
V427:HIGHEST DELTA-V—"C5" = 6
V428:HIGHEST DELTA-V—"C6" = 0
V429:HIGHEST DELTA-V—"D" = 40
V430:SECOND DELTA-V—"L" = 999
V431:SECOND DELTA-V—"C1" = 99
V432:SECOND DELTA-V—"C2" = 99
V433:SECOND DELTA-V—"C3" = 99
V434:SECOND DELTA-V—"C4" = 99
V435:SECOND DELTA-V—"C5" = 99
V436:SECOND DELTA-V—"C6" = 99
V437:SECOND DELTA-V—"D" = 9999
V438:CDC'S DOC/NOT CODED = No
V439:VEHICLE DISPOSITION = Towed due to veh
V440:ORIGINAL WHEELBASE = ****
V503:RECORD NUMBER = Interior Damage
V504:VERSION NUMBER = Version 2
V505:VEHICLE NUMBER = Vehicle #1

V506:PASS COMPART INTEGRITY = Side window
V507:DOOR/GATE/HATCH OPN—LF = D/g/h closed &
V508:DOOR/GATE/HATCH OPN—RF = D/g/h jam shut
V509:DOOR/GATE/HATCH OPN—LR = D/g/h closed &
V510:DOOR/GATE/HATCH OPN—RR = D/g/h closed &
V511:DOOR/GATE/HATCH OPN—TG = No door/gate/hat
V512:DOOR/GATE/HATCH DAM—LF = No d/g/h or door
V513:DOOR/GATE/HATCH DAM—RF = No d/g/h or door
V514:DOOR/GATE/HATCH DAM—LR = No d/g/h or door
V515:DOOR/GATE/HATCH DAM—RR = No d/g/h or door
V516:DOOR/GATE/HATCH DAM—TG = No d/g/h or door
V517:IMPACT GLAZING DAM—WS = In place & crack
V518:IMPACT GLAZING DAM—LF = No glazing damag
V519:IMPACT GLAZING DAM—RF = Glazing disinteg
V520:IMPACT GLAZING DAM—LR = No glazing damag
V521:IMPACT GLAZING DAM—RR = No glazing damag
V522:IMPACT GLAZING DAM—BL = No glazing damag
V523:IMPACT GLAZING DAM—RO = No glazing
V524:IMPACT GLAZING DAM—OT = No glazing damag
V525:CONTACT GLAZING DAM—WS = No occ contact,
V526:CONTACT GLAZING DAM—LF = No occ contact,
V527:CONTACT GLAZING DAM—RF = Unk if contacted
V528:CONTACT GLAZING DAM—LR = No occ contact,
V529:CONTACT GLAZING DAM—RR = No occ contact,
V530:CONTACT GLAZING DAM—BL = No occ contact,

V531:CONTACT GLAZING DAM—RO = No occ contact,

V532:CONTACT GLAZING DAM—OT = No occ contact,

V533:TYPE OF GLAZING—WS = AS-1 Laminated

V534:TYPE OF GLAZING—LF = N/contact, n/dam,

V535:TYPE OF GLAZING—RF = AS-2 Tempered

V536:TYPE OF GLAZING—LR = N/contact, n/dam,

V537:TYPE OF GLAZING—RR = N/contact, n/dam,

V538:TYPE OF GLAZING—BL = N/contact, n/dam,

V539:TYPE OF GLAZING—RO = N/contact, n/dam,

V540:TYPE OF GLAZING—OT = N/contact, n/dam,

V541:WIN PRECRASH STAT—WS = Fixed

V542:WIN PRECRASH STAT—LF = N/contact, n/dam,

V543:WIN PRECRASH STAT—RF = Closed

V544:WIN PRECRASH STAT—LR = N/contact, n/dam,

V545:WIN PRECRASH STAT—RR = N/contact, n/dam,

V546:WIN PRECRASH STAT—BL = N/contact, n/dam,

V547:WIN PRECRASH STAT—RO = N/contact, n/dam,

V548:WIN PRECRASH STAT—OT = N/contact, n/dam,

V603:RECORD NUMBER = Interior Damage

V604:VERSION NUMBER = Version 2

V605:VEHICLE NUMBER = Vehicle #1

V606:INTRUSION LOCATION (1) = Front row—righ

V607:INTRUDING COMPONENT (1) = Door panel

V608:INTRUSION MAGNITUDE (1) = > = 6in but <12

V609:CRUSH DIRECTION (1) = Lateral

V610:INTRUSION LOCATION (2) = Front row—righ

V611:INTRUDING COMPONENT (2) = Instrum panel r

V612:INTRUSION MAGNITUDE (2) = > = 6in but <12

V613:CRUSH DIRECTION (2) = Longitudinal

V614:INTRUSION LOCATION (3) = Front row—righ

V615:INTRUDING COMPONENT (3) = Side panel rear

V616:INTRUSION MAGNITUDE (3) = > = 6in but <12

V617:CRUSH DIRECTION (3) = Lateral

V618:INTRUSION LOCATION (4) = Front row—righ

V619:INTRUDING COMPONENT (4) = A-pillar

V620:INTRUSION MAGNITUDE (4) = > = 1 in but <3

V621:CRUSH DIRECTION (4) = Lateral

V622:INTRUSION LOCATION (5) = No intrusion

V623:INTRUDING COMPONENT (5) = No intrusion

V624:INTRUSION MAGNITUDE (5) = No intrusion

V625:CRUSH DIRECTION (5) = No intrusion

V626:INTRUSION LOCATION (6) = No intrusion

V627:INTRUDING COMPONENT (6) = No intrusion

V628:INTRUSION MAGNITUDE (6) = No intrusion

V629:CRUSH DIRECTION (6) = No intrusion

V630:INTRUSION LOCATION (7) = No intrusion

V631:INTRUDING COMPONENT (7) = No intrusion

V632:INTRUSION MAGNITUDE (7) = No intrusion

V633:CRUSH DIRECTION (7) = No intrusion

V634:INTRUSION LOCATION (8) = No intrusion

V635:INTRUDING COMPONENT (8) = No intrusion

V636:INTRUSION MAGNITUDE (8) = No intrusion

V637:CRUSH DIRECTION (8) = No intrusion

V638:INTRUSION LOCATION (9) = No intrusion

V639:INTRUDING COMPONENT (9) = No intrusion

V640:INTRUSION MAGNITUDE (9) = No intrusion

V641:CRUSH DIRECTION (9) = No intrusion

V642:INTRUSION LOCATION (10) = No intrusion

V643:INTRUDING COMPONENT (10) = No intrusion

V644:INTRUSION MAGNITUDE (10) = No intrusion

V645:CRUSH DIRECTION (10) = No intrusion

V646:STEERING COLUMN TYPE = Fixed column

V647:STEERING COL COLLAPSE = No move, comp, col

V648:SC VERTICAL MOVEMENT = No sc movement

V649:SC LATERAL MOVEMENT = No sc movement

V650:SC LONGITUD MOVEMENT = No sc movement

V651:RIM/SPOKE DEFORMATION = No deformation

V652:RIM/SPOKE DEF LOCATION = No steering rim

V653:ODOMETER READING = 64

V654:INSTRUMENT PANEL DAMAGE = No

V655:KNEE BOLSTERS DEFORMED = Not present

V656:GLOVE COMPART DOOR OPEN = No

V703:RECORD NUMBER = Occ assess rec

V704:VERSION NUMBER = Version 2

V705:VEHICLE NUMBER = Vehicle #1

V706:OCCUPANT NUMBER = 1

V707:AGE = 22

V708:SEX = Male

V709:HEIGHT = 70

V710:WEIGHT = 170

V711:ROLE = Driver

V712:SEAT POSITION = Front seat—lef

V713:POSTURE = Normal posture

V714:EJECTION = No ejection

V715:EJECTION AREA = No ejection

V716:EJECTION MEDIUM = No ejection

V717:MEDIUM STATUS = No ejection

V718:ENTRAPMENT = Not entrapped

V719:MANUAL BELT AVAILABILITY = Lap and shoulder

V720:MANUAL BELT USE = None used, not a

V721:MANUAL BELT PROPER USE = None used or not

V722:MANUAL BELT FAILURE = N/used-n/availab

V723:AUTO RESTRAINT AVAILABLE = N/equip-n/availa

V724:AUTO RESTRAINT FUNCTION = N/equip-n/availa

V725:AUTO RESTRAINT FAILURE = N/equip-n/availa

V726:PAR RESTRAINT USE = None used

V727:HEAD RESTRAINT TYPE/DAM = Adjustable-n/dam

V728:SEAT TYPE = Bench

V729:SEAT PERFORMANCE = No failure

V730:CHILD SEAT MAKE/MODEL = No child safety

V731:CHILD SEAT TYPE = No child safety

V732:CHILD SEAT ORIENTATION = No child safety

V733:CHILD SEAT HARNESS USE = No child safety

V734:CHILD SEAT SHIELD USE = No child safety

V735:CHILD SEAT TETHER USE = No child safety

V736:INJURY SEVERITY = C-possible inj

V737:TREATMENT/MORTALITY = Hospitalized

V738:TYPE OF MEDICAL FACILITY = Hospital

V739:HOSPITAL STAY = 1

V740:WORKING DAYS LOST = 2

V741:TIME TO DEATH = Not fatal

V742:CAUSE OF DEATH—MED REP = 000000

V743:NUM RECORDED INJURIES = 2

V744:MAXIMUM KNOWN AIS = Moderate injury

V745:INJURY SEVERITY SCORE = 5

V803:RECORD NUMBER = Occupant injury

V804:VERSION NUMBER = Version 2

V805:VEHICLE NUMBER = Vehicle #1

V806:OCCUPANT NUMBER = 1

V807:INJURY NUMBER = 1

V808:INJURY   DATA   SOURCE   =
   Emergency room r

V809:OIC/AIS = HPLI1

V810:OIC—BODY REGION = H—Head—
   skull

V811:OIC—ASPECT = P—Posterior (b

V812:OIC—LESION = L—Laceration

V813:OIC—SYSTEM   ORGAN   =   I—
   Integumentar

V814:AIS SEVERITY = Minor injury

V815:INJURY SOURCE = Right side inter

V816:CONFIDENCE LEVEL = Possible

V817:DIRECT/INDIRECT   INJURY   =
   Direct cont inj

V818:INTRUSION NUMBER = 1

4
Anthropomorphic Test Devices

Harold J. Mertz

Introduction

Anthropomorphic test devices, commonly referred to as dummies, are mechanical surrogates of the human body used in the automotive industry to estimate the effectiveness of occupant restraint systems used in new-vehicle car designs. These human surrogates are designed to mimic pertinent human physical characteristics such as size, shape, mass, stiffness, and energy dissipation so that their mechanical responses simulate corresponding human responses of trajectory, velocity, acceleration, deformation, and articulation when the dummies are exposed to simulated accident conditions. They are instrumented with transducers to measure exterior and interior loading of their body parts. Analyses of these measurements are used to assess the effectiveness of the restraint-system design for the accident conditions that are simulated.

The efficacy of these assessments is dependent on three factors: (1) the degree to which pertinent human physical characteristics are incorporated in the dummy design, called "biofidelity," (2) the measurement of dummy responses that are related to potential injury concerns, and (3) the degree of correlation that exists between the measured responses and the associated injury concerns. A deficiency in any one of these factors can greatly affect the accuracy of the assessment. For example, if pertinent human physical characteristics are not incorporated in a dummy design, then that dummy will not respond in a humanlike manner when exposed to simulated accident conditions, so occupant protection assessments will be highly questionable. Also, if the dummy is not instrumented to measure a response that is correlated to a specific injury concern, or if the correlation between a measured response and an injury concern is not known, then assessing protection for that injury concern cannot be done.

Dummies are classified according to their physical size. The midsize adult male dummy, the most-utilized size in automotive restraint testing, approximates the median height and weight of the U.S. adult male population. The small female and large male dummies approximate the height and weight of the fifth-percentile adult female and 95th-percentile adult male. Child dummies' heights and weights approximate median heights and weights of children of the specified age group without regard to sex.

Early versions of dummies were developed to assess the integrity of restraint systems during simulated frontal collisions. These dummies were quite durable in construction and mimicked human shape and weight. Their major deficiencies were that they were not designed to mimic human impact response and they were not instrumented to measure responses associated with many of the potential injury concerns.

The most notable of these early dummies is the Hybrid II dummy, which was developed by General Motors in 1972 to assess the integrity of lap/shoulder belt systems.[1] This dummy mimicked the size, shape, mass, and ranges of arm and leg motion of the 50th-percentile adult male. It was instrumented to measure the orthogonal linear accelerations of the center of gravity of its head and a point prescribed in its thoracic spine. Its femurs were instrumented to measure axial-shaft loading. It had acceptable levels of durability and serviceability to be used in routine restraint-system integrity testing. In 1973, the Hybrid II dummy was specified in Federal Motor Vehicle Safety Standard (FMVSS) 208 as the dummy to be used for compliance testing of vehicles equipped with passive restraints.[2] Testing with the Hybrid II dummy provided assurance that a given restraint system would not fail under the specified simulated collision conditions. However, it was not possible to obtain reliable estimates of restraint effectiveness because the Hybrid II had limited impact response biofidelity and measurement capacity.[3-8] These deficiencies led to the development of dummies with improved biofidelity and greater measurement capacity.

This chapter provides descriptions of the physical characteristics, biofidelity levels, and measurement capabilities of some of the more advanced dummies that are used in the automotive industry. For frontal-collision simulations, descriptions are given of adult, child, and infant dummies. For lateral-collision simulations, the three side-impact dummies, SID, EUROSID-1, and BIOSID, are described. Injury-assessment reference values that have been suggested as guidelines for assessing restraint-system designs are noted.

Dummies for Frontal-Collision Simulations

Midsize Male Hybrid III Dummy

In the early 1970s, a number of dummy-development programs[3,9-23] were undertaken to address the biofidelity and measurement deficiencies of the Hybrid II dummy. The most notable of these programs was the development of the Hybrid III dummy by General Motors.[3] The Hybrid III dummy, shown in Figure 4.1, was designed to approximate the size, shape, and mass of the 50th-percentile

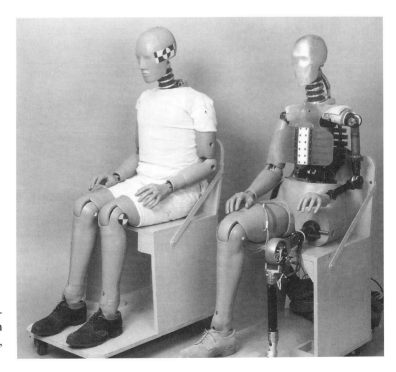

FIGURE 4.1. Hybrid III mid-size adult male dummy shown with and without its head, torso, arm, and leg skins.

adult male. The dummy's "skeleton" is composed primarily of metal parts to give it structural strength. This structure is covered by a vinyl skin and foam to give the desired external human shape. Vinyl was chosen for the skin because it is easily repaired by applying heat. The Hybrid III features a curved, rubber lumbar spine that provides the desired automotive seated posture. Constant-torque joints are used in the shoulders and knees to minimize the time needed to set joint resistance. The shoulder structure was designed to carry shoulder-belt loads and to improve the belt-to-shoulder interface, which was a problem with the Hybrid II dummy. The Hybrid III head acceleration response mimics human head acceleration response for forehead and side-of-the-head impacts.[3,13,14,24,25] The fore–aft and lateral bending response of its neck mimics human response.[3,4,25,36] Its chest structure mimics human force-deflection response for blunt, distributed sternal impacts[3,5] and its

knees were designed to mimic human knee impact data.[3,6,8,27] The original Hybrid III described by Foster et al.[3] used pin-joints for both the knee and ankle joints. As a result of knee-bolster testing the knee joint was modified to allow humanlike fore–aft translation of the tibia relative to the femur[28] and the ankle joint was changed to a ball-joint to allow humanlike lateral rotation of the foot relative to the tibia. In addition, the tibial shaft was instrumented to assess a variety of possible leg injuries.[29] Recently, Begeman and Prasad[30] presented cadaver data that suggest that the dorsiflexion angle of the ankle joint should be increased from 30 degrees to 45 degrees. A prototype ankle joint incorporating this proposed increased in angle has been developed and is currently being evaluated. However, it is not yet part of the standard Hybrid III dummy.

A summary of the standard instrumentation for the Hybrid III dummy is given in Table 4.1.

TABLE 4.1. Standard instrumentation for frontal impact, adult-size dummies.

	No. data channels			
	H-II	H-III–type dummies[a]		
Body region Measurements	Midsize male	Small female	Midsize male	Large male
Head				
Triaxial acceleration	3	3	3	3
Head/neck interface				
Shear & axial forces	0	3	3	3
Bending & twist moments	0	3	3	3
Chest				
Triaxial acceleration	3	3	3	3
Sternal deflection (D_x)	0	1	1	1
Pelvis				
Triaxial acceleration	3	3	3	3
Femur				
Axial force	2	2	2	2
Knee				
Tibia-to-femur displacement	0	2	2	2
Med. & lat. clevis forces	0	4	4	4
Tibia				
Up. bending moments (M_x, M_y)	0	4	4	4
Lo. bending moments (M_y)	0	2	2	2
Lo. shear & axial forces (F_x, F_z)	0	4	4	4
Totals	9	34	34	34

[a] For Hybrid III type dummies, external head impact force can be calculated using head acceleration and neck-load data.

TABLE 4.2. Optional instrumentation available for H-III–type small female, midsize male, and large male dummies.[a]

Body region Measurements	Data channels
Head	
Angular accelerations	3
Neck/chest interface	
Shear & axial forces	3
Bending moments (M_x, M_y)	2
Lumbar/pelvis interface	
Shear & axial forces	3
Bending moments (M_x, M_y)	2
Pelvis	
Angular acceleration (α_y)	1
Ant.-sup. iliac lap-belt load	2
Iliac crest lap-belt transducer	2
Femur	
Shear forces (F_x, F_y)	4
Bending moments (M_x, M_y, M_z)	6
Totals	28

[a] Deformable face available for use in assessing facial bone fracture potential.[74] Deformable abdomen available for assessing abdominal injury potential if lap-belt submarining occurs.[72,73]

It consists of 34 data channels, 25 more data channels than were specified for the Hybrid II dummy. Optional transducers available for use with the Hybrid III dummy are listed in Table 4.2.

The Hybrid III dummy has proven to be a very repeatable, reproducible, durable, and serviceable test device. In addition, its increased measurement capabilities and impact biofidelity allow much better assessment of restraint-system effectiveness than can be obtained from Hybrid II data. For these reasons in 1983 General Motors petitioned the National Highway Traffic Safety Administration (NHTSA) to allow the use of the Hybrid III dummy as an alternative test device for FMVSS 208 compliance testing of passive restraints.[31] After a rather lengthy comment period, its use was allowed in 1986, 9 years after the Hybrid III became commercially available.

General Motors provided NHTSA with a set of reference values that GM used as guidelines to assess injury potentials associated with the various Hybrid III measurements.[32] These Injury Assessment Reference Values (IARV) are summarized in Appendix A with two exceptions. The IARV for sternal deflection for distributed chest loading produced by air bag or steering-hub interactions has been lowered to 65 mm based on a recent statistical analysis of cadaver data that indicated that the original IARV of 75 mm posed too great a risk of significant thoracic injury.[33] The IARV for sternal deflection of 50 mm for shoulder-harness loading was not changed since the recent analyses of Mertz et al.[34] and Horsch et al.[35] supported this value. The other exception is that the Viscous Criterion for assessing the risk of thoracic organ injury proposed by Viano and Lau[33] has been added. Mertz notes[32] that each IARV refers "to a human response level below which a specified significant injury is considered unlikely to occur for a given individual." He cautions that being below all the IARVs does not assure that the significant injury could not occur since IARVs are not specified and the dummy is not instrumented to measure the responses associated with all the types of injuries that an occupant might experience in the collision being simulated. Further, exceeding an IARV does not necessarily imply that a person would be injured if exposed to the collision being simulated since the IARVs are lower bounds for injury thresholds.

On November 13, 1990, General Motors petitioned the NHTSA to make the Hybrid III dummy the only allowable dummy for FMVSS 208 compliance testing.[36] To date there has been no formal action by NHTSA on the GM petition.

Small Female and Large Male Hybrid III–Type Dummies

While the Hybrid III dummy provides excellent assessments of the effectiveness of automotive restraint systems for the midsize adult male occupant, it provides no information concerning restraint effectiveness for large- or small-size adult occupants. To fill this void, the Center for Disease Control (CDC) awarded a grant in 1987 to Ohio State University (OSU) to develop a multisized Hybrid III–based dummy family. To support the OSU effort the Mechanical Human Simulation Subcommittee of the Human Biomechanics and Simulation Standards Committee of the Society of Automotive Engineers (SAE) formed a Task Force of biomechanics, test dummy, transducer, and restraint-system experts. They defined the specifications for an adult-size small female dummy and an adult-size large male dummy having the same level of biofidelity and measurement capacity as the Hybrid III dummy.[37] Key body-segment lengths and weights were selected for each dummy based on the anthropometry data for the extremes of the U.S. adult population.[38] Geometric- and mass-scale factors were developed to assure that each body segment had the same mass density as the corresponding Hybrid III body segment. Other pertinent dimensions were scaled from their corresponding Hybrid III dimensions using the corresponding geometric-scale factors.

The Hybrid III biomechanical response requirements for the head, neck, chest, and knee were scaled using the appropriate scale factors giving corresponding biofidelity response requirements for each size dummy.[37]

The Hybrid III design drawings were scaled using these geometric-scale factors to produce design drawings for each dummy. This procedure assured that each-size dummy made according to its scaled drawings would meet its scaled biofidelity requirements. The dummies were instrumented identically to the Hybrid III dummy (Tables 4.1 and 4.2). Both are commercially available.

The SAE task force noted that IARVs for each dummy could be obtained by assuming constant failure stress and scaling the Hybrid III IARVs using the appropriate scale factors. The resulting IARVs are given in Appendix A.

Child Dummies

There are a number of different types and sizes of child dummies that are commercially available. Most of these child dummies were designed to evaluate only the integrity of child restraints. Like the Hybrid II dummy, they mimic appropriate weight and size characteristics but lack the necessary impact response biofidelity and measurement capacity needed to assess injury potential. Three child dummies were designed to specifically assess injury

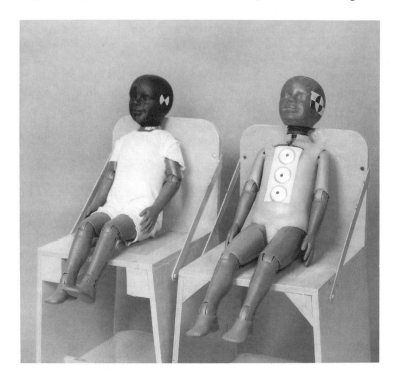

FIGURE 4.2. Three-year-old child dummy for use in passenger air-bag evaluation shown with and without its torso skin.

potential. Descriptions of these three child dummies are given.

Three-Year-Old "Air-bag" Dummy

A primary concern in the development of a passenger air-bag system is the possibility that a child could be in the path of a deploying cushion. General Motors developed a specially instrumented 3-year-old child dummy to evaluate the injury potentials associated with such interactions.[39] A test program was conducted to identify the types of injuries that could occur to children.[40] The dummy, shown in Figure 4.2, was designed to provide measurements that could be associated with those injuries. Dummy features include a biofidelic neck and a load transducer located at the head–neck interface to measure the potential for neck injuries due to cushion "membrane" forces. Three uniaxial accelerometers are mounted to

the front surface of the torso to measure the injury potential to thoracic and abdominal organs due to cushion "punch-out" forces. Dummy instrumentation is listed in Table 4.3. An analysis was done to correlate child-dummy responses to observed injuries for identical exposure environments.[41] Based on analyses of these results injury risk curves were developed. Appendix B gives Injury Assessment Reference Values corresponding to 1, 10, and 25% risks of life-threatening injuries for the various child-dummy measurements. In 1986, an SAE task force was convened for the purpose of developing a formal set of specifications for the GM child dummy, and the first commercial dummy became available in 1987.

Six-Month-Old Infant Dummy

A second concern with passenger air-bag design is the injury potential associated with

TABLE 4.3. Child and infant dummy instrumentation.[a]

Body region Measurements	CRABI 6-month	"Air-bag" 3-year	H-III–type 6-year
Head			
Triaxial acceleration	3	3	3
Angular acceleration (α_y)	1	1	0
Head/neck interface			
Shear & axial forces	3	2 (F_x, F_z)	3
Bending & twist moments	3	1 (M_y)	3
Neck/torso interface			
Shear & axial force	3	0	3
Bending & twist moments	3	0	2 (M_x, M_y)
Chest			
Triaxial acc. of c.g.	3	0	3
Triaxial acc. of upper spine	0	3	0
Triaxial acc. of lower spine	0	3	0
Sternal acc.; upper, mid, lower (A_x)	0	3	0
Sternal deflection (D_x)	0	0	1
Lumbar spine/pelvis interface			
Shear & axial forces	3	0	3
Bending & twist moments	3	0	2 (M_x, M_y)
Pelvis			
Triaxial acceleration	3	0	3
Ant.-sup. iliac lap-belt load	0	0	2
Femur			
Shear & axial forces	0	0	6
Bending moments	0	0	4
Totals	28	16	38

[a] Acc., acceleration; c.g., center of gravity.

the interaction of the deploying cushion and rearward-facing infant restraints that are placed in the front seat. Potential for head, neck, and thoracic injury due to high head acceleration, neck loads, and torso acceleration are of particular concern. An SAE task force was convened with the specific purpose of developing instrumented 6-month- and 1-year-old infant dummies to assess these injury potentials. The first prototype 6-month-old infant dummy became available September 1991 and is currently being evaluated. The dummy is called CRABI-6mo where CRABI refers to Child Restraint Air-Bag Interaction. The dummy features a biofidelic neck and a neck-load transducer. Table 4.3 provides a list of the instrumentation.

Six-Year-Old Child Dummy

As part of their CDC grant, Ohio State University, with the cooperation of the SAE task force, is developing a 6-year-old child dummy with the same level of biofidelity as the Hybrid III dummy. To date, scaling and biofidelity response corridors have been developed. Agreement has been reached on its instrumentation (Table 4.3). The first prototype dummy should be available for evaluation by October 1992.

Side-Impact Dummies

There are three side-impact dummies that are commercially available: SID, EUROSID-1, and BIOSID. All three dummies were designed to be representative of the physical size and weight of the midsize (50th percentile) adult male. SID was developed in 1979–82 by the Highway Safety Research Institute (HSRI) of the University of Michigan under a contract with NHTSA.[42–45] In the same time period, three side-impact dummies, APROD82, MIRA, and ONSER50, were being developed in Europe. A special task force of the SAE Human Biomechanics and Simulation Subcommittee was convened for the purpose of evaluating the SID and APROD dummies. The U.S. experts noted many deficiencies in

the two dummies.[46] In Europe, the European Economic Commission (EEC) sponsored a program to evaluate the SID and three European-prototype side-impact dummies. The European experts concluded "that none of the existing dummies or even its components are in a sufficient advanced stage of development to be used directly in a regulation test procedure."[47] Since none of the available side-impact dummies were found adequate for European side-impact regulation, the European Experimental Vehicle Committee (EEVC) of EEC sponsored the development of EUROSID, which was developed in the 1983–85 time frame.[48,49]

Concurrently, the International Standards Organization (ISO) took on the task of developing a full-scale side-impact test procedure. In order to select a dummy for the test procedure, ISO developed a set of impact-response requirements for the head, neck, chest, shoulder, abdomen, and pelvis to assess the biofidelity of side-impact dummies.[50–55] The biofidelity requirements for the thorax and pelvis specified by NHTSA for SID[45] were included in the more comprehensive ISO requirements.[52,55] Both SID and EUROSID were evaluated relative to these requirements.[56–61] Based on these results, the ISO experts concluded that neither SID nor EUROSID in its present state of development had sufficient biofidelity to be used in the ISO full-scale side-impact test procedure.[62]

In response to the ISO conclusion, an SAE task force was formed with the mission to identify and implement changes to either SID or EUROSID or Hybrid III to make its responses more compatible with the ISO biofidelity requirements. The result of the SAE task force efforts was BIOSID.[25,63] The EEVC modified EUROSID and the modified dummy was called EUROSID-1. Both dummies were evaluated by ISO and were found to have acceptable biofidelity and measurement capacity to be used in full-scale side-impact testing.[64–66] Since SID was not modified, the ISO reaffirmed its position that SID did not have an acceptable level of biofidelity, nor was it adequately instrumented to be used in side-impact testing.[64–66] ISO transmitted all their

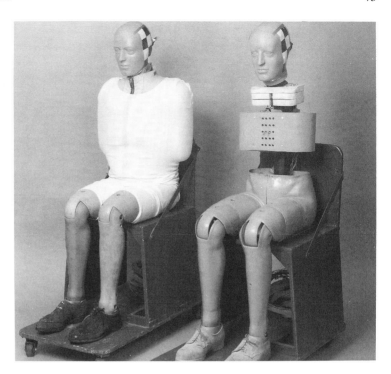

FIGURE 4.3. SID shown with and without its torso skin.

data and findings regarding SID, EUROSID-1, and BIOSID to NHTSA for consideration in their side-impact rule-making. The NHTSA opted to use SID as the dummy for MVSS 214 testing, noting that "BIOSID and EUROSID are under development."[67] Further, NHTSA commented that "if ongoing studies demonstrate that one or both of these dummies compare satisfactorily to SID, the agency will consider proposing such dummies as alternative devices in the future."[68] For this reason, descriptions of all three dummies are given.

SID

The SID dummy[42-45] is essentially a Hybrid II dummy with different chest, shoulder, and arm structures (Fig. 4.3). The chest structure consists of a very heavy rib structure whose displacement relative to the spine is controlled by a hydraulic damper. The arm and shoulder are simulated with soft foam. SID instrumentation is listed in Table 4.4. The NHTSA specifies performance limits for the thorax and pelvis for MVSS 214 compliance testing.[69] For the thorax, NHTSA defines a performance cri-

terion called the Thoracic Trauma Index, TTI.[45] The TTI is calculated by taking one-half the sum of the greater of the upper or lower peak rib acceleration and the peak lower spine acceleration with both accelerations expressed in gravity units, G. MVSS 214 gives two limits for TTI. For passenger cars with four side doors, the TTI limit is 85 G and for cars with two side doors the limit is 90 G. The performance criterion for the pelvis is the peak lateral acceleration and the limit is 130 G.

The SID dummy has a number of deficiencies. The chest structure does not have any lateral elastic stiffness. Because of this its chest compliance does not mimic the human chest response over a range of impact velocities. Interior padding that may meet the TTI limit may not prevent crushing thoracic injuries.[70] The lateral load-carrying capacity of the shoulder is not simulated in the SID. Interiors that are designed to transfer part of occupant loading to the shoulder area cannot be fairly evaluated with the SID. Armrest interaction, one of the main sources of liver/spleen injuries in side-impact collisions, cannot be assessed with the SID since its lateral abdominal region

TABLE 4.4. Side-impact dummy instrumentation.[a]

| Body region | No. data channels | | |
Measurements	SID	EUROSID-1	BIOSID
Head			
Triaxial acceleration	(3)	3	3
Head/neck interface			
Shear & axial forces	0	0	3
Bending & twist moment	0	0	3
Neck/torso interface			
Shear & axial forces	0	0	3
Bending & twist moment	0	0	3
Shoulder			
Force (F_x, F_y, F_z)	0	0	3
Deflection (D_y)	0	0	1
Acceleration (A_y)	0	0	1
Chest			
Upper-spine acceleration (T_1)	(3)	3	3
C.g. acceleration (T_4)	(3)	(3)	3
Lower-spine acceleration (T_{12})	3	(3)	3
Rib accelerations (A_y)	2	3	3
Rib deflections (D_y)	(2)	3	3
Abdomen			
Force (F_y)	0	3	0
Deflection (D_y)	0	0	2
Acceleration (A_y)	0	0	2
Lumbar spine/pelvis interface			
Shear & axial forces	0	0	3
Bending moments (M_y, M_x)	0	0	2
Pelvis			
Acceleration	3	3	3
Sacrum force (F_y)	0	0	1
Pubic symphysis force (F_y)	0	1	1
Iliac wing force (F_y)	0	1	1
Femur			
Shear & axial forces	(6)	(6)	6
Bending & twist moments	(6)	(6)	6
Knee			
Med. & lat. clevis forces	0	0	4
Tibia			
Up. bending moments (M_x, M_y)	0	0	4
Lo. bending moments (M_x)	0	0	2
Lo. shear & axial forces (F_y, F_z)	0	0	4
Totals	8 + (23)	20 + (18)	76

[a] Numbers in parentheses are channels that could be or have been used with the dummy.

is not biofidelic and it is not instrumented to measure armrest interaction with the abdomen.

EUROSID-1

The EUROSID-1 dummy is a modified version of the EUROSID dummy shown in Figure 4.4. It was designed to have lateral-impact response

biofidelity for the head, neck, shoulder, thorax, abdomen, and pelvis.[48,49] Its head is the Hybrid III head and its lower extremities are Hybrid II. The dummy features a shoulder structure that is designed to "roll forward" when impacted. The chest structure is designed to mimic human lateral force-deflection compliance. This is accomplished using hydraulic dampers and springs. An abdominal insert is

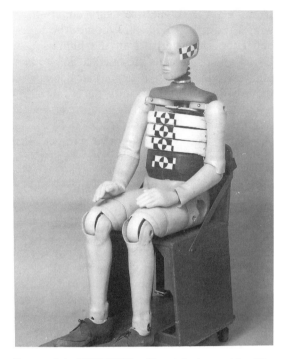

FIGURE 4.4. EUROSID without its torso skin. The lower portion of the arm and hand are removed for the EUROSID-1 design.

used to give humanlike abdominal compliance. The pelvis was designed so that pubic symphysis loads can be measured. EUROSID-1 instrumentation is listed in Table 4.4. Assessments of head, thorax, abdomen, and pelvis injury potentials can be made. Proposed IARVs for measurements made with the various transducers are given in Appendix C. Three deficiencies of EUROSID-1 are: (1) the maximum rib-to-spine displacement is limited to 50 mm of travel, (2) the shoulder is unstable when loaded laterally, and (3) the load distribution function of the humerus is not simulated in the arm structure.

BIOSID

The BIOSID dummy, shown in Figure 4.5, was designed to have lateral-impact response biofidelity for the head, neck, shoulder, thorax, abdomen, and pelvis[63–65] and was instrumented to assess the potential for head, neck, shoulder, thoracic, abdominal, pelvic, and leg injuries.[25,64,65] The dummy uses the Hybrid III head, neck, and legs along with the associated Hybrid III instrumentation. The chest uses the "far side" mounted rib concept of Lau et al.[71] This concept allows 75 mm of rib

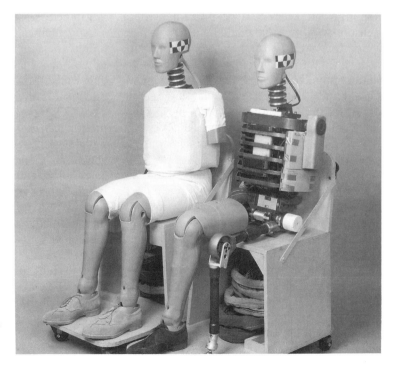

FIGURE 4.5. BIOSID shown with and without its torso, pelvic, and leg skins.

deflection without permanent deformation of the rib. The same concept was used to support the arm and for the abdominal region. Only the upper portion of the arm is simulated with BIOSID. The arm incorporates the load-distribution function of the humerus and can be positioned at any desired angle relative to the torso. The pelvis is a modification of the EUROSID pelvis and is instrumented to measure sacrum, iliac wing, and pubic symphysis loads. BIOSID instrumentation is given in Table 4.4 and some proposed IARVs are given in Appendix C.

A concern of the BIOSID design is the need to replace the foam block pelvis insert after each test. Such a crushable insert was needed to meet the biofidelity impact requirement for the pelvis.

Future Dummy Development

Early versions of dummies were used to assess the load-carrying capacity of restraint systems. For this purpose, they only needed to simulate a prescribed human weight and size. To address the question of level of occupant protection offered by a restraint system, dummies needed to be designed to mimic human impact response and needed to be instrumented to measure responses that could be used to assess injury potential. Examples of these more sophisticated dummies are the Hybrid III family that includes the 6-year-old child, small adult female, midsize male and large male dummies; the 6-month-old infant and 3-year-old air-bag dummies; and the EUROSID-1 and BIOSID side-impact dummies. Even these sophisticated dummies have deficiencies in biofidelity and/or measurement capability. For example, Rouhana et al.[72,73] have developed crushable foam abdominal inserts for the Hybrid III midsize male and small female dummies. The force-deflection characteristics of the inserts were selected to mimic appropriate human abdominal response to lap-belt loading. The residual crush of the insert produced if lap-belt submarining occurs provides a measure of abdominal injury potential. Melvin and Shee[74] have replaced the facial structure

of the Hybrid III midsize male dummy head with a crushable foam that mimics the force-deflection characteristics of the human face. Facial impacts to this modified head produce humanlike loadings that can be calculated from the existing Hybrid III transducer measurements and can be used to assess facial bone fracture potential.

Future dummy development projects will address perceived deficiencies of current dummies. Experience has shown that two types of deficiencies are used to justify dummy-development projects. The current dummy does not mimic critical human impact responses or is not instrumented to assess potential injury concerns. All the sophisticated dummies that have been described were developed because the dummies that they replaced had one or both of these deficiencies.

The difficulty in dummy-development projects is seldom the selection of mechanical concepts. The difficulty is reaching agreements among interested parties (government regulators, car manufacturers, university researchers, insurance companies, safety advocates on (1) the need for a dummy-development project, (2) the impact response requirements that are to be used to judge acceptable dummy biofidelity, and (3) the injury potentials that are to be assessed with the dummy.

An example of determining the need for a dummy-development project is the ISO evaluation of the available side-impact dummies, SID and EUROSID. The ISO needed to select a dummy for their side-impact test procedure. The ISO experts reviewed the available biomechanical literature and developed a set of biofidelity requirements for the head, neck, chest, shoulder, abdomen, and pelvis.[50–55] They also agreed on a procedure for determining an overall biofidelity rating for each dummy.[64] A prioritized list of desired dummy measurements was developed as well as a method to assign an overall measurement rating.[65] These requirements were used by ISO to judge the acceptability of SID and EUROSID. Because neither dummy met the requirements the ISO requested that interested parties modify the dummies or develop a new dummy to meet the ISO requirements. The

BIOSID development program was initiated by SAE because of the reluctance of the developers of SID and EUROSID to modify their dummies. Belatedly, EUROSID was modified, resulting in EUROSID-1. Unfortunately, the SID design was not modified by NHTSA.

Developing impact biofidelity requirements is a very difficult task. The question of what constitutes an acceptable biomechanical database is the main problem. Most biomechanical data are taken from cadaver impact studies. There are three principal problems that need to be addressed when assessing the usefulness of cadaver data. First, cadaver subjects are not uniform in size, shape, and mass. Scaling techniques[75,76] have to be applied to cadaver data to account for these differences. Second, most cadavers have been tested under very severe impact conditions that resulted in extensive damage to the cadavers. Such cadaver data may be inappropriate for setting biofidelity requirements for dummies that are to be used to assess restraint systems that are designed to prevent such severe loading. Third, the cadaver response may not mimic the human response. This is especially true for responses that involve muscle tone such as the neck bending,[26] chest deflection,[5] and extremity joint articulation. For future dummy-development projects, these deficiencies of cadaver data need to be resolved in order to develop impact biofidelity requirements that are agreeable to all interested parties.

Reaching agreement on dummy instrumentation can be a relatively easy process. The process used by ISO for the side-impact dummy can be used as an example. A meeting was convened of appropriate experts to identify potential side-impact injury concerns. For each injury concern, possible dummy measurements were noted. Then each expert assigned an importance level to each measurement. The individual expert ratings were combined to give a rank ordering to the list of measurements. This ranking can be used to assess the acceptability of existing dummy instrumentation or as a guideline for instrumentation to be added to an existing or new dummy. The question of acceptable levels for occupant protection should not be addressed during the process of measurement selection since such levels are not relevant to the question of what constitutes an acceptable dummy.

A final observation is that it is extremely important that any future dummy development involve the *participation* of *all* interested parties. If this does not happen, then there may be a group of people who will not support the dummy that is developed. A process must be found where the input from all interested parties can be voiced and consensus decisions can be made on an international basis. The ISO can provide this forum, but all interested parties must be willing to participate and abide by the consensus decisions reached by the participants.

References

1. Mertz HJ. Anthropomorphic models. In *The biomechanics of trauma*. Appleton-Century-Crofts, Norwalk, CT, 1985.
2. Code of Federal Regulations. Title 49, Chapter V, Part 572—Anthropomorphic test dummy. Federal Register 38(147) August 1, 1973.
3. Foster JK, Kortge JO, Wolanin MJ. Hybrid III—a biomechanically-based crash test dummy. Twenty-First Stapp Car Crash Conference. SAE 770938, October 1977.
4. Mertz HJ, Neathery RF, Culver CC. Performance requirements and characteristics of mechanical necks. In *Human impact response—measurement and simulation*. Plenum Press, New York, 1973.
5. Lobdell TE, Kroell CK, Schneider DC, Hering WE. Impact response of the human thorax. In *Human impact response—measurement and simulation*. Plenum Press, New York, 1973.
6. Horsch JD, Patrick LM. Cadaver and dummy knee impact response. SAE 760799, October 1976.
7. Kroell CK, Schneider DC, Nahum AM. Comparative knee impact response of Part 572 dummy and cadaver subject. Twentieth Stapp Car Crash Conference. SAE 760817, October 1976.
8. Hering WE, Patrick LM. Response comparisons of the human cadaver knee and a Part 572 dummy knee to impacts by crushable materials. Twenty-First Stapp Car Crash Conference. SAE 770939, October 1977.
9. McElhaney HJ, Mate PI, Roberts VL. A new crash test device—Repeatable Pete. Seven-

teenth Stapp Car Crash Conference. SAE 730983, November 1973.

10. Haslegrave CM, Croke MD. *Performance measurements of the OPAT dummy*. MIRA Publication, January 1974.

11. Tennant JA, Jensen RJ, Potter RA. GM-ATD 502 anthropomorphic test dummy—development and evaluation. Fifth International Technical Conference on Experimental Safety Vehicles. London, England, June 1974.

12. Warner P. The development of UK standard occupant protection assessment test dummy. SAE 740115, March 1974.

13. Hubbard RP, McLeod DG. A basis for crash dummy skull and head geometry. In *Human impact response—measurement and simulation*. Plenum Press, New York, 1973.

14. Hubbard RP, McLeod DG. Definition and development of a crash dummy head. Eighteenth Stapp Car Crash Conference. SAE 741193, December 1974.

15. Hodgson VR, Mason MW, Thomas LH. Head model for impact. Sixteenth Stapp Car Crash Conference. SAE 720969, November 1972.

16. Hodgson VR. Head model for impact tolerance. In *Human impact response—measurement and simulation*. Plenum Press, New York, 1973.

17. McElhaney JH, Stalnaker RL, Roberts VL. Biomechanical aspects of head injury. In *Human impact response—measurement and simulation*. Plenum Press, New York, 1973.

18. McLeod DG, Gadd CW. An anatomical skull for impact testing. In *Human impact response—measurement and simulation*. Plenum Press, New York, 1973.

19. Culver CC, Neathery RF, Mertz HJ. Mechanical necks with humanlike responses. Sixteenth Stapp Car Crash Conference. SAE 720959, November 1972.

20. Melvin JW, McElhaney JH, Roberts VL. Evaluation of dummy neck performance. In *Human impact response—measurement and simulation*. Plenum Press, New York, 1973.

21. Melvin JW, McElhaney JH, Roberts VL. Improved neck simulation for anthropometric dummies. Sixteenth Stapp Car Crash Conference. SAE 720958, November 1972.

22. Foster K. Analysis of a slanted-rib model of the human thorax. In *Human impact response—measurement and simulation*. Plenum Press, New York, 1973.

23. Stalnaker RL, McElhaney JH, Roberts VL, Trollope ML. Human torso response to blunt trauma. In *Human impact response—measurement and simulation*. Plenum Press, New York, 1973.

24. Mertz HJ. Biofidelity of the Hybrid III head. SAE 851245, February 1985.

25. Beebe MS. What is BIOSID?. SAE 900377, February 1990.

26. Mertz HJ, Patrick LM. Strength and response of the human neck. Fifteenth Stapp Car Crash Conference. SAE 710855, November 1971.

27. Nyquist GW. Static force-penetration response of the human knee. Eighteenth Stapp Car Crash Conference. SAE 741189, December 1974.

28. Viano DC, Culver CC, Haut RC. Bolster impacts to the knee and tibia of human cadavers and an anthropomorphic dummy. Twenty-Second Stapp Car Crash Conference. SAE 780896, October 1978.

29. Nyquist GW, Denton RA. Crash test dummy lower leg instrumentation for axial force and bending moment. ISA Transaction, 18(3) 1979.

30. Begeman PC, Prasad P. Human ankle impact response in dorsiflexion. Thirty-Fourth Stapp Car Crash Conference. SAE 902308, November 1990.

31. NHTSA Docket 74-14, Notice 32. General Motors Submission USG 2284, Appendix E. December 19, 1983.

32. Mertz HJ. Injury assessment values used to evaluate Hybrid III response measurements. NHTSA Docket 74-14, Notice 32, Enclosure 2 of Attachment I of Part III of General Motors Submission USG 2284. March 22, 1984.

33. Viano DC, Lau IV (1988) A viscous tolerance criterion for soft tissue injury assessment. Biomech 21(5):387–399.

34. Mertz HJ, Horsch JD, Horn G. Hybrid III sternal deflection associated with thoracic injury severities of occupants restrained with force-limiting shoulder belts. SAE 910812, February 1991.

35. Horsch JD, Melvin J, Viano D, Mertz H. Thoracic injury assessment of belt restraint systems based on Hybrid III chest compression. Thirty-Fifth Stapp Car Crash Conference. SAE 912895, November 1991.

36. NHTSA Docket 74-14, Notice 66. General Motors Submission USG 2842, Appendix A. November 13, 1990.

37. Mertz HJ, Irwin AL, Melvin JW, Stalnaker RL, Beebe MS. Size, weight and biomechanical impact response requirements for adult size small female and large male dummies. SAE 890756, March 1989.

38. Schneider LW, Robbins DH, Pflug MA, Snyder RG. Development of anthropometrically based design specifications for an advanced adult anthropomorphic dummy family. Volume 1,

NHTSA Contract No. DTNH22-80-C-07502, December 1983.

39. Wolanin MJ, Mertz HJ, Nyznyk RS, Vincent JH. Description and basis of a three-year-old child dummy for evaluating passenger inflatable restraint concepts. Ninth International Technical Conference on Experimental Safety Vehicles. November 1982. (Republished as SAE 826040, *Automatic occupant protection systems*, SP-736, 1988.)

40. Mertz HJ, Driscoll JD, Lenox JB, Nyquist GW, Weber DA. Responses of animals exposed to deployment of various passenger inflatable restraint systems concepts for a variety of collision severities and animal positions. Ninth International Technical Conference on Experimental Safety Vehicles. November 1982. (Republished as SAE 826047, *Passenger car inflatable restraint systems*, PT31, 1987.)

41. Mertz HJ, Weber DA. Interpretations of the impact responses of a three-year-old child dummy relative to child injury potential. Ninth International Technical Conference on Experimental Safety Vehicles. November 1982. (Republished as SAE 826048, *Automatic occupant protection systems*, SP-736, 1988.)

42. Melvin JW, Robbins DH, Benson JB. Experimental application of advanced thoracic instrumentation techniques to anthropomorphic test devices. Seventh International Technical Conference on Experimental Safety Vehicles. NHTSA, June 1979.

43. Morgan RM, Marcus JH, Eppinger RH. Correlation of side impact dummy cadaver tests. Twenty-Fifth Stapp Car Crash Conference. SAE 81008, September 1989.

44. Donnelly BR, Morgan RM, Eppinger RH. Durability, repeatability and reproducibility of NHTSA side impact dummy. Twenty-Seventh Stapp Car Crash Conference. SAE 831624, October 1983.

45. Eppinger RH, Marcus JH, Morgan RM. Development of dummy and injury index for NHTSA's thoracic side impact protection research program. SAE 840885, May 1984.

46. Nyquist GW, Brinn J, Daniel R, Kortge J, Mertz H. An evaluation of APR and SID side impact anthropomorphic dummies. ISO/TC22/SC12/WG5 Document No. N99. June 1983.

47. Maltha J, Janssen EG. EEC comparison testing of four side impact dummies. EEC Biomechanics Seminar. ISO/TC22/SC12/WG5 Document No. N98. June 1983.

48. Neilson L, Lowne R, Tarriere C, Bendjellal F, Gillet D, Maltha J, Cesari D, Bouquet R. The EUROSID side impact dummy. Tenth International Technical Conference on Experimental Safety Vehicles. NHTSA, June 1985.

49. Lowne RW, Neilson JD. The development and certification of EUROSID. Eleventh International Technical Conference on Experimental Safety Vehicles. NHTSA, May 1987.

50. ISO TR9790-1. Road vehicles—anthropomorphic side impact dummy—lateral head impact response requirements to assess the biofidelity of the dummy. American National Standards Institute, New York, 1988.

51. ISO TR9790-2. Road vehicles—anthropomorphic side impact dummy—lateral neck impact response requirements to assess the biofidelity of the dummy. American National Standards Institute, New York, 1988.

52. ISO TR9790-3. Road vehicles—anthropomorphic side impact dummy—lateral thoracic impact response requirements to assess the biofidelity of the dummy. American National Standards Institute, New York, 1988.

53. ISO TR9790-4. Road vehicles—anthropomorphic side impact dummy—lateral shoulder impact response requirements to assess the biofidelity of the dummy. American National Standards Institute, New York, 1988.

54. ISO TR9790-5. Road vehicles—anthropomorphic side impact dummy—lateral abdominal impact response requirements to assess the biofidelity of the dummy. American National Standards Institute, New York, 1988.

55. ISO TR9790-6. Road vehicles—anthropomorphic side impact dummy—lateral pelvic impact response requirements to assess the biofidelity of the dummy. American National Standards Institute, New York, 1988.

56. Irwin AL, Pricopio LA, Mertz HJ, Balser JS, Chkoreff WM. Comparison of the EUROSID and SID impact responses to the response corridors of the International Standards Organization. SAE 890604, February 1989.

57. Janssen EG, Vermissen AC. Biofidelity of the european side impact dummy—EUROSID. Thirty-Second Stapp Car Crash Conference. SAE 881716, October 1988.

58. Bendjellal F, Tarriere C, Brun-Cassan F, Foret-Bruno J, Caillibot P, Gillet D. Comparative evaluation of the biofidelity of EUROSID and SID side impact dummies. Thirty-Second Stapp Car Crash Conference. SAE 881717, October 1988.

59. ISO/TC22/SC12/WG5. The biofidelity test results on SID and EUROSID. Document No. N213, Submitted by JAMA, October 1988.

60. ISO/TC22/SC12/WG5. Summary tables for SID and EUROSID evaluation relative to bio-

mechanical impact response requirements of ISO/DP9790-1 to 6. Document No. N216 (Revised June 1989), October 1988.

61. ISO/TC22/SC12/WG5. Summary of WG5 evaluation of SID and EUROSID. Document No. N218 (Revised June 1989), October 1988.

62. ISO/TC22/SC12/WG5. Resolution 3. Document No. N219, October 1988.

63. Beebe MS, BIOSID update and calibration requirements. SAE 910319, 1991.

64. Mertz HJ, Irwin A. Biofidelity ratings of SID, EUROSID and BIOSID. ISO/TC22/SC12/WG5 Document No. N288, October 1990.

65. Mertz HJ. Rating of measurement capacity of side impact dummies. ISO/TC22/SC12/WG5 Document No. N281, July 1990.

66. ISO/TC22/SC12/WG5. Resolution 1. Document No. N298, November 1990.

67. Code of Federal Regulations. Part 572—Anthropomorphic test dummies, sub-part F—anthropomorphic test dummy; side impact protection. November 29, 1990.

68. Federal Register 49 CFR. Part 572, Anthropomorphic Test Dummy; Side Impact Protection. 55(210):45757–45768, Tuesday, October 30, 1990.

69. Code of Federal Regulations. Part 571, Paragraph 571.214. November 29, 1990.

70. Lau IV, Capp JP, Obermeyer JA. A comparison of frontal and side impact: crash dynamics, countermeasurers and subsystems. Thirty-Fifth Stapp Car Crash Conference, SAE 912896, November 1991.

71. Lau IV, Viano DC, Culver CC, Jedrzejczak E. Design of a modified chest for EUROSID providing biofidelity and injury assessment. SAE 890881, Side impact: injury causation and occupant protection, SP-769, February 1989.

72. Rouhana SW, Viano DC, Jedrzejczak EA, McCleary JD. Assessing submarining and abdominal injury risk in the Hybrid III family of dummies. Thirty-Third Stapp Car Crash Conference. SAE 892440, October 1989.

73. Rouhana SW, Jedrzejczak EA, McCleary JD. Assessing submarining and abdominal injury risk in the Hybrid III family of dummies: Part II—development of the small female frangible abdomen. Thirty-Fourth Stapp Car Crash Conference. SAE 902317, November 1990.

74. Melvin JW, Shee TR. Facial injury assessment techniques. Twelfth International Technical Conference on Experimental Safety Vehicles. NHTSA, 1989.

75. Mertz HJ. A procedure for normalizing impact response data. SAE 840884, May 1984.

76. Krause P. Normalization of side impact cadaver dynamic response data utilizing regression techniques. SAE 840883, May 1984.

77. SAE Recommended Practice. Rules for SAE use of SI (metric) units. J916, May, 1991.

Appendix A: Injury-Assessment Reference Values for Hybrid III–Type Adult Dummies

Table 4.A1 lists the IARVs that have been suggested as guidelines for assessing injury potentials associated with measurements made with Hybrid III–type adult dummies. A curve indicating the risk of life-threatening brain injury as a function of HIC is given in Figure 4.A1. For neck tension, compression, and shear forces and for axial compressive femur force, time-dependent injury assessment curves are specified and are shown in Figures 4.A2, 4.A3, 4.A4, and 4.A5, respectively. The IARVs given for the midsize male are the values submitted to NHTSA by General Motors[32] with two exceptions. The IARV for sternal deflection produced by a well-distributed load such as an air bag has been lowered to 65 mm based on a reanalysis of the cadaver data used to establish the original 75-mm value.[33] The other exception, the Viscous Criterion proposed by Viano and Lau,[33] has been added to the list. The IARVs for the small female and large male were scaled from the midsize male values using appropriate scale factors[37] and assuming constant failure stress.

The cautions noted by Mertz[32] for use of the IARVs bear repeating. Each IARV refers "to a human response level below which a specified significant injury is considered unlikely to occur for the given size individual." Being below all the IARVs does not assure that significant injury could not occur since IARVs are not specified and the dummy is not instrumented to measure all responses that are associated with all possible types of injuries. Further, exceeding an IARV does not necessarily mean that a person would be injured if exposed to the collision being simulated since the IARVs are lower bounds for injury thresholds.

TABLE 4.A1. Injury assessment reference values for Hybrid III–type adult dummies.[32–35,37]

Body region Injury-assessment criteria[a]	Small female	Midsize male	Large male
Head			
HIC; $(t_2 - t_1) \leqslant 15$ ms	1,113	1,000[b]	957
Head/neck interface			
Flexion bending moment (Nm)	104	190	258
Extension bending moment (Nm)	31	57	78
Axial tension (N)	Fig. 4.A2	Fig. 4.A2	Fig. 4.A2
Axial compression (N)	Fig. 4.A3	Fig. 4.A3	Fig. 4.A3
Fore/aft shear (N)	Fig. 4.A4	Fig. 4.A4	Fig. 4.A4
Chest			
Spine box acc.; (3 ms, G)	73	60	54
Sternal deflection due to:			
— Shoulder belt (mm)	41	50	55
— Air-bag & steering-wheel hub (mm)	53	65	72
Viscous criterion (m/s)	1	1	1
Femur			
Axial compression (N)	Fig. 4.A5	Fig. 4.A5	Fig. 4.A5
Knee			
Tibia-to-femur translation (mm)	12	15	17
Med./lat. clevis compression (N)	2,552	4,000	4,920
Tibia			
Axial compression (N)	5,104	8,000	9,840
Tibia index, $TI = M/M_c + F/F_c$	1	1	1
Where,			
M_c—critical bending moment (Nm)	115	225	307
F_c—critical comp. force (kN)	22.9	35.9	44.2

[a] Units are SI notation.[77]
[b] See Fig. 4.A1 for injury risk curve.

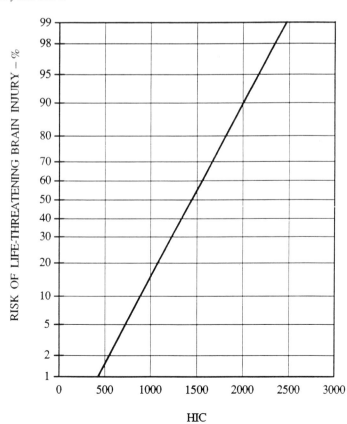

FIGURE 4.A1. Injury risk curve for HIC for $t_2 - t_1 \leqslant 15$ ms.[32]

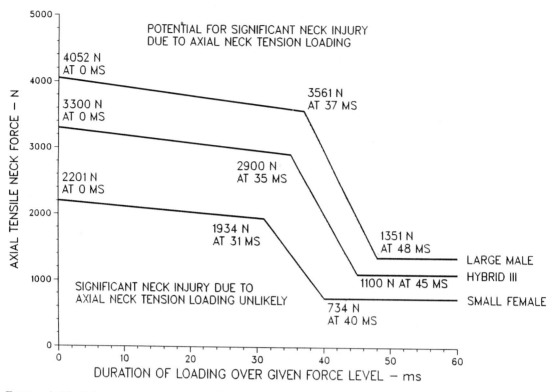

FIGURE 4.A2. Injury-assessment curves for axial neck tension measured with Hybrid III–type adult dummies.[32,37]

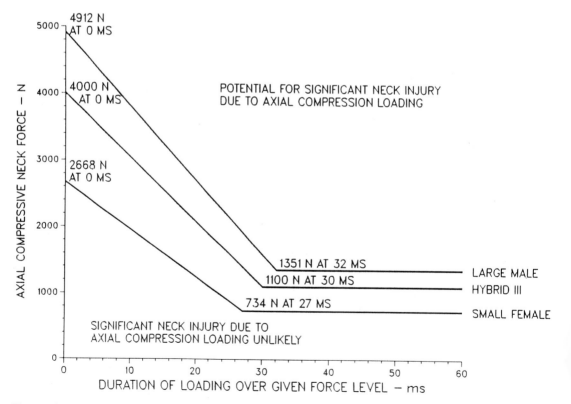

FIGURE 4.A3. Injury-assessment curves for axial neck compression measured with Hybrid III–type adult dummies.[32,37]

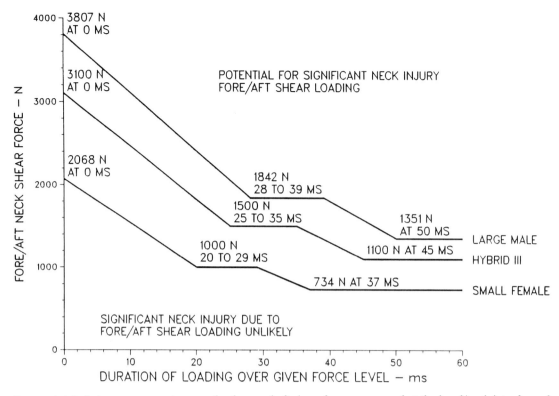

FIGURE 4.A4. Injury-assessment curves for fore and aft shear forces measured at the head/neck interface of Hybrid III–type adult dummies.[32,37]

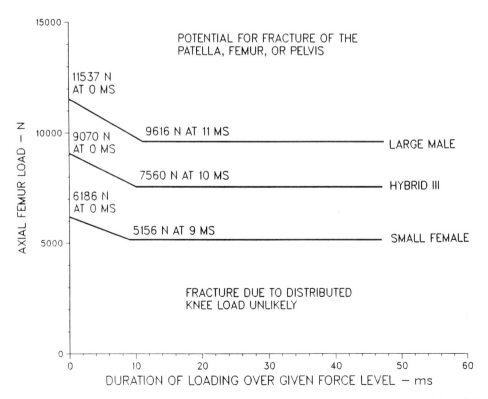

FIGURE 4.A5. Injury-assessment curves for axial compressive femur force measured with Hybrid III–type adult dummies.[32,37]

Appendix 4B. Injury-assessment reference values (IARV) corresponding to various injury-risk levels for measurements made with the 3-year-old child "air-bag" dummy.[39–41]

Body region Injury-assessment criteria[a]	IARV		
	1% risk	10% risk	25% risk
Head HIC; $(t_2 - t_1) \leq 15$ ms	1,480	1,530	1,570
Neck Neck tension (N)	1,060	1,125	1,160
Thorax Upper-spine acc. (G)	55	59	62
Upper & midsternal ΔV (km/h) (for Δt windows ≤ 4 ms)	9	16	19
Abdomen Lower spine acc. (G)	34	42	45
Lower sternal ΔV (km/h) (for Δt windows ≤ 4 ms)	19.5	19.9	20.4

[a] Units are SI notation.[77]

Appendix 4C. Injury-assessment reference values proposed for side-impact dummy measurements.[48,69]

Body region Injury-assessment criteria[a]	SID	EUROSID-1	BIOSID
Head HIC; $(t_2 - t_1) \leq 15$ ms	—	—	1,000
HIC; $(t_2 - t_1) \leq 36$ ms	—	1,000	—
Chest Lat. rib to spine def. (mm)	—	42	42
TTI for, Coupe (G)	90	90	90
Sedan (G)	85	85	85
Viscous criterion (m/s)	—	1	1
Abdomen Lateral compression (mm)	—	—	39
Lateral force (kN)	—	4.5	—
Pelvis Lateral acceleration (G)	130	130	130
Pubic symphysis force (kN)	—	10	10
Iliac wing force (kN)	—	10	10

[a] Units are SI notation.[77]

5
Radiologic Analysis of Trauma

Mini N. Pathria and Donald Resnick

Diagnostic imaging plays an important role in the detection, management, and follow-up of skeletal and soft-tissue injuries. The use of routine radiography to identify fractures constituted one of the earliest applications of this technique. Fractures represent incomplete or complete breaks in the continuity of bones that may result from a single episode of excessive stress applied to normal bone, multiple episodes of excessive stress applied to normal bone, or normal or excessive stress applied to abnormal bone. Injuries may be due to direct trauma, load applied directly upon the osseous structures, or more commonly, to indirect forces applied through muscles or tendons. The configuration of the fracture is dependent upon the magnitude, type, and site of applied force.[32] Bone may fail secondary to tension, compression, bending, torsion, or combined loading.[3,21]

The location and configuration of a fracture not only are dependent upon the mechanism of injury but also depend upon the age of the patient and the presence of any predisposing factors that might alter the bones or soft tissues.[25] The sites most frequently injured are the physeal and metaphyseal regions in children, the epiphyses in teenagers, the diaphyses in young adults, and in the elderly, the subarticular area and diaphyses of the tubular bones (Fig. 5.1).[25]

The fatigue type of stress fracture results from repeated application of abnormal stresses on normal bone. The insufficiency type of stress fracture occurs when abnormally weakened bone encounters physiological stresses. Diseases associated with insufficiency fractures include a variety of metabolic bone disorders such as osteoporosis, osteomalacia, and hyperparathyroidism. Pathological fractures specifically refer to fractures occurring in areas of bone replacement by tumor.[32] These fractures typically are transverse and show little comminution since the preexisting abnormality impairs the bone's ability to absorb energy and the fracture occurs with minimal loading (Fig. 5.2).[3]

This chapter will emphasize imaging abnormalities associated with acute and stress fractures. A discussion of diagnostic imaging of pathological fractures is beyond the scope of this chapter.

Conventional Radiography

The evaluation of complications of trauma represents the most common indication for skeletal radiographs.[25] Plain-film radiography is well suited to the assessment of skeletal injuries because it is sensitive to osseous injury, has excellent spatial resolution, and is widely available. Examination of injuries of the extremeties should include at least two views at right angles to each other of the site of involvement. The joints at either end of the bone should be evaluated if the shaft of a long bone is fractured to exclude a concomitant dislocation (Fig. 5.3). If the suspected injury involves only the metaphyseal or epiphyseal

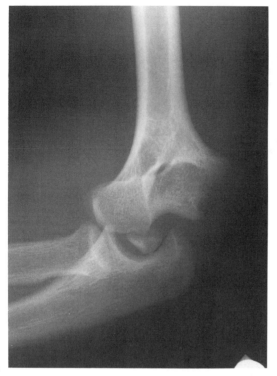

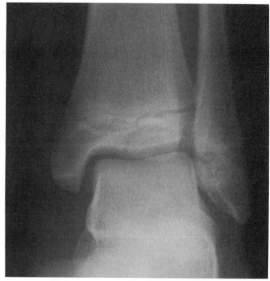

A

FIGURE 5.1. Injuries of the immature skeleton typically involve the physeal region. Avulsion of the medial epicondyle (A) is the most common bony injury associated with elbow dislocations in chil-

dren. The epicondyle is displaced into the joint in this case. The Tillaux fracture of the distal tibia (B) is an avulsion of the anterolateral epiphysis seen in the setting of partial physeal fusion.

area, then only that area and the adjacent joint should be examined to provide optimal detail.[32] Oblique views often are necessary for assessment of articular injuries.

Indirect evidence of skeletal injuries may be noted in the overlying soft tissues. The soft tissues themselves may be the primary site of injury and should be carefully assessed in all cases of trauma. Radiographic findings associated with trauma include nonspecific soft-tissue swelling, blurring or displacement of the normal fat stripes that outline the fascial planes, and focal masses representing hematomas or fracture blisters. The presence of soft-tissue gas or radioopaque foreign bodies implies that a penetrating injury has occurred.[27] Articular trauma typically produces joint effusions that are readily identified in the knee, ankle, and elbow but are difficult to detect in other locations such as the wrist, hip, and shoulder.

It generally is believed that the presence of intraarticular fluid is strong evidence of an occult fracture, particularly if the effusion contains fat.[30] Some authors state that a radiographically evident lipohemarthrosis, most commonly seen in the knee on cross-table radiographs, is virtually pathognomonic of an intraarticular fracture (Fig. 5.4).[15,27]

Most fractures are readily apparent on good-quality radiographs. In order to determine the mechanism of injury and appropriate management, it is essential to understand the forces that produce the typical fractures encountered in daily practice. The conventional radiographic appearances of fractures produced by tensile, compressive, rotary, and angular forces are well known.[3,21,27,32] A brief review of these classic injuries is presented here but one must be aware that many injuries result from a complex combination of these forces.

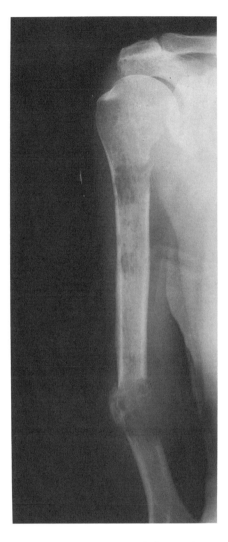

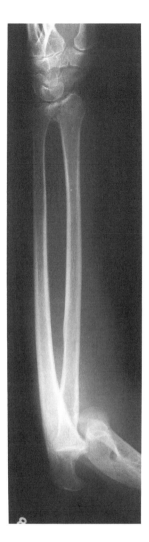

FIGURE 5.2. Multiple areas of bone destruction secondary to multiple myeloma are evident in the humerus. There is a pathological fracture in the distal humerus with angular deformity.

FIGURE 5.3. The importance of radiographing the entire length of an injured bone is apparent. There is a distal radial fracture and a complete elbow dislocation involving the same extremity. Multiple injuries are not uncommon and may be easily overlooked if adequate radiographs are not obtained.

Complete fractures occur when the entire circumference of a tubular bone has been disrupted. Incomplete fractures, where the break does not extend completely through the bone, typically occur in the resilient, elastic bones of children and young adults (Fig. 5.5).[25]

Fractures produced by tensile loading generally occur in the cancellous bone of the metaphysis at sites of major tendinous or ligamentous attachment.[3] Avulsion fractures due to the pull of a muscle or tendon typically are transverse and result from tension loading.[32] Common sites for this type of injury include the base of the fifth metatarsal bone, the calcaneus adjacent to the attachment of the Achilles tendon, and the patella.[21] Cortical bone rarely fails in pure tension so this type of fracture is unusual in the diaphysis of a long tubular bone.[26]

Compression fractures may involve either cancellous or cortical bone. Because normal

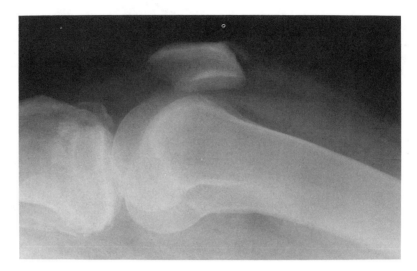

FIGURE 5.4. A cross-table lateral radiograph demonstrates a fat-fluid level within the knee joint. The lucent fat is layered above the denser fluid component of the effusion producing a straight horizontal fluid interface. There is a fracture of the tibial plateau.

cancellous bone can absorb significant energy in compression, substantial force is required to produce these fractures in nonosteoporotic individuals. A very common example of this type of injury is the compression fractures seen in the vertebrae, particularly in the osteoporotic person.[3] Compressive loading of the diaphyses of long bones mainly produces oblique fractures through the osteons.[21] Other examples of compression fractures include the T-shaped or Y-shaped fracture of the proximal aspect of the tibia or distal portion of the femur and longitudinal or long oblique shaft fractures without significant displacement.[32] Compressive loading also can be produced by abnormally strong contraction of the surrounding muscles. An example of this mechanism is the presence of bilateral subcapital fractures of the femoral neck following electric-shock therapy (Fig. 5.6).[21]

Torsion occurs when a load is applied to a structure in a manner that causes it to twist about an axis.[21] The fracture pattern associated with torsion characteristically consists of a spiral fracture that is oriented at 45° to the shaft with the fracture ends being sharpened and pointed.[32] Such injuries are common in the humerus, femur, and tibia, and the adjacent articulations must be evaluated carefully for rotary deformities.

Bending or angular forces applied to the bone produce transverse fractures that are frequently associated with comminution of the cortex on the concave side of the injury.[32] Large butterfly fragments may be produced when axial loading is combined with bending (Fig. 5.7).[3] In adult bone, failure begins on the side subjected to tension since adult bone is weaker in tension than in compression.[21] Immature bone may fail first in compression, producing an incomplete buckle fracture on the compressive side.[21]

Direct trauma to the bone results in transverse fractures that become increasingly more comminuted with progressively greater force.[32] Characteristic sites of fractures produced by a direct blow include the distal portion of the ulna and the tibial shaft. Highly comminuted fractures typically are associated with extensive soft-tissue injury and indicate a large amount of energy dissipation in conjunction with a rapid loading rate.[3]

The cortical disruption seen with acute fractures is typically not present in patients presenting with stress fractures because the initial failure in these persons takes place in the medullary bone. Knowledge of the clinical history of exercise-induced pain and awareness of the common sites of these fractures and their typical appearance are essential as they may be

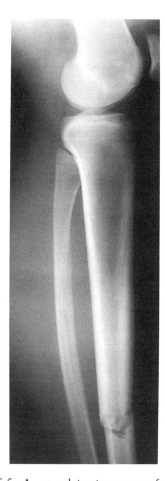

FIGURE 5.5. A complete transverse fracture of the tibial diaphysis is associated with a bowing deformity of the fibula. Plastic deformation of the fibula has occurred without the development of a frank fracture. This phenomenon occurs in young individuals, particularly children.

mistaken for infection or tumor on the basis of their radiographic appearance alone (Fig. 5.8). Radiological findings in fatigue and insufficiency fractures depend on the duration of the injury and the site of the fracture. The initial radiographs are frequently are normal and remodeling changes that render the injury apparent may not be present for several weeks. Periosteal reaction, endosteal thickening, and medullary sclerosis generally are identified prior to the development of a cortical radiolucent area (Fig. 5.9).[28] Scintigraphy and magnetic resonance imaging are more sensitive than conventional radiography in the identification of fatigue and insufficiency fractures.

There are situations in which ancillary radiographic studies are required for either the detection or the characterization of skeletal injury but these studies constitute a small percentage of all examinations.[10] Stress radiographs refer to conventional radiographic images obtained at the extremes of range of motion or during manual application of distraction of angular stress to the site of suspected injury.[10] Their purpose is to identify articular instability that is not apparent on either or both the physical examination and the unstressed radiographs. The technique is most frequently applied to the acromioclavicular knee and ankle joints (Fig. 5.10). Both acute and chronic ligamentous disruption is manifest by asymmetric, abnormal widening of an articulation. Comparison with the uninjured side is mandatory because there is considerable

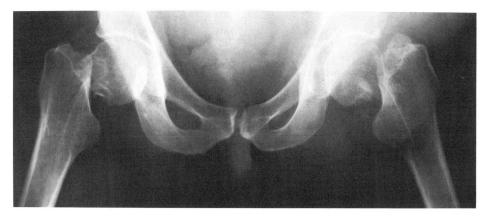

FIGURE 5.6. Bilateral displaced subcapital fractures were present following a prolonged seizure. This patient subsequently developed avascular necrosis of both femoral heads.

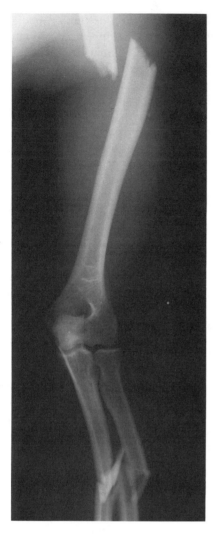

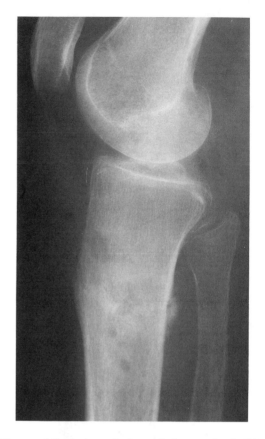

FIGURE 5.8. A lateral view of the proximal tibia illustrates periostitis, medullary sclerosis, and endosteal thickening. The patient underwent a biopsy of the area because of persistent pain and an abnormal bone scan obtained prior tc the development of these radiographic abnormalities. This x-ray, obtained 2 weeks after the biopsy, shows a thin, irregular lucency and cortical disruption consistent with a stress fracture.

FIGURE 5.7. Fractures of the humerus and both forearm bones occurred during a motorcycle accident. The fractures are short oblique or transverse and the forearm injuries show comminution and butterfly fragments laterally.

variability in joint laxity in normal persons.[10] Stress views should be acquired following sedation or anesthesia of the patient to ensure that an adequate examination has been obtained because pain may lead to spasm that masks the injury.[10] Flexion and extension views of the spine obtained at the extremes of active motion are a form of stress radiography. These views may demonstrate ligamentous injuries when no discernible abnormalities

are seen on the examination obtained in the neutral position.[23]

A variety of specialized radiographic techniques are occasionally used for the assessment of trauma. These techniques rarely are necessary for initial diagnosis of skeletal injury but are helpful in the identification or confirmation of subtle fracture lines that are difficult to see on the plain films or in the delineation of the orientation of a recognized fracture.[25] Magnification radiographs are obtained by decreasing the distance between the x-ray tube and the object while maintaining

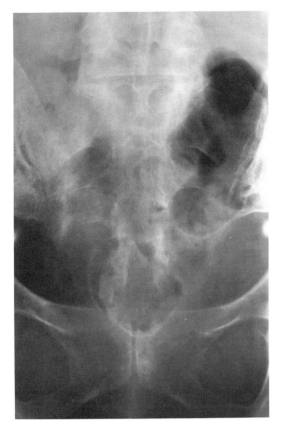

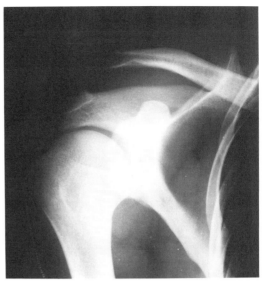

FIGURE 5.10. An AP view of the acromioclavicular joint obtained with weights shows widening of the AC joint, superior displacement of the clavicle, and an increase in the coracoclavicular distance. These features indicate a grade 3 AC separation. Without weights it was difficult to determine whether the injury involved the coracoclavicular ligaments.

FIGURE 5.9. An abnormal linear band of sclerosis is present in the right sacrum adjacent to the arcuate lines. The location and appearance are typical of an insufficiency fracture occurring at one of its characteristic sites.

the distance between the x-ray tube and the film. The enlargement of the imaged structures may be helpful for assessment of injuries in small body parts such as the fingers and toes. Xeroradiography, low-kilovoltage radiography, and stereo radiography are other specialized techniques that are rarely utilized currently but that may be helpful if magnetic resonance (MR) imaging (MRI), computed tomography, and ultrasound are unavailable.

Conventional Tomography

Conventional tomography is the only specialized radiographic technique that we use regularly at our institution. The technique was developed to better demonstrate internal anatomy by minimizing the superimposition of structures that obscure the area of interest on standard radiography. Synchronous motion of the radiographic film and x-ray tube produces blurring of objects outside the selected focal plane, reducing radiographic contrast.[12,32] Conventional tomography increases the radiation exposure to the patient but still has applications in the assessment of complex skeletal trauma (Fig. 5.11). Fractures that are undisplaced may be identified with conventional tomography in the presence of normal initial radiographs even though the imaging planes are identical. The presence of a lipohemarthosis and normal radiographs is strongly suggestive of an occult fracture of the knee, particularly in the osteopenic patient.[15] In this situation, conventional tomography is extremely helpful in evaluating the osseous structures.[1] The major indications for conventional tomography at our institution include analysis of tibial plateau fractures, horizontally oriented spinal fractures, and complex injuries involving the carpus or tarsus.

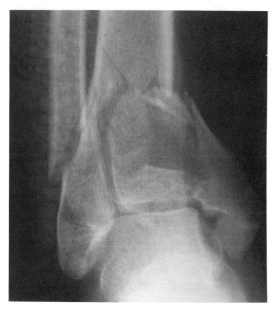

A

FIGURE 5.11. The conventional radiograph (A) and tomogram (B) of a comminuted intraarticular fracture of the distal tibia illustrate some of the advantages of tomography. The overlying cast de- grades the plain film far more than on the tomogram because of superimposition. The deformity of the tibial plafond is much easier to appreciate on the tomogram.

Computed Tomography

Computed tomography (CT) is an important adjunct to conventional radiography in the evaluation and diagnosis of trauma, particularly in complex anatomic areas. Both osseous and soft-tissue injuries are well depicted. It has replaced conventional tomography at most institutions because it requires less patient movement, is easier to perform, and has a far lower radiation dose.[4] Unlike conventional tomography, CT also demonstrates the soft tissues with excellent contrast resolution. The images generally are limited to the transaxial plane though direct coronal and sagittal images of the extremities may be obtained. Large metallic objects produce extensive artifact on CT and limit the use of this technique in the presence of extensive orthopedic hardware.[32]

Computed tomography has been widely used in the assessment of spinal trauma. The transaxial plane is extremely useful in the identification of retropulsed bone fragments that may be difficult to detect with conventional radiography. Posterior element fractures are far easier to visualize on CT than on plain films.[23] Intervertebral malalignment may not be identified on the transaxial scans but sagittal or coronal reformations can aid in the documentation of minor degrees of vertebral subluxation (Fig. 5.12). Horizontal fractures of the spine, such as odontoid and Chance

FIGURE 5.12. The AP radiograph of the spine (A) demonstrates an angular deformity and a complex fracture of L2. There is widening of the inter- pediculate distance consistent with a burst frac- ture. The transaxial CT (B) shows fractures of the vertebral body, pedicles, spinous process, and left transverse process. Note the presence of retropulsed bone within the spinal canal. The 2D sagittal reformations (C) show the malalignment and retropulsed bone to better advantage.

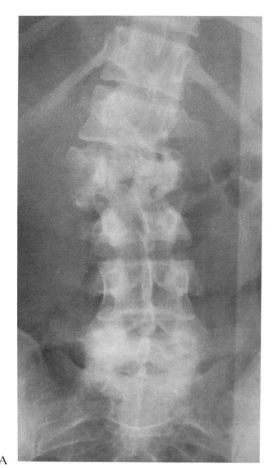

A

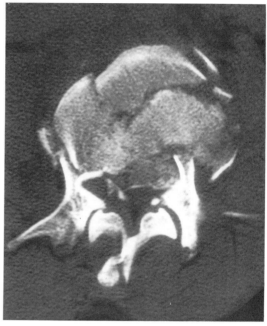

B

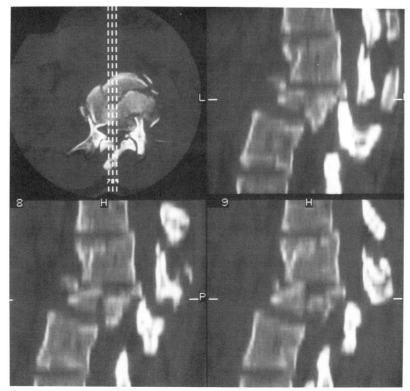

C

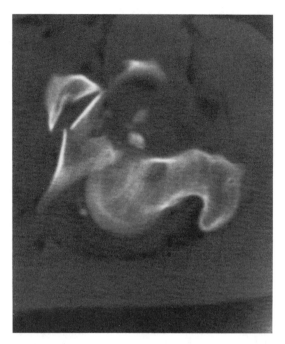

FIGURE 5.13. An axial CT scan through the left hip joint shows a posterior dislocation of the femoral head associated with a complex acetabular fracture. Disruption of the quadrilateral plate and posterior column of the acetabulum is present. Comminution of the posterior rim is associated with the presence of intraarticular bodies.

fractures, may be overlooked unless thin overlapping CT sections are obtained.

Fractures of the pelvis also are a major indication for CT examination. Computed tomography is superior to plain films in the identification of fractures of the sacrum, acetabular roof, posterior acetabular lip, and quadrilateral plate.[11] Plain films and CT are comparable in diagnostic accuracy for fractures of the iliac wing, pubic rami, and anterior and posterior column of the osseous pelvis.[11] Mild sacroiliac-joint diastasis may be difficult to detect with conventional radiography but is usually apparent with CT. Intraarticular bodies in the hip associated with acetabular fractures or dislocations can be readily identified (Fig. 5.13). Computed tomography is superior to conventional radiography in the determination of the stable fragment and greatly aids in

determining the precise pattern of acetabular injury.[17]

Analysis of areas of complex anatomy such as the sternoclavicular joint, shoulder, and hindfoot are other frequent indications for CT.[4] We routinely perform CT for complex intraarticular calcaneal and talar fractures and find the technique invaluable. Articular-surface malalignment and fracture displacement are accurately identified. The role of CT in the evaluation of extraarticular fractures is less clear. In this setting, CT has been utilized for assessment of nonunion and infection complicating trauma. The technique can indicate that a fracture is pathological when cortical erosions or expansion are present at the fracture site. In most instances, however, plain films are adequate in the analysis of nonarticular injuries.

The transaxial images obtained by CT can be reformatted into sagittal or coronal two-dimensional images that allow each structure to be visualized in at least three planes.[18] More recently, CT units that reformat the transaxial data into simulated three-dimensional (3D) images have been developed. These reformatted 3D images allow the viewer to study the object from a variety of perspectives as the image is rotated through space (Fig. 5.14). While the images are beneficial for characterization and integration of abnormalities, no additional data are generated by the 3D reconstruction. Rather, the existing data are displayed in a manner that is easier to understand, particularly by persons with limited experience with transaxial imaging.[22] This technique is most useful in areas of complex anatomy such as the pelvis, spine, shoulder region, and facial bones.[18,22]

Angiography

The indications for arterial angiography in patients suffering blunt or penetrating trauma in proximity to large vessels remain controversial. While there is no doubt that angiography prior to or during vascular exploration is mandatory in patients with clinical evidence

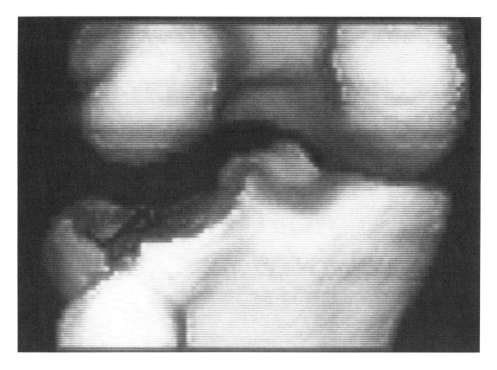

FIGURE 5.14. A 3D CT of a lateral tibial plateau fracture demonstrates depression of the posterior articular surfaces and displacement of the fracture fragments.

of vascular injury, its role in patients with a clinically normal vascular examination is far less clear.[24] Penetrating wounds and fractures in the region of the distal portion of the femur and around the knee constitute the most frequent indication for angiography after trauma. The mechanisms leading to vascular injury include laceration by a sharp bone fragment, compression secondary to hematoma or swelling within a tight fascial compartment, shearing injuries, and arterial entrapment within fracture fragments.[25] The vessels that are injured most commonly are in close proximity to bone and held in a relatively fixed position by fascial or muscular attachments.[25] Angiographic abnormalities indicating vessel trauma include small-vessel extravasation, pseudoaneurysm, arteriovenous fistula, intimal tears, and vessel laceration.[8,24] Angiography may be utilized as an adjunctive therapeutic method in patients with extensive posttraumatic hemorrhage in which vascular embolization may be performed.

Ultrasonography

Applications of diagnostic ultrasound (US) to musculoskeletal trauma are largely limited to the assessment of soft tissues. The US beam is completely reflected at the interface between bone and soft tissue; therefore, the technique is not suitable for the study of osseous structures.[14,32] The advantages of US include its widespread availability, low cost, rapidity, and portability. The lack of ionizing radiation makes this technique particularly advantageous in children or when repetitive examinations are necessary. Considerable operator experience, however, is necessary for this technique to yield reliable information.

Ultrasonography is a useful technique in the detection and serial evaluation of muscular hematomas. Hemorrhage produces focal or diffuse muscle enlargement and may be associated with muscle tears. The echo characteristics of hematomas are highly variable and are dependent upon the age of the collection.[31]

The US appearance is quite nonspecific, and it may be difficult to distinguish hematomas, muscle ruptures, and rhabdomyolysis from inflammatory processes and neoplasms.[31]

One of the major applications of US is in the assessment of traumatic tendon abnormalities such as partial or complete tears, tendinitis, and infection following puncture wounds.[14] The rotator cuff, biceps, patellar, and quadriceps tendons and those of the hand have been evaluated with this technique.[14] In the United States, MRI is replacing US as the imaging method of choice for assessment of tendon injuries owing to its superior accuracy.

Scintigraphy

Bone scanning with technetium-99M-labeled phosphate or diphosphonate compounds plays an important role in the imaging assessment of the traumatized patient. Scintigraphy can be useful in the injured patient with a confusing clinical picture and normal radiographs, in evaluation of incidentally discovered radiographic changes of uncertain clinical significance, and in providing objective evidence of bone injury in highly competitive athletes.[2] Finally, scintigraphy may be necessary to determine the age of a fracture, often for medicolegal purposes. It often is difficult to determine whether a fracture is acute when the underlying bone is osteopenic, a common situation when there are compression fractures of the thoracolumbar spine.

Following the intravenous administration of the radiopharmaceutical agent the movement of the tracer occurs in three phases: the flow phase (1–2 minutes), when the tracer is intravascular; the blood pool phase (5–10 minutes), when the tracer is in the extravascular extracellular space; and the delayed or osseous phase (2–4 hours), when the tracer is incorporated into bone.[13] Images of the injured area are obtained during each of these phases, and in the delayed phase the remainder of the skeleton also can be evaluated. Tomographic bone imaging with single-photon-emission computed tomography (SPECT) often supplements the conventional bone scan; SPECT

images provide improved image contrast and spatial resolution, particularly in deep structures such as those in the spine.[13]

Clinical examination and standard radiography are adequate for almost all uncomplicated acute fractures.[19] Less than 3% of patients at two large sports-medicine centers were referred for bone scans.[29] A normal bone scan enables the clinician to rule out the diagnosis of a significant osseous injury provided that the examination is obtained following an adequate delay from the time of injury, particularly in the elderly patient. The bone scan is abnormal in 95% of patients younger than 65 years of age at 24 hours after a fracture and in 100% by 72 hours. In older persons, 80% of scintigrams are positive at 24 hours and 95% at 72 hours.[19]

The scintigraphic appearance of a fracture changes over time. In the acute stage, persisting for approximately 2–4 weeks following the injury, there is diffuse uptake about the fracture site. Undisplaced fractures, such as those of the scaphoid and the femoral neck, particularly when they occur in the osteoporotic patient, may not be evident on early radiographs but demonstrate focal areas of increased uptake at the fracture site with scintigraphic techniques (Fig. 5.15).[19] In the subacute stage, present for approximately 8–12 weeks, a well-defined linear area of increased activity is seen at the site of the fracture. The fracture will usually be apparent radiographically during this stage owing to resorption and healing. The healing stage is heralded by a gradual diminution in the intensity of the scintigraphic uptake until the scan eventually returns to normal.[25] Over 90% of fracture sites are scintigraphically normal after 2 years. When healing does not result in normal anatomical alignment, continued biomechanical stress results in continuous remodeling, and increased uptake of the radionuclide may persist indefinitely.[13]

Stress fractures are seen with scintigraphy prior to the development of radiographic abnormalities. The need for an early diagnosis of stress fractures is greatest in the femoral neck because continued activity can result in overt cortical fractures necessitating major surgery.[29] In Marine recruits, stress fractures

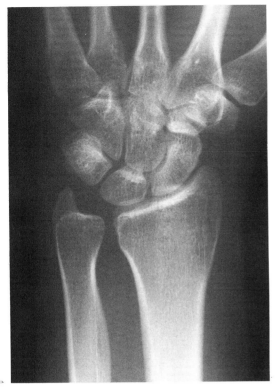

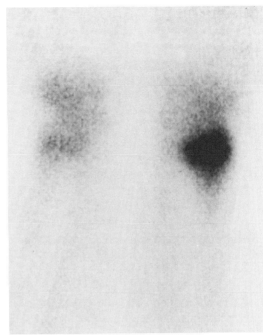

B

FIGURE 5.15. A normal PA radiograph (A) of the wrist was obtained on an osteopenic woman following a fall. A bone scan (B) obtained 2 days later shows diffuse increased activity in the distal radius on this supinated image. Follow-up radiographs showed an undisplaced distal radius fracture.

predominate in the lower extremity with the tibia and the calcaneus representing the most frequently involved sites.[9] Approximately half of scintigraphic foci of increased activity in military recruits never show any radiographic abnormalities.[9,20] In one large study, only 28% of 839 abnormal sites of stress at scintigraphy showed correlative radiographic abnormalities. With delayed evaluation after 2–6 weeks, 54% of these sites developed radiographic changes consistent with stress fractures.[9] Multifocal abnormalities, such as bilateral pubic rami or calcaneal uptake, are frequent.[20]

The spectrum of scintigraphic abnormalities associated with bone stress includes both ill-defined and sharply marginated sites of radionuclide uptake. Ill-defined areas of increased scintigraphic activity may represent sites of increased metabolic turnover in areas of stress and do not necessarily indicate the presence of a stress fracture. These nonspecific foci of abnormal activity do not result in any radiographic abnormalities and presumably represent sites of focal microscopic periosteal, subchondral, or intraosseous trauma.[13] The classic scintigraphic appearance of a stress fracture consists of a sharply marginated oval or fusiform area of increased radioactivity.[28] These well-defined focal areas of markedly increased uptake of radiopharmaceutical agent resolve slowly after the cessation of the offending physical activity.[28]

Magnetic Resonance (MR) Imaging

Assessment of musculoskeletal trauma, particularly soft-tissue injury, is a major application of MR imaging. The major advantages of

MRI are that the technique is noninvasive, has multiplanar capability, and provides excellent contrast and spatial resolution. Its major disadvantages include high cost, long examination time, claustrophobia experienced by the patient within the narrow bore of the magnet, and limited availability. Patients with pacemakers, surgical clips for cerebral aneurysm surgery, and ocular metallic foreign bodies cannot be imaged. Despite the relatively recent development and limited availability of MR, the appearance of a wide spectrum of osseous and soft-tissue injuries with this technique has already been described.

Normal bone marrow in adults demonstrates high signal intensity on both T1- and T2-weighted images owing to the predominance of fat. Fluid-containing structures, such as areas of edema and inflammation, are dark on T1-weighted spin-echo sequences and demonstrate high signal intensity of T2-weighted sequences. Cortical bone has very low signal on all imaging sequences and its presence is inferred by the signal void it creates. Early reports suggested that MR imaging was poorly suited to the evaluation of cortical bone, but recent advances in software allow the radiologist to detect most displacements and discontinuities of the cortex. Although the mineralized bone is not as well seen as with CT, the adjacent medullary changes render MRI equally sensitive in cases of osseous trauma. Newly developed techniques that suppress bone-marrow fat, such as short tau inversion recovery (STIR) or fat-saturation techniques, are more sensitive than conventional spin-echo imaging for detection of intramedullary abnormalities.[5]

The MR abnormalities of a variety of different osseous injuries have been described. The bone "bruise" is a commonly encountered abnormality associated with a variety of major knee injuries such as cruciate or collateral ligament tears.[5] This abnormality produces an intramedullary area with low signal on T1-weighted and high signal on T2-weighted spin-echo images, consistent with marrow edema. Although the cortical bone and cartilage are intact, there presumably are trabecular microfractures that produce edema.[33] This situation

is probably analogous to the ill-defined areas of scintigraphic uptake seen in such patients.[13] The abnormalities typically resolve rapidly and no reported case of progression of a bone bruise has been documented.[5] This relatively benign entity must be distinguished from osteochondral injuries that result in disruption of the overlying cartilage and osseous surfaces.

Magnetic resonance imaging also can detect numerous acute fractures that either are radiographically inapparent or demonstrate very subtle abnormalities that are missed on prospective interpretation (Fig. 5.16).[2,6,33] The detection of these radiographically occult fractures is particularly significant with injuries in areas of major weight-bearing such as the femoral neck and the tibial plateau. While both scintigraphy and MR imaging will allow detection of these abnormalities, the latter examination generally is more specific because it actually outlines the anatomic extent of the fracture line; MR can also be performed acutely whereas scintigraphy must be obtained after a 48–72-hour delay in the elderly patient. In one study evaluating 23 elderly patients with posttraumatic hip pain and normal radiographs, MR detected nine unrecognized fractures and correctly excluded injury in the remainder.[6]

Two MR-imaging patterns of stress fractures have been described. Amorphous stress fractures are clinically similar to a bone bruise but may be differentiated on the basis of the patient's history.[5] The more common abnormality of a stress fracture that is seen on T1-weighted spin-echo images is a linear band of decreased intensity oriented perpendicular to the cortex, surrounded by a more poorly defined low signal area. The linear component remains dark on T2-weighted spin-echo images but the surrounding zone, presumably representing edema, becomes brighter on T2-weighted spin-echo images.[5,16] Insufficiency fractures also produce linear or oblique lines of low signal on T1-weighted spin-echo images surrounded by edema.

Magnetic resonance imaging is an excellent technique for the assessment of soft-tissue injury. Both plain films and scintigraphy are relatively insensitive for soft-tissue abnormal-

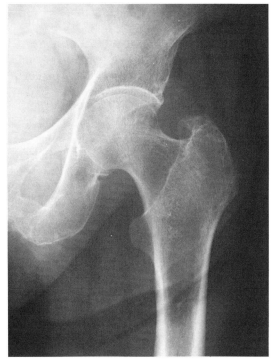

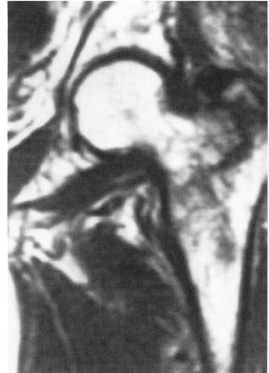

B

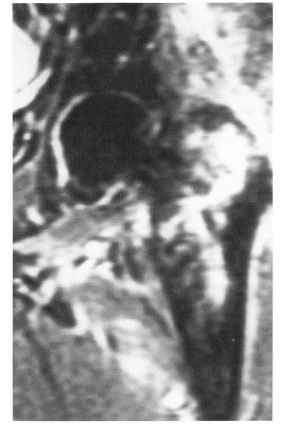

FIGURE 5.16. The AP radiograph (A) in an elderly woman with a history of a fall is normal. A T1-Weighted MR image (B) demonstrates an occult intertrochanteric fracture. The fracture produces loss of the normal bright signal of the fatty marrow. The STIR MR image (C) shows high signal at the fracture site due to adjacent edema and hemorrhage.

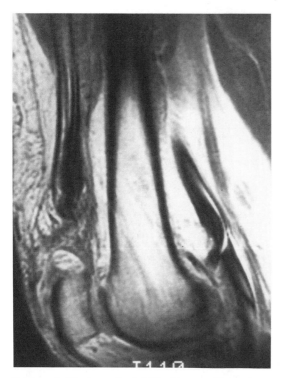

FIGURE 5.17. A sagittal MR image of the knee shows complete disruption of the quadriceps tendon. The normal dark tendon is disrupted, inhomogeneous, and retracted proximally, with a large gap between the tendon and the patella.

ities. While CT allows detection of hematoma and soft-tissue edema, far-more-accurate assessment of soft tissues is afforded by MR imaging because of its higher contrast resolution. Soft-tissue injuries are most conspicuous on T2-weighted spin-echo images, which optimize contrast between edema and/or hemorrhage and normal structures.[5] A variety of injuries involving muscles, ligaments, and tendons have been described.[5,7] Injuries to muscle typically result in high signal areas within the muscle on T2-weighted spin-echo images. Muscle edema, contusion, rupture, and intramuscular hematomas all have been described, largely in anecdotal form or in small series of patients.[5] The specific diagnosis of subacute hematomas can be made with high accuracy because they are one of the few soft-tissue masses that have high signal on both T1- and T2-weighted spin-echo sequences.

Normal ligaments and tendons are devoid of signal on all imaging sequences. Tears of these structures produce retraction and gaps within their substance that typically contain areas of high signal on T2-weighted spin-echo images (Fig. 5.17). Injuries of the rotator cuff, quadriceps, patellar, and Achilles tendons have received the most attention. Anecdotal reports also indicate that MR imaging may be a useful technique for evaluation of compartment syndromes associated with lower-extremity fractures. Unilateral swelling and a slight increase of muscle intensity on T2-weighted spin-echo images in the involved compartments have been described.[7]

Conclusion

Numerous different imaging methods are used for accurate diagnosis in the traumatized patient. Many of these techniques, particularly MR imaging and CT, have been available for only a short time and their roles are still evolving. Other techniques, such as conventional tomography and ultrasonography, are being supplanted by these newer methods. All of these techniques have advantages, disadvantages, and inherent limitations. It is hoped that this brief review will help our collegues select and interpret imaging examinations for their traumatized patients.

Acknowledgments. A special thanks to Marcia Earnshaw and Gale Hurley for their assistance in preparing this manuscript.

References
1. Apple JS, Martinez S, Allen NB, et al (1983) Occult fractures of the knee: tomographic evaluation. Radiology 148(2):383–387.
2. Berger PE, Ofstein RA, Jackson DW, et al (1989) MRI demonstration of radiographically occult fractures: what have we been missing? Radiographics 9(3):407–436.
3. Carter DR. Biomechanics of bone. In Nahum AM, Melvin J (ed) *The biomechanics of trauma.* Appleton-Century-Crofts, Norwalk, CT, pp 135–166, 1985.

 4. Dalinka MK, Boorstein JM, Zlatkin MB (1986) Computed tomography of musculoskeletal trauma. Radiol Clin North Am 24(2):933–944.
 5. Deutsch AL, Mink JH (1989) Magnetic resonance imaging of musculoskeletal injuries. Radiol Clin North Am 27(5):983–1002.
 6. Deutsch AL, Mink JH, Waxman AD (1989) Occult fractures of the proximal femur: MR imaging. Radiology 170(1):113–116.
 7. Ehman RL, Berquist TH (1986) Magnetic resonance imaging of musculoskeletal trauma. Radiol Clin North Am 24(2):291–319.
 8. Goodman PC, Jeffrey RB, Zawadzki MB (1984) Digital subtraction angiography in extremity trauma. Radiology 153(1):61–64.
 9. Greaney RB, Gerber FH, Laughlin RL, et al (1983) Distribution and natural history of stress fractures in U.S. Marine recruits. Radiology 146(2):339–346.
10. Guerra Jr J. Radiography and other imaging modalities in the diagnosis of trauma. In Nahum AM, Melvin J (eds) The biomechanics of trauma. Appleton-Century-Crofts, Norwolk, CT, pp 205–224, 1985.
11. Harley JD, Mack LA, Winquist RA (1982) CT of acetabular fractures: comparison with conventional radiography. AJR 138(3):413–417.
12. Ho C, Sartoris DJ, Resnick D (1986) Conventional tomography in musculoskeletal trauma. Radiol Clin North Am 24(2):929–932.
13. Holder LE (1990) Clinical radionuclide bone imaging. Radiology 176(3):607–614.
14. Kaplan PA, Anderson JC, Norris MA, et al (1989) Ultrasonography of post-traumatic soft-tissue lesions. Radiol Clin North Am 27(5): 973–982.
15. Lee JH, Weissman BN, Nikpoor N, et al (1989) Lipohemarthrosis of the knee: a review of recent experiences. Radiology 173(1):189–191.
16. Lee JK, Yao L (1988) Stress fractures: MR imaging. Radiology 169(1):217–220.
17. Mack LA, Harley JD, Winquist RA (1982) CT of acetabular fractures: analysis of fracture patterns. AJR 138(3):407–412.
18. Magid D, Fishman EK (1989) Imaging of musculoskeletal trauma in three dimensions: an integrated two-dimensional/three-dimensional approach with computed tomography. Radiol Clin North Am 27(5):945–956.
19. McDougall IR, Rieser RP (1989) Scintigraphic techniques in musculoskeletal trauma. Radiol Clin of North Am 27(5):1003–1011.
20. Meurman KOA, Elfving S (1980) Stress fracture in soldiers: a multifocal bone disorder. Radiology 134(2):483–487.
21. Nordin M, Frankel VH. Biomechanics of whole bones and bone tissue. In Glass L (ed) Basic biomechanics of the skeletal system. Lea and Febiger, Philadelphia, pp 15–16, 1980.
22. Pate D, Resnick D, Andre M, et al (1986) Perspective: three-dimensional imaging of the musculoskeletal system. AJR 147(9):545–552.
23. Pathria MN, Petersilge CA (1991) Spinal trauma. Radiol Clin N America 29:847–865.
24. Reid JDS, Redman HC, Weigelt JA, et al (1988) Wounds of the extremities in proximity to major arteries: value of angiography in the detection of arterial injury. AJR 151: 1035–1039.
25. Resnick D, Goergen TC, Niwayama G. Physical injury. In Diagnosis of bone and joint disorders. 2nd ed. WB Saunders, Philadelphia, 5:2756–3008, 1988.
26. Rogers LF. Skeletal biomechanics. In Radiology of skeletal trauma. Churchill Livingstone, New York, pp 15–22, 1982.
27. Rogers LF. Classification of fractures. In Radiology of skeletal trauma. Churchill Livingstone, New York, pp 31–66, 1982.
28. Roub LW, Gumerman LW, Hanley EN, et al (1979) Bone stress: a radionuclide imaging perspective. Radiology 132(8):431–438.
29. Rupani HD, Holder LE, Espinola DA, et al (1985) Three-phase radionuclide bone imaging in sports medicine. Radiology 156(1):187–196.
30. Swischuk LE, Hayden CK, Kupfer MC (1984) Significance of intraarticular fluid without visible fracture in children. AJR 142(6): 1261–1262.
31. Vincent LM (1988) US of soft tissue abnormalities of the extremities. Radiol Clin North Am 26(1):131–144.
32. Weissman BNW, Sledge CB. General principals. In Orthopedic radiology. WB Saunders, Philadelphia, 1–70, 1986.
33. Yao L, Lee JK (1988) Occult intraosseous fracture: Detection with MR imaging. Musculoskel Radiol 167(3):749–752.

6
A Review of Mathematical Occupant Simulation Models

Priya Prasad and C.C. Chou

Introduction

With the advent of computers, mathematical modeling became part of CAE (computer-aided engineering) in engineering and many areas of the physical sciences. Almost 28 years have elapsed since McHenry[1] proposed one of the first mathematical simulation models to describe the dynamic response of a vehicle occupant involved in a collision event in 1963. Since then, many more sophisticated models have been developed for simulating occupant kinematics in crashes. During the past decades, a great deal of emphasis has been placed on the use of mathematical models in research and development in the field of automotive safety.

A review of several *gross-motion simulators* was made by King and Chou[2] in 1975. Two of the models reviewed, namely, CAL3D and MVMA2D, have gone through extensive use and development, and a third model called MADYMO 2D/3D was developed by TNO in Holland in 1979. A detailed description of the basic features of the three occupant simulation models is contained in a review by Prasad,[3] who also further comparatively evaluated the MVMA2D and the MADYMO2D occupant simulation models (as reported in ref. 4). Further developments in these gross-motion simulators and others like UCIN3D,[5] SOMLA,[6] and some one-dimensional and special-purpose restraint system models were reported by Prasad and Chou.[7]

All the mentioned reviews concentrated on mathematical models derived on the basis of rigid body dynamics. Although the SOMLA program had integrated an occupant model with a finite element seat model for light aircraft, use of finite element analysis in occupant simulation was limited in the past due to lack of software and fast computing capabilities. Recent developments in finite element analysis[8] and coupling of finite element analysis codes with rigid body dynamics codes have opened a new era in occupant dynamics simulation. Finite element codes are now available in which the entire occupant or parts of the occupant can be modeled using finite elements, making it possible to model the deformations in occupants due to contact loadings more accurately than with rigid body dynamics codes. Although a majority of the studies so far have concentrated on modeling dummies, in the long run, the use of mathematical models to explore injury criteria and countermeasures will be feasible.

This chapter reviews the state of the art in occupant modeling, keeping in mind that the field is rapidly evolving. The chapter discusses occupant models ranging from simple to the more complex. For completeness, some discussions presented in ref. 7 will be repeated in this chapter.

Simple Occupant Models

Many simple occupant simulation models, including two-dimensional models for frontal impact simulations and one- and two-dimensional models for side impact studies, are available. Some of these models will be briefly discussed:

2D/Frontal Impact Simplified Models

A number of two-dimensional simplified-occupant-but-detailed-steering-column-and-air-bag models are available.[9–12] Models that can be mentioned are:

- DRACR (*DR*iver *A*ir *C*ushion—*R*otation)[9]
- PAC (*P*assenger *A*ir *C*ushion)[10]
- PADS (*P*assenger *A*nd *D*river *S*imulation)[11]
- SCORES (*S*teering *C*olumn and *O*ccupant *RE*sponse *S*imulation)[12]

They were originally developed under the sponsorship of the National Highway Traffic Safety Administration (NHTSA) by Fitzpatrick Engineering. In addition, Fitzpatrick Engineering also developed DRISIM (*DRI*ver *SIM*ulation), PASSIM (*PAS*senger *SIM*ulation),[13,14] as well as PASSIM-PLUS.[15] These models are available on personal computers (PCs). The main features are that the occupant is two-dimensional and represented by three to four masses. The steering column hardware and air-bags are detailed as shown in Fig. 6.1. Methodology using the DRISIM model and design of experiment for an air-bag restraint system design were proposed by Dickson et al.[16] PAC[17] and PASSIM-PLUS were the first models capable of modeling out-of-position occupant responses due to "bag-slap" effects. Figure 6.2 shows the PASSIM-PLUS schematic. Several studies using these models and their variations have been reported.[10–12]

The PADS occupant simulator was developed by MGA Research Corp.[18] primarily for simulations of the driver and steering assembly interaction. It is a two-dimensional model with a four mass (head/neck, torso, lower body, and sternum) occupant and compartment geometry defined by seven contact planes and steering assembly as shown in Fig. 6.3. Fessahaie et al.[19] used PADS for simulation of unrestrained drivers of light trucks and vans in a frontal collision study, while Naab and Stucki used it in the development and test of steering assembly countermeasures for driver impacts.[20]

Sieveha et al.[21] developed the PADPREP processor, which accepts a standard PADS input file. Sieveha and Pilkey[22] have also implemented the PADS into the Safety Systems Optimization Model.[23]

One- and Two-Dimensional Side Impact Models

In order to study occupant and vehicle dynamics in car-to-car side impacts, a number of one-dimensional combined occupant and structural models have been developed by Trella and Kanianthra.[24] In these models, the occupant is represented by four masses—pelvis, chest, rib, and head. These masses are connected by nonlinear springs and dampers. The structure of the car is represented by several masses, representing door, body, rocker panel, and the barrier. These masses are again connected by nonlinear springs. The software used to generate these models is known as CRUSH (*C*rash *R*eproduction *U*sing *S*tatic *H*istory), developed by Ford Motor Co. and publicly available in the revised SSOM (*S*afety *S*ystem *O*ptimization *M*odel) program by the University of Virginia.[23] Even though these models are one-dimensional, because of their ease of use, they are very useful in studying the interaction between side structure and the occupant.

To account for occupant rotational effects in side impact, a two-dimensional model of the side impact dummy has been suggested by Hasegawa et al.[25]

Gross-Motion Simulators

Gross-motion simulators are a class of mathematical models formulated to describe a vehicle occupant in planar or three-dimensional motion in a crash environment. The "occupant" is generally assumed to be a set of rigid bodies with prescribed masses and moments of inertia, linked by various types of joints in an open loop system known as a "tree structure." In some models, the number of rigid bodies used to describe the occupant is fixed. In others, any number of rigid bodies can be used to

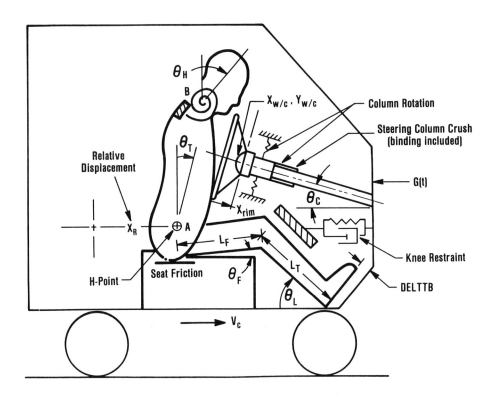

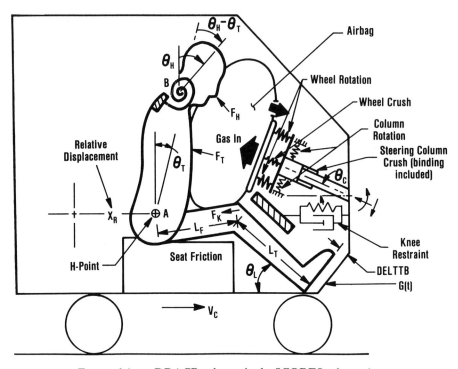

FIGURE 6.1. a. DRACR schematic. b. SCORES schematic.

FIGURE 6.2. PASSIM-PLUS schematic.

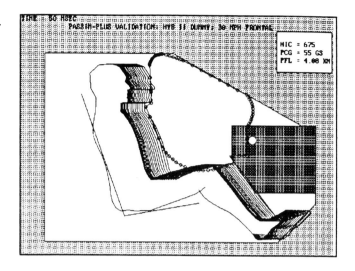

FIGURE 6.3. PADS occupant, compartment, and steering assembly.[20]

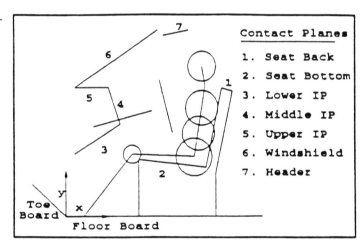

describe the occupant, resulting in simple to complex models of the occupant. The governing equations of motion of such a collection of rigid bodies are derived in closed form or automatically using the Lagrangian or the Newtonian approach.

The shapes and surfaces of the rigid body links are described by ellipses in the MVMA2D, by ellipses or hyperellipses in the MADYMO2D version and by ellipsoids in the CAL3D, MADYMO3D, and UCIN3D. Hyperellipsoids can also be used in the CAL3D and the MADYMO3D to describe the shapes. In the UCIN3D elliptical cylinders or frustums of elliptical cones are used to describe the

shapes of the links. In all models the relative rotation between links are resisted by nonlinear torsional springs, viscous dampers, and/or Coulomb frictions.

With the exception of the UCIN3D model, which uses springs for contact force generation, the human body linkage system in other models interacts with the environment through contact planes or ellipsoids that develop resistive forces on the segments in contact. In most of the models (except UCIN3D), the ellipses or ellipsoids/hyperellipsoids are used to sense contacts. The amount and rate of penetration between ellipsoids into planes or ellipsoids into ellipsoids are used to develop nonlinear spring forces, viscous damping (in MADYMO only) and frictional forces on the link in contact.

Additionally, restraint systems, e.g., belts or supplemental air bags, also provide coupling of the occupant to the vehicle. In general, the belts are represented by nonlinear springs connecting belt anchor locations and various segments of the occupant. Even in the two-dimensional models, the three-dimensional geometry of the belt system is simulated to produce realistic belt loads. Slipping of the belts across the occupant and through rings attached to the vehicle are simulated.

The airbag is modelled by a fluid filled container of a geometrically describable final shape. As the occupant contacts and penetrates the airbag, the instantaneous volume of the bag is calculated based on volumes intersected by contacting occupant ellipsoids and/or vehicle interior. The instantaneous volume, temperature, and the remaining fluid mass in the bag is used to calculate the instantaneous pressure in the bag using ideal gas equations. The calculated pressure and membrane forces from the bag are applied to the contacting segments of the occupant.

The resulting equations of motion are solved numerically using Runge–Kutta techniques in the MVMA2D, the MADYMO and the UCIN3D models, and by a vector exponential integrator in the CAL3D model.

The following sections in this chapter describe the various features of the four models mentioned above and various studies using these models reported in the literature. No attempt to select the best of the above is made. It is believed that all the models discussed can simulate a variety of impact conditions depending on the experience of the modeler. In fact, even though they were developed for vehicle occupant or pedestrian simulations, they can be used to simulate the dynamics of many other systems of rigid bodies.

MVMA2D

Historical Review

The origins of the MVMA2D occupant simulation model can be traced to a model developed at the Cornell Aeronautical Labs by McHenry and Naab[26] in 1966. Further improvements in the model were carried out under AMA sponsorship and the resulting model was released by Segal[27] and was called ROS (Revised Occupant Simulation Model). Improvements to the ROS were made at G.M. by Danforth and Randal,[28] and the new model was named MODROS. MODROS was released to the MVMA in 1972. Further developments to the MODROS were undertaken at the HSRI by Robbins, Bennett and Bowman. Between 1972 and 1974, three versions of the MVMA2D model were developed. Version 3 was the first reported in 1974,[29] and Version 4 was released in 1979. Since 1974 various additions and debugging have been carried out at G.M. and HSRI, the most notable being in the advanced belt simulation algorithm. Attempts at the development of an advanced air bag algorithm and a driver air bag system incorporating a supplemental air bag and an energy-absorbing steering column have been made. These algorithms are currently inoperable and future efforts to enhance the model may be in completing the above algorithms. In 1985, an "ellipse man" Calcomp plot program postprocessor was added in Version 5.[30]

Many of the features in the MVMA2D model regarding the treatment of joints, contact detection, resistive moments and forces, and belt and airbag models have been adopted by other codes developed later. Hence, they will be discussed in this chapter.

Analytical Formulation

The linkage system used to describe an occupant is shown in Fig. 6.4. As can be seen, there are ten segments and nine masses. The mass of the neck is lumped partially in the head and partially in the upper torso. The neck is modelled by an extensible link with two articulations—one at the head/neck junction and the other at the upper torso/neck junction. The shoulder is also modelled by an extensible element. These two features of the MVMA2D formulation of the occupant are unique when compared with other occupant simulators.

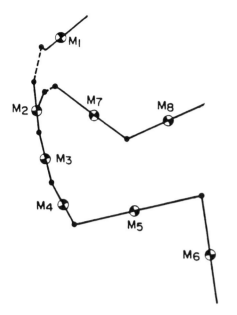

FIGURE 6.4. MVMA2D occupant simulation linkage system.

The equations of motion of the linkage system are derived using the Lagrangian technique explicitly as opposed to other models, like the MADYMO, the CAL3D or the UCIN3D, in which they are generated automatically.

Current Features

Joints

There are eight hinged joints used in the model. Torques generated in the joints are of the elastic, viscous damping, coulomb friction types, and a nonlinear and nonlinear energy-dissipating type for the joint stop. Figure 6.5 shows a general representation of the linear and nonlinear joint torque. A unique feature of this model is its attempt to simulate bio-dynamic muscle tension into the joints. Use of the muscle tension model has been demonstrated by Schneider and Bowman[31] in a study of the dynamic response of the head and neck of volunteers subjected to $-G_x$ acceleration, and by Bowman et al.[32] in a study of lateral head and neck response of human volunteers.

Contact Model

Occupant interaction with vehicle interior surfaces is sensed by ellipses fixed to body links. The contact ellipses can be arbitrary in number and dimensions, and can be deformable or rigid. The reaction forces on the occupant linkage system are generated as a function of the penetration of these ellipses into vehicle contact planes, e.g., seat, instrument panel, windshield, etc. Additionally, ellipses can contact other ellipses, e.g., head into chest or knees, etc. In order to save computer time, ellipse–ellipse or ellipse–plane contacts can be inhibited.

The stiffness characteristics of the contact planes or deformable ellipses are described in a tabular form. Inertia spikes to account for rate effects can also be simulated. Hysteresis of the

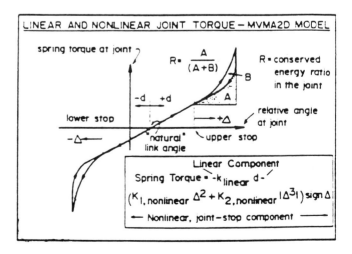

FIGURE 6.5. Joint torque model.

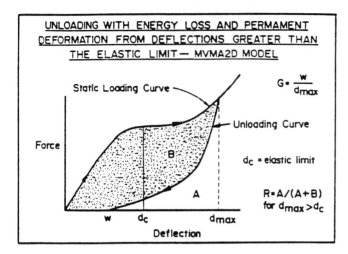

FIGURE 6.6. Contact hysteresis model.

contact surfaces or ellipses are described by R and G factors shown in Fig. 6.6. By specifying the location of the contact planes as a function of time, intrusion can be simulated, e.g., instrument panel intrusion into the occupant compartment.

Restraint Systems

Simple Belt System

The simple belt system essentially consists of an upper torso strap, a lower torso strap and a one-piece lap belt. Since most automotive belt systems are three-dimensional in nature, the usefulness of this system is limited.

Advanced Belt Restraint System

This system allows for a more realistic simulation of the belt system in today's vehicles. It consists of up to seven belt segments acting independently or in pairs. Friction between the upper torso, the pelvis, and the belt system can be simulated. Inertia reels at three of the four anchor locations can be simulated. Figure 6.7 shows a side view of a five-segment advanced belt system. The three-dimensional aspect of the belt system is simulated by specifying lateral dimensions as shown in Figure 6.8. Note that the coordinates of the inboard and outboard anchors can be different.

Air Bag

The supplemental air bag model used in the MVMA2D was developed at the Cornell Aeronautical Laboratory by Hammond.[33] The air bag is cylindrical in shape. The mass inflow rate and the temperature of the gas entering the bag are input parameters to the model along with other thermodynamic properties of the gas. Deflation membranes can be simulated.

The bag attachment point in the air bag model is a fixed point in the vehicle. As

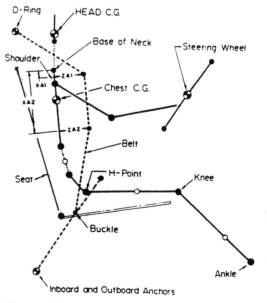

FIGURE 6.7. Side view: advanced belt simulation.

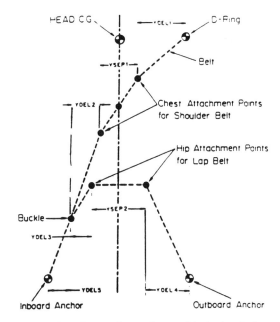

FIGURE 6.8. Front view: advanced belt simulation.

a result, an air bag mounted on an energy-absorbing steering column cannot be simulated. Efforts at developing a model of a driver supplemental air bag mounted on a collapsible steering column were made by Chou et al.[34] Due to problems with the steering column model, Chou's model becomes unstable under general input conditions. The air bag model itself has been identified as having instabilities under certain input conditions.

Steering Column

The steering column model incorporated in the MVMA2D was developed by Segal for the ROS model.[27] This portion of the MVMA2D needs extensive improvement to become a useful tool.

Special Features

Although not generally used for occupant simulation, a force can be applied directly to any point on the head. This force—both in magnitude and direction—can be time dependent. This special feature of the model was used to empirically derive the composite lateral bending stiffness of the human neck for small deformations.[35]

Other Applications

Even though the MVMA2D model was developed for simulating occupants of vehicles in frontal or rear impacts, with careful choice of input parameters, other crash modes can be simulated. Robbins and Becker[36] have developed baseline data for describing response of occupants in side impacts, and pedestrian impacts using the MVMA2D. Backaitis and Robbins[37] have also reported a study on side impact using this model. Robbins and Viano[38] have reported a simulation of occupant response in vehicle rollover.

Further application of the model include its use in vehicle accident investigation,[39] head/neck response of helmeted and nonhelmeted motorcyclists,[40] simulations of falling people striking hard or soft surfaces,[41] driver environment design parameter study,[42] computer modeling in new vehicle design,[43] and study of influence of vehicle deceleration curve on dummy injury criteria.[44] Shimamura et al.[45] investigated the occupant movement due to belt characteristics variations.

Experimental Verification

Alem et al.[46] have reported the results of sled tests with three-point belted cadavers and their comparisons with simulations using the MVMA2D. Considering the variations in the cadaver anthropometry and joint character-istics, the model results compared well with the test results. It was pointed out that a more general joint model is required for cadaver simulations. Ideally, tabular specification of joint torque loading curves is required.

Comparison of sled test results with the Hybrid II dummy and the MVMA2D model simulations have been reported by Viano et al.[47] Various modifications to the advanced belt routine were made during this study to incorporate the lateral locations of the belt anchor points. The belt loads predicted by the model agreed poorly with the test results. It was felt by the authors that a five-segment belt simulation would improve the simulations. It should be noted here that since then, further improvements in the advanced belt routine have been made. Shimamura et al.,[45] Henson,[48] and Henson et al.[49] have shown good correlation between test results and simulations.

Oho et al.[50] recently carried out a verification study between simulated unrestrained passenger dummy responses with sled test data in 15 mph and 30 mph frontal impact simulations. Through parametric studies they investigated the effects of crash pulse, location and characteristics of the instrument panel and cross car beam, and the position of seat frame on the occupant injury. Countermeasures to reduce injury parameters were developed on the basis of the parametric study, and were further verified by tests.

User Convenience

The model is documented in three volumes of the user manual covering the analytical formulation, card-by-card description, and description of the subroutines used in the program.[51,52] A "Validation Command Language" program was developed to perform many postprocessing operations on MVMA2D generated data and to add a capability of quantifying comparisons between the test and simulated results. To facilitate the learning process in using the model, a Tutorial System has been developed. It consists of a Self-Study Guide and an Audio-Visual program.[35,53] The Self-Study Guide contains text, illustrations and example problems. The Audio-Visual program includes narration text and figures on 35-mm slides.

An interactive program that positions the MVMA2D occupant in approximate equilibrium has been developed by Bowman[52] for General Motors. Later, O'Leary[54] developed a program for the MVMA2D model in seating the occupant to establish initial equilibrium. Printer plots of the occupant, vehicle interior, and the restraint system are standard options in the model output. An occupant display package in use at General Motors has been reported by Danforth and Prisk.[55] An interactive occupant display package has been developed at Ford Motor Company by Huang.[56] Sieveha et al.[21] developed a MVMA occupant simulator processor, called MVMAPREP, for automating the task of generating files for large parametric studies.

It should be mentioned that a spin-off model called PRAKIMOD (*P*eugeot/*R*enault *A*ccidents *KI*nematic *MOD*el), which is based on the very first version of MVMA2D model, was developed by Peugeot/Renault Associations for safety related studies.[57] Three applications of PRAKIMOD were presented by Lestrelin et al.[58] Simulations of side impacts using PARKIMOD were reported by Steyer et al.[59]

MADYMO

Historical Review

The MADYMO occupant simulation program package consists of a two-dimensional and a three-dimensional version. The formulation of the two packages are nearly identical and were completed in 1975 at TNO, Netherlands. Since 1975, the simulation program package has gone through considerable refinement and optimization at TNO. The first reference to the package in the literature was made by Wismans, Maltha, et al. in 1979[60] where model responses were compared with sled test results using a child dummy and child cadavers. The review of MADYMO by Prasad[3] was based on Version 3, released in 1983. Version 4.2 with six volumes of documentation was completed in 1988, and has been implemented at Ford Motor Company and at a few other locations in the USA, Canada, Japan, and Europe. From Version 3 to Version 4.2, a major development has been in the restructuring on the input by introducing keywords. The following modifications and added features were made in Version 4.2:

- An optional 2D air bag module: an ellipsoid or an elliptical cylinder
- A second hysteresis model: for flexibility in defining the unloading curve
- Multiple null systems: up to 15 null systems can be specified for simulating passenger compartment intrusions.
- Kelvin spring-damper element: a non-linear spring in parallel with a damper with a velocity dependent damping coefficient
- Calculations of injury parameters, such as HIC, the Gadd Severity Index (GSI) and the 3 msec Chest Gs, as output

- Calculation of the origin of point-restraint coordinate system per user's request
- Improved slip algorithm in the belt model
- A provision for retractor locking due to a specified acceleration level
- Specification of accelerometer coordinate systems
- Outputs of relative velocity and displacement
- Expansion of the kinematic output file
- Provisions for providing comments in the input file

The currently available version, referred to as Version 4.3,[61] was released in April 1990. New features in Version 4.3 included the following:

- 2D airbag model extensions including:
  arbitrary bag shape
    bag elasticity as a stretch factor
    variable discharge coefficients
  calculation of inflator properties based on tank pressure test data using a pre-processor, called MTA
  triggering airbag using a calculated acceleration which exceeds a user's pre-scribed value
- Maxwell element model for simulating a spring and damper in series, with non-linear spring and velocity dependent damping characteristics
- Contact model extensions including:
  nonlinear damping coefficients as a function of the penetration velocity
  nonlinear friction specified as a function of the normal force
- Belt model extensions including:
  seat belt rupture
  location of belt attachment points in inertial space
  retractor locking based on a calculated acceleration
- Initial conditions with respect to different coordinate systems
- Dynamic amplification factor
- Interface program for converting GEBOD (*GE*nerator of *BO*dy *D*ata) 3D output into a format for MADYMO 2D/3D data
- MADYMO3D air bag model[62] using a 3-node membrane elements with simple gas dynamic, linear elastic isotropic material

bag properties and the central difference method for time integration
- New output features:
  limit the amount of output as specified by users
  penetration in contact models written to a new output file
  (relative) elongation output for belt segments, Kelvin elements and the spring of the Maxwell elements
  (relative) angles (available in MADYMO2D)
  point-restraint output including the co-ordinates in and the components of cal-culated resultant force with respect to the point restraint coordinate system
  2D pin joint, Cardan joint, and flexion torsion joint outputs from joint models.

Analytical Formulation

The equations of motion for multiple tree structures composed of rigid bodies connected by joints (hinge or ball- socket type) are derived using Lagrangian methods. As a result, constraint equations of the type used in the CAL3D formulation for joints are not required. The memory requirement depends on the number of elements and contacts used for a particular simulation. MADYMO uses a Runge–Kutta method either a fourth order with a fixed time step or a fifth order with a variable time step. Generally speaking, the solution time is longer when a variable time step is used than with a fixed time step.

Current Version Features

There are no limitations on the number of rigid bodies for the human surrogate, its environ-ment, i.e. the car interior or exterior, belt systems, etc. Closed chains or paths are not allowed. However chains may be closed by using the point restraint feature whereby a point on one element is tied to a point on a second element by a stiff spring. Programmers have to use their own editing software to set some key dimensions based on the number of elements, belt systems, contacts, etc. This allows for the minimum memory requirement for any given simulation.

Types of Joints

Two types of joints are permitted. They are:

1. Hinged joints in two-dimensional version
2. Ball and socket joints in three-dimensional version. Two joint models are available, namely, the Cardan joint model and the flexion-torsion joint model. Joint torques are described in tabular forms as opposed to polynomial forms in the MVMA2D and the CAL3D models.

Standard Force Interaction Models

Four interactions are permitted as follows:

1. Acceleration forces
2. Contact forces from ellipsoids (ellipses in 2D) interacting with planes
3. Contact forces from ellipsoids (ellipses in 2D) interacting with ellipsoids (ellipses in 2D)—Planes can be attached to the vehicle or the occupant ellipses. Also, ellipses can be attached to the vehicle.
4. Hyperellipsoids to avoid edge effects.

The contact forces can be of the nonlinear spring, viscous damping, or frictional type. Note that the viscous type of contact force is not allowed in the MVMA2D or the CAL3D models. An interesting feature of this model is that penetration used to calculate contact forces is taken relative to the initial penetration, e.g. from the initial penetration of the pelvis into the seat cushion as a result of normal seat compression. This assumes a state of equilibrium of the system at the initiation of the simulation. Hysteresis is simulated by unloading slopes as opposed to the R and G factors used in the MVMA2D and the CAL3D models.

Restraint Systems

Two restraint systems can be modelled. They are:

1. Simple belts—these are basically springs.
2. Advanced belts—more realistic belt model accounting for the spatial geometry of a belt system. Locations of belt anchorage points can be specified in the inertial space co-ordinates. Slip between belt segments is possible, e.g., as between the lap belt portion and shoulder harness portion of a three point belt system. For belt systems with a retractor, "film spool effect" can be simulated if the data are available, e.g., applied belt load versus length of belt spooled out of the retractor. The acceleration-sensitive retractor locking mechanism can now be simulated using Version 4.3.

2D Air Bag Model

The air bag model, released in 1986, is available in MADYMO 2D version only.[63] Theoretical formulation follows that used in the MVMA2D. Required air bag input parameters are bag size, bag location, gas properties and mass inflow rate. The air bag can be assumed to be either as an ellipsoid or an elliptical cylinder for a better representation of a driver-side bag and passenger-side bag, respectively. Deflation can be simulated through mechanisms such as vent holes and/or bag porosity.

An inflator model for generating the required mass inflow rate into an air bag model using the tank test pressure information was implemented under a contract from Ford.[64]

The air bag can be attached to any element of any system. Air bag rotation can be simulated by using a joint connecting the bag-attached element to another element. A driver-side supplemental air bag can be mounted on a collapsible steering column system, which is modeled via a point-restraint system. No multi-bag configuration can be simulated. However, multi-inflators are allowed.

Special Features

The point-restraint system, the spring-damper model and the hysteresis model are available in MADYMO. These are discussed below:

Point-Restraint Model

This is basically a combination of three spring-damper elements in 3D (two such elements in 2D) that limit the relative motion of a point in another system. A slip joint can be simulated using two point-restraints. Dynamic steering collapse can be effectively modeled with this feature.

Spring-Damper Model

This model allows a nonlinear spring to be either in parallel or in series with a damper, representing the Kelvin and the Maxwell viscoelastic model, respectively. Damping coefficients of the damper can be non-constant, expressed as a function of the relative velocity across the damper. The Kelvin element has been used in simulating the chest response of an EUROSID/DOT SID dummy subjected to lateral impacts.

Hysteresis Model

This feature provides a provision of simulating an energy dissipating capability. The basic formulation used in the hysteresis model is similar to that used in CRUSH.[23] Two hysteresis models are currently available depending on whether the unloading curve passes through the origin or not (see Fig. 6.9).

Experimental Verification

Comparisons of the two-dimensional model responses with sled test results for a child dummy and cadaver in a harness type child restraint system have been reported by Wismans et al.[60] Satisfactory agreement between model and test results were obtained in terms of peak responses and shapes of the response-time histories. Prasad[4] also reported that the simulation results agreed well with the test results in his MADYMO2D-Test comparisons with the Hybrid II dummy. Prasad has also reported excellent model correlation with sled test results with the Hybrid III dummy at the 1988 SAE International Congress and Exhibition, Detroit, Michigan. Comparative evaluation of the dynamic responses between the Hybrid II and Hybrid III dummies between the MADYMO simulations and sled test data was presented by Prasad.[65] An advanced 50th percentile Hybrid III dummy database was established and reported in refs. 66 and 67.

Verification of the 3D model has been made using data from three sled test runs at dif-

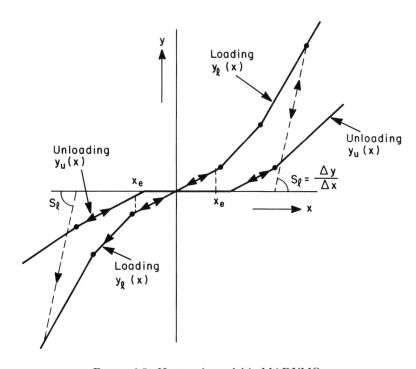

FIGURE 6.9. Hysteresis model in MADYMO.

ferent impact severity levels by Ford Motor Company. Part of the effort was to develop MADYMO Hybrid III input data based on dummy characteristics measured by the Wright Paterson Air Force Base.[68] A good agreement between the simulated and experimental results was found for most of the parameters (head acceleration, chest acceleration, belt load, etc.) compared in the study.[69] Matsumoto et al.[70] have conducted a parametric evaluation of vehicle crash performance and used the results to provide design guidance.

Validation studies of the 2D air bag model have been conducted by Chou and Wyman on Tempo supplemental air bag system,[71] and by Heinz et al. from Porsche.[72]

Side impact simulations with the Part 572 dummy and their correlations with rigid wall tests are described by Wismans et al.[73] Mathematical models of the various dummy thoraxes developed for side impact have been reported by Wismans and Wittebrood.[74]

Pedestrian simulations using two-dimensional models and a fifteen segment three-dimensional model and their comparisons with two tests at 30 and 40 km/h are reported by Wijk et al.[75] The model predictions are within or close to the range of experimental responses.

Dynamic simulations of a belted occupant with submarining are reported by Bosio[76] for passenger dummy in 2D study and by O'conner and Rao[77] for rear seated dummy in 3D simulation. In O'Cooner and Rao's study, a linkage system with a sliding contact was used between the pelvis and the lap belt in the dummy model to allow the simulation of submarining. Model predictions were verified by comparing with the results from Hyge sled tests for both rear seated Hybrid II and Hybrid III dummies. The times of the occurrence of submarining and the trends in dummy accelerations matched fairly well between the simulated and sled test results.

Other Applications

The versatility of the program package is demonstrated by the design and optimization of a new concept child restraint system using the MADYMO.[78] The MADYMO two-dimensional package has also been used in the design of an abdominal section for use in side impact dummies[79] and in the analysis of thoraxes of side impact dummies.[74] In addition, it has been adopted by Wiecher et al.[80] in a study regarding two dimensional thoracic modeling consideration. Other usages of MADYMO have also been demonstrated in wheelchair occupant protection systems by Kooi et al.,[81] and in a flight safety application by Wismans et al.[82] Recently, design of experiments methodology has received attention for use with MADYMO occupant simulations. In these regards, Bosio and Lupkar[83] have carried out a design of experiments (DOE) for a MADYMO 2D airbag and 3-point belt simulation study of the design factors that affect the head HIC in a 30 mph frontal barrier crash test, while Rieken and Fleming[84] used DOE to design a rear 3-point belt restraint system using a Hybrid III. Other advances in MADYMO crash simulations are documented by Lupkar et al. in ref. 85, including:

- EUROSID dummy database
- Frontal car crash with multiple occupants
- kicking soccer players
- multibody side-impact model
- unrestrained truck driver
- accident involving a trailer and a cyclist.

Current studies performed at Ford by the authors have shown that, with the availability of new generalized hysteresis algorithms, it is possible to model lumped and distributed mass responses of vehicle structure in the frontal and side impacts. The results of these studies will be published later. A 3D SID (Side Impact Dummy) model with a detailed thoracic configuration, developed by Low and Prasad at Ford, is shown in Figure 10. Side impact simulations using MADYMO will be discussed next.

Side Impact Studies

Low and Prasad[86] have conducted a series of rigid wall tests at three impact velocities to quantify the dynamic responses of the SID for the verification of the 3D mathematical SID model as shown in Fig. 6.11. This model uses

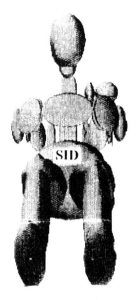

FIGURE 6.10. A 3D SID dummy model.

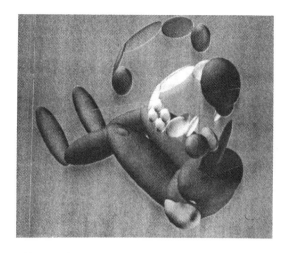

FIGURE 6.11. DOT-SID model: exploded view.

the mass distribution and the linkage system of the current Part 572 Hybrid II dummy which forms the basic platform of the SID. The unique chest construction of the dummy is modeled by two systems of linkages simulating the rib cage and the jacket as illustrated in Fig. 6.12. The internal hardware of a damper, rib stopper, and a clavicle simulator at the upper spine are also included. Model verifications were carried out at the component levels by comparing model and dummy certification results, and at the whole dummy levels by comparing the simulated outputs with rigid wall and APR padding test results. The study showed that the model simulations matched the test data very well in most responses, including TTI values.

Prasad, Low, Chou, Lim and Sundararajan[87] in their side impact studies developed a 3D lumped-mass structure and dummy model to simulate barrier-to-car side impacts (see Fig. 6.13). A series of static crusher tests were conducted to develop model input data. The model results compared very well with crash test results from a series of six barrier-to-car tests as given in ref.[87] The model, shown in

MODEL SCHEMATIC OF DOT SID CHEST

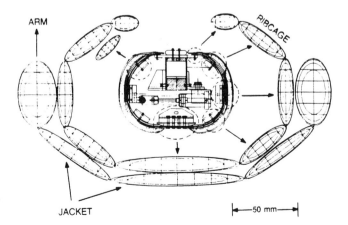

ARM

RIBCAGE

JACKET

|←—50 mm—→|

FIGURE 6.12. Actual ribcage layout vs. model segments.

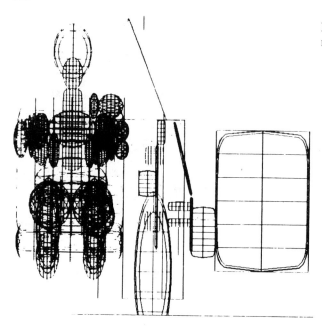

FIGURE 6.13. MADYMO 3D side impact model.

Fig. 6.13, is further extended to a more generic model including crabbed MDB (*Moving Deformable Barrier*), a target vehicle and a driver SID.[88] The results of this have been presented at the ASME Winter Annual Meeting in Atlanta, Georgia, in December 1991.

User Convenience

The user manual is written clearly with actual examples of simulations, making it easy for use by an inexperienced programmer. A graphics package for the representation of three-dimensional kinematics is included in the latest version.

TNO has developed a pre-processor of the MADYMO 2D program on an IBM PC system. allowing the user to prepare/edit/plot an input file through an interactive mode. A post-processor, MADPOST, for the MADYMO analysis package was developed by H.W. Structures[89] for VAX mainframe computer and Tektronic graphic terminals. This post-processor generates animation and graphs of simulation results. This processor has full color control with enhanced 3D hidden line and hyperellipsoid plotting. The post-processor capability including graphic package has been

further enhanced by the Ford CAE activity. Recently, a new menu driven *MADYMO Pre-* and *Post-*processor (MAPP), is being developed by TNO.[85]

New Developments

Coupling with FEM Packages

An interface has been developed coupling the MADYMO 3D and the PISCES finite element structures/gas flow program. The combined program is useful for simulating interactions between a 3D MADYMO rigid body dummy with a FE airbag. Details of this development will be discussed in Section VI. The MADYMO3D has also been coupled with PAMCRASH and DYNA3D Finite element codes.

Foam/Contact Model

Recently, a theoretical ellipsoid/plane contact model for simulating an ellipsoid impacting a flat foam bolster has been developed by Chou, Lim, and Mitchell.[90] Equations and algorithms have been developed for computing the contact force based on a uniaxial characteristic of a foam. A test program is being conducted to validate the contact model, which will be incorporated into the MADYMO program for simulation of occupant/bolster interaction.

CAL3D

History

Around 1970, the CALSPAN Corporation of Buffalo, New York began the development of a mathematical model for simulating the three-dimensional response of a vehicle occupant in a crash environment. The resulting model described by Bartz[91] and Bartz et al.[92] was known variously as the CAL3D occupant simulation model or the CVS (Crash Victim Simulator) model. In this model, the occupant was described by 15 segments with forty degrees of freedom and a contact model was developed for generating the external forces acting on the occupant. Restraint systems such as the belts and air bags were included. The early programs were known as Versions I and II of the CAL3D.

Further developments at CALSPAN by Fleck et al. resulted in an Improved Three-Dimensional Crash Victim Simulation Program known as CVS Version III.[93] The earlier version of the model was generalized to an arbitrary number of segments to describe an occupant. In addition, the concept of "null joints" was introduced so that disjointed sets of segments interacting against one another could be simulated. The vehicle and the ground were designated as additional segments, thus making it easier to model pedestrian impacts. Additionally, in this version, two symmetry modes could be specified—a two-dimensional symmetry and mirror type symmetry. As a result of the improvements, Version III can be regarded as a general purpose program for simulating three-dimensional motion of sets of connected or disjointed rigid elements.

Between 1974 and 1982 several modifications and features were developed by Fleck and Butler under contracts from NHTSA and Air Force Aerospace Medical Research Laboratory (AFAMRL).[94,95] The AFAMRL CAL3D version is also known as ATB (Articulated Total Body) Program. Further

additions and improvements have also been reported by Diggs.[96]

The latest versions of this model is known as ATB40A. However, the most recent version of the program available for public use is Version 37. The major developments are the following:

- A new, more efficient integration technique
- Automatic equilibrium routine for a seated occupant
- An advanced harness-belt routine that treats interaction of belts connected at a common junction point, belt slippage on deformable segments and rate-dependent belt forces
- Aerodynamic forces
- Incorporation into the main program integrator of the air bag equations and vehicle equations.
- The ability to specify the motion of up to six segments
- Principal axes may be different from the geometric axes of a segment
- Slip joint, and the ball and socket with globalgraphic torque and damping specification.
- Hyperellipsoid and edge effect option
- Hybrid III dummy parameters
- GEBOD (GEnerator of BOdy Data) for generating data on off size dummies by scaling from the 50th-percentile-male occupant.

This chapter reviews the latest version and relies on four volumes of available documentation[97] released in 1982 covering the analytical formulation, validation effort, user's manual, and a programmer's manual, along with published works on improvements.[96,98-104]

Analytical Formulation

The analytical treatment for deriving the equations of motion of sets of rigid bodies used in this model is neither Newtonian nor Lagrangian. It is similar to the Newtonian method, since the constraint forces are explicitly contained in the equations of motion without employing Lagrange multipliers. However, constraint relations of the type used in the Lagrange method augmented by compatibility relations as a direct consequence of Newton's third law are used. The authors have demonstrated the equivalence of the method used in the model to the classical Lagrange method in Appendix 2 of ref. 97, Volume 1.

Current Version Features

The capability of Version 20 is 30 segments plus the vehicle and ground, with 21 joints and 20 other types of constraints. With proper dimensioning, the capability may be increased.

Segments, if connected by joints, have to have "tree structures," i.e., there may be no closed paths which leave a segment via a joint and return to the same segment through another joint.

Types of Joints

Five types of joints are permitted in this model. They are:

1. Locked
2. Pinned
3. Ball and socket
4. Euler Joint—based on Euler angles using three axes of rotation
5. Slip joint—linear separation allowed on one axis.

The ball or pinned joints can be locked. The Euler joints can be locked on any combination of its principal axes (eight possible conditions including no lock on any axis). The ball and socket joint can work with either global-graphic constraints or globalgraphic torque and damping specification.

For computing joint torques, a separate coordinate system is defined for the joint, described by yaw, pitch, and roll angles relative to segment principal axes. Joint coordination are defined for both segments attached to the joint, and the joint torques are computed based on a relative angular orientation and velocity of the two coordinate systems. The joint torques can be spring, viscous or friction types and are described similar to those in the MVMA2D.

Contact Forces

Contact forces are specified similar to those in the MVMA2D. Five contact force systems are permitted as follows:

1. Ellipsoids with planes
2. Ellipsoids with ellipsoids
3. Hyperellipsoids with planes
4. Hyperellipsoids with hyperellipsoids
5. Impulsive forces.

Restraint System

The model permits the use of two restraint systems as follows:

1. Belts—simple and advanced. Harness belts are not working at tie point
2. Air bag—stored gas type. Improvements for accepting tabular mass inflow rate have been made by General Motors (see New Development below).

Other Constraints

Four other constraints are allowed. They are:

1. Zero distance constraint—a point on one segment be the same as a point on another segment
2. Fixed distance constraint—a specific point on one segment to be a fixed distance from a specified point on another segment.
3. Sliding constraint
4. Rolling constraint.

Special Elements

The model permits the use of two special elements and a slip joint as follows:

1. Tension only—for muscle simulation
2. Flexible element—for possible use in simulating neck, torso, and trunk
3. Slip joint—for simulating steering column collapse and Hybrid III dummy chest deflection.

Integration of Equations of Motion

Integration is done by a Vector Exponential Integrator that has proven to be more accurate and time efficient than the integrator in CVS III. Three-dimensional rotational equations are integrated using quaternions (also known as Euler Parameters).

The efficiency of the numerical integration strategy and its accuracy for three-dimensional rigid body motion is demonstrated by simulating a single rotating segment for a case where the exact analytical solution is known.[97]

Experimental Verification

Experimental verification of the model has been attempted by the authors for two sled test conditions using the a Part 572 dummy restrained by a three-point belt restraint system and a preinflated supplemental air bag restraint system. A major portion of this effort consisted of developing input data to describe the physical characteristics and impact responses of the Part 572 dummy by actual laboratory measurements, pendulum tests, and simulations of the various pendulum tests. The dummy is described in the model by 15 rigid segments and 14 joints. Three types of joints are used:

1. Ball joints—neck and the lumbar spine
2. Pin joints—knees
3. Euler joints—hips, ankles, shoulders, and elbows.

A complete description of the dummy segment geometrical and initial properties and joint properties are reported in Part II of the engineering manual. Also reported in this manual are the effective belt/chest stiffness and air bag properties.

The sled test results and model results are well documented in Part II of the engineering manual. The important model responses compare well with the test results in magnitude and pulse shapes. It is left up to the user to decide whether the fidelity of model simulation is adequate or not.

Using the CAL3D, an analytical study of the interaction between the seat belt and a Hybrid III dummy in sled tests was conducted by Deng[105] in 1988.

Studies Using the CAL3D

Pedestrian Impact

Since the introduction of the model in 1974, several studies using the model have been reported. The majority of the earlier usage of the model has been in studying the pedestrian impact problem. Padgaonkar et al.,[106] Niederer and Walz,[107] Kruse,[108] and Fowler et al.[109] were the early users of this model for pedestrian impact simulation. The current version was used by Verma and Repa[110] for pedestrian impact simulations.

Side Impacts

In the earlier versions of the model, vehicle hardware simulation planes could not be intruded into the passenger compartment. Thus side impact simulations were not attempted. Padgaonkar and Prasad[111,112] used Version III of the model and the option of using disjointed sets of ellipsoids to simulate car-to-car side impacts. Newman et al.[113] and Segal[114,115] have used the latest version to simulate side impact by using the option of prescribed motion to ellipsoids. Robbins[116] has also reported using the CVS for side impacts. But in the course of the study, the contact model was modified extensively. The final report on this project has not been released. In 1987, Deng[117] developed a car-to-car side impact model with a more detailed vehicle side structure representation and a two-segment thorax. He also studied the effects of door padding in side impacts in different computer simulated "test" methods.[118]

Rollover Simulation

Rollover accident simulations were made possible with an improved option that allows specification of vehicle angular motion. Kaleps et al.[119] and Obergefell et al.[120] conducted simulations of rollovers lasting up to 4 sec.

Others

Whole body ejection problems from high speed aircraft have been studied by Frisch.[121] Hubbard and Begeman[122] used the CAL3D in evaluation of biomechanical performance of a new head/neck support development for race car driver helmet.[122] Although the validation of the model was done using the advanced harness routine by the authors, only the experience of Newman et al.[123] of British Leyland is reported in the literature. It appears that

Newman made extensive changes in the routine for simulating frontal impacts with three point belt systems. It is not known whether the current version incorporates the changes made at British Leyland. Recently, Deng[104] has made some improvements in the belt model (see New Development below).

New Developments

A CAL3D Steering System Impact Model

Recently, Wang and Lin[99] developed an energy absorbing steering system model and integrated it into the CAL3D CVS program. The steering column has the capability of simulating the impact response of essential components of the steering column to render it useful as a product engineering design tool. Two special features, namely, a slip joint and an enhanced spring-damper element, were developed and incorporated into a GM proprietary version of CVS. The slip joint option allows the connected segments to move along the axis of joints, thus simulating the column collapse. The EA steering column model has been validated with data obtained from a drop tower test and a mini-sled test.

A New CAL3D Airbag Inflation Model

In 1988, Wang and Nefske[100] replaced the original stored-gas model with a general gas inflator model, which has provisions for accepting tabular input of mass inflow rate and taking the gas temperature into account. This model has been integrated into an advanced version of CAL3D. An application of this model to a driver supplemental air bag system study indicated that the simulated occupant responses were adequately predicted when compared with data from an actual barrier test. Further enhancements in modeling of pyrotechnic inflators for inflatable restraint systems were made by Wang[101] using dual-pressure (i.e., tank pressure and inflator pressure) method.

Airbag Models

Two developments can be mentioned. One made recently by Wang and Ngo[102] was an

algorithm allowing use of multi-contact ellipsoids to represent a complex passenger side airbag as shown in Fig. 6.14. Use of the model was illustrated by examples, and validations were also conducted using two sled test data. The complex bag shape algorithm was implemented by J & J Technologies, Inc into the CAL3D code, and will not be publicly available.

The other development made by Rangarajan[103] was algorithms for passenger airbag model for deployment and occupant interaction into the ATB code under a DOT contract with NHTSA in 1988. This passenger side airbag model has the following enhancements:

- Provisions for a more general deployment history of the bag including arbitrary mass inflow rate and bag geometry changing in time. Venting can also be simulated
- Provision for general bag shape, specifically for ellipsoidal cylinders
- Effects of bag motion during deployment
- Improvements of contact between the bag and external rigid segments and planes.

An Improved Belt Model

In 1990, Deng[104] improved the CAL3D "Harness Model" by incorporating a reference

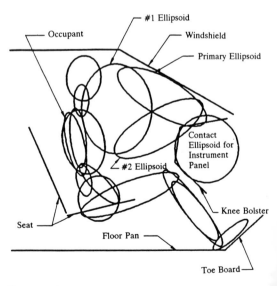

FIGURE 6.14. A passenger side tear-drop shape airbag.[102]

point generation scheme and a new belt slip algorithm. These improvements resulted in more accurate belt geometry representation and satisfactory predictions without the convergence problem as encountered previously in the older version. Using the improved belt model, simulations of the Hybrid III dummy response in a barrier test were found to have good correlation with the test results.

User Convenience

A user convenience package has been developed by McGrath and Segal.[123] This package allows a user to generate an input data deck and post process response variables. It also contains plotting and occupant kinematics display packages.

An occupant display package called VIEW has been developed at AFAMRL and its extensive use has been reported by Kaleps and Marcus.[124] The commercially available PC version (known as DYNAMAN) has excellent pre-and post-processing capabilities- occupant display, plots, tables, etc. The airbag graphic enhancement for VIEW to process airbag information was recently made by Latouf et al.[125] in their CAL3D simulation of occupant neck response to airbag deployment in frontal impacts.

Shaibani[126] developed the SJSATBPC package by implementing the ATB crash victim simulation program in microcomputer environment.

UCIN3D

Historical Review

The UCIN3D man model,[5] developed by Huston, Passerello, et al. at the University of Cincinnati in 1974, is composed of 12 body segments connected by hinges and ball-and-socket joints. It has 34 degrees-of-freedom. The body segments are represented by elliptical cylinders, ellipsoids, and frustums of elliptical cones. The neck is modelled by a spring and a damper between the head and upper torso. This paper reviews the model primarily based on information available in refs. 5 and 127.

Analytical Formulation

The dynamic analysis of the UCIN3D model is based on a virtual work type principle called "Lagrange's form of d'Alembert principle," which is claimed by the developers to have the advantages of both the Lagrangian and the Newtonian methods without the associated disadvantages. The governing equations of motion are solved by a fourth-order Runge Kutta integration method.

Type of Joints

Two types of joints are allowed in the model. They are:

1. Hinge
2. Ball and socket.

The model has bilinear and flexural viscous damping at the joints. Angle-stops, modelled by one-way dampers, can be specified as constraints for limiting body motion.

Restraint System

Up to 10 simple belt restraints can be used in the model. They can be attached at arbitrary points between the vehicle interior and the bodies of the occupant. Linear springs are used to characterize the belts.

Contact Forces

Contact forces are modelled by springs for seat cushion and seat back. Modifications to incorporate the contact force features, as discussed in the aforementioned models, into the model are needed to render it more practical and useful.

Intrusion Surfaces

These surfaces are used to simulate vehicle interiors for interaction indications only without generating contact forces. It requires some improvement in this area.

Special Features

Some special features in the model are:

- The provision for the arbitrary specification of external forces and moments on each of its body segments

- The provision of a "stretching" or extending neck.

Studies Using the UCIN3D

The UCIN3D model has been used in simulating a belted restrained occupant in a front collision environment.[128] The model has been applied to the study of the influence of the three-point belt restraint system on the driver occupant movement under various accident configuration.[129]

The dynamic analysis of UCIN3D was also applied to the development of a head/neck model for predicting their respective accelerations resulting from contact and/or impact forces.[130]

Other Application

The UCIN man model has been utilized in the study of human attitude control,[131] and in an aircraft-occupant analysis.[132]

Experimental Verification

Only limited verification runs were attempted,[127] more are still needed.[133]

CVS Interaction with FEA Model

In most CVSs, as described in refs. 3 and 4, occupant interactions with vehicle interior surfaces are sensed by ellipses/ellipsoids attached to body links. Contact surfaces are represented by either a line segment in 2D or a plane in 3D simulation. The contact forces on the occupant linkage system are generated as a function of the penetration of these ellipses/ellipsoids into vehicle contact lines/planes representing seat, instrument panel, windshield, etc, of which the stiffness characteristics are described in a tabular form by a user.

Vehicle interior surfaces are part of vehicle structures, and their structural characteristics can be obtained by a finite element analysis approach. A pioneer model along this line is SOMLA (*Seat Occupant Model: Light Aircraft*).

SOMLA

SOMLA is a computer modelling program developed under the sponsorship of the Federal Aviation Administration (FAA)[134] to provide an engineering analysis tool for aircraft seat designs, and later for use in the analysis of light aircraft crashworthiness.[135] Descriptions of the original model were published by the FAA in 1975.[136] Since then a number of modifications have been made to the model to improve simulation quality and to provide increased capability and additional desirable output.[136–138]

SOMLA is a 3D model of an aircraft seat, occupant and restraint system for light aircraft crashworthiness analysis. The program combines a three-dimensional occupant model and a finite element seat model to interact dynamically. They are discussed separately below.

Occupant Model

The 3D occupant model, shown in Fig. 6.15, is a 29 degrees-of-freedom system consisting of 12 rigid segments representing the head, neck, upper and lower torso, and left and right upper legs, lower legs, upper arms, and lower arms. Two types of joints are used: a ball-and-socket type for the mid-torso, lower neck, shoulder, and hip joints and a hinge type for the upper neck, elbow, and knee joints.

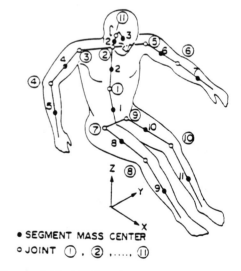

FIGURE 6.15. SOMLA 3D occupant model (twelve segments).

The Lagrangian formulation is used in the analytical treatment for deriving the equations of motion of sets of rigid bodies, which are expressed as functions of 29 independent generalized coordinates that define the position of the occupant system. The numerical integration is carried out by the Adams–Moulton predictor–corrector method with variable time step using the starting values provided by the fourth order Runge–Kutta method. The external forces are generated through contact or restraint system.

Contact Model

In the early version, ellipsoids are used to sense contact between the occupant and the contact surfaces other than the seat to provide computation of relative velocity of impact only.[138] Contact forces through the seat are provided by the seat model to be described later. The new version[135] uses ellipsoids attached to body segments, similar to the other occupant simulation model reviewed above, and determines the penetration of the ellipsoids into the contact planes. The contact forces are calculated using an exponential model expressed as

$$F = A(e^{b\delta} - 1)$$

where δ = deflection, and A and b are empirical constants.

A damping term, which is proportional to the deflection rate, is applied to each normal contact force. In addition, the friction force, which is generated opposite to the tangential component of relative velocity between the body segment and the contact plane, can be generated.

Restraint System Model

The restraint system consists of a lap belt with or without a shoulder harness. Lap and shoulder belt tie-down straps can also be included. The belt loads are applied at body-attachment points on the ellipsoidal surfaces fixed to the upper and lower torso segments as shown in Fig. 6.16. More recently, this capability has been extended to include double shoulder belts (i.e., a diagonal shoulder belt over left shoulder and a diagonal shoulder belt over the right shoulder), and to introduce a parameter for simulating various buckle connections, shown in Fig. 6.17.[137] All force-deflection characteristics for restraint system webbings are approximated by three linear segments as shown in Fig. 6.18.

Special Features

The program allows the point of application of the resultant belt loads to move relative to the ellipsoidal surfaces of the torso segments. This enables simulation of potential submarining under the lap belt as described in ref. 135. A unique feature available in this model is that friction force between the shoulder belt and the occupant chest can be simulated.

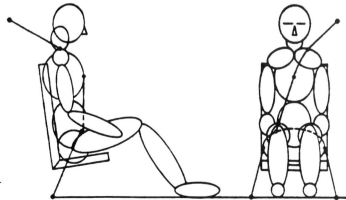

FIGURE 6.16. Restraint system configuration.

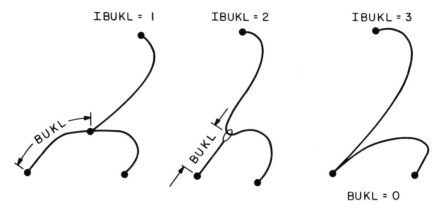

I = Shoulder belt fixed to buckle

2 = Shoulder belt and one length of webbing

3 = Shoulder belt and lap belt attached
     to fixed point

FIGURE 6.17. Types of buckle connections.

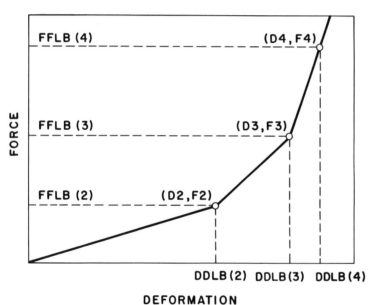

FIGURE 6.18. Force-deflection characterization for restraint system webbing.

Seat Model

Using conventional linear finite element analysis techniques, the original seat model[138] consisted of the seat pan and back modelled by membrane elements and the seat supporting frame structures by beam elements, shown in Fig. 6.19. Limitations of linear program have resulted from inadequacies in element formu-lation, material representation, or solution procedures. The WRECKER II program,[139] a nonlinear code for automotive crash simula-tion, was adopted and modified to provide needed capabilities in large displacements, nonlinear material behavior, and local buckling for the seat model.[135]

Triangular plate, three-dimensional beams and spring elements are available. The large

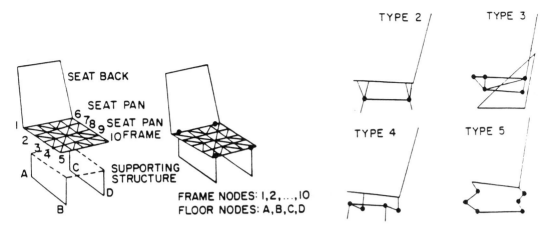

FIGURE 6.19. Seat model components.

displacements and rotations are treated by a decomposition of the element displacement into a rigid body rotation and translation associated with a local coordinate system that moves with the element, and small element distortions relative to the current position of the element coordinate system. A detailed description of the theoretical formulation, can be found in ref. 139. Nonlinear material behavior is based on a uniaxial elastic–plastic stress-strain law which is approximated by three-linear segments.

Local Buckling Model

A simple local buckling model for thin-walled tubes under the action of axial compression and/or bending loads was developed. This provides a capability for simulating the reduction in bending rigidity of the tube as the cross section buckles locally. Figure 6.20 shows

the ovalization of a thin-walled circular tube during a buckling process.

Special Feature

Using the beam element for the seat model, conditions including axial force, shear, moment, and torque releases can be made to allow simulations of collapse in any element/ direction.

Experimental Verification

Several dynamic tests of transport aircraft seats were conducted by the Federal Aviation Administration Civil Aeromedical Institute for validating the model during each revision of the SOMLA program.[6,134,135] An extensive program was also carried out by static and dynamic testings of various existing aircraft seating systems to determine the loading conditions causing the seats to collapse structurally and the specific modes of collapse. Predictive capability of the seat structural analysis was verified by comparing simulated results with data from a test in which significant structural deformation was involved.[140] Occupant (human body or dummy) responses had also been verified under a range of impact conditions as reported in ref. 141. However, verification of the seat model using plate elements has yet to be carried out.

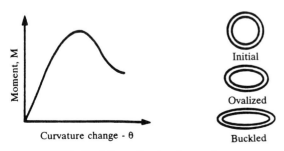

FIGURE 6.20. Buckling of a circular section.

Finite Difference and Finite Element Air Bag Models

The current "gross-motion simulators" discussed in Section III have simplified airbag models. All the calculations regarding volume changes in the bag are based on the final shape of the bag without occupant or vehicle interactions. This shape and volume of the bag has to be known a priori through deployment experiments, adding uncertainties. In reality, the shape of the bag changes with occupant or vehicle interior interactions. Two-dimensional airbag models developed by Fitzpatrick in PASSIM-PLUS have attempted to circumvent this limitation. Additionally, only the Fitzpatrick models have attempted to account for the inertia effects of the bag fabric. The current limitations in the airbag models in the gross-motion simulators preclude the simulation of the following effects judged to be important in many circumstances:

- Deployment of an air bag with a general bag shape including unfolding and wrinkling of the bag, and bag material properties
- "Bag-slap" effect, due to air bag inertia forces and gas blow forces during the deployment process
- An asymmetric tethered bag whose shape is controlled by internal restraining straps of different lengths.

In order to circumvent these limitations, a new approach to the air bag restraint modelling has been to resort to finite element (FE) analysis. Published works along this line include

The PISCES (now known as MSC/DYTRAN) air bag model[142,143] based on finite difference and finite element techniques
The PAM-CRASH air bag model[8] based on finite element techniques
The MVMA/DYNA3D air bag model[144,145] based on finite element techniques
The WSU-2D air bag model[146] based on finite element techniques.

All the above codes assume uniform pressure and temperature within the bag at each time step. However, within the PISCES code it is also possible to model the spatial distribution of gas mass, pressure and temperature within the bag. The PISCES, PAM-CRASH and MVMA/DYNA3D air bag models are three-dimensional, while the WSU air bag is only two dimensional. These four FE air bag models will be reviewed next.

PISCES (MSC-DYTRAN) Air Bag Model

This air bag model was developed by PISCES International using the PISCES finite difference code 3D-ELK to work in tandem with the MADYMO occupant model. A preliminary feasible model developed thus far couples the Lagrange/shell element for bags and the Euler discretization for gas for simulation of a deploying air bag interacting with an impacting rigid body. The bag shape is assumed to be an ellipsoid as reported, in this model. Straps, when used inside the airbag, can be modelled by springs with a velocity constraint. The PISCES gas dynamic model uses an Eulerian mesh with an appropriate material model to define the gas.

Figure 6.21 shows an undeployed air bag represented by two ellipses retained by a rigid support. A gas-filled cylinder is modelled to allow gas flow into the air bag during the deployment process as shown in Fig. 6.22. As an example, the time history of the interaction

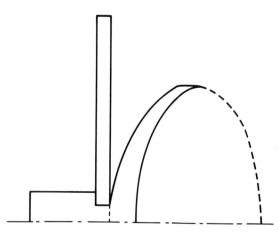

FIGURE 6.21. An undeployed airbag—PISCES air bag model.

FIGURE 6.22. Deployment of the PISCES air bag models.

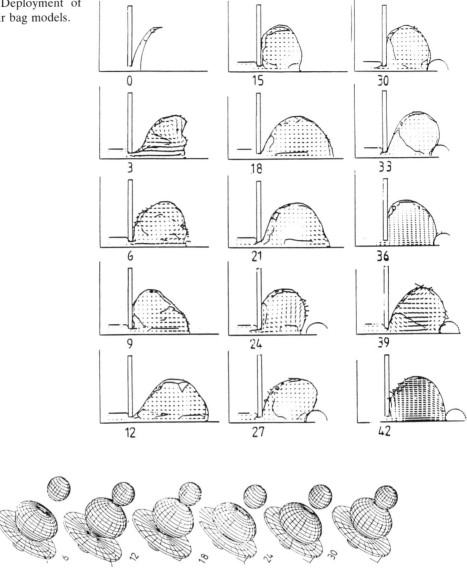

FIGURE 6.23. Time history of dynamic interaction between the air bag and a rigid body.

between the air bag and the impacting rigid body is shown in Fig. 6.23. Numerical simulation of an unfolding airbag has been reported by Florie and Buijk.[147] Fig. 6.24 displays the unfolding of a driver side airbag for a 30-msec duration. For sealed bags, correlation of the simulated results with test data has been conducted by TNO under a MVMA sponsorship. Detailed results have been published in refs. 62, 148. This model has been integrated with the MADYMO occupant simulation (CVS) program to be discussed in Section VI.

PAM-CRASH Air Bag Model

This finite element air bag model was developed by the ESI (*E*ngineering *S*ystems *I*nternational) using the PAM-CRASH program to aid designs of an air bag system. This model has the following features:

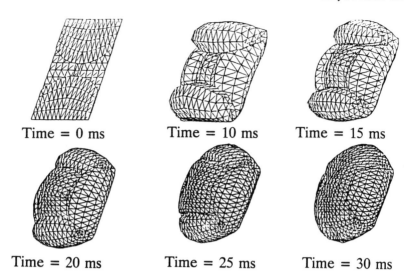

Time = 0 ms   Time = 10 ms   Time = 15 ms

Time = 20 ms   Time = 25 ms   Time = 30 ms

FIGURE 6.24. Unfolding of a driver side airbag.[147]

- Simulation of unfolding and deployment of an air bag, and provisions for interaction with an occupant during the unfolding and deployment process, thus permitting analysis of "bag-slap"
- Simulation of 3D arbitrary bag shape including internal retaining straps
- Modelling of bag stretch, wrinkling, and deformation
- Simulation of bag conformation to the shapes of vehicle interiors and occupant profile.

Current Version Features

The PAM-CRASH air bag model consists of the following submodels:

- Air bag FE-discretization submodel—use of shell finite elements to model the air bag. The initially folded bag geometry can be modelled. The volume of the air bag at a given time step can be determined more accurately by calculating the volume enclosed by the discretized bag elements.
- Material submodel—this allows not only simulations of nonlinear fabric material properties, but also the bag fabrications including wrinkling. A tissue material model

incorporated in an nonlinear membrane element is used.
- Gas dynamic submodel—this submodel assumes an ideal gas and uses the equations of states and energy conservation along with a prescribed mass inflow rate function and the equations for computing mass outflow rate through vents. The approach is similar to many other air bag models described in Section III.

Analytical Formulation

Using the PAM-CRASH program, the air bag model was discretized spatially using finite elements. An explicit central difference is used to integrate the nonlinear discrete equations of motion.

Special Features

Special features available in this model are:

- Self-contact algorithm—this allows air bag skin-to-skin contact between folds in a folded fashion and during the early stage of deployment.
- Nonlinear membrane element—this element incorporates a material model to account for the nonlinear and orthotropic properties of the air bag fabric.

SIDE VIEW

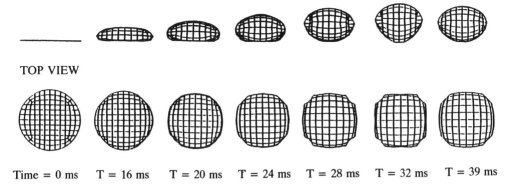

TOP VIEW

Time = 0 ms   T = 16 ms   T = 20 ms   T = 24 ms   T = 28 ms   T = 32 ms   T = 39 ms

FIGURE 6.25. Deployment of an initially flat air bag.

Illustrated Examples

The capability of the PAM-CRASH air bag model has been illustrated in three cases:

- Deployment of a flat airbag (see Fig. 6.25)
- Deployment of a folded air bag (see Fig. 6.26)
- Impacting of a rigid body block with a deploying air bag (see Fig. 6.27).

Experimental Verification

The model was developed to demonstrate the feasible application of a finite element approach to supplemental air bag restraint modelling. To date, only validation of a fully folded driver side airbag deployment has been done in correlating the reaction force at the airbag base attachment and the pressure in the airbag as reported by Lasry et al.[149] Further validation of the model has yet to be established.

MVMA/DYNA3D Air Bag Model

The DYNA3D[150] is an explicit finite element program for solving three dimensional, in-elastic, large deformation structural dynamic problems. One of the primary applications of DYNA3D is vehicle crash simulations. The original DYNA3D program developed at Lawrence Livermore National Laboratory is available in the public domain. Current

DYNA3D contains some improvements sponsored by GM, that will remain proprietary. In mid-1989, Hallquist[144,145,151–153] initiated the development of this FE air bag model under a MVMA sponsorship. This work is continued and expected to be completed at the end of 1991. The development

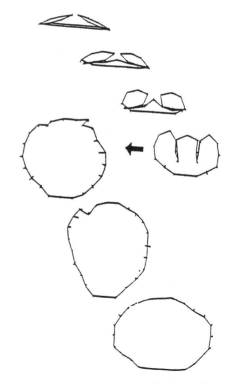

FIGURE 6.26. Deployment of a folded air bag.

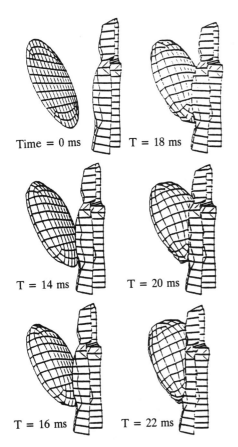

Time = 0 ms   T = 18 ms

T = 14 ms   T = 20 ms

T = 16 ms   T = 22 ms

FIGURE 6.27. Interaction between a rigid body block and an air bag.

sponsored by MVMA is currently available only to the members of the organization, and will be made available to the public in the future. The review of this model is based on material provided in ref. 153.

Current Version Features

The MVMA/DYNA3D air bag model consists of the following submodels:

- Fabric material submodel—the material submodel is based on an orthotropic material with inadmissible compressive stresses. The fabric behavior is modeled using an idealized modulus-strain relation for a fabric material.
- Equation of state (EOS) submodel—this submodel relates the pressure to the current gas density (volume) and the specific

internal energy of the gas. The pressure in the airbag corresponding to the control volume is determined from this submodel.

- Airbag inflation submodel—this submodel follows the work by Wang and Nefske.[85] The mass flow rate and the temperature of the gas into the bag are provided as tabulated functions of time.

Analytical Formulation

Using the DYNA3D, the air bag is modeled using quadrilateral shell, triangular shell or quadrilateral membrane elements. Particular development in the formulation includes:

- Airbag folding algorithm—it is used to create finite element model of a folded airbag as shown in Fig. 6.28. Two types of folds, namely, small radius and large radius folds, are allowed.
- Airbag unfolding-contact algorithm—it allows the airbag to unfold due to mass inflow of gas and treats multiple surface contacts among the airbag folds.

Special Features

- Airbag propellant burn submodel—this deflagration reactive flow model is a unique feature of MVMA/DYNA3D air bag model. It requires an unreacted solid equation of state, a reaction product equation of state, a reaction rate law and a mixture rule for the two or more species.
- Occupant submodel—using rigid body mechanics and spherical joint capabilities in DYNA3D, a MADYMO3D-type Hybrid III dummy model is created with the mesh

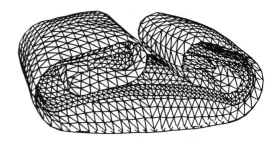

FIGURE 6.28. Finite element model of a folded airbag.[153]

FIGURE 6.29. MVMA/DYNA3D Hybrid III dummy submodel—a MADYMO3D-type.

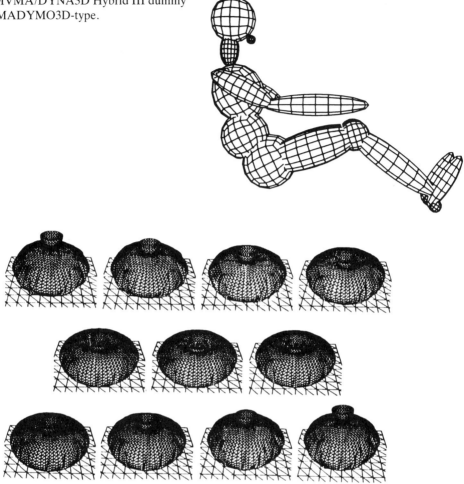

FIGURE 6.30. Deformed shapes at 10-msec intervals for the airbag using material model with coarse meshing.

generator, INGRID. This submodel is shown in Fig. 6.29.

Illustrated Example

Figure 6.30 shows an semi-spherical impactor interacts with an airbag using material submodel with coarse meshing (3,696 elements in the airbag). In addition, a propellant burn problem is also illustrated using the driver airbag propellant supplied by ICI (Imperical Chemical Industries) Corporation.

Experimental Verification

The MVMA/DYNA3D air bag modeling capabilities are validated against data obtained from experimental tests conducted by TNO sponsored by MVMA under a separate project. The finite element model of the TNO airbag experiment is shown in Fig. 6.31. The model includes the six internal tethers, the flat plate support and the spherical impactor. The model used a total of 3696 C^0 triangular shell elements.

Four simulation runs were conducted using spherical and circular plate impactors with various mass at different impact velocities as used in the TNO experiments. Typical outputs from the finite element model, consisting of impactor's displacement, velocity and acceleration as a function of time, and impactor's force vs. displacement, are shown in Figure 6.32.

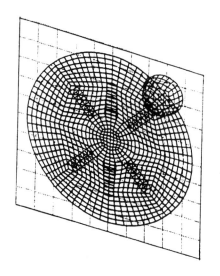

FIGURE 6.31. MVAM/DYNA3D finite element model of the TNO airbag experiment.

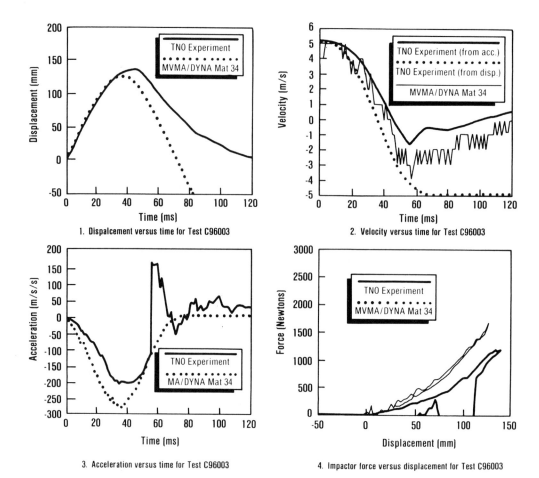

FIGURE 6.32. Comparisons of MVMA/DYNA3D airbag simulation results with TNO test data a. Displacement history. b. Velocity history. c. Acceleration history. d. Force vs. displacement.

FIGURE 6.33. Comparison of MVMA/DYNA3D simulated pressure history result with TNO test data.

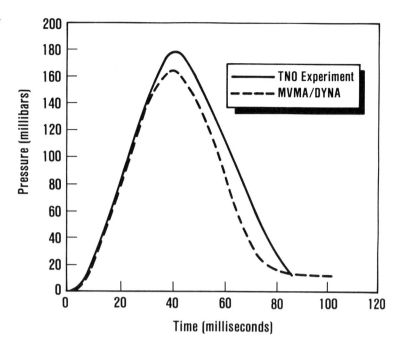

A comparison of airbag pressure history between the MVMA/DYNA3D simulation and TNO test result is presented in Fig. 6.33. Further development and validation are still needed to make the airbag capability useful to the engineering community.

WSU-2D Air Bag Model

This finite element air bag was developed by Yang et al. at Wayne State University under a grant from Ford University Research Fund. It is a 2D simulation of the inflation process during unfolding and deploying. It was intended to develop a geometric model that could be either coupled with commonly available CVS programs such as CAL3D, MADYMO or implemented in PAM-CRASH.

Since the model is 2D, only the sagittal section of an airbag is analyzed. Figure 6.34 shows the magnified initial folding pattern and full deployment of an airbag. The first unfolding process was pivoted about the turning point "C". The following assumptions were postulated:

- The fabric elasticity is neglected
- The mass of airbag is negligible

- The inertia effect of the deploying bag is accounted for by a weighted coefficient
- The bag pressure remains at atmospheric unit until full deployment if there is no contact, or its surfaces are fully stretched by "out-of-position" contact
- An adiabatic process is assumed
- The ideal gas equation is used.

Two different mass inflow rates were used to demonstrate an airbag deployment. The deployment patterns due to these inputs are shown in Fig. 6.35.

Experimental Verification

The preliminary WSU-2D air bag is validated using compressing air and a targeted beach ball. Images of the targets from a high speed video indicated that their movement in the experiment was very similar to the pattern predicted by the model. Further verification is needed for an actual airbag deployment.

Coupling with CVS

In coupling a FE airbag model with a CVS program, an interface software is needed to

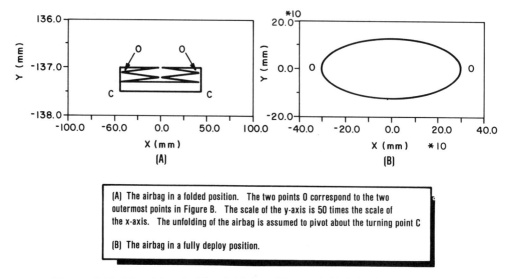

FIGURE 6.34. The airbag in (a) a folded position and (b) fully deployed position.

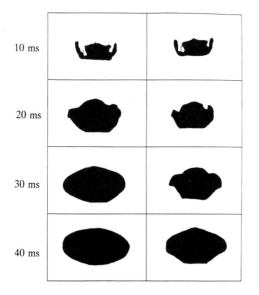

FIGURE 6.35. Airbag deployment patterns due to two different mass inflow rates.

establish a means of sharing information. This is a two-way coupling in which the results of the airbag model analysis are used by the CVS program, and vice-versa. A schematic illustrating the interaction between the two programs is shown in Fig. 6.36. First, the positions and velocities of the occupant body segments are updated with the CVS program. The information describing the outer surfaces of the occupant is fed into the airbag model. The finite airbag program then updates the positions and velocities of the nodal points and determines whether any nodal points interact with the body segments. Once the interaction has occurred, the contact force and moment are calculated and input as external force and moment into the CVS model. This process is continued until the simulation is terminated.

PISCES, PAM-CRASH, DYNA3D, and WSU2D air bag models have been or are currently being coupled with CVS models. These couplings include:

- PISCES with MADYMO3D
- PAM-CRASH with MADYMO3D and ATB/CAL3D
- DYNA3D with MADYMO3D-type dummy
- WSU2D with CAL3D

Each of these efforts will be presented below.

PISCES with MADYMO3D

Efforts toward coupling the PISCES airbag model with MADYMO model have been reported in refs. 62, 147, 154. For two-dimensional applications, Nieboer et al.[62] reported their work on coupling the PISCES-2D-ELK

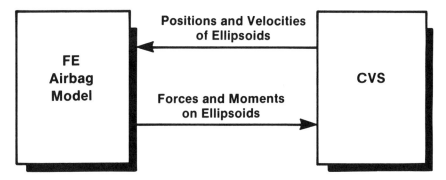

FIGURE 6.36. Schematic overview of coupling between an finite element airbag model and a CVS.

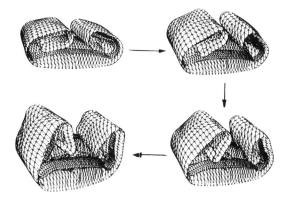

FIGURE 6.37. Unfolding of an airbag.[147]

airbag model with the MADYMO2D occupant simulation model. Initial folded geometry and unfolding of an airbag were developed by Florie and Buijk.[147] Figure 6.37 shows the unfolding of an airbag during deployment up to 30 msec.

The coupling of the PISCES-3D-ELK airbag model and the MADYMO3D occupant simulation model was carried out in ref. 154.

Experimental Verifications

Bruijs[154] conducted some experimental for validation tests using a pendulum and a Hybrid III dummy impacting against both the driver and passenger airbags. Good correlation was obtained for the driver airbag simulations, but not for the passenger counterparts. Further validation of the PISCES/MADYMO3D model has been carried out for MVMA by Nieboer et al.[154,156] Advanced Vehicle

Engineering Technology of Ford is currently evaluating this model for feasible application.

PAM-CRASH with MADYMO3D and ATB/CAL3D

An interface package, called PAM-CVS (PAM-CRASH to *C*rash *V*ictim *S*imulator), was developed by Hoffmann and Lasry[155] for the coupling between the PAM-CRASH FE airbag model and the rigid body program MADYMO3D. This package controls initialization, time advancement of solution from the PAM-CRASH and the occupant simulator, and directs the information exchange between the airbag and the occupant programs as well as the output phases as shown in Fig. 6.38. The ESI graphic package DAISY is used for postprocessing the simulation results.

The feasibility of the coupling capability was demonstrated by simulating a gross motion of a Hybrid III dummy interacting with an airbag as shown in Fig. 6.39.

An illustration of predicted kinematics of an unbelted child dummy impacting with a deploying passenger airbag is depicted in Fig. 6.40.[149] In addition to airbag coupling, a description of MADYMO interaction with the PAM-CRASH finite element analysis of kneebolster was also reported by Hoffmann et al.[156]

Recently, ESI developed PAM-SAFE[157] for safety analysis using finite element methods based on PAM-CRASH. PAM-SAFE provides:

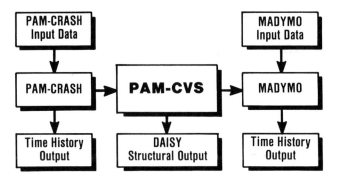

FIGURE 6.38. The interface program PAM-CVS.[155]

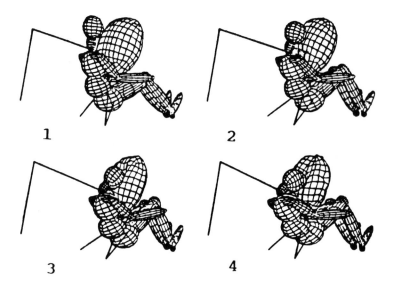

FIGURE 6.39. Gross motion of the dummy in interaction with the airbag.[155]

- Capabilities for modeling arbitrary airbag designs, and folded and unfolded airbags
- Coupling to occupant simulation models such as MADYMO and ATB/CAL3D.

Experimental Verifications

In a joint study between ESI and VW, Hoffmann et al. reported that the dummy accelerations measured in the head, thorax and pelvis compared well with the experimental data.[149] Ford has conducted a similar study resulted in less degree of success in correlating the head acceleration.

DYNA3D with MADYMO3D-type dummy

Various versions of DYNA3D exist including MVMA/DYNA3D,[145] OASYS DYNA3D,[158] and LS-DYNA3D.[159]

Instead of coupling the MADYMO3D with DYNA3D, Hallquist[145] initiated the development of a dummy model based on body segment sizes and inertial properties of Hybrid III reported by Wismans et al.[69] However, dummy joint stiffnesses and damping characteristics have not been modeled. Figure 6.41 depicts a sequence of airbag deployment and

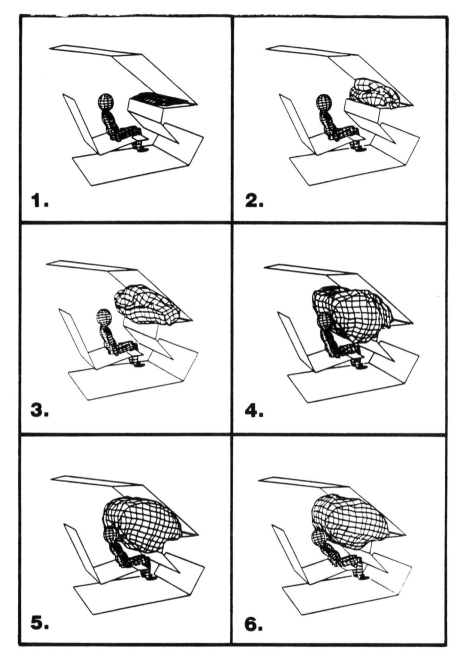

FIGURE 6.40. Predicted child dummy kinematics during a passenger airbag deployment.

its interaction with the dummy. This work is still continuing by Livermore Software Technology Corporation under MVMA sponsorship.

Along this line in OASYS DYNA3D, a Hybrid III dummy model was developed using the discrete elements to represent occupants as rigid body mechanisms consisting of lumped

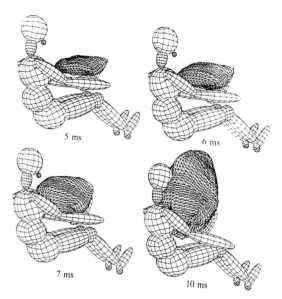

FIGURE 6.41. MVMA/DYNA3D airbag/dummy model.

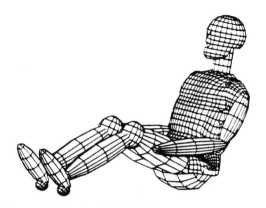

FIGURE 6.42. A Hybrid III Dummy Model in OASYS DYNA3D.

masses and rotational spring/dampers as shown in Fig. 6.42.

However, a link has been established between LS-DYNA3D and CVS programs such as MADYMO and CAL3D.[160]

Future Trends

All the mathematical models reviewed above are pertinent to simulations of occupant responses in a crash environment. Computer models also exist that can simulate the structural response to a crash event. These models separately simulate the structural crash performance from the occupant response, whereas in actual crash event these responses occur concurrently and interactively. Therefore, it is necessary to model simultaneously the occupant and the structure in a crash analysis. This has stimulated new trends in approaches by integrating structural/occupant simulation models for safety/crashworthiness analysis.

Vehicle crash simulation modeling offers several advantages over the traditional full vehicle crash testing to determine occupant responses to contact with interior compartment and restraint systems. These include:

- Providing early design guidance
- Evaluation of design alternatives
- Optimization of structure and package efficiency
- Reduced prototype test requirements
- Shortening vehicle design/development time.

Two approaches seen evident by:

Extending the CVS program capability to model structural response

Developing FE dummy and restraint systems within a non-linear FE code.

Within CVS Program

Early studies by Padgaonkar and Prasad[111,112] used CAL3D to demonstrate the feasibility of simultaneously modeling the structure and the dummy occupant in three-dimensional car-to-car side impacts. A more detailed structure and occupant model in CAL3D has also been reported by Deng.[161] Prasad and Low[86,87] have shown the feasibility of using MADYMO to simultaneously model the occupant and the structure during side impact in greater detail than in previous studies. Recently, the authors extended the MADYMO3D side impact model further by including a door structural model.[88] Integrated MADYMO 2D/3D front end structural/occupant models are also being developed by the authors. An integrated MADYMO2D model is shown in Fig. 6.43.

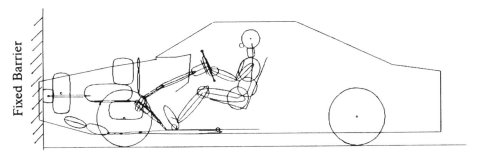

FIGURE 6.43. An integrated MADYMO2D model.

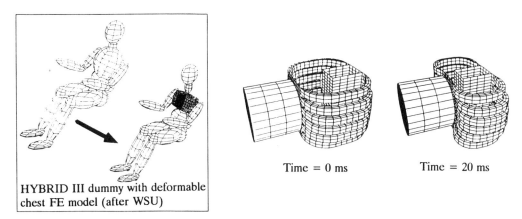

HYBRID III dummy with deformable chest FE model (after WSU)

Time = 0 ms   Time = 20 ms

FIGURE 6.44. A deformable Hybrid III finite element model (PAM-SAFE).

Within FE Codes

In the past decades, finite element approaches were primarily used for vehicle structural and NVH analyses in automobile industry. Due to the availability of super computers and "super-mini" computers in the last few years, considerable efforts have been concentrated on the simulation of occupant dynamics via finite element methods. Recent efforts at modelling human responses to blunt impacts have been reported by Tong et al.[162] and Lighthill et al.[163] for the brain, and by Plank and Eppinger[164] for the human thorax. With increased availability of fast computers, it appears that integration of the above models with models of other parts of the human body will be possible in the future.[165] This integration can lead to the exploration of injury criteria[166,167] and better dummy designs.

Reviews of various finite element airbag models are presented in Section V, and the coupling of airbag models with CVS programs are given in Section VI. Some recent development of dummy models and belt restraint system models will be discussed below.

FE Dummy Model

Numerous FE dummy models have been developed using either two-dimensional or three-dimensional approach. In 1989, Yang and King developed a simplified finite element based two dimensional human surrogate for side impact simulation.[168] Pan at Wayne State University developed a deformable Hybrid III thoracic model using PAM-CRASH and verified the model using pendulum test data.[169] This thoracic model has been implemented into PAM-SAFE as a submodel for deformable finite element Hybrid III dummy model as shown in Fig. 6.44.

Traditional representation of dummy occupant body segments was done through the use of ellipsoids/spheres. OASYS,[158] recently generated in DYNA3D a dummy model by digitizing the head, shoulder and torso geometries from an actual Hybrid III dummy as shown in Fig. 6.42.

Seat Belt Model

A series of seat belt routines have been developed within the OASYS DYNA3D[170] for modelling a seat belt in conjunction with OASYS Hybrid III dummy model as shown in Fig. 6.45.

Seat Belt Model

A series of seat belt routines have been developed within the OASYS DYNA3D[172] for modelling a seat belt in conjunction with OASYS Hybrid III dummy model as shown in Fig. 6.46. This model allows:[172]

- Nonlinear webbing materials
- Belt pay-out prior to retractor locking
- Pre-tensioning of belt
- Slip behavior
- Movement of belt over occupant shoulder/torso/pelvis areas.

PAM-SAFE[157] has also has a belt modelling capability as shown in Fig. 6.47.

Integrated Structural/Occupant FE Method (FEM)

An integrated occupant-car crash simulation with the finite element method (FEM) was presented by Schelkle et al.[171] with the Porsche Hybrid III dummy and airbag models using DYNA3D. The kinematics of a Hybrid III dummy interactin with an airbag and vehicle interior is shown in Fig. 6.48. This approach provides a more detailed representation of occupant and vehicle interior interactins.

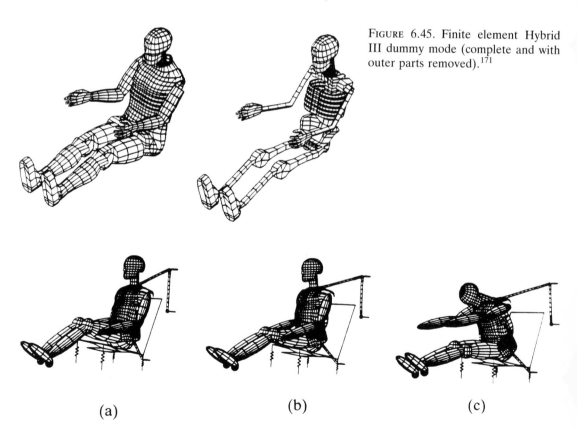

FIGURE 6.45. Finite element Hybrid III dummy mode (complete and with outer parts removed).[171]

(a)   (b)   (c)

FIGURE 6.46. Occupant and seat belt model [OASYS DYNA3D].

FIGURE 6.47. PAM-SAFE occupant and seat belt model.

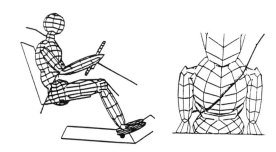

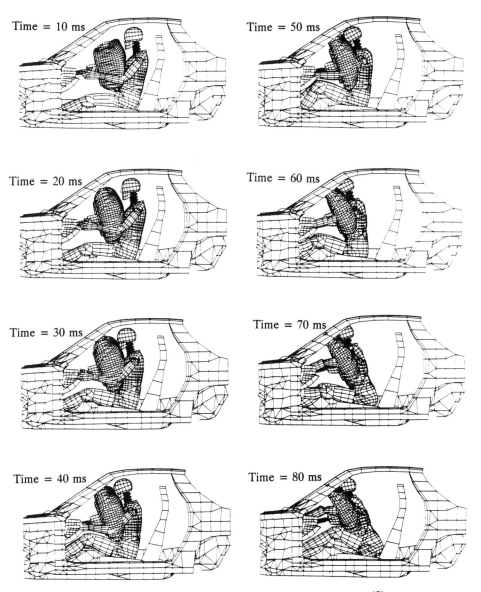

FIGURE 6.48. An integrated vehicle/occupant FE model.[171]

Others

Other efforts in the integration of different analysis types between particular FE codes, which requires data translators, are also reported.[173,174] MacNeal-Schwendler markets an integrated FEA code called MSC/DYTRAN that combines MSC/DYNA and MSC/PISCES fluid-mechanical package. In this coupling, the Lagrangian processor in DYNA accepts forces calculated from the Eulerian processor in PISCES as loads on a DYNA FE model structure. On the other hand, the motion of the Lagrangian mesh acts as a boundary flow for fluid model. PISCES models simulating driver and passenger airbags, which are supported by the steering column/wheel and instrument panel structural models, respectively, are developed at Ford using MSC/DYTRAN.

Both of the CVS and FE approaches discussed above have advantages and disadvantages. The CVS approach is fast in terms of model preparation and computer run times. As a result, many design alternatives can be evaluated in relatively short time. However, the model input parameters, e.g., stiffnesses, need to be translated into vehicle design parameters, e.g., size, shape, material and thickness, by other design tools. The finite element approach yields vehicle design parameters readily, but the model preparation and computer run times are relatively long. Limited experience of the authors with a recently introduced finite element dummy model indicates that the computer run time for similar size problem is approximately nine times that with the CVS models. It is, however, felt that advances in finite element model preparation will take place to reduce some modeling time. Additional experience with the finite element techniques will also lead to the development of simpler models that can run faster. As a result of the foregoing discussion, it is obvious that trade-offs are required and the use of either the CVS approach or the finite element approach will involve the immediate needs of the analyst.

Summary and Recommendations

It is obvious that, rather than providing an exhaustive description of existing occupant simulation models, only a group of selective models, which have been or can be used for occupant/pedestrian, structural response and air bag supplemental restraint system simulations, were reviewed. An attempt was made at describing historical development and the salient features of these models.

Due to their ease of use, two-dimensional simplified occupant models such as DRACR, PAC, PADS and SCORES are useful for detailed steering column and air bag supplemental restraint system studies. One-dimensional combined occupant and structural models developed by Kanianthra et al. have been used in studying the interaction between side structure and the occupant.

Among the gross motion simulation models reviewed, the MVMA2D, the MADYMO2D/3D and the CAL3D have already gained acceptance in the automotive and aircraft industries. Since the review made by the first author, these models have been improved in many analytical capabilities and applied to simulate occurences in a variety of crash environments. Developments of these models are expected to be continued in the future. A few areas of developments are suggested:

- Air bag models capable of simulating "bag slap" effects and out-of-position occupants. MSC/DYTRAN or MSC/PISCES airbag is now capable of simulating out-of-position airbag. Verification of these need to be carried out further.
- Pyrotechnic belt retractors
- Contact algorithm for generating force when the corner of a hyperellipsoid interacting with a plane
- Seat cushion models
- Foam models for side impact padding design and selection
- Pre- and post-processor capabilities and user friendliness
- Continued integrated structural/occupant model development. Structural model should concentrate on development of kinematic models capable of simulating dash panel and steering column intrusions.
- Injury model
- Simulation of human response

The SOMLA program has been used for aircraft crash simulation and seat design for some time, and its application to automotive safety and structural research has yet to be seen. A better and reliable non-linear finite element code may be incorporated to improve the structural response predictive capability.

Recently finite element air bag models are promising for future supplemental air bag restraint system design and development. In order to render such models useful analytical design tools for such a system, these models have been coupled to major CVS models to demonstrate feasibility and will be continued in many prove-out studies in the future.

References

1. McHenry RR (1963) Analysis of the dynamics of automobile passenger-restraint systems. In Proceedings of the 7th Stapp Car Crash Conference.
2. King AI, Chou CC (1976) Mathematical modelling, simulation and experimental testing of biomechanical system crash response. AIAA Paper 75-272, Presented at the AIAA 11th Annual Meeting and Technical Display, Washington DC, February 24–26, 1975. Also in J Biomechan 9:301–317.
3. Prasad P (1984) An overview of major occupant simulation models. In Mathematical Simulation of Occupant and Vehicle Kinematics. SAE Publication P-146. SAE Paper No. 840855.
4. Prasad P (1985) Comparative evaluation of the MVMA2D and the MADYMO2D occupant simulation models with MADYMO-test comparisons. In Proceedings of the Tenth International Technical Conference on Experimental Safety Vehicles, Oxford, England, July 1–5.
5. Huston RI, Passerello CE, Harlow MW (1978) UCIN vehicle-occupant/crash victim simulation model. Structural Mechanics Software Series, Vol II, University Press of Virginia, pp 131–150.
6. Laananen DH (1986) Simulation of passenger response in transport aircraft accidents. In Tong P, et al. (ed) Symposium on Vehicle Crashworthiness Including Impact Biomechanics, AMD-Vol 79, BED-Vol 1, ASME, pp 47–56.
7. Prasad P, Chou CC (1989) A review of mathematical occupant simulation models. In Crashworthiness and Occupant Protection in Transportation systems, AMD-Vol 106/BED-Vol 13, The American Society of Mechanical Engineers, pp 96–112.
8. Hoffmann R, Pickett AK, Ulrich D, Haug E, Lasry D, Clinkemaillie J (1989) A finite element approach to occupant simulation: the PAM-crash airbag model. SAE Publication SP-782, pp 79–88. SAE Paper No. 890754.
9. Fitzpatrick MU (1980) Development of DRACR and PAC occupant—air bag models. NHTSA Contract No. DTNH22-80-C-07120, Draft Report, U.S. DOT, August.
10. Fitzpatrick MU (1982) PAC User's Manual. Contract No. DTNH22-80-C-07550, September.
11. Stucki L, Cohen D, Rogland R (1985) Evaluation of frontal occupant protection using the passenger/driver simulation model. Proceedings of the 10th International ESV Conference, Oxford.
12. Stucki L, Fitzpatrick MU (1982) A computer model for simulating an unrestrained driver in frontal collisions. SAE Paper No. 820469.
13. Fitzpatrick Engineering (1984) Crash simulation models (DRISIM version 6.67 and PASSIM version 4.35), 3452 Lake Lynda Drive, Suite 185, Orlando, Florida 32817.
14. Fitzpatrick Engineering (1983) Component test procedures. DRISIM and PASSIM Software Training Manual, 3452 Lake Lynda Drive, Suite 185, Orlando, Florida.
15. Fitzpatrick KU, Thompson KE (1991) PASSIM-PLUS, a multi-element, passenger airbag model. SAE Paper No. 910151.
16. Dickson KR, Afzal N (1990) Airbag restraint system design by crash simulation modeling and design of experiments. SAE Paper No. 901718.
17. Fitzpatrick M (1980) Development of deploy computer math model for the investigation of various airbag and crash parameters on the out-of-position occupant. Contract No. DTNH22-80-C-07120, December.
18. McGrath M, Segal D (1984) The development and use of the PADS (passenger/driver simulation) computer program. Final Report, NHTSA Contract No. DTNH22-80-R-07017, March.
19. Fessahaie O, Guglielmi J, Crane D, Stucki L (1991) Collection fo properties, development of input sets and modeling for simulation of unrestrained drivers of light trucks and vans in fronta collisions. Front Crash Safety

Technologies for the 90's. SAE Publication No. SP-852, pp 77–98, SAE Paper No. 910810.

20. Naab KN, Stucki L (1990) Development and test of steering assembly countermeasures for driver impacts. Vehicle Crashworthiness and Occupant Protection in Frontal Collisions. SAE SP-807, pp 125–139. SAE Paper No. 900546.

21. Sieveka EM, Pilkey WD, Hollowell WT (1989) Occupant simulator pre-processors: parameter studies made easy. The 12th International Technical Conference on ESV, Goteborg, Sweden, May 29–June 1.

22. Sieveka EM, Pilkey WD (1988) Implementation of the PADS program in the safety systems optimization model. Final Report, NHTSA Contract No. DTRS-57-85-00103.

23. Contact Prof. Pilkey WD (1971) Division of Applied Mechanics, University of Virginia, Thornton Hall, McCormick Road, Charlottesville, Virginia 22901.

24. Trella TJ, Kanianthra JN (1987) Analytical simulation of the effects of structural parameters on occupant responses in side impacts of passenger cars. In: Proceedings of the 11th International ESV Conference, Washington DC.

25. Hasewaga J, Fukatsu T, Katsumata T (1989) Side impact simulation analysis using an improved occupant model. 12th International Technical Conference on ESV, Goteborg, Sweden, March 29–June 1, pp 1071–1076.

26. McHenry RR, Naab KN (1966) Computer simulation of the automobile crash victim in a frontal collision—a validation study. Cornell Aeronautical Laboratory, Inc., Report No. YB-2126-V-1R.

27. Segal DJ (1971) Revised computer simulation of the automobile crash victim. Cornell Aeronautical Laboratory, Inc., Report No. VJ-2759-V-2, January.

28. Danforth JP, Randall CD (1972) Modified ROS Occupant Dynamics Simulation User Manual. General Motors Corporation Research Laboratories, Publication No. GMR-1254, October.

29. Robbins DH, Bowman BM, Bennett RO (1974) The MVMA two-dimensional crash victim simulation. SAE 741195, Proceedings of the 18th Stapp Car Crash Conference, SAE, Warrendale, Pennsylvania, December.

30. Bowman BM, Bennett RO, Robbins DH (1985) MVMA-two-dimensional crash victim simulation, Version 5, Vols. 1–3, UMTRI-85-

24-1 to 3, Transportation Research Institute, University of Michigan, June 28.

31. Schneider LW, Bowman BM (1978) Prediction of head/neck dynamic response of selected military subjects to—G_x acceleration. Aviation Space Environm Med, Vol 49, Jaunary.

32. Bowman BM, Schneider LW, Foust DR (1975) Simulated occupant response to side-impact collisions. SAE 751155, Proceedings of the 19th Stapp Car Crash Conference, SAE, Warrendale, Pennsylvania.

33. Hammond RA (1971) Digital simulation of an inflatable safety restraint. SAE 710019, Automotive Engineering Congress, Detroit, Michigan, January.

34. Chou CC, Lev A, Lenardon DM (1980) MVMA2D air bag/steering assembly simulation model. SAE 800298, Congress and Exposition, Detroit, Michigan, February.

35. Bowman BM, Robbins DH, Bennett RO (1977) MVMA two-dimensional crash victim simulation: self-study guide. UM-HSRI-77-18-1, Highway Safety Research Institute, University of Michigan, April.

36. Robbins DH, Becker JM (1981) Baseline data for describing occupant side impacts and pedestrian front impacts in two dimensions. UM-HRSI-81-29, Project No. 1151 for MVMA, University of Michigan, June.

37. Backaitis S, Robbins DH (1982) The effects of lateral collision speeds, vehicle side stiffness and occupant spacing to the vehicle door upon initial impact speed of the occupant. In Proceedings of the 9th International Technical Conference on Experimental Safety Vehicles, Kyoto, Japan.

38. Robbins DH, Viano D (1984) Occupant rollover simulation. Presented at Mathematical Modelling Workshop Sponsored by NHTSA at Washington DC, January 11–13.

39. Robbins DH, Melvin JW, Huelke DF, Sherman HW (1983) Biomechanical accident investigation methodology using analytical techniques. SAE 831609, Proceedings of the 27th Stapp Car Crash Conference, SAE, Warrendale, Pennsylvania.

40. Bowman DM, Schneider LW, Rohr PR, Mohan D (1981) Simulation of head/neck impact responses for helmeted and unhelmeted motorcyclists. SAE 811029, Proceedings of the 25th Stapp Car Crash Conference, SAE, Warrendale Pennsylvania.

41. Foust DR, Bowman BM, Snyder RG (1977) Study of Human impact tolerance using investigations and simulations of free-falls.

SAE 770915, Proceedings of the 21st Stapp Car Crash Conference, SAE, Warrendale, Pennsylvania.

42. Cooper GA (1989) A driver environment parameter study. SAE Paper No. 840865.

43. Fischer R, Haertle JA (1984) Computer modeling in new vehicle design. Mathematical Simulation of Occupant and Vehicle Kinematics, SAE Publication No. P-146, pp 107–112. (SAE Paper No. 840863).

44. Ishii K, Yamanaka I (1988) Influence of vehicle deceleration curve on dummy injury criteria. SAE Paper No. 880612.

45. Shimamura M, Omura H, Isobe H (1987) An occupant movement analysis using improved input data for MVMA-2D simulation. SAE Paper No. 870332.

46. Alem NM, Bowman BM, Melvin JW, Benson JB (1978) Whole-body human surrogate response to three-point harness restraint. SAE Paper No. 780895, Proceedings of the 22nd Stapp Car Crash Conference, SAE, Warrendale, Pennsylvania.

47. Viano DC, Culver CC, Prisk B (1980) Influence of initial length of lap-shoulder belt on occupant dynamics—a comparison of sled testing and MVMA-2D modeling. SAE 801309, Proceedings of the 24th Stapp Car Crash Conference, SAE, Warrendale, Pennsylvania.

48. Henson SE (1982) Computer modeling of occupant dynamics in very severe frontal crashes. The Ninth International Technical Conference on ESV, Kyoto, Japan, Nov. 1–4.

49. Henson SE, Dueweke JJ, Huang M (1983) Computer modeling of intrusion effects on occupant dynamics in very severe crashes. SAE Paper No. 830613.

50. Oho K, Sugamori I, Yamasaki K (1989) Effect of internal fittings on injury value of unrestrained occupant. Twelfth International Technical Conference on Experimental Safety Vehicles, Proceedings Vol 2, Goteborg, Sweden, May 29–June 1, pp 1205–1208.

51. Bowman BM, Bennett RO, Robbins DH (1974) MVMA two-dimensional crash victim simulation, Version 3, Volumes 1–3, HSRI, University of Michigan, Ann Arbor, Michigan, June.

52. Bowman BM, Robbins DH, Bennett RO (1977) MVMA two-dimensional crash victim simulation: audio-visual program. UM-HRSI-77-18-2, Highway Safety Research Institute, University of Michigan, April.

53. Bowman BM, Pope ME (1982) MVMA-2D occupant positioning for approximate initial equilibrium. GMR-4198, General Motors Corporation Research Laboratories, Warren, Michigan, September.

54. O'Leary ED (1987) Establishing initial equilibrium positions for crash victim simulations. SAE Paper No. 871111.

55. Danforth JP, Prisk BC (1979) Occupant restraint system modelling using MVMA two-dimensional occupant dynamics model. In Proceedings of the 23rd Conference of the AAAM, American Association for Automotive Medicine, Morton Grove, Illinois.

56. Huang M (1984) Graphics and animation related to MVMA-2D model. Presented at the Mathematical Modelling Workshop, Sponsored by NHTSA at Washington DC, January 11–13.

57. Schuller F, Mack P, Brun-Cassan F, Tarriere C (1988) PRAKIMOD: Peugeot/Renault accidents kinematics model—theory, validation and applications. International IRCOBI Conference on the Biomechanics of Impacts, held in Bergisch Gladback (F.R.G), September 14–16.

58. Lestrelin D, Fayon A, Tarriere C, Mack P (1984) Three applications of a mathematical model, PRAKIMOD, in frontal collisions. Mathematical Simulation of Occupant and Vehicle Kinematics, SAE P-146, pp 15–22; SAE Paper No. 840857.

59. Steyer C, Mack P, DuBois P, Renault R (1989) Mathematical modelisation of side collisions. Twelfth International Technical Conference on Experimental Safety Vehicles, Proceedings Vol 2, Goteborg, Sweden, May 29–June 1, pp 1032–1043.

60. Wismans J, Maltha J, Melvin JW, Stalnaker RL (1979) Child restraint evaluation by experimental and mathematical simulation. SAE Paper No. 791017, Proceedings of the 23rd Stapp Car Crash Conference, SAE, Warrendale, Pennsylvania.

61. MADYMO User's Manual 2D/3D, Version 4.3 (1990) Department of Injury Prevention, TNO Road-Vehicle Research Institute, April.

62. Nieboer JJ, Wismans J, de Coo PJ (1990) Airbag modelling techniques. In Proceedings of the 34th Stapp Car Crash Conference Proceedings, SAE P-236, pp 243–258. SAE Paper No. 902322.

63. Nieboer JJ, Wismans J, Fraterman E (1988) Status of the MADYMO 2D Airbag Model. In Proceedings of the 32nd Stapp Car Crash

Conference, Atlanta, Georgia, October, pp 223–235.

64. Nieboer JJ (1988) Determination of the inflator characteristics for airbag simulation using tank test results. TNO Technical Report No. 751760081-a, April.

65. Prasad P (1990) Comparative evaluation of the dynamic responses of the Hybrid II and the Hybrid III Dummies. In Proceedings of the 34th Stapp Car Crash Conference, SAE P-236, pp 175–183. SAE Paper No. 902318.

66. Heinz M, Pletschen B, Wester H, Scharnhorst T (1991) An advanced 50th percentile Hybrid III dummy database. Frontal Crash Safety Technologies for the 90's. SAE Publication No. SP-852, pp 35–50. SAE Paper No. 910658.

67. Phillippens M, Nieboer JJ, Wismans J (1991) An advanced database of the 50th percentile Hybrid III dummy. Frontal Crash Safety Technologies for the 90's. SAE Publication No. SP-852, pp 121–129. SAE Paper No. 910813.

68. Kaleps I, Whitestone J (1988) Hybrid III Geometrical and Inertial Properties. SAE Paper No. 880638.

69. Wismans J, Hermans JHA (1988) MADYMO 3D simulations of hybrid III dummy sled tests. SAE Paper No. 880645.

70. Matsumoto H, Sakakida M, Kurimoto K (1990) A parametric evaluation of vehicle crash performance. Vehicle Crashworthiness and Occupant Protection in Frontal Collisions. SAE Publication SP-807, pp 73–84. SAE Paper No. 900465.

71. Chou CC, Wyman MH (1989) 1988 Tempo driver air bag simulation study. The Bioengineering Center 50th Anniversary Symposium Proceedings, Wayne State University, College of Engineering, Nov. 10, pp 67–75.

72. Heinz M, Hoefs R (1989) Vehicle occupant crash simulation using MADYMO Porsche airbag 2D. SAE publication SP-782 Automotive Frontal Impacts. SAE Paper No. 890755.

73. Wismans J, Maltha J, van Wijk JJ, Janssen EG (1982) MADYMO—a crash victim simulation computer program for biomechanical research and optimization of designs for impact injury prevention. AGARD Meeting Kooln, Germany, April.

74. Wismans, J, Wittebrood LJJ (1983) The MADYMO Crash Victim Simulation Package and Its Application in Analyzing Thoraxes of Side Impact Dummies. Seminar on The Biomechanics of Impacts in Road Accidents, Commission of the European Committees, Brussels, 21st–23rd March.

75. van Wijk J, Wismans J, Maltha J, Wittebrood L (1983) MADYMO Pedestrian Simulations. SAE 830060, Pedestrian Impact Injury and Assessment, P-121, SAE, Warrendale, Pennsylvania.

76. Bosio AC (1990) Simulation of submarining with MADYMO Proceedings of the second International MADYMO user's meeting, pp 135–170, May.

77. O'Conner CS, Rao MK (1990) Dynamic simulations of belted occupants with submarining. SAE Paper No. 901749.

78. Stalnaker RL, Maltha J (1980) MADYMO used for computer aided design of a dynamic acting child restraint scat. In Proceedings of the 5th IRCOBI Conference on the Biomechanics of Impacts, Birmingham.

79. Maltha J, Stalnaker RL (1981) Development of a dummy abdomen capable of injury detection in side impacts. SAE 811019. In Proceedings of the 25th Stapp Car Crash Conference, SAE, Warrendale, Pennsylvania.

80. Wiecher JF, Guenther DA (1989) Two dimensional thoracic modeling considerations. SAE Paper No. 890605.

81. Kooi J, Janssen EG (1988) Wheelchair occupant protection systems: safety during transport. No. 3, June.

82. Wismans J, Griffioen JA (1988) A flight safety application. Proceedings of the AGARD specialists meeting on energy absorption of aircraft structures as an aspect of crashworthiness, Luxembourg.

83. Bosio AC, Lupkar HA (1991) Design of experiments in occupant simulation. SAE Paper No. 910891.

84. Rieken A, Fleming P (1990) Co-ordinated approach to restraint system design using MADYMO occupant simulation & Taguchi methods. Presented at the second International MADYMO Users' Meeting, held at Noordwijk, Holland, May 14–15.

85. Lupkar HA, de Coo JA, Nieboer JJ, Wismans J (1991) Advances in MADYMO crash simulations. Side Impact Occupant Protection Technologies, SAE SP-851, pp 135–146. SAE Paper No. 910879.

86. Low TC, Prasad P (1990) Dynamic response and mathematical model of the side impact

dummy. In Proceedings of the 34th Stapp Car Crash Conference, SAE P-236, pp 233–242.

87. Prasad P, Low TC, Chou CC, Lim GG, Sundararajan S (1991) Side impact modeling using quasi-static crush data. SAE Paper No. 910601.

88. Low TC, Prasad P, Lim GG, Chou CC, Sundararajan S (1991) A MADYMO 3D side impact simulation model. Accepted for presentation at and publication in Crashworthiness and Occupant Protection in Transportation System, 1991 ASME Winter Annual Meeting, to be held in Atlanta, Georgia, Dec. 1–6.

89. MADYMO Post Processor (1988) H. W. Structures Newsletter, Wingter.

90. Chou CC, Lim GG, Mitchell JO (1990) Theoretical development of an ellipsoid/plane contact model. P&MES Technical Report No. EM-90-10, Ford Motor Company, December.

91. Bartz JA (1971) A three-dimensional computer simulation of a motor vehicle crash victim, phase 1—development of the computer program. Calspan Report Number VJ-2978-V-1, July.

92. Bartz JA, Butler FE (1972) A three-dimensional computer simulation of a motor vehicle crash victim, phase 2—validation study of the model. Calspan Report No. VJ-2978-V-2, December.

93. Fleck JT, Butler FE, Vogel SL (1974) An improved three-dimensional computer simulation of motor vehicle crash victims, Volume I–IV, Report Nos. DOT-HS-801507, -508, -509, -510, July.

94. Fleck JT, Butler FE (1975) Development of an improved computer model of the human body and extremity dynamics. Report No. AMRL-TR-75-14, July.

95. Butler FE, Fleck JT (1980) Advanced restraint system modeling. Report No. AFAMRL-TR-80-14, May.

96. Digges KH (1988) Recent improvements in occupant crash simulation capabilities of the CVS/ATB Model. SAE Paper No. 880655.

97. Fleck JT, Butler FE (1981) Validation of the crash victim simulator, Volumes 1–4, Report No. ZS-5881-V-1, DOT-HS-6-01300, December.

98. Fleck JT (1987) Improvements in the CVS/ATB occupant simulation model. SAE Paper No. 871110.

99. Wang JT, Lin Kuang-Huei (1988) A CAL3D steering system impact model. SAE Paper No. 880650.

100. Wang JT, Nefske DJ (1988) A new CAL3D airbag inflation model. SAE Paper No. 880654.

101. Wang JT (1989) Recent advances in modeling of pyrotechnic inflators for inflatable restraint systems. Crashworthiness and Occupant Protection in Transportation Systems, AMD-Vol 101/BED-Vol 13, The American Society of Mechanical Engineers, pp 89–93.

102. Wang JT, Ngo T (1990) Modeling of passenger side airbags with a complex shape. Vehicle Crashworthiness and Occupant Protection in Frontal Collisions. SAE Publication SP-807, pp 117–123. SAE Paper No. 900545.

103. Rangarajan N (1988) Passenger airbag model of deployment and occupant interaction. Report under a DOT contract with NHTSA-Contract No: DTNH22-88-C-07477. By GESAC, Inc. (8484 Georgia Ave. Suite 704, Silver Spring, MD 20910, (301) 585-7166).

104. Deng Y-C (1990) An improved belt model in CAL3D and its application. Vehicle Crashworthiness and Occupant Protection in Frontal Collisions. SAE Publication SP-807, pp 155–164. SAE Paper No. 900549.

105. Deng Y-C (1988) Analytical study of the interaction between the seat belt and a Hybrid III dummy in sled tests. SAE Paper No. 880648.

106. Padgaonkar AJ, Krieger KW, King AI (1977) A three-dimensional mathematical simulation of pedestrian–vehicle impact with experimental verification. J Biomechan Engin (ASME), 99K:116–123.

107. Niederer P, Walz F (1976) Stability considerations in the mathematical reconstruction of traffic accidents. SAE 760775, Mathematical Modeling Biodynamic Response to Impact, SAE SP-412, Warrendale, Pennsylvania.

108. Kruse WL (1976) Calspan–Chrysler research safety vehicle front end design for property and pedestrian protection. In Proceedings of the 6th International Technical Conference on Experimental Safety Vehicles, Washington DC.

109. Fowler JE, Axford RK, Butterfield KR (1976) Computer simulation of the pedestrian impact—development of the contact model. In Proceedings of the 6th International Technical Conference on Experimental Safety Vehicles, Washington DC.

110. Verma MK, Repa BS (1983) Pedestrian impact simulation—a preliminary study. SAE 831601. In Proceedings of the 27th Stapp Car Crash Conference, SAE, Warrendale, Pennsylvania.

111. Padgaonkar AJ, Prasad P (1979) Simulation of side impact using the CAL3D simulation model. SAE 791007. In Proceedings of the 23rd Stapp Car Crash Conference, SAE, Warrendale, PA.

112. Padgaonkar AJ, Prasad P (1982) A mathematical analysis of side impact using the CAL3D simulation model. In Proceedings of the 9th International Technical Conference on Experimental Safety Vehicles, Kyoto, Japan, November.

113. Newman KF, Grew ND, Dowzall G (1981) CAL3D: its use in BL cars limited. In Proceedings of the CAL3D Uses Conferences Sponsored By MVMA and NHSTA, May.

114. Segal DJ (1983) Computer modeling of side impact penetration of dummies of various sizes into padding. MGA Report G 37-V-3, DOT-NH-22-82-C-07047, August.

115. Segal DJ (1984) Side impact modelling using lumped mass and CAL3D CVS simulations. SAE publication P-146, Mathematical Simulation of Occupant and Vehicle Kinematics, pp 51–63, 1984. SAE Paper No. 840859.

116. Robbins DH, Becker JM, Bennett RO, Bowman BM (1980) Accident data simulation, pedestrian and side impact—3D. HSRI Report No. UM-HSRI-80-75, December, prepared for MVMA.

117. Deng Y-C (1987) Side impact simulation and thoracic injury assessment. Presented at the 11th International Technical Conference on ESV, Washington DC, May 15.

118. Deng Y-C (1989) The importance of the test method in determining the effects of door padding in side impact. In Proceedings of the 33rd Stapp Car Crash Conference, SAE Publication P-227. pp 79–85, SAE Paper No. 8924290.

119. Kaleps I, Obergefell LA, Ryerson J (1983) Simulation of restrained occupant dynamics during vehicle rollover. Final Report for DOT Interagency Agreement DTNH22-83-X-07296.

120. Obergefell LA, Kaleps I, Johnson AK (1986) Prediction of an occupant's motion during rollover crashes. In Proceedings of the 30th Stapp Car Crash Conference, October. SAE Paper No. 861876.

121. Frisch GD (1983) Simulation of occupant–crew station interaction during impact. Impact Injury of the Head and Spine, edited by Ewing et al, Charles C Thomas, Publisher, Springfield, Illinois.

122. Hubbard RP, Begeman PC (1990) Biomechanical performance of a new head and neck support. In Proceedings of the 34th Stapp Car Crash Conference Proceedings, SAE P-236, pp 83–91. SAE Paper No. 902312.

123. McGrath MT, Segal DJ (1984) CAL3D user convenience package—version II. DOT. NH-22-82-A-37046 Report, January.

124. Kaleps I, Marcus JH (1982) Predictions of child motion during panic braking and impact. SAE 821166. In Proceedings of the 26th Stapp Car Crash Conference, SAE, Warrendale, Pennsylvania.

125. Latouf BK, Yang KH, King AI (1989) CAL3D simulation of occupant neck response to airbag deployment in frontal impacts. The Bioengineering Center 50th Anniversary Symposium Proceedings, Wayne State University, College of Engineering, Nov. 10, pp 76–82.

126. Shaibani SJ (1990) The SJSATBPC package: mainframe-quality results with the crash victim simulation in the microcomputer environment. Seventh Annual International Workshop on Human Subject for Biomechanical Research, Washington DC, October 4.

127. Huston RL, Hessel RE, Winget JM (1976) Dynamics of a crash victim—a finite segment model. AIAA Journal, Vol 14, No. 2, February, pp 173–178.

128. Huston RL, Hessel RE, Passerello CE (1974) A three-dimensional vehicle–man model for collision and high acceleration studies. SAE Paper No. 740275.

129. Huston RL, King TP (1988) An analytical assessment of three-point restraints in several accident configuration. SAE Paper No. 880398.

130. Huston JC, Advanti SH (1976) Three dimensional model of the human head and neck for automobile crashes. Mathematical Modeling Biodynamic Response to Impact, SP-412, Society of Automobile Engineers, pp 9–20. SAE Paper No. 760769.

131. Passerello C, Huston RL (1971) Human attitude control. J Biomechan 4:95–102.

132. Huston RL, Passerello CE, Harlow MW, Winget JM (1975) The UCIN-3D aircraft-occupant. In Saczalski et al (eds) Aircraft Crashworthiness. University Press of Virginia, Charlottesville.

133. Huston RL (1985) Three-dimensional, gross-motion crash–victim simulators, Dept.

of Engineering Analysis, University of Cincinnati.

134. Chandler RG, Laananen DH (1979) Seat/occupant crash dynamic analysis verification test program. SAE Paper No. 790590.

135. Bolukbasi AO, Laananen DH (1983) Application of the nonlinear finite element method to crashworthiness analysis of aircraft seats. AIAA Publication No. 83-0929.

136. Laananen DH (1975) Development of a Scientific Basis for Analysis of Aircraft Seating Systems. Dynamic Science, Division of Ultra-systems, Inc., Phoenix, Arizona, FAA-RD-74-130.

137. Laananen DH, Bolukbasi AO (1982) Program SOM-LA (seat/occupant model—light aircraft), final briefing at federal aviation administration technical center, September 29–30.

138. Laananen DH (1977) Mathematical simulation for crashworthy aircraft seat design. AIAA Aircraft Systems & Technological Meeting, Seattle, Washington, August 22–24. AIAA Paper No. 77-1250.

139. Yeung KS, Welch RE (1977) Refinement of finite element analysis of automobile structures under crash loading, Vol II (Technical Final Report), DOT HS-803 466, October.

140. Bolukbasi AO, Laananen DH (1986) Computer simulation of a transport aircraft seat and occupants in a crash environment, Volume I—Technical Report (Draft), Simular Inc. Report TR-84430, March, Federal Aviation Administration Technical Center, Atlantic City Airport, NJ.

141. Laananen DH (1985) Validation of SOMLA occupant response. Crash Dynamics of General Aviation Aircraft, SP-622, Society of Automotive Engineers, Warrendale, PA, April, pp 1–12.

142. Anom (1982) Airbag simulation with finite elements. Technical Report, Physics International Scientific Codes and Engineering Service.

143. Buijk A (1988) 2D-calculations of a body impacting on an inflated airbag compared to experimental results. Technical Note: TN-8813, PISCES International bv, September.

144. Hallquist JO (1990) DYNA3D development and application. Presented at 1990 SAE International Congress and Exhibition, February 28.

145. Hallquist JO (1990) MVMA/DYNA3D and user's manual. Presented at MVMA quarterly meeting, March 9.

146. Yang KH, Wang H, Wang H-C, King AI (1990) Development of a two-dimensional driver side airbag development algorithm. In Proceedings of the 34th Stapp Car Crash Conference Proceedings, SAE P-236, pp 259–266. SAE Paper No. 902323.

147. Florie CJL, Buijk AJ (1981) Numerical simulation of unfolding airbags (date unknown).

148. Nieboer C, Wismans J (1980) Computer simulation of airbag contact with rigid body. TNO report to MVMA.

149. Hoffman R, Ulrich D, Protard J-B, Wester H, Jaehn N, Scharnhorst T (1990) Finite element analysis of occupant restraint system interaction with PAM-CRASH. In Proceedings of the 34th Stapp Car Crash Conference, held in Orlando, Florida, No. 4–7, pp 289–300 (SAE Paper No. 902325).

150. Hallquist JO, Benson DJ (1989) DYNA3D—an explicit finite program for impact calculations. Crashworthiness and Occupant Protection in Transportation Systems. ASME Publication AMD-Vol 106/BED-Vol 13, pp 95–112.

151. Hallquist JO, Hughes TJR, Stillman DW (1990) MVMA airbag development. Status report to MVMA, July 24.

152. Hallquist JO (1990) MVMA/DYNA3D user's manual (nonlinear dynamic analysis of structures in three dimensions). LSTC Report 1007, Rev. 1, February (sponsored by MVMA)

153. Hallquist JO, Stillman DW, Hughes TJR, Tarver C (1990) Modeling of airbags using MVMA/DYNA3D. Final report to MVMA, July 31.

154. Bruijs WEM, Buijk AJ, de Coo PJA, Sauren AAHJ (1990) Validation of coupled calculations with MADYMO and PISCES airbag. Presented at the Second User's Conference at TNO, May 14–16.

155. Hoffman R, Lasry D (1989) Design for passive safety using numerical simulation techniques. The Bioengineering Center 50th Anniversary Symposium Proceedings, Wayne State University, College of Engineering, Nov. 10, pp 61–66.

156. Lasry D, Hoffman R, Protard J-B (1991) Numerical simulation of fully folded airbags and their interaction with occupants with PAM-SAFE. SAE Paper No. 910150.

157. Lasry D (1990) Advances in crash, occupant & restraints simulation. Presented by Engineering Systems International at EASI, Auburn Hills, Michigan, Nov. 16.

158. OASYS DYNA3D Version 5.0 User Manual (1991) OASYS Ltd, 13 Fibzroy St., London W1P 6BQ, England.

159. Halloquist JO (1990) LS-DYNA3D 902 user manual. Livermore Software Technology Corporation.

160. Stillman D (1991) Personal communication, October.

161. Deng YC (1988) Design considerations for occupant protection in side impact—a modeling approach, SAE Paper No. 881713. In: Proceedings of the Thirty-Second Stapp Car Crash Conference, Atlanta.

162. Tong P, Eppinger R, Marcus J, Galabraith C (1989) Finite element modeling of head injury caused by internal loading. 12th International Technical Conference on ESV, Goteborg, Sweden, May 29–June 1, pp 617–627.

163. Lighthall JW, Melvin JW, Ueno K (1988) Toward a biomchanical criterion for functional brain injury. 12th International Technical Conference on ESV, Goteborg, Sweden, May 29–June 1, 1988, pp 627–633.

164. Plank G, Eppinger R (1989) Computed dynamic response of the human thorax from a finite element model. 12th International Technical Conference on ESV, Goteborg, Sweden, May 29–June 1, pp 665–672.

165. Walker BD, Dallard PRB (1991) An integrated approach to the simulation of vehicle crashworthiness and occupant protection systems. SAE Paper No. 910148.

166. Bush IS, Challener SA (1988) Finite element of modelling of non-penetrating thoracic impact. 1988 International IRCOBI Conference on the Biomechanics of Impacts, Sept. 14–16, Bergisch Gladbach (F.R.G.), pp 227–238.

167. Yang KH, Wang H, Jou JS (1991) Responses of human and dummy chests due to lateral impacts. Proceedings of Third U.S.A.–China–Japan Conference on Biomechanics,

held in Atlanta, Georgia, August 25–29, pp 193–194.

168. Sievaka E, Brazell J, Digges K, Pilkey W (1991) Impact injury simulation research. Symposium Proceedings of Injury Prevention Through Biomechanics, Bioengineering Engineering Center and Department of Orthopaedic Surgery, Wayne State University, April 12, pp 63–76.

169. Yang KH, King AI (1989) Development of a finite element based two dimensional human surrogate. The Bioengineering Center 50th Anniversary Symposium Proceedings, Wayne State University, College of Engineering, Nov. 10, pp 52–57.

170. Pan H (1991) Finite element modelling of the Hybrid III dummy chest. Thesis for the Degree of Master of Science, Wayne State University, April.

171. Schelkle E, Remensperger (1991) Integrated occupant-car crash simulation with the finite element method: the Porsche Hybrid III dummy and airbag model. SAE Paper No. 910654.

172. Miles JC (1991) Applications of DYNA3D to crashworthiness, metalforming and other non-linear problems. Presented at Japan Research Institute Conference 91, Tokyo, Japan, August.

173. Puttre M (1991) FEA programs band together. Mechanical Engineering, September, pp 77–80.

174. Buijk AJ, Florie CJL (1972) Numerical simulation of deploying airbags and their interaction with vehicle occupants. Report by the MacNeal-Schwendler Company B.V., Groningenweg 6, 2803 PV Gouda, The Netherlands.

175. Robbins DH (1989) Restraint systems computer modeling and simulation—state of the art and correlation with reality. SAE Paper No. 891976.

7
Development of Crash Injury Protection in Civil Aviation

Richard F. Chandler

Historical Background

Before World War I

It was not until the late 19th century that manned flight in heavier-than-air craft became a reality. One of the leading aeronauts of that time was Otto Lilienthal, a German engineer, who designed and built several manned gliders between 1891 and his death in a glider crash in 1896. He made over 2,000 gliding or soaring flights, mostly from a specially constructed hill at Lichterfelde, near Berlin. Lilienthal authored several works on the theory and practice of flight. These provided important data and guidance for aspiring aeronauts. Octave Chanute, a railway and bridge engineer and mentor of several hopeful aviators in the United States, provided extensive details of Lilienthal's work in his book *Progress in Flying Machines*.[28] Lilienthal's belief in quick escape in case of emergency was presented as a rule: "The aviator must be so affixed to his apparatus that he can detach himself instantly should the machine take a sheer."[28] When Chanute sponsored glider tests, he followed Lilienthal's advice, specifying:

The operator should in no wise be attached to the machine. He may be suspended by his arms, or sit upon a seat, or stand on a running board, but he must be able to disengage himself instantly from the machine should anything go wrong, and be able to come down upon his legs in landing.[34]

This guidance, perhaps appropriate for the early small gliders that flew just a few feet above the surface of the earth, also set a precedent for powered aircraft. The Wright brothers had studied the efforts of Lilienthal and Chanute in preparation for their experiments. They also chose not to restrain the operator in their gliders or early airplanes. Although they experienced several minor mishaps during their experiments, there were no serious injuries until 1908. The Wright brothers had accepted a contract with the U.S. Army to provide a "heavier-than-air" flying machine. Among the specifications were requirements that it carry two persons and sufficient fuel for a flight of 125 miles. Orville Wright began flight demonstrations of the aircraft at Fort Meyer, Virginia, on September 3, 1908, and carried his first passenger on September 12. A flight on September 17, with Lt. Thomas Selfridge as a passenger, ended in a crash caused by a faulty propeller. Selfridge sustained a depressed skull fracture from impact with one of the wooden uprights of the aircraft framework, and died a few hours later. This death was the first of an occupant of a powered heavier-than-air aircraft. Orville Wright escaped the crash with a fractured leg, four broken ribs, and three pelvic fractures, one with dislocation. The pelvic injuries were not discovered until 12 years after the crash. He suffered from the aftermath of these injuries for the rest of his life. The tragedy of this crash was widely mourned in the aeronautical community. Unfortunately, it did little to spur interest in protection from crash injuries other than a limited concern about the use of crash helmets.

At the time of Orville Wright's crash, Wilbur Wright was demonstrating the Wright aircraft in Europe. The press coverage that resulted form these demonstrations caused a resurgence of European activity in flying. Numerous enthusiasts attempted flight, some with copies of the Wright aircraft, but most with aircraft designed and built in Europe. These new participants did not exhibit the caution of the Wright brothers in their enthusiasm. In the next year (1909), there were three aviation fatalities. In 1910, there were 30 fatal crashes, with 32 fatalities.

It was during this time that pilots began to discover turbulence in the air, then described as "holes in the air" or "air pockets." Also, the cause of an occasional accident was attributed to the pilot sliding out of the seat or falling into the controls during flight. Most pilots responded to this risk by wrapping their legs around airframe structure or by simply "holding on," but a few pilots began to strap themselves into the seat (Fig. 7.1). These safety belts were not intended to offer protection in a crash. The racing fuselage of the French Antoinette monoplane used a "rigid" belt to hold the aviator in place, but it usually broke on impact or held fast and caused internal injuries to the occupant.[97] The R.E.P. monoplane was equipped with an "elastic" safety belt that stretched in a crash and did not protect the pilot (o.c.).

Adolphe Pégoud, a French pilot known for the risks he took in flying, exhibited upside-

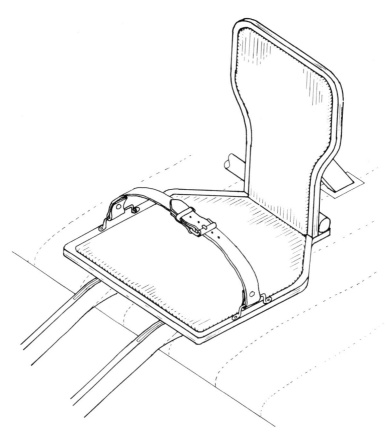

FIGURE 7.1. Early lap belt. Early installations of safety belts in airplanes were intended to keep the occupant in place during flight turbulence or or maneuvers. The first safety belt in a U.S. Army airplane was adapted from a leather trunk strap by the local harness maker for the Calvary.

down flying and "looping the loop" in 1913. He flew a specially reinforced Blériot monoplane equipped with a torso restraint system to keep him within the plane during inverted flight. This restraint system consisted of a leather chest belt, with straps going over each shoulder and passing under the seat structure. Straps were also connected from the chest belt to the bottom-fuselage longerons just behind the pilot. While effective for acrobatic maneuvers by holding the pilot in the aircraft during inverted flight, the restraint was not intended for crash protection and lacked quick-release capability.

Most pilots still had strong objections to strapping themselves into their seats. The fear of being trapped in a burning aircraft was strong, even though fire played a small part in actual crash deaths. This fear was fortified by frequent failures of the aircraft fuel systems that often drenched the pilot with gasoline. Quick-release mechanisms were developed for safety belts, but these were most often used to release the belt just before landing so there would be no risk of entrapment.

"Passive" means of crash protection were occasionally encountered in these early aircraft. Lilienthal had incorporated a "prellbügel" in some of his gliders. This elastic ring, made of willow wood, surrounded the pilot and acted as a resilient bumper on landing. Lilienthal credited this device with saving his life in a crash in 1894. His fatal crash in 1896 was in a glider without a Prellbügel. The structure supporting the forward elevators in the first Wright airplanes provided some measure of energy absorption as it twisted and cracked in a crash. When the pilot was enclosed in the fuselage, the forward edge of the cockpit cutout was padded to protect his head during a crash.

World War I

The first widespread organized use of airplanes took place in World War I. This provided the opportunity to show that a systematic policy of "accident prevention" would save lives and aircraft. Even before the war it was understood that ordinary carpenters or mechanics lacked

the skills necessary to produce reliable repairs on aircraft. The military had the resources to specially train and assign capable technicians for this work. Techniques of inspecting and "signing" repairs were developed to promote quality work. Pilots received graded instruction, moving through basic training, acrobatics (where they learned to routinely do maneuvers that were dangerously impossible only 2 years before), and simulated combat training. The design of aircraft and engines became more formal and was more often the responsibility of trained engineers. Large military aviation training centers and combat area aerodromes required that techniques for safe management of airports be developed. The traditionally structured military organization also provided the rudiments of an air-traffic control system.

One of the more dramatic advances in accident prevention was made in the field of aviation medicine. During the first year of the war, the British found that, out of every 100 aviators killed, two met death at the hands of the enemy, eight were lost to a fault of the engine or the airplane, and the remaining 90 were lost because of failure of the flyer himself. Of these 90, 60 were caused by physical defects.[12] Germany had completed studies in 1910 and published a definite procedure for medical examination and selection of applicants for military pilot training. They established a specially trained medical service to provide required monthly medical examinations for pilots. The British established a similar program, organizing a "Care of the Flyer Service." At the end of the second year of the war, fatalities due to physical defects had been reduced to 20%. At the end of the third year, they were further reduced to 12%.

Restraint systems were more widely used during the war. Safety belts were often 5–6 inches wide for increased strength and to distribute the restraint load over the abdomen. However, one design widely used in British aircraft had a narrow quick-release buckle that extended on either side of the belt and caused frequent internal injuries in survivable crashes (Fig. 7.2a). Some safety belts used a "simple rubber shock absorber" to anchor the belt in the aircraft (Fig. 7.2b). This "decidedly

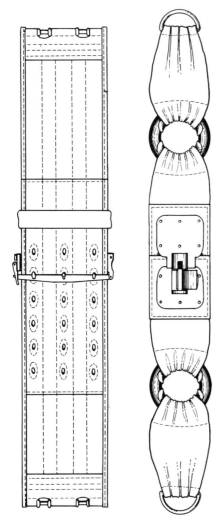

FIGURE 7.2. Safety belts in World War I. Mass production of aircraft for the First World War resulted in some standardization of safety-belt designs. The left belt was often found in airplanes used by the British Commonwealth countries. The long, narrow, quick-release buckle was a frequent cause of injuries if the restraint was worn during a crash. The right belt was a design often used in French and German airplanes. The large rubber rings served as a rudimentary shock absorber that decreased belt forces transmitted to the occupant and aircraft structure during a crash. While this design reduced belt injuries and structural failures, it also allowed the occupant to move forward, thus increasing the risk of injury.

reduced" injuries to the upper abdomen and ribs.[6] The "gunner's belt" (essentially an industrial safety belt with a quick-release buckle) was used when the aircraft machine-gun operator would have to stand to aim the gun or get up from his seat to reload the gun. Similar designs are still in use. Simple changes in the airplane were sometimes made to reduce crash injuries. Medical officers had observed that more than half of the injuries sustained in crashes were caused by striking the head against the cowl. Cutting the cowl so as to give 8 more inches of room in front of the pilot was found to "practically eliminate" head injuries in one aircraft.[6]

The cruciform type of torso restraint was used in highly maneuverable scout airplanes by both sides in the war to keep the pilot in the cockpit during maneuvers and to assist him in controlling the airplane. The British "Sutton" restraint (Fig. 7.3) is perhaps the simplest of this type, and certainly one of the most lasting. (Derivatives of the Sutton harness remained in service on some aircraft through the 1950s, even though earlier accident reports and research had shown that it did not provide good protection in crashes.[98,61]) This restraint consisted of four straps, one over each shoulder and over each thigh. Eyelets in the straps were threaded on a cone-shaped pin which was positioned over the abdomen. When all four straps were in place, they were secured in position by a split pin placed through a hole in the cone pin. The restraint system was released by tugging on a thong attached to the split pin, thus pulling the pin out of the hole, allowing the straps to slide freely over the cone pin. Variations of this concept used webbing or leather straps, adjustment devices along the straps instead of holes in the straps, and different forms of release mechanisms.

The quick-release mechanism was a vital part of the restraint system, since many pilots continued the practice of releasing the restraint system before landing in the belief that their chances of survival in a crash would be better if they were not strapped into the airplane. However, data from formal accident investigations contradicted this belief, so that when the *General Rules and Regulations Governing*

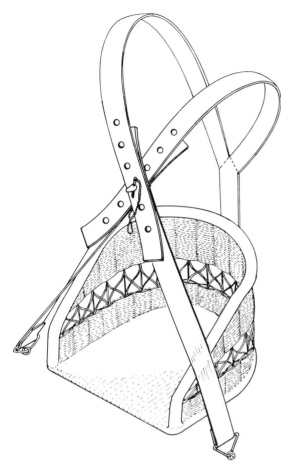

FIGURE 7.3. The "Sutton" restraint. The cruciform type of restraint was used in scout airplanes by both sides during the First World War. This restraint served to keep the pilot in place during acrobatic combat maneuvers. It was not an efficient restraint during crashes because of injuries sustained when the pilot submarined under the lower straps. The British "Sutton" restraint, shown here, made of improved materials, with shoulder-belt adjustors and occasionally modified by additional shoulder straps attached toward the tail of the airplane, remained in service well past World War II.

Flying on Individual Fields became effective on October 21, 1918, they included the following requirements:

17. All machines must be equipped with safety belts for pilot and passenger.
18. Always use safety belts. In case of accident, do not release belt until after accident. It will probably save injury, especially if the machine turns over.[7]

The effectiveness of this requirement has not been determined. It should be noted that the rule addressed safety belts, not shoulder harnesses, and that the primary benefit offered is the retention in the aircraft in the event it overturns, an action similar to being thrown from the aircraft in turbulence. Even if the belts were worn during a crash, their effectiveness was reduced by the limited strength of the belts and their installation. Typically, the restraint system would withstand a load of only a few hundred pounds.

Between the Wars

After World War I, the United States found itself with hundreds of airplanes and thousands of pilots and no real use for most of them. The airplanes, mostly Curtiss JN-4 trainers (the "Jenny") and De Haviland D.H. 4 "battle-planes," and spare engines were sold on the surplus market for less than 10% of their cost. Former military pilots bought these planes and attempted to earn a living by flying. These planes were mostly used for "barnstorming" exhibition flights and for occasional skywriting, crop dusting, aerial photography, and aerial surveying. An attempt to develop a scheduled passenger service in the United States failed in 1924. In 1924, 124 fixed-base operators provided some sort of air service, including nonscheduled passenger flying. The number dropped to 60 in 1925, despite a booming economy in other business sectors of the United States. Accidents increased as the public demanded more and more "death-defying" acts of the barnstormers, and as airplane maintenance deteriorated. In 1924, private fliers experienced a fatal accident every 13,500 miles flown. (In contrast, the U.S. government Air Mail Service had experienced only one fatal accident for every 463,000 miles.) By that time the supply of surplus aircraft had been largely depleted, and new untried and often unsafe airplanes were being marketed. Private aviation insurance became prohibitively expensive because of losses in crashes caused by irresponsible fliers or by unsafe airplanes. Several states had passed laws that governed flying within their borders.

These laws were often inconsistent with and sometimes contradicted the laws of neighboring states.

Investors in the United States compared this situation with that of Europe, where well-regulated, profitable air commerce had been developing since the end of the war. They brought pressure on the federal government to bring order to private flying so that it could be profitably developed. They also saw the need for federal support and direction to promote a system of safe airways and airports, just as had been done for roadways, railways, and harbors.

Congress responded to these pressures with the Kelly Air Mail Act (1925) and the Air Commerce Act of 1926. The Kelly Air Mail Act authorized the post office to contract for the transportation of air mail and thus provided economic support for operators and manufacturers of new airplanes. The Air Commerce Act empowered the secretary of commerce to develop a comprehensive system of commercial aviation for the United States. While the specific goal of this act was to foster air commerce, improved safety was an inherent

part of that goal. Improved safety was accomplished in a number of ways that included the development of a system of air routes with check points marked by light beacons (and later radio guides). There was also support for local development and management of airports as well as regulation and licensing of aircraft, airmen, and mechanics. In addition, a system of reporting accidents was started. In effect, this program established a nation-wide aviation accident-prevention program.

As this new regulatory system developed, the results of the act became evident. The new aviation industry prospered and flying was safer (Fig. 7.4). The accident-prevention efforts were working. However, crash injury prevention was not emphasized. The first (1926) Air Commerce Regulations required "[s]afety belts or equivalent apparatus for pilots and passengers in open-cockpit airplanes carrying passengers for hire or reward."[16] This rule suggests that safety belts were still regarded solely as protection when flying in turbulent air. The absence of similar protection for people flying in a "not-for-hire" airplane is also apparent. Additional protection was

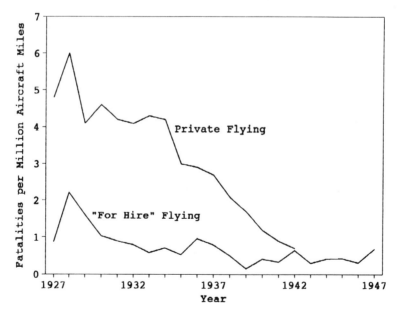

FIGURE 7.4. Aviation fatality rate: 1927–1947. The accident-prevention program created by the Air Commerce Act of 1926 resulted in significant reductions of fatalities associated with both private and commercial ("for hire") flying. Accident data were not uniformly reported in 1927, the first year of the act, so the low fatality rate indicated for that year is probably in error. Private aviation was drastically curtailed by the Second World War, so the fatality data for those years are not reported here.

provided in 1928, when the rules were expanded by requiring

[s]afety belts or equivalent for pilots and passengers in all airplanes. Seats or chairs in cabin planes shall be firmly secured in place. Safety belts and their attachments shall be capable of withstanding a load of 1,000 pounds applied in the same manner as a passenger's weight would be applied in a crash. The attachment shall be capable of carrying the loads through to the main structure.[17]

This new requirement may have resulted from research conducted by the military. Investigations of military airplane accidents found several cases where pilots, and one case where passengers, lost their lives as a result of seat and safety belt failures. The Assistant Secretary of War for Aeronautics issued a general order covering investigations of the strength properties of airplane seats, safety belts, flooring, and seat supports. In support of that order, the Air Corps Material Division developed a dynamic test procedure for evaluating seating and restraint systems and initiated tests. An early test of the system installed in the Fokker C2-A transport airplane found that the safety belt broke under the equivalent of a 100-pound tension load.[100] Ultimately, these tests led to a redesign of the floor, seat, and safety belt, which showed no failures in 8g tests. It was "believed that acceleration, or rather deceleration greater than 8g in a forward thrust would probably be injurious to the average man." No documentation has been discovered that required that these improvements be installed in operational airplanes.

These tests attempted to simulate a crash in which the airplane nosed over into the ground. It was believed that in such a crash, the crash forces would result in an upward and forward inertial load from the occupant. The seat was not stressed by downward crash loads. This concept of a survivable crash was adapted for civil aircraft in 1934, when the regulations were changed to require that "[s]afety belts and their attachments shall be capable of withstanding a design load of 1,000 pounds per person applied upwardly and forwardly at an angle of approximately 45° with the floor line."[18]

The results of military-aircraft accident investigations continued to show injuries to the face and head even when the seat and safety belt did not fail in a crash. Vertical scale instruments were developed that allowed space on the instrument panel for a crash pad directly in line with the pilot's head.[8] However, no documentation of the application of results of this instrument-panel crash pad has been found. In 1936, Lt. Col. M.C. Grow, chief flight surgeon of the Army Air Corps, initiated development of a modified restraint with shoulder belts. Captain H.G. Armstrong conducted impact tests of this restraint with human volunteer test subjects at decelerations up to 15g, the limit of the test equipment.[5] As a result of these tests, it was estimated that one could live through a deceleration of between 30 and 50gs when using the combined safety-belt and shoulder-belt restraint.

Predictions that the shoulder belt would soon be in use in all airplanes in the country fell short of reality. The introduction of shoulder belts was accomplished very slowly, even in military airplanes. In an accident study released late in 1943, Capt. G.M. Hass commented that the "shoulder harness is now coming into general use in most types of aircraft used for the training of cadets."[64] Hass felt that "the shoulder harness has disadvantages and should not be regarded as anything more than a temporary substitute for safety in design." He concluded

[f]inally, and most important, a method should be devised so that an occupant of an aircraft could pull a lever and be ejected mechanically from the aircraft while still strapped in the seat. An attached parachute should be opened automatically by the action of a cord attached to the aircraft from which the seat had been ejected.

Such a system had already been placed in service by the German Luftwaffe.

The Beginning of Crash Injury Reduction

CIR

In 1917, Hugh De Haven, then a young cadet flying with the Canadian Royal Flying Corps, was rammed by another plane during combat practice. Both planes crashed. De Haven suffered two broken legs as well as a ruptured liver, pancreas, and gallbladder. After a 6-month recovery, he returned to duty and was assigned as a headquarters clerk in a pilot-training squadron near Toronto. He observed the frequent crashes at this airfield and began to sense a relationship between the injuries to the occupants and features of the aircraft. He concluded that his own internal injuries were caused by the safety belt, which he described as being "5 to 6 inches wide with a narrow pointed 6 inch high buckle in the middle."[41] When De Haven attempted to point out the causes of injury to his superiors, he was informed that flying was dangerous, crash injuries were a matter of fate, and the only way to prevent those injuries was to stay on the ground. The end of the war concluded De Haven's military career and temporarily ended his interest in the causes of injury in crashes.

A minor automobile accident in 1935 caused De Haven to recall his earlier findings and realize that no progress had been made in reducing crash injuries. In 1936, he urged the U.S. Bureau of Air Commerce to undertake a program in which doctors, engineers, and safety groups could work together to reduce crash injuries in aircraft. After several meetings with James Edgerton, chairman of the Special Committee for Aviation Medicine (a group established to define human capabilities and limitations for substratosphere flight), he was able to present his ideas to the committee. The committee took a dim view of the prospects for his plan. They pointed out that there was no money to build a deceleration facility. (They were looking for resources to support their substratosphere research facility.) They also expressed concern that the threat of legal involvement would prevent the use of federal accident investigations to study injury, and doctors would not discuss the injuries sustained by their patients because of ethical considerations.

De Haven attempted to interest other groups in his plan, but without much success. Pilots and aircraft operators still were fatalistic about survival in aircraft crashes and felt that

any money spent on injury prevention would have been better spent on accident prevention. Engineers believed that changes to improve survival in crashes would result in unacceptable weight-and-cost penalties. De Haven did obtain the cooperation of a few accident investigators and, from 1938 to 1941, personally investigated aircraft crashes in which there were both fatalities and survivors. He found that he was unable to estimate the forces involved in the crashes or in producing the injuries.

Looking for other areas where the impact conditions might be easier to estimate, De Haven obtained the cooperation of Bellevue Hospital in New York City and began to study impacts that caused skull fracture. This led to his study of falls, and suicide attempts by jumping, from heights of 50–150 ft. In 1941, De Haven used the findings of this study to argue that crash protection was feasible for small airplanes.[35] Even at this early date, he had found that "proper positional distribution of pressure" could ensure survival of major impact forces with minimal injuries. He urged that research on crash safety for light airplanes be initiated.

Doctor J.F. Fulton of the Yale School of Medicine, a member of the National Research Council Committee on Aviation Medicine (NRC/CAM), recommended that a special committee be formed to study crashes, report on the character of injures sustained in both fatal and nonfatal crashes, and take steps to redesign structures that cause recurring injuries. This committee was to consist of De Haven, a pilot, and a physician. Fulton also made several "recommendations," including what was apparently a widely held belief regarding seat belts: "(iii) Seat belts are highly dangerous and have been known to cause fatal lower abdominal injuries even to cutting a person in two; their only conceivable value is to hold an individual in the seat during a sharp down draft or inverted flight."[59] Doctor Eugene F. DuBois, chairman of the NRC/CAM and head of the Department of Physiology at the Cornell University Medical College, with the support of Jerome Lederer, recently appointed chief of the Aviation Safety

Bureau of the Civil Aeronautics Board, obtained funding for the project from the U.S. Office of Scientific Research and Development. The Crash Injury Research (CIR) Project was begun in 1942 at Cornell University Medical College. De Haven was director of the CIR Project. He was supported by a staff of three (an assistant, a secretary, and an analyst-librarian). To supplement this meager staff, De Haven provided the opportunity for others to participate in the project in accordance with their talents. De Haven's assistant resigned in 1947, and lack of funds prevented filling the position until 1949, when A. Howard Hasbrook joined the staff. Hasbrook, a pilot since 1934, had extensive pilot experience. Like De Haven many years before, Hasbrook had recently been seriously injured in a crash. After serving as De Haven's assistant, Hasbrook became director of accident investigation for the CIR in 1950. In 1953, the CIR Project was divided into Aviation Crash Injury Research (AvCIR) and Automobile Crash Injury Research (ACIR). De Haven served as Director of ACIR until his retirement in 1954, when the post was taken over by John Moore. Hasbrook became the first director of AvCir. The work of these people provided the foundation for crash injury protection in all forms of transportation.

At the inception of the Crash Injury Research Project in 1942, aircraft accident investigators were concerned almost exclusively with determining the cause of the accident. Investigators of the Civil Aeronautics Board were provided CIR forms on which details of the crash, injuries, and their causes could be documented. Similar investigations were undertaken by some states and the military. By November 1943, De Haven had published the results of the investigations of the first 30 crashes.[37] By 1945, this database had been expanded to include 110 crashes with fore and aft seating arrangements and 75 crashes with side-by-side seating.[38] These studies found that the occupants head was the first and often the only vital part of the body exposed to injury, and that severe injuries of the head, extremities, and chest were increased by failure of safety-belt assemblies or anchorages.

The 1,000-pound (tension load) safety belt, or the belt anchorages, failed in 94 cases among the 260 survivors of the crashes. Only seven of the survivors showed evidence of injury to abdominal viscera and only two of these injuries were considered serious. Among the survivors, strained neck muscles and fractures of the cervical or dorsal spines were rare. De Haven expressed his concern about pilot acceptance of shoulder harnesses and his belief in the benefits of improved designs, which we would now call "passive protection":

It is, however, very doubtful that the methodical wearing of this additional gear (shoulder harness) will be the popular answer to greater safety in casual use of personal aircraft. The reasons are primarily psychological. Fortunately, evidence indicates that, in many dangerous mishaps typical of popular flying, a stronger seat belt, and improved cabin installations can provide a higher degree of protection of occupants in a plane in an emergency.

Concern about the acceptance of shoulder harnesses was justified in a later study of surplus military airplane crashes.[41] The shoulder harness had been removed in 68% of the crashes investigated. The harness was used in only 23% of the crashes and was ineffective in one-third of those because the pilot had failed to lock the harness take-up reel. Nevertheless, the study showed statistically significant reductions in injuries when the shoulder belt was effectively used, until such a point when crushing injuries were sustained due to collapse of the structure surrounding the pilot.

The early CIR studies reflect some of the problems that were encountered in promoting crash protection. The widely held belief was that "1,000-pound" belt assemblies in common use were sufficient because the human body could not withstand higher forces. This belief was one of the first obstacles to overcome. In 1947, the accident database, which had grown to include 833 cases of injury, was reviewed to determine the frequency of abdominal injury due to the safety belt. Three hundred fifty four of these injuries were in severe but survivable crashes, but only three survivors and five fatalities showed any evidence of internal abdominal injury.[40]

Continued concern over possible injuries from the safety belt resulted in a special grant from the Civil Aeronautics Administration to study and report on the problem. The study reviewed injuries of 1,039 survivors of airplane crashes. Of these survivors, 79.9% had injuries to the head, 6.1% had injuries to the neck (including the cervical spine), 19.8% had injuries to the upper torso (including the dorsal spine), 23.9% had injuries to the lower torso (including the lumbar spine), 15.8% had injuries to the spine, and 59.1% had injuries to the extremities. Thirty-nine survivors were not using the safety belt. Of the remaining 1,000 survivors, only nine (0.9%) had dangerous (life threatening) lower-torso injuries for which the safety belt could reasonably be considered a direct cause.[46]

While De Haven was attempting to obtain support for improvements in design and use of seat belts, a report of injuries sustained in the crash of a Viking transport airplane was made public. A conclusion of this report was that "[t]he immediate cause of death in more than half the victims was acute flexion over the safety-belt."[93] While the apparent intent of this report was to encourage the adoption of rear-facing seats in transport airplanes, the conclusion regarding sefety belts was extensively quoted in the United States (e.g., ref. 4). This publicity threatened to nullify the attempts being made for improved design and use of safety belts and shoulder harnesses for small aircraft as well as for transport airplanes.

DuBois responded to the report, concluding that the injuries were due to causes other than safety belts and that the victims did not have the typical signs of injury due to safety-belt contact.[50] Of course, this response did not receive the widespread distribution of the original report. The CIR published several reports that emphasized the benefits resulting from proper forward-facing-seat-and-restraint systems.[43,62] Proponents of rearward-facing seats were quick to respond (e.g., ref. 58), continuing a conflict that still has not been conclusively resolved in favor of either seat position.

De Haven had not neglected development of improved restraint systems. As early as April 1942, he conceived, designed, fabricated, and tested a restraint harness concept using what we would now call a "powered retractor."[36] De Haven apologized that the harness was built with "totally inadequate materials" since the retractor was actuated by a basketball that was rapidly inflated by a blank cartridge. (Research engineers with the du Pont company stated that this technique was entirely new.) Nevertheless, this harness was able to check dummy motion without striking the cockpit structure under force conditions sufficient to bend portions of the fuselage. While this development was not carried further, De Haven continued to seek a practical restraint harness that might be acceptable to the average pilot.

The Army Air Forces found that the shoulder harness was not well accepted by military pilots because it hindered their movement and ability to see out of the cockpit during flight. A spring-and-plunger device was developed to fit between the harness and the airframe in order to allow the pilots to move. This early "retractor" was provided with a manual lock that was to be actuated by the pilot during landing, takeoff, and acrobatic flight. However, it was found that pilots often "forgot" to lock the restraint. Early in 1943, Drs. J.C. Hinsley and William A. Geohegan of Cornell University Medical School worked under the CIR project to develop an "inertia lock" for the manual locking retractor. This device was actuated by the impact of an aircraft crash. About this time, the Army changed from the spring-and-plunger-type retractor to a reel-and-cable-type system to avoid the progressive increase in force (and discomfort) produced by the spring-and-plunger mechanism. By June 1943, Dr. Geohegan had developed an inertia lock system for the reel-and-cable-type retractor, and, after a few changes, submitted prototype inertia locking retractors to the Army for field evaluation.[3,54] The reels became available for installation late in 1944 (Fig. 7.5). They were set to lock automatically under an impact of 2–3g. No documentation has been found to give the reason for this 2–3g locking range. However, it is noted that human muscular control of body motion was considered poss-

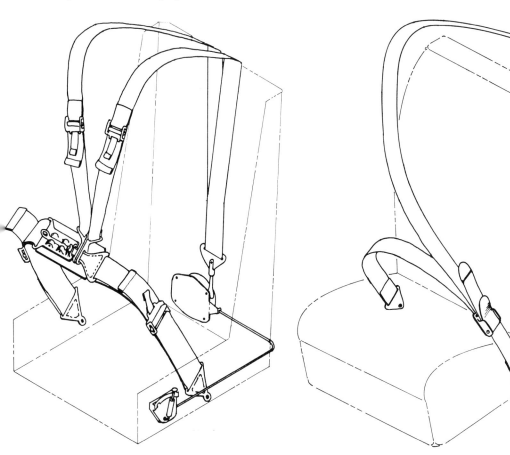

FIGURE 7.5. Military airplane restraint system. Shoulder-harness-type restraint was introduced to American Military pilots late in the second World War. A manually locked rod-and-spring-type retractor was provided with the restraint system to overcome pilot objections that the shoulder belts restricted necessary mobility during flight. The manual lock was seldom used, and was replaced by a cable-and-reel automatically locking retractor, shown here. The reel would lock in response to aircraft deceleration of 2–3 g. Auxiliary manual locking and unlocking was also incorporated in this retractor.

FIGURE 7.6. The CIR-Griswold restraint. In 1950 De Haven and Griswold developed a simplified restraint system consisting of a combined diagonal and safety belt. The one-piece diagonal and safety-belt strap can slide through the buckle, which is locked onto a short strap to adjust and position the restraint.

ible at these decelerations, so the reel would lock before muscular control of the body was exceeded.

In 1950, De Haven and Mr. Roger Griswold developed a new safety harness, shown in Fig. 7.6. Fundamentally, this CIR-Griswold harness consisted of

a long strap with one end attached behind the pilot ... and the other end attached to one of the safety belt anchorages. A buckle ... is slideably mounted on this long strap. A short "stub" strap is attached to the other safety belt anchorage. This stub strap is easily and quickly threaded through the buckle like a conventional airline safety belt; it can be loosened, taken off, or tightened by using only one hand.[42]

De Haven considered this belt and harness combination to have desirable features:

- The chest strap lies across the strong central portion of the chest and shoulder.
- The harness does not tend to pull the seat belt up into the abdomen.

- The combination belt and harness can be put on and taken off as easily and simply as an airline safety belt.
- The safety belt cannot be used (comfortably) without wearing the shoulder strap.
- The harness (and belt) can be quickly tightened or released in one motion by one hand.
- The combination is comfortable to wear and does not give a trussed-up binding on the shoulders. By pivoting centrally on the single strap, the user can reach forward with either arm and shoulder.
- The use of right- or left-hand sets of harness, depending on which side of the cabin it is being installed in, provides protection for the upper torso and head under conditions of severe side loads in cartwheeling accidents.
- The single strap has an important advantage over the double-strap harness in that women can wear it comfortably.
- It adjusts itself, and fits, persons of various sizes without readjustment.
- Cost-wise, the combination should not greatly exceed that of an ordinary safety belt, since there is a minimum of extra weight and no additional hardware.

While the harness incorporated the *metal-to-webbing buckle* in common use at the time, De Haven also noted that the *tongue-and-hook type of buckle* could be used as well if independent adjustment was provided in the safety-belt portion of the restraint. An inertia reel would be used for taking up slack in the chest strap in this system, shown in Fig. 7.7. In 1953, De Haven described applications of CIR research findings to operational airplanes.[45] This report illustrated the use of the CIR-Griswold restraint harness in two production airplanes, the Helioplane Courier and the Meyers 145.

The other aircraft featured in that report used different restraint systems but were nevertheless noteworthy developments in aviation crashworthiness. The Beech Bonanza and Twin Bonanza were postwar designs using all-metal construction and incorporated numerous crash safety features. The CAA-sponsored AG-1 experimental agricultural

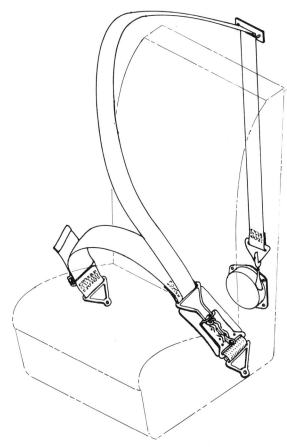

FIGURE 7.7. An alternate CIR-Griswold restraint. De Haven suggested an alternate form of simplified restraint to provide a snug seat belt and a diagonal belt that attached to an automatic-locking retractor. This configuration would provide the security of the conventional seat belt during turbulence and still allow the freedom of shoulder movement desired during normal operations.

airplane incorporated both operational and crashworthy features that were subsequently adopted by many manufacturers.

The First Prototype Crashworthy Airplane—the AG-1

The National Flying Farmers Association had, since the late 1940s, been urging the Department of Agriculture and the CAA to provide assistance in developing an airplane especially suited to agricultural uses. In 1949, the CAA agreed to provide a grant of $50,000 to Texas A&M College to develop such an airplane. Fred E. Weick, a noted aircraft designer who had just joined the college, was put in charge of the project.[103] Weick was well acquainted with De Haven and had just met Hasbrook, who was recovering from injuries resulting from a crash in an agricultural aircraft. Together, they worked on the crashworthy features of the new airplane. De Haven and Hasbrook made 10 recommendations for making the AG-1 crashworthy:

- Design forward fuselage and cabin structure to resist nominal crash loads as well as flight and landing loads.
- Design aircraft structures to absorb energy by progressive collapse.
- Design tubular structure to bend and fail outwardly away from the occupants.
- Locate the passengers and pilot seats as far aft in the fuselage as possible behind the wing.
- Locate fuel tanks in or on the wings, not between the fire wall and the instrument panel.
- Provide space between the instrument panel and fire wall or nose section to permit forward displacement of the panel and the instrument casings.
- Design the instrument panel to be free of sharp rigid edges in the range of the pilot's head.
- Fabricate the instrument panel of ductile material and/or use an energy-absorbing shield on the panel face.
- Mount instrument cases on shear pins as low on the panel as possible.
- Provide shoulder harnesses, safety belts, seats, and seat anchorages of sufficient strength to resist failure up to the point of cabin collapse.

The AG-1 conformed to these recommendations except that the fuel tanks were located in the fuselage above and behind the engine. This was done to provide a simple gravity-fed fuel system and reduce the potential for fuel-feed failure as an accident cause.

The AG-1 used a restraint system capable of withstanding an 8,000-pound static load. As originally designed, each shoulder strap had a loop at the lower end to slip over the safety belt buckle when fastening in place. However, it was found that many crop-duster pilots would not use the shoulder harness, even though it was available. The design was changed so that each shoulder strap was permanently fastened to the safety belt near the buckle, so that the shoulder harness had to be donned when the safety belt was used. An inertia reel, just becoming available for civil aircraft, was used with the shoulder harness to increase comfort.

The still-experimental version of the AG-1 was flown to the February 1951 National Agricultural Aviation Conference for demonstration. Modifications and improvements continued until July, when the plane was taken on a demonstration tour through most of the agricultural area of the United States. The airplane was well received by pilots; it obtained a 98% satisfactory rating. Demonstrations, improvements, and modifications continued until June 26, 1953, when the crashworthiness features were accidently evaluated. In a sharp turn during a demonstration flight that day, the aircraft hit a utility pole with its left wing, flipped over, and crashed inverted. The pilot was unhurt except for a sore thumb on the hand that was on the control stick.

Technical data, design reports, specifications, and blueprints for fabrication of the AG-1 were made available in 1952 (at a cost of only $50). These data, and the wreckage of the AG-1, were purchased by George Wing, who modified the design and produced the Ag-2 agricultural airplane. In 1953, Weick began development of an agricultural aircraft with improved performance (the Ag-3) under contract with Piper Aircraft. Weick later joined Piper Aircraft, and the Ag-3 prototype was developed into the Piper Pawnee agricultural aircraft. The AG-1 design concept also served as a prototype for the Leland Snow S-1 and S-2 aircraft (later to become the North American Rockwell Thrush) the Grumman Ag-Cat, and the Cessna Ag-Wagon.

The Beech Bonanzas

In 1951, Beech Aircraft Corporation introduced the new model C35 Bonanza single-engine and model 50 Twin-Bonanza (two-engine) airplanes. These aircraft incorporated many safety features that were advocated by the CIR project:

- A long, crushable structure ahead of the occupied area that could provide energy absorption in a crash.
- Reinforcement under the fuselage to reduce the tendency to "dig in" during a crash and to reduce fuselage crushing from below.
- Concentration of mass forward and below the cabin, to reduce the problem of cabin intrusion by high-mass structure.
- Reinforced cabin structure to maintain interior space during a crash.
- Instrument panel mounted on shock mounts designed to shear during a severe crash so that the panel could move forward, out of head-strike range.
- Thin, crushable sheet-metal shields around the instrument panel to absorb localized impact energy.
- The control wheel was provided with a broad, flat surface to support the body and reduce chest and lung injuries in a crash.
- Seats were mounted on basic structure, and front seat backs were designed to swing forward out of the head-strike range of occupants in the rear seat.
- A "Beech Hi-Strength Safety Harness" available for all seats.

The Beech safety harness provided dual-shoulder belts that passed from a common point at the top-center of the seat back through the safety-belt fittings on either side of the seat bottom and were then buckled near the center of the body to form the safety belt.

As Beech announced these safety features, they launched a campaign to inform their customers about the safety benefits of their new aircraft, and particularly the benefits of the new restraint system. This campaign included production of a 10-minute movie, *Elmer Gets A Workout*, which included the dynamic tests conducted by Beech in developing the safety harness. Despite these valiant efforts, the safety features were not enthusiastically received by most customers. The "passive" safety features of the aircraft

were generally accepted without complaint, but customers objected to the safety harness (even though the restraint could also be used as only a simple safety belt, with the shoulder straps fitting smoothly against the seat back). Some owners demanded that the restraint system be removed from their airplanes and that conventional seat belts be installed instead. This negative customer reaction became well known throughout the industry and served to discourage action by industry or the government to implement the general use of shoulder belts.

ACIR

In a 1946 editorial written for the *Journal of the American Medical Association*, De Haven urged that physicians help in obtaining data on the nature, location, and severity of injuries sustained by victims of survivable automobile crashes.[39] He described the benefits already found for safety belts, shoulder harnesses, instrument panels made of a ductile structure that would distribute the force and absorb the energy in impacts, and control wheels with broad surfaces that would support the chest and cause lesser injuries under extreme crash conditions. He proposed that these findings were equally applicable to automobile accidents.

A student attending De Haven's lecture at the Northwestern University Traffic Institute in 1949, Corporal Elmer C. Paul, of the Indiana State Police, was impressed by the success of the CIR studies of the causes of injury in aircraft crashes. Shortly thereafter, Hasbrook was visiting with Paul to coordinate aircraft accident investigation procedures when it was learned that a police officer had been killed in an automobile crash. Hasbrook's comment that the aircraft investigation procedures could be successfully applied to automobile crashes motivated Paul to seek support from his superiors for an automobile-crash injury study. This was expanded to a state-wide project to collect data on rural fatal accidents involving motor vehicles.

De Haven used the early results from the Indiana study in a 1952 paper to show how the aviation developments could enhance crash protection in automobiles.[44] He also suggested adding padding in the head-strike zone and improving door strikes and hinges to hold doors closed during a crash. His comment that shoulder harnesses, which did an "amazing job" of protecting the occupant, would not be accepted in automobiles for "psychological reasons" proved to be prophetic.

Sensing that the automobile industry was ready to move ahead with improvements in crash injury protection, De Haven hosted a conference at Cornell Medical College in December 1952. As a result of this meeting, an Automotive Crash Injury Research project (ACIR) was begun as a special division of the CIR project. The ACIR effort extended the Indiana automobile crash study to 30 states; it collected detailed information and photographs on accidents and injury data on survivors as well as fatalities. The results of these studies supported the expansion of auto-industry studies of crashes, which ultimately resulted in automobiles with specific crash-injury-protection features being offered to the public.

AvCIR

The rapid growth of the ACIR program after 1952 caused the CIR project to outgrow its facilities at Cornell University Medical College. In March 1954, the aviation and automotive divisions were physically separated, with the Aviation Crash Injury Research project (AvCIR) attached to the Cornell–Guggenheim Aviation Safety Center with the Flight Safety Foundation, an organization founded in 1945 by De Haven and Lederer for the promotion of flight safety. Hasbrook was appointed director of the AvCir project. By the time Hasbrook resigned this position to join the FAA Civil Aeromedical Institute in 1960, he had authored or co-authored over 60 reports dealing with various aspects of accident investigation and crash injury protection. It was also during this period that AvCIR began to publish a *Crash Survival Design Manual*. This manual was composed of a series of loose-leaf inserts that covered topics such as human tolerance to

impact, seat anchorages, inadvertent release of seat-belt buckles, seat pans and cushions, shoulder harness tie-down, instrument panels and delethalization, and the effectiveness of the tie-down chain. Later, an extensive expansion of this beginning work resulted in the first crash-survival design guide.

AvSER

With most of its support provided by military organizations, the direction of AvCIR's work became more and more directed toward the needs of the services. Administration of AvCIR was transferred to the Flight Safety Foundation (FSF) in April 1959, and the name was changed to Aviation Safety Engineering and Research (AvSER) in May 1963. The name change reflected a change in emphasis of activity toward the engineering aspects of crashworthiness design. A summary of the military aspects of the AvSER project has been reported elsewhere.[27]

A major achievement of this program was the development of a *Crash Survival Design Guide* (*CSDG*). This report provides design data and guidance that can be used to incorporate crashworthiness features in airplanes and helicopters. First published in 1967, the *CSDG* has gone through a number of revisions and expansions, and presently contains five volumes:[11]

Volume 1: *Design Criteria and Checklist*
Volume 2: *Aircraft Design Crash Impact Conditions and Human Tolerance*
Volume 3: *Aircraft Structural Crash Resistance*
Volume 4: *Aircraft Seats, Restraints, Litters, and Cockpit/Cabin Delethalization*
Volume 5: *Aircraft Postcrash Survival*

The *CSDG* was, however, only a guide. It was not required for use in any aircraft and was not in a format that could easily be incorporated into military contracts. Military specifications and standards were developed so that they could be used in procurement of crashworthy seats and helicopters.[9,10] These were used in developing the first U.S. Army helicopter that was designed to be crashworthy, the Sikorsky UH-60 Blackhawk.

AvSER Crash Tests of Transport Airplanes

Although the major programs conducted by AvSER during the 1960s were funded by and directed toward military applications, AvSER also continued to work on civil crash problems. In 1963, AvSER was awarded a contract by the FAA to conduct two full-scale crash tests using large transport-type aircraft. These tests still provide the most useful test data available for understanding the crash environment in severe, but survivable, crashes of large transport airplanes.

The tests, conducted in April and September of 1964, used a Douglas DC-7 airplane [77] and a Lockheed model 1649A Constellation airplane.[78] The airplanes, under their own power, were guided by a 4,000-ft rail to a prepared crash site, where they first hit barriers designed to break landing gear, propellors, and wing structure, and then crashed into a specially prepared earthen hill with an initial slope of 8 (first test) or 6 degrees and a final slope of 20 degrees. The initial impact velocity in the two tests was 71 m/sec and 58 m/sec, respectively.

Numerous seat and restraint experiments were carried on the airplanes. Failure of the attachment of seats to the airplane, failure of seat backs, structural failure due to overload, and indications of head impact with the seat backs or interior were observed in many of the experiments. Seats located over the wing structure and toward the rear of the aircraft appeared more successful in withstanding the crash environment. Preinflated air bags used (with seat belts) restrained occupants even though the seat backs that supported the air bags broke forward. Seat backs of military rearward-facing seats failed in the first test, releasing the occupants, but performed well in the second test. In the second test, a dummy was successfully restrained in a passenger seat equipped with a three-point restraint having an energy absorber in the shoulder-belt retractor.

Both crashes contained child-restraint experiments. In the first test, a child dummy was restrained in a passenger seat by a vest-type restraint even though the seat was damaged due to vertical load. However, it appeared that the child dummy had been subjected to considerable flailing. In the second test, a child dummy was restrained in an aft inboard seat by a harness-type child restraint system that was attached to the floor by a single strap that passed between the seat back and seat pan. Also, weighted infant dolls were placed in two airline-type bassinets. A bassinet with a nylon net to restrain the doll was attached to the forward wall of a cloak closet located in the tail. The other bassinet, with crossover straps to restrain the doll, was placed on the floor of the closet, with its side against the forward wall. Both bassinets retained the dolls and remained in position, although the bassinet on the floor turned completely over.

NACA and NASA Studies

After the war, De Haven and DuBois urged that crash tests be performed with surplus airplanes to measure the forces generated in survivable crashes and to document the events on film. The National Advisory Committee on Aeronautics (NACA) responded by initiating a comprehensive study of airplane crash problems at the Lewis Flight Propulsion Laboratory in Cleveland, Ohio. The laboratory had developed a *ground-to-ground* technique for crashing airplanes as part of a study of aircraft fires.[14] This technique was used for crash tests of light airplanes,[51] low-wing jet fighter airplanes,[1] and transport airplanes.[75]

The accelerations measured in the transport airplane crash tests were analyzed to determine impact pulse shapes for design purposes.[74] Typically, the crash deceleration consisted of a primary-impact pulse of low magnitude and long duration, with a superimposed secondary pulse of short duration and high magnitude. A second crash pulse, which brought the aircraft to a final stop, was frequently observed. The data shown in Table 7.1 were considered to be representative of severe crashes. A simple linear spring-mass model was developed to study the seat response to a crash pulse, and experimental seats were tested to

TABLE 7.1. Data from NACA crash tests of large airplanes[a]

	First crash deceleration							
	Transport (low wing)				Cargo (high wing)			
Velocity change, m/sec	15	25	40	55	15	25	40	55
	Primary pulse							
Maximum g's	12	18	20	20	4	8	10	10
Pulse duration, seconds	0.20	0.20	0.25	0.30	0.50	0.38	0.46	0.58
Rise time, seconds	Since	0.06	0.045	0.03	Since	0.10	0.08	0.06
	Secondary pulse							
Maximum g's	10	15	20	25	7	10	12	15
Pulse duration, seconds	0.20	0.03	0.04	0.03	0.06	0.04	0.04	0.03
	Secondary crash deceleration							
Primary pulse, g's	9	9	7	1	4	4	3	1
Secondary pulse g's	8	7	7	1	6	5	4	1

These test data indicated that crash environment could be represented by a fairly long, low-amplitude acceleration with a superimposed high-acceleration secondary pulse. In addition, a second deceleration of lower magnitude was evident.

verify the model predictions. The conclusions were:

- Slack in the seat or restraint system will have unfavorable consequences. Slack could be caused by loose restraints, restraints that slip or stretch under low loads, and soft or deep seat cushions. A proper seat-pan cushion should compress completely under the weight of the occupant and bring his buttocks substantially in contact with the seat pan.
- The practice of fastening seats to both the airplane fuselage wall and the floor exposes the seat to failure when the airplane structure distorts during a crash.
- Floor structure that flexes in a crash can seriously alter the seat's natural frequency and reduce the ability of the seat to support the passenger.
- Higher landing and takeoff speeds increase the probability that more than one principal deceleration pulse will be experienced in a crash. Seats should have residual strength after exposure to the design crash deceleration pulse.

Martin Eiband's summary of the literature pertaining to human tolerance to impact is perhaps the best known of the reports gen-erated by the NACA program.[52] He consolidated data from both animal and human tests and presented the data on the basis of a standardized trapezoidal-shaped impact pulse for impact accelerations directed toward the spine, sternum, head, and tail.

The results of Eiband's survey indicated that adequate torso and extremity restraint was the primary variable in establishing tolerance limits. Only when adequate restraint was provided did the variables of impact direction, magnitude, and rate of onset govern maximum tolerance and injury levels. Survival of impact forces increased with increased distribution of force to the entire skeleton, for all impacts from all directions. The major portion of the impact force should be transmitted directly to the pelvic structure. Restraints should be designed to support the vertebral column and pelvic girdle to maintain the normal standing alignment as nearly as possible. Restraining straps that apply forces to soft abdominal tissue should be avoided.

Following this guidance, Eiband suggested that the rear-facing seats would offer maximum body support with minimum objectionable harnessing, but cautioned that such a seat, "whether designed for 20, 30 or 40 G dynamic loading," should include lap strap, chest strap, a winged back (to increase headward and lateral *g* protection), full-height integral head rest, load-bearing armrests with recessed handholds and provisions to prevent the arms from slipping either laterally or beyond the seat back, and leg support to keep the legs from being wedged under the seat. For forward-facing seats, he suggested that proper restraint would require lap, shoulder, and thigh straps, lap-belt tie-down strap, and a full-height seat back with integral head support.

Eiband's summary plot for headward acceleration is shown in Fig. 7.8. This plot is typical of the presentation of data in the report. It will be noted that the plot combines data from tests of human subjects (to define the area of voluntary exposure) with data from animal tests (to define the area of serious injury). No corrections for size or species differences

were attempted. Also, in this figure, the area representing "limits upon which current ejection seats are designed" is taken from a 1944 translation of a German ejection seat study that described the area as limits of static and dynamic tolerance of vertebra.[60]

As this first NACA/NASA program was being completed, Pinkel used the data to compare the potential performance of forward- and rearward-facing passenger seats for transport airplanes.[74] His analysis indicated that forward-facing seats would have significantly greater strength than rear-facing seats of the same weight in crashes with durations greater than 0.125 seconds, and might be better in crashes that didn't involve fire or ditching. However, in crashes involving fire or ditching, passengers should survive the crash with only minor injuries so that they can rapidly evacuate

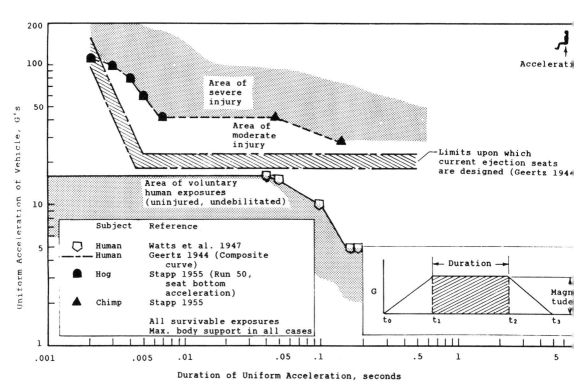

FIGURE 7.8. Eiband's curve for vertical acceleration tolerance. This figure shows four levels of tolerance. The lowest level represents the uninjured experience of human voluntary test exposure. A slightly higher zone represents the design level for equipment such as ejection seats that would be voluntarily

used in emergency situations. Above this zone is the area of moderate injury, where full recovery is possible. Finally, the highest zone represents the area of severe injury as defined by animal testing. Aircraft structure is generally incapable of sustaining the forces represented by this highest zone the airplane without assistance. Rearward-facing seats appeared to have an advantage under those conditions.

The next major aircraft crashworthiness program by the National Aeronautics and Space Administration (NASA) began in 1973. In August of the previous year, a hurricane caused extensive flooding of the Piper Aircraft Corporation facility at Lock Haven, Pennsylvania, submerging many new and almost-completed airplanes. Since these airframes could not be made airworthy, they were offered to the government for nonflight research purposes. These 35 low-wing airframes and four high-wing Cessna 172 airframes were used in a joint NASA–FAA crash dynamics program conducted at the NASA Langley Research Center in Virginia.

The objectives of this program were to determine the effects of impact speed, flight-path angle, roll angle, and ground condition on the dynamic response of airplane structures, seats, and occupants during crashes in which the airplane structure retained sufficient volume and integrity to permit occupant survival. The airframes were swung from a large gantry onto concrete or soil impact surfaces at speeds ranging from 12 to 40 m/sec. Twenty-eight tests were completed.[19,94] Data from these tests are summarized in Table 7.2.

The horizontal slide-out distance following the major impact was found to be important in assessing the longitudinal impulse data. A coefficient of friction of 0.42 was found to represent the slide-out distance found in the concrete impacts with gear retracted or broken off. Slide-out distances in the soil impacts (tests 11 and FAA 4) were very short and resulted in high longitudinal decelerations.

The program of controlled crash tests was supplemented by development efforts to improve seat and floor-structure performance. A "corrugated beam–notched corner" energy-absorbing subfloor concept was developed that could reduce floor decelerations as much as 50% in some crashes and also reduce intrusion into the cabin space. Three types of prototype energy-absorbing seats were installed in the crashed airframes: a seat with S-shaped legs similar in concept to an earlier Piper Aircraft

seat;[96] a tube-guided, vertically stroking seat similar to earlier helicopter seats;[56] and a seat with legs having a stroking diagonal link for energy absorption.[19] These seats absorbed some energy as they stroked but showed problems with seat-leg breakage, seat and restraint incompatibilities, and floor deformation causing eccentric loading on the seats. A sled test program, in cooperation with the FAA Civil Aeromedical Institute, was then initiated to continue seat development.[2,53] Seats suspended from the ceiling by energy absorbers that were similar to earlier troop seats used in military helicopters[79] were found unsuitable for small airplanes because of the tendency of the roof structure to collapse under certain crash loads. Seats with parallelogram-linkage-type seat legs, and an energy absorber that could stroke into the seat-back structure, were found to provide good energy absorption. A "tilting" seat design that used a rigid seat bucket intended to rotate from an upright position to a reclined position during a crash exhibited a number of hardware malfunctions and was not further developed.

FAA Studies

The Federal Aviation Administration (FAA) now holds responsibility for most governmental functions pertaining to civil aviation, including fostering air commerce; use of airspace; provision of air navigation facilities and air traffic control; and the certification of airmen, aircraft, and aviation operations. Provision of a safe environment for civil aviation is an inherent goal of all the functions within the FAA. Traditionally, the safety goals of these functions have been linked by the concept of "accident prevention." The importance of accident prevention was readily accepted by most manufacturers, owners, and operators of aircraft, so accident prevention became a widely practiced industry goal.

The early success of accident prevention in aviation has already been described. After the Second World War, the aviation accident-prevention program met with continued success (Figs. 7.9 and 7.10). The transport aviation industry, in particular, was rewarded

TABLE 7.2. Data from NASA crash tests of small airplanes.[a]

Test No.	Aircraft and impact surface	Crash velocity, m/sec			Aircraft pitch angle, degrees	Primary aircraft crash pulse					
						Maximum $-g$		Duration (ms)		Velocity change (m/sec)	
		V_R	V_V	V_H		z	x	z	x	z	x
1	t; u; l; c	12.7	3.6	12.1	−12	N. R.		N. R.		N. R.	
3	t; u; l; c	26.7	7.4	25.6	−12	20	19	89	60	8.5	6
4	t; u; l; c	26.2	8.4	24.8	−18	28	18	50	44	8.7	4.3
	t; u; l; c	27.4	7	26.5	4	16	7	102	101	8.5	5
5	t; u; l; c	26.1	9.1	24.4	−19.5	N. R.		N. R.		N. R.	
6	t; u; l; c	26.9	7.6	25.8	14	18	8	110	110	10.4	3.1
7	t; u; l; c	28.6	21.1	19.3	−47.25	20	8.8	174	144	20.7	4.6
8	t; u; l; c	27.6	13.8	23.9	−31	18	16	135	110	13	6
9	t; u; l; c	26.3	7.3	25.3	−13	N. R.		N. R.		N. R.	
10	t; u; l; c	27.8	8.6	26.4	−14	N. R.		N. R.		N. R.	
11	s; u; l; s	25	12.9	21.4	−27	12	28	132	138	10	17.7
12	s; u; l; c	25	6.5	24.1	9	12	4	149	60	9.5	1.2
13	s; u; l; c	25	12.1	21.9	−26	27	11	49	93	13	5
14	t; p; l; c	32.7	9.5	31.4	−11.75	N. R.		N. R.		N. R.	
15	t; p; l; c	41.4	12.7	39.3	−12	46	16	64	58	17	5
16	t; u; l; c	40	10.4	38.6	−4	46	12	54	62	15	4
17	t; p; l; c	40	20	34.6	−38	42	22	97	68	19	10
18	t; u; l; c	27.9	13.9	24.2	−31	27.2	15.2	83	90	11.3	8.2
19	t; u; l; c	27	7	26.1	−17.7	16	5.5	120	88	10.6	4
20	t; u; l; c	26.6	7.1	25.6	2	31	6.4	57	52	9.1	1.9
21	t; u; l; c	27.1	13.6	23.5	−29.5	29.9	14	96	112	12.3	10.5
22	t; l; p; c	33.7	8.7	32.6	0	N. R.		N. R.		N. R.	
23	t; l; p; c	36.4	9.4	35.2	1.2	N. R.		N. R.		N. R.	
24	t; l; p; c	37.9	9.8	36.6	2.5	N. R.		N. R.		N. R.	
Additional FAA-sponsored tests											
1	s; h; u; c	25	12.5	21.6	−32	21	22	120	110	11	8
2	s; h; u; c	23	6.7	22	13.5	7	3.5	160	60	6	1.5
3	s; h; u; c	25.9	14.7	21.3	−39	18	17	120	130	13.8	12
4	s; h; u; s	25.3	13.9	21.4	−34.5	18	45	130	100	14.8	21.5

[a] Notation in the second column of this table represent twin (t) or single (s) engine aircraft, low (l) or high (h) wings, pressurized (p) or unpressurized (u) fuselage design, and impacts on concrete (c) or soil (s). The vertical (V_V) and horizontal (V_H) components of the resultant impact velocity (V_R) are shown in the third column. Data for the primary aircraft crash pulse as measured along the normal (z) and longitudinal (x) aircraft axis are shown in the last columns. N. R., Not reported.

with an outstanding safety history, and the perfect record of "zero annual fatalities" became an achievable goal.

The success of the accident-prevention program led many to discount the potential for a general program of injury prevention in those crashes that still took place. The arguments against injury prevention were pervasive in a system that was satisfied with its safety performance:

- The costs of an injury-prevention program would be excessive and those resources could be more beneficially applied to further improving the already-successful accident-prevention efforts.
- The techniques for crash injury protection would add excessive weight to the airplane. This would decrease performance and thus increase the potential for accidents.
- Head injury was the most serious threat in

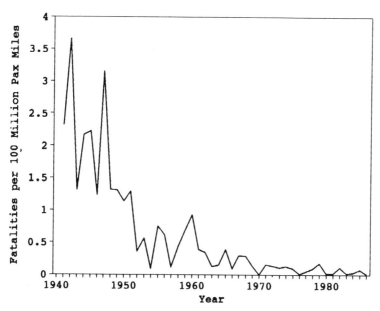

FIGURE 7.9. Recent fatality rates in scheduled domestic air travel. The continued success of the accident-prevention program is shown in this figure. The fatality rate approaches zero in several years. While this outstanding success speaks well for the accident-prevention program, it makes it difficult to justify improved crash-injury-prevention technology in large transport airplanes unless the costs of incorporating that technology are minimal.

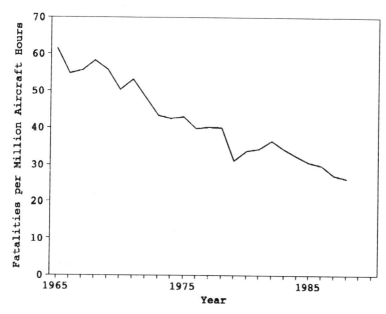

FIGURE 7.10. Recent fatality rates in small aircraft. The downward trend of the fatality rate in small aircraft again shows the success of the accident prevention program. However, the fatality rate has not yet approached the zero level.

crashes. The most practical way to prevent head injury was to use a shoulder harness. But pilot error was already a major cause of accidents. Pilots who were so insensitive to safety issues as to cause the accident wouldn't wear the shoulder harness either. The pilots who cared about safety wouldn't be involved in accidents, and wouldn't need crash protection.

- Crash injury protection was not important to people who bought airplanes. They wouldn't pay for crash-injury-protection features, even if offered.

Arguments such as these, the continued success of the accident-prevention program in reducing aviation-related deaths (Figs. 7.9 and 7.10), and the lack of any broad-based support for mandatory requirements for crash injury protection did not prompt regulatory action in this area until recently. However, the FAA did provide continuing (but relatively modest) support for medical research.

The need for improved crash injury protection has long been advocated in the civil aviation medical service. In 1947, William R. Stovall, medical director for aeronautics, proposed improvements of aircraft seats and restraint systems:[65]

- Strength requirements for seatbelts and their fastenings should be increased to resist forces of 200 pounds at $40g$.
- Seat tie-downs should resist thrust loads of at least $20g$ before tearing away from their moorings.
- Shoulder harnesses should be provided for all members of a flight crew.

No evidence of a formal response to these proposals has been found.

In this same year, a civil aviation medical-research program began with the appointment of Dr. Barry King as research executive for the CAA Aviation Medical Service. A research laboratory was established in Oklahoma City under the direction of John Swearingen, a former aviation physiologist with the navy. While the major effort of the research program was to review the physical standards for pilot certification, Stovall also directed that inves-

tigations of hazardous features of aircraft design be accomplished. Unfortunately, 1948 and 1949 were years of budget tightening, and aeromedical research was not among the CAA's top priorities. Funds for a new laboratory could not be found, and Swearingen operated out of a vacant building at the Aeronautical Center in Oklahoma City.

King continued to press for improvements in injury protection for aircraft. In 1949 he submitted a proposal to a CAA-CAB subcommittee (set up to evaluate proposals for Civil Air Regulations) that the regulations be changed so that:

After June, 1950, new aircraft are required to have provisions for anchoring shoulder harness or equivalent restraining protection against the pilot's head being allowed to go forward and striking structure or equipment of the airplane. In the manual of the aircraft the shoulder harness or restraining devices should be described so that the owners can procure them and install them at their own discretion.[29]

Stovall continued to press for shoulder belts, recommending in 1950 that:

on all airplanes manufactured after 1 June 1951 having a seating capacity of six persons or less, the aircraft structures which carried safety belts or harness loads be capable of withstanding inertial forces of $3g$'s upward, $9g$'s forward, and $1.5g$'s sideward; . . . and that all airplanes manufactured after that same date were to have built-in provisions (attachments) for the installation of CAA approved shoulder harnesses for each occupant.[65]

In 1951, Stovall also recommended installation of shoulder harnesses for crew members on transport airplanes. These recommendations seem to have had little effect other than to provide a source of friction between Stovall and the regulating authorities.

Swearingen began studies of windshield strain patterns, pilot comfort, measurements for cockpit design, protection against explosive decompression, and impact protection. Sensing the need for a crash test dummy with more humanlike characteristics than the hinged rigid-mass dummies then available, he designed and built one of the first anthropomorphic dummies.[90] This dummy was used by Beech Aircraft in developing the restraint system for the Bonanza airplanes and served as a prototype for the dummy provided by the air force for use in the NACA crash tests described earlier. De Haven had stressed the ideas of protecting against head injury in crashes by providing adequate head clearance or by the use of energy-absorbing structure to distribute the impact forces over the head. Swearingen defined the strike paths for the head and trunk under simulated crash forces.[91]

A study of human voluntary tolerance to vertical impact while standing with knees locked, standing with knees bending, squatting, seated in a rigid chair, and seated in an energy-absorbing chair was conducted in cooperation with the navy.[92] This study provided human impact data on short-duration exposures up to 250g and demonstrated the effectiveness of energy-absorbing seats in increasing voluntary tolerance. Studies of aircraft crashes confirmed that head injuries remained the major source of injury and death. Data from automobile crashes and laboratory tests of cadaver head impact provided measures of the tolerance of the human face to crash impact. Tests were performed to evaluate the impact hazards of aircraft instrument panels, airline seat backs, and the protection offered by padding materials or crushable structure. Continued investigations of crashes involving small airplanes and agricultural airplanes served to emphasize both the problems and potential for crash injury protection.[48]

Other investigators in the Civil Aeromedical Research Laboratory were also studying problems of crash impact. Hasbrook joined the Laboratory and continued crash investigations, most notably documenting evacuation problems in transport airplanes.[63] R.G. Snyder studied free-falls to obtain survival data under extreme impact loads [82-84] and led a cooperative project with the air force to investigate injury patterns with a variety of restraint systems.[85-88] These studies provided some of the first evidence of the effectiveness of airbags in impacts using living (animal) subjects and on impact injuries during pregnancy.

After Swearingen's retirement in 1971, the Civil Aeromedical Institute (CAMI) Protection and Survival Laboratory was placed under the direction of R.F. Chandler, an engineer who had been involved with dynamic testing since 1956 at the Aeromedical Laboratory at Holloman Air Force Base and with the U.S. Bureau of Standards. Chandler, new to the civil aviation industry and to the FAA, organized the laboratory along program lines, with sections responsible for transport-aircraft emergency evacuation and cabin safety, protective breathing systems (oxygen and smoke protection), aircraft accident investigation, flotation systems, physical anthropology, and crash injury protection. He then began an informal assessment of the use of research findings by the FAA and the aviation industry. In the area of crash injury protection, he found that there was little concern except for the agricultural aircraft applications. (The agricultural aircraft were the exception because crashes were considered a regular hazard of agricultural aircraft applications.) The "Beech experience" of having customers reject the installation of shoulder harnesses had not been forgotten. Kits for optional installation of shoulder harnesses had been designed for several airplanes, but they were almost never requested by new airplane buyers or owners of existing airplanes. A few examples of what we would now call "passive" protection were being used: some control wheels had broad contact surfaces that would help distribute chest impact loads, some instrument-panel glare shields would fold over the panel when impacted by the head, and seat backs in transport airplanes were often constructed of lightweight sheet aluminum, which crushed and absorbed energy when impacted by the passenger in a crash. Several manufacturers of passenger seats for transport airplanes had offered seats with energy-absorbing features in the early 1960s, but these had not been demanded by customers and were generally dropped from production in favor of lighter-weight, less-expensive designs.

There were no "injury reduction" performance standards for these attempts, and no one knew how effective they would be. These designs usually resulted from the efforts of one or two individuals responsible for interior design. Typically, these people were highly motivated and well intentioned, and had the support of their management, but they had neither the resources nor the time to become specialists in sophisticated designs for crash injury protection. Most seat and restraint system designs were based on traditional static load analysis, and only two manufacturers had minimal dynamic test capability for seat and restraint systems.

Even though statistics showed a trend of decreasing fatalities in civil aircraft, the industry was becoming increasingly perplexed by the issue of *crashworthiness litigation*. The responsibility for accident prevention had long been accepted, but the concept of being held strictly liable for injury without regard to the cause of an accident was new and unfamiliar. one result of this sensitivity was an increasing reluctance to freely discuss problems pertaining to crashworthiness or the solutions to those problems. Nevertheless, attempts were being made to develop better seat, restraint, and interior systems. Engineers pursuing those improvements were generally receptive to constructive private discussions.

By this time, it was generally acknowledged within the FAA that shoulder belts would improve crash protection in airplanes. In 1969, the FAA had amended its rules to require (in newly certified small airplanes) protection from head impact by a shoulder harness, high seat back (for rear-facing seats), or elimination of injurious objects within the striking radius of the head. A "Notice of Proposed Rulemaking" was being developed that would have required shoulder harnesses in all seats in newly certified small airplanes unless injurious objects were removed from within the head-strike zone. (Substantial opposition to the restraint system requirements of this proposal resulted in a rule that required shoulder harnesses only in the front seats of small airplanes manufactured after July 18, 1978. In 1985, the rules were finally changed to require shoulder harnesses for all occupants of small airplanes manufactured after December 12, 1986.) Unfortunately, there were no test procedures

or measurable performance requirements to evaluate the effectiveness of the installations, so neither the industry nor the FAA knew if an adequate system would be certified under these rules.

Chandler was also aware of the significance of the creation of the National Highway Safety Bureau (now the National Highway Traffic Safety Administration, NHTSA) just a few years earlier. Funding for this agency alone had resulted in a ninefold increase in all federal funding for biomechanics crashworthiness projects.[12] At least as important as the magnitude of the funding was the fact that these new resources were to be under the control of a single government agency, rather than split among several military and civilian groups having diverse interests and priorities. Furthermore, the *compliance testing* regulatory approach taken by the NHTSA (as opposed to the *certification* methods used by the FAA) would encourage the automobile industry to devote even more resources to crashworthiness research and product development. It was apparent that progress in the biomechanics of crash injury would now rest largely in the laboratories of those engaged in automobile research. While that progress would be directed toward automobile applications, it was expected that many of the findings would be equally applicable to the problems of injury reduction in civil aircraft.

As the assessment of the role of crashworthiness in civil aircraft continued, Chandler refurbished the CAMI dynamic test facility and initiated a test program that stressed cooperation with manufacturers of civil aircraft and other government agencies that were pursuing crash-injury reduction techniques that might be applicable to civil aviation. This program had several goals. Dynamic test results would provide a more realistic assessment of equipment performance. This could lead to improvements in the crash protection equipment offered to the public. By participating in the testing, engineers from industry would become more familiar with dynamic testing techniques and be more willing to use those techniques in developing seat, restraint, and interior systems. The FAA could become more familiar with the ability of the industry to develop improved systems. Test techniques developed for crashworthy military aircraft would be used in evaluating military systems, and the military test procedures could then be adapted for use in tests of civil aircraft systems. Advanced military seat and restraint technology could be evaluated for potential applications in civil aircraft.

This program was well received and proved effective. Typical results included the demonstration of practical improvements in civil aircraft seat and restraint systems,[20,21,23] energy-absorbing seat concepts for both military and civil aircraft,[53,96,66,80,49,22,31] and conventional and inflatable restraint systems.[81,71,20,21,23] Many of the improvements developed through this program have been placed in service. A major cooperative program with Cessna Aircraft Company had begun just before the start of the General Aviation Safety Panel effort to improve small-airplane-occupant crash protection. This program was to provide the prototype seat and restraint system for that effort.

Development of Regulations for Injury Reduction

The General Aviation Safety Panel

In 1982, FAA Administrator J. Lynn Helms requested the formation of an independent panel to recommend regulatory and non-regulatory ways by which the FAA could promote general aviation safety. A panel of 13 people representing the senior management from aircraft manufacturers, operators, and insurers, organizations representing owners, pilots, home builders, aircraft safety foundations, and publishers dedicated to the general aviation community was formed. The group, which became known as the General Aviation Safety Panel (GASP), made specific recommendations to the FAA on February 9, 1983. These recommendations included establishment of night weather minimums, better dissemination of weather information and

safety data, yearly recurrent training for pilots, and improved crashworthiness for small airplanes.

The GASP recommendations for improved crashworthiness included the following three action items:

- Require that all newly manufactured small airplanes be equipped with shoulder harness or some other form of upper-torso restraint, and that they be used.
- Promote the installation and use of shoulder harnesses on all part 23 (general aviation) aircraft.
- Establish a joint FAA–NASA program office to establish an industry group to coordinate research and use of crashworthiness data, to monitor dynamic tests to determine the capability of typical production seats, to serve as a clearinghouse for all existing crashworthiness data, to accelerate research to confirm or revise regulatory criteria to account for dynamic loads, and to collect meaningful accident data on the effectiveness of seat and restraint systems.

In response, the FAA indicated that action would be taken on the first two recommendations as part of existing regulatory and accident prevention projects, but requested an extension of the GASP to undertake the third action item. Accordingly, a technical working group was formed by the GASP. Aircraft manufacturers and suppliers, FAA CAMI and regulatory activities, the NTSB, NASA, the U.S. Army, and organizations representing flight safety, owners and pilots, and developers of experimental aircraft participated in this working group, which became known as GASP-1.

The group met formally at 1-month intervals beginning in September 1983. The group agreed that a dynamic test procedure involving the seat, restraint, occupant, and interior "system" of the aircraft should be developed. The two dynamic test configurations outlined in the U.S. Army Crash Survival Design Guide (CSDG) had proven effective in CAMI tests of military systems and were used as a basis for the test procedure to be developed. The first of these tests generated forces that drove the occupant down and forward relative to the airframe. The primary purpose of this test was to evaluate the performance of seat and restraint systems in crashes that produced large vertical loads and the need for energy-absorbing seat design to limit spinal compression injuries. The second test generated forces that drove the occupant forward and laterally relative to the airframe. This test is primarily a test of the structural integrity of the seat and restraint system. A requirement for "floor deformation" was adapted from the static test requirements outlined in the CSDG and made a part of the dynamic tests. This requirement is intended to limit excessive seat structural rigidity and to assure that seat deformation and energy absorption could take place without breaking the seat attachment to the aircraft. Occupant head-strike envelopes (displacements and velocities) from both tests generated conditions for interior delethalization of the aircraft.

The deceleration-time conditions for these two system tests were based on extensive discussions within the GASP-1 group. Test pulses in the CSDG for military-helicopter seats, the results of the NASA crash tests of small airplanes (previously discussed), the findings of an FAA-sponsored study of civil helicopter accidents[32,33] and an NTSB study of small-airplane crashes,[30,67-69] and the suggestions of working-group participants were considered. Twenty-four tests of seats provided by six manufactures of small airplanes were conducted at CAMI to assess the performance of typical seats under tentatively selected test conditions.[25] A more detailed discussion of these deliberations has been previously documented.[27]

Reduced decelerations (80%) were suggested for seats behind front seats. In addition, it was recommended that static tests, with forces equivalent to those generated by a 215-pound occupant (95th-percentile male), should be used to demonstrate seat and restraint system performance throughout the aircraft's entire design performance envelope. It was also recommended that the FAA develop advisory material to define acceptable methods and criteria for *floor warping* in the

dynamic tests, for secondary impact of the occupant with the interior of the airplane, and for acceptable variations in the shape of the impact pulse.

Performance requirements were also being developed in the discussions. Perhaps the most difficult to resolve was the problem of a criteria for spinal injury. Spinal compression loading has long been considered a problem in aircraft crashes that can generate high vertical forces. The air force had developed the *Dynamic Response Index* (DRI) as a means of evaluating the likelihood of spinal injury during seat or capsule ejection from combat aircraft.[15] The DRI represents the maximum response of a single degree-of-freedom, damped, spring-mass system forced into oscillation by the acceleration of the seat. The procedure is well known in the aviation industry. The DRI had been used at CAMI in several cooperative programs with the military services. However, CAMI found it difficult to apply the DRI in tests of civil aircraft seats because the flexible lightweight construction of most seats made it difficult to define a single seat acceleration measurement that could be used with the DRI model. In addition, the DRI could not consider spinal column loading which might result from the shoulder harness. This is a problem with some aircraft installations in which the shoulder-harness anchorages are low because of the airframe design. Finally, the DRI does not show the advantages of rearward-facing seating in reducing spinal-column loading. An earlier test program at CAMI made use of a load cell inserted at the base of the lumbar spine in the dummy.[31] This technique was then used in a CAMI–USAF program in which both the DRI and the axial loads acting on the dummy's spine were measured. This provided a direct comparison between the DRI and the compression load.[25] This comparison suggested a lumbar column compression load of 6,670 N (1,500 lbf) measured in a Hybrid II dummy would correspond to a DRI of about 19. (Ejection-seat experience would indicate a 9% probability of detectable spinal column injury in seats that produced a DRI of 19.) This force was selected as a performance criteria for their recommendations.

Other performance criteria selected by the GASP-1 group included a 7,780-N (1,750 lbf) limit on the tension force in a diagonal shoulder belt and a 8,900-N (2,000 lbf) limit on the combined tension in a dual shoulder-belt system. These limits were intended to limit injuries resulting from the diagonal strap[55] as well as to require the measurement of this load for future use in airframe design. The Head Injury Criterion (HIC) was chosen as a limit for head injury in the tests because of its long history of use and acceptance in the automobile industry. Prohibitions against submarining under the safety belt and "rolling out" of a (diagonal belt) upper-torso restraint were also included.

The proposed tests were evaluated by the NTSB in light of their studies of small-airplane crashes. They estimated that fatal injuries would decrease by 20% and serious injuries would decrease by 34% in survivable accidents of aircraft that incorporated the proposed criteria.

The GASP proposal was formally submitted to the FAA on May 2, 1984.[70] It was supported by the General Aviation Manufacturers Association at the Review Conference for the Small Airplane Airworthiness Review Program held in St. Louis Missouri in October 1984. The GASP proposal, along with several other proposed changes in rules pertaining to general aviation airplanes, was included by the FAA in a "Notice of Proposed Rulemaking" (NPRM) issued in December 1986. After receiving and considering public comments regarding the NPRM, the FAA issued the final rule on August 15, 1988. This rule incorporated the GASP recommendations, with minor changes, as a requirement for general-aviation airplanes carrying no more than nine passengers that would be certified after September 14, 1988. The requirements are shown in Table 7.3.

Coincident with the work by the General Aviation Safety Panel on improved occupant crash protection, Cessna Aircraft Company proceeded with a program for developing a crew seat for the new Caravan 1 airplane.[76] The Caravan 1 is a large single-engine turbo-prop airplane designed for diverse private,

commercial, and utility applications. The project began in early 1983 and continued into 1984. As the GASP proposed new criteria, the seat design and dynamic testing program was adjusted to meet the new criteria. In effect, the Caravan 1 Crew Seat Project became a demonstration project for the GASP recommendations.

The final version of the seat incorporates a four-point restraint system attached entirely to the seat. This restraint system uses two shoulder belts, attached to the center of the top of the seat back through an inertial reel. The lower ends of the belts were attached to the seat pan at the seat-belt attachment points. A conventional seat belt was also used. An aluminum seat pan was used to limit elastic deformation under the cushion and thus to better restrain the occupant and reduce submarining. Each set of seat legs was made of a four-bar linkage arrangement with C-shaped front links. The C-shaped front legs would bend to provide energy absorption. The final tests of this seat were done in accordance with the recommendations of the GASP.

One of the recommendations of the GASP was that the FAA issue revised specifications for restraint systems with shoulder harnesses that would be consistent with the minimum dynamic performance standards being developed. No major revision had been made to the (then) current standard for aircraft restraint systems since it was issued in 1948. To assist in this effort, the FAA requested that the Society of Automotive Engineers (SAE) develop an Aerospace Standard that could serve as a basis for a new FAA standard. To do this work, the SAE established an Ad Hoc Committee on Upper Torso Restraint.

The first meeting of the committee was held at the FAA CAMI in February 1984. The first draft of the proposed Aerospace Standard was completed in May 1984 and submitted to committee members and other interested parties for comments and approval. The final draft was submitted to the SAE in September 1985 and issued as SAE Aerospace Standard 8043, Torso Restraint Systems, in March 1986. The FAA adopted the Standard as "FAA

TABLE 7.3. Recent FAA requirements for improved aircraft-seat strength and occupant crash injury protection.[a]

Category	Test parameter	Test 1	Test 2	Criteria for pass or fail
SMALL AIRPLANES, 9 or fewer passengers U.S. 14 CFR Part 23, § 23.562 (Amendment 23–36)				• HIC must be ≤1,000 during head impact
First row of seats	Minimum velocity change	31.0 ft/s (9.45 m/s)	42.0 ft/s (12.94 m/s)	• The ATD must be restrained
	Maximum rise time	0.05 s	0.05 s	• Seat may deform if intended by design
	Minimum deceleration	19.0 g	26.0 g	• Attachment between seat/restraint system and test fixture must be maintained
	Floor track misalignment, pitch/roll	0°/0°	10°/10°	• Shoulder belt(s) must remain on the ATD's shoulder(s)
Seats behind first row	Minimum velocity change	31.0 ft/s (9.45 m/s)	42.0 ft/s (12.94 m/s)	• Safety belt must remain on the ATD's pelvis
	Maximum rise time	0.06 s	0.06 s	• Individual shoulder-strap force must be ≤1,750 lb (7,784 N), with total (dual) shoulder-strap force ≤2,000 lb (8,896 N)
	Minimum deceleration	15.0 g	21.0 g	• The compression force between the pelvis and lumbar spine of the ATD must be ≤1,500 lb (6,672 N)
	Floor track misalignment, pitch/roll	0°/0°	10°/10°	
TRANSPORT AIRPLANES U.S. 14 CFR Part 25, §25.562 (Amendment 25–64)	Minimum velocity change	35.0 ft/s (10.67 m/s)	44.0 ft/s (13.42 m/s)	As for small airplanes, plus:
	Maximum rise time	0.08 s	0.09 s	• If leg impact occurs, femur force must be ≤2,250 lbs (10,008 N)
	Minimum deceleration	14.0 g	16.0 g	• Seat deformation must not impede rapid evacuation of the airplane
	Floor track misalignment, pitch/roll	0°/0°	10°/10°	
NORMAL CATEGORY ROTORCRAFT U.S. 14 CFR Part 27, §27.562 (Amendment 27–25)	Minimum velocity change	30.0 ft/s (9.15 m/s)	42.0 ft/s (12.94 m/s)	As for small airplanes, except:
	Maximum rise time	0.031 s	0.071 s	• The seating device may experience separation if part of design
TRANSPORT CATEGORY ROTORCRAFT U.S. 14 CFR Part 29, §29.562 (Amendment 29–29)	Minimum deceleration	30.0 g	18.4 g	• The shoulder harness must remain on or in the vicinity of the ATD's shoulder
	Floor track misalignment, pitch/roll	10°/10°	10°/10°	

[a] "U.S. 14 CFR" refers to the U.S. Code of Federal Regulations; "Title 14; Aeronautics and Space." "ATD" means a 50th-percentile anthropomorphic test device (dummy) in accordance with U.S. 49 CFR 572, Subpart B, adapted for the aircraft seat tests by the installation of a lumbar spinal column compression force transducer.

Technical Standard Order C114, Torso Restraint Systems," in March 1987.

Seat/Restraint Systems for Helicopters

While the preceding discussion has addressed the requirements developed for occupant crash protection in small airplanes with less than 10 occupants, the GASP-1 working group also served as a forum for developing occupant crash protection requirements for helicopters. Data from the helicopter crash investigation studies (o.c.)[32,33] were supplemented by crashworthiness studies and design developments by Bell Helicopter Textron[56,57] and by input from the Crashworthiness Project Group of the Rotorcraft Airworthiness Requirements Committee of the Aerospace Industries Association for establishing the helicopter requirements. The dynamic test requirements established by the FAA for helicopters are shown in Table 7.3.

Seat/Restraint Systems for Large Transport Airplanes

In February 1979, the FAA Civil Aeromedical Institute initiated a program to evaluate the performance of passenger seat/restraint systems used on civil transport airplanes.[24] The purpose of the study was to compare occupant protection and failure modes of several different passenger-seat designs. Following the positive results of the GASP initiative, it was inevitable that rulemaking for improved performance of passenger seats in transport airplanes would follow. The small CAMI program was greatly expanded in 1984 by the participation of the Aerospace Industries Association (AIA) and the Air Transport Association (ATA).

This project provided a means for transport-airplane seat manufacturers, airframe manufacturers, and airline operators to participate in dynamic testing, define the limits of existing designs, and understand how dynamic testing could be used as a practical technique for improving the performance of seats in transport airplanes. A program was developed to investigate the effects of pulse shape, the interaction of deceleration level and impact velocity, two vs. three occupants in triple-seat assemblies, the effects of floor deformation, the effects of impacts with vertical load components, and the effects of multiple-row seating.[102] The test configurations and methodology developed in the earlier GASP project were adapted for the multiple-occupancy passenger-seat tests. The forces generated at the attachment of the seat legs to the aircraft floor tracks were measured in the dynamic tests and compared to the allowable floor loads for a typical narrow-bodied passenger aircraft. Test conditions were selected so that the tests produced force reactions at the floor that were within allowable limits for existing airplane designs. This compatibility would enable the new seats to be used on existing airplanes without the delays that would be encountered if increased floor strength was also required. Because of the close proximity of seats in some passenger airplanes, a requirement for limiting femur force was added to the performance requirements established in the GASP program.

As this test program was being conducted, seat manufacturers began submitting a variety of prototype seats for testing. Although several of the prototype seats failed to complete the tests in the first attempt, the experience gained in these programs and the data obtained from measurements of forces introduced into the seat structure during the dynamic test enabled successful designs to be developed. Several seat manufacturers soon announced that they were able to supply seats capable of passing a 16g dynamic test and accommodating floor deformation.[101] The Federal Aviation Administration issued a "Notice of Proposed Rulemaking" for improved seat safety standards for transport airplane seats in July 1986. Seat manufacturers announced that they could comply with the proposed requirements, and airframe manufacturers and airline operators began to reference the proposed rule as an additional requirement when purchasing seats. A new FAA rule that required dynamic testing for seats in newly certified large transport airplanes was issued in May 1988. The requirements of this rule are summarized in Table 7.3.

Federal Aviation Administration regulations provide only the minimum requirements for a system, and do not detail the technical process for demonstrating conformity to those requirements. Additional documents (Advisory Circulars or "Technical Standard Orders") are developed to guide both the industry and the government on techniques that can be used by the manufacturers in demonstrating that their systems conform to the requirements.

An "Advisory Circular" is a document that provides information with which to better understand the intent or technological basis for an aviation system. While "Advisory Circulars" are strictly information documents and have no regulatory stature, they often provide an avenue for both the aviation industry and the government to follow in the certification process. Since both the dynamic testing of aircraft seats, restraints, and interiors and the performance standards for occupant crash injury protection were new concepts for the industry and the FAA, a draft "Advisory Circular" was written to describe dynamic test procedures, instrumentation, dummy modifications, and data interpretation that would be applicable to the new rule.[26] After considering the comments received on this draft, "Advisory Circular AC No: 25.562-1, Dynamic Evaluation of Seat Restraint Systems & Occupant Protection on Transport Airplanes," was issued by the FAA in March 1990.

A "Technical Standard Order" (TSO) describes a formal process that can be used to demonstrate one method of conformity with the regulations. Certification of seats for large transport airplanes is usually accomplished under the TSO process. An ad hoc committee of the Society of Automotive Engineers was formed in 1987 for the purpose of developing an Aerospace Standard (AS) that could be used by the FAA as a basis for a TSO for certification of seats under the new rule. "Aerospace Standard AS 8049, Performance Standard for Seats in Civil Rotorcraft and Transport Airplanes," was published in July 1990. This comprehensive document includes both static and dynamic test procedures, general design guidance and requirements, strength requirements, and detailed criteria for determining if the seat system passed or failed the various tests. The FAA has issued notice that they intend to adopt this AS as a TSO.

Conclusion

At the present time, most aircraft newly certified in the United States must meet requirements for occupant crash protection. Requirements are being prepared for commuter-category airplanes (small transport airplanes), the only class of production aircraft not yet covered by the regulations. Most airlines are requiring new passenger seats to meet the new crash protection requirements as they refurbish airplane interiors. Regulations have been proposed that would require the installation of crashworthy seats in all operational large transport airplanes.

While these new requirements are, at last, a move in the right direction, much additional work remains to be done. The ability of a person to rapidly evacuate a transport airplane is essential for survival in crashes that produce postcrash fires. Non-life-threatening injuries that impair this ability, such as simple fractures of the arms or legs or short-duration unconsciousness, can result in death. Data to assess the significance of this problem are not yet available, since deaths that are documented under those circumstances are usually attributed to the postcrash fire rather than the crash injuries.

The use of "air-bag" restraint might reduce these injuries. Special applications of air bags (such as at a bulkhead or galley in front of a row of seats) might prove practical, but general use throughout a passenger airplane seems unlikely at this time because of cost and weight problems. The widespread use of rearward-facing passenger seats would be the most practical means of reducing these injuries (if problems with retention of overhead bins and contents are resolved). In 1986, Weber Aircraft initiated a program to develop a rear-facing triple passenger seat for the air force that was capable of withstanding the dynamic test loads.[13] The military required this seat to be designed for 250-pound occupant weights and to have folding legs and seat backs to meet stowing and stacking requirements. Nevertheless, the total weight of the seat assembly was only 93 pounds. On the basis of seat/occupant weight, this was less than many forward-facing passenger seats. Plastic deformation of the seat legs in dynamic tests at CAMI limited the force acting on the floor to levels equivalent to a $12g$ static load. While work such as this seems to demonstrate the practicality of rearward-facing seats, their widespread use would be contrary to the well-established tradition of forward-facing seats in civil transport airplanes and is expected only if an unprecedented public demand for improved crash protection materializes.

A more rudimentary limitation on improved standards is the lack of a suitable test dummy with biofidelity in response to dynamic axial compression and bending of the spinal column. Attempts by the military to develop such a dummy have been accompanied by costs that place the product far beyond practical use in tests of civil aircraft systems. Yet improved attempts to reduce spinal column injury will be thwarted until the time when such a dummy is available and appropriate injury criteria have been defined.

Field crash experience has been limited, so the effectiveness of systems meeting the new requirements cannot be firmly established. There has been only one significant crash of a large transport airplane that was equipped with seats that "nominally" met the new requirements.[95] In this crash, the B-737 airplane hit the side of a roadway cut at an angle of about 32 degrees with an estimated impact velocity of between 44 and 49 m/sec. Analysis indicated that the peak longitudinal deceleration of the cabin midsection was on the order of $26g$, and peak normal decelerations was on the order of $23g$. Several sections of the fuselage were destroyed by the crash, but the fuselage and floor remained relatively intact in the area of the wing and near the tail. In those areas where the floor was not destroyed, the seats remained attached to the floor and the occupants of those seats generally survived the crash. This singular experience seems to indicate that the seats performed well, even though the crash environment was significantly greater than the test environment.

References

1. Acker LW, Black DO, Moser JC. Accelerations in fighter airplane crashes. NACA RM E57G11, NACA Lewis Flight Propulsion Laboratory, Cleveland, OH, 1957.
2. Alfaro-Bou E, Fasanella EL, Williams MS. Crashworthy design considerations for general aviation seats. SAE 850855, Society of Automotive Engineers, Warrendale, PA, 1985.
3. Anon (1944) The shoulder harness. Air Surgeon's Bulletin 1:8–9.
4. Anon (1951) The dangerous safety belt. Sci Am V:185–186.
5. Armstrong HG. *Principles and Practice of Aviation Medicine*. Williams and Wilkins, Baltimore, 1939.
6. Army. *Air Service Medical*. War Department, Washington DC, 1919.
7. Army. *Aviation Medicine in the A.E.F.* Document No. 1004, Office of the Director of Air Service, War Department, Washington DC, 1920.
8. Army. Handbook of instructions for airplane designers. 4th ed. Engineering Division, Army Air Service, Dayton, Ohio, 1925.
9. Army. Military Specification: General Specification for Seat System: Crash Resistant, Non-Ejection, Aircrew. Mil-S-58095 (AV), 1971.
10. Army. Military Standard: Light Fixed and Rotary Wing Aircraft Crashworthiness. Mil-STD-1290 (AV), 1974.
11. Army. Aircraft crash survival design guide, USAAVSCOM TR 89-D-22A thru E. U.S. Army Aviation Research and Technology Activity, Ft. Eustis, VA, 1989.
12. Bauer LH. *Aviation Medicine*. Williams & Wilkins, Baltimore, MD, 1926.
13. Bilezikjian V (1989) Aft facing transport aircraft passenger seats under 16G dynamic crash simulation. SAFE J, Winter Quarter, 19:6–10.
14. Black DO. Facilities and methods used in full scale airplane crash fire investigation. NACA RM E51L06, NACA Lewis Flight Propulsion Laboratory, Cleveland, OH, 1952.

15. Brinkley JW. Development of aerospace escape systems. Air University Review, July/August, pp 34–39, 1968.

16. CAA. Air commerce regulations effective December 31, 1926, U.S. Department of Commerce, Aeronautics Branch, Washington DC, 1926.

17. CAA. Airworthiness requirements of air commerce regulations. Aeronautics Bulletin No. 7-A, Effective July 1, 1929, Department of Commerce, Aeronautics Branch, Washington DC, 1929.

18. CAA. Airworthiness requirements for aircraft: Aeronautics Bulletin No. 7-A, effective October 1, 1934. Bureau of Air Commerce, Washington DC, 1934.

19. Carden HD. Full scale crash-test evaluation of two load-limiting subfloors for general aviation airframes. NASA Technical Paper 2380, Langley Research Center, Hampton, VA, 1984.

20. Chandler RF, Trout EM. Evaluation of seating and restraint systems and anthropomorphic dummies conducted during fiscal year 1976. FAA-AM-78-6, Federal Aviation Administration, Washington DC, 1978.

21. Chandler RF, Trout EM. Evaluation of seating and restraint systems conducted during fiscal year 1978. FAA-AM-79-17, Federal Aviation Administration, Washington DC, 1979.

22. Chandler RF. Dynamic test of joint Army/Navy crashworthy armored crew seat. Memorandum Report AAC-119-80-2. Protection and Survival Laboratory, FAA Civil Aeromedical Institute, Oklahoma City, OK, 1980.

23. Chandler RF. Crash injury protection research at CAMI. SAE 830746, Society of Automotive Engineers, Warrendale, PA, 1983.

24. Chandler RF, Gowdy RV. Loads measured in passenger seat tests. Memorandum report AAC-119-81-8A, Protection and Survival Laboratory, FAA Civil Aeromedical Institute, Oklahoma City, OK, 1985a.

25. Chandler RF. Data for the development of criteria for general aviation seat and restraint system performance. SAE 850851, Society of Automotive Engineers, Warrendale, PA, 1985b.

26. Chandler RF. Draft advisory circular: dynamic testing of seat/restraint and occupant protection for transport airplanes. Memorandum No. AAM-119-88-1, Protection and Survival Laboratory, FAA Civil Aeromedical Institute, Oklahoma City, OK, 1988.

27. Chandler RF. Occupant crash protection in military air transport. AGARD-AG-306, North Atlantic Treaty Organization Advisory Group for Aerospace Research and Development, Neuilly-Sur-Seine, France, 1990.

28. Chanute O. Progress in flying machines, New York, 1894. (Republished by Lorenz and Herweg, Long Beach, CA, 1976.)

29. Child L. Memorandum for file: crash injury research and development. W-146, 1949.

30. Clark JC. Summary report on the national transportation safety board's general aviation crashworthiness project findings. SAE 871006, Society of Automotive Engineers, Warrendale, PA, 1987.

31. Coltman JW. Design and test criteria for increased energy-absorbing seat effectiveness. FAA-AM-83-3, Federal Aviation Administration, Washington DC, 1983.

32. Coltman JW, Bolukbasi AO, Laananen DH. Analysis of rotorcraft crash dynamics for development of improved crashworthiness design criteria. DOT/FAA/CT-83/48, Federal Aviation Administration, Washington DC, 1984.

33. Coltman JW, Neri LM. Analysis of U.S. civil rotorcraft accidents for development of improved design criteria. B-86-SE-26-H000. Proceedings of the Meeting on Crashworthiness Design of Rotorcraft, Georgia Institute of Technology, Atlanta, GA, 1986.

34. Crouch TD. *A Dream of Wings*. Smithsonian Institute Press, Washington DC, 1989.

35. De Haven H (1941) Miraculous safety, air facts. 4(3):21–26.

36. De Haven H. Report on crash injury research project. April 1st to May 1st 1942, to Dr. Eugene F. Du Bois, Cornell University Medical School, NY, 1942.

37. De Haven H. Injuries in thirty light-aircraft accidents: medical data and crash details from field investigations of the civil aeronautics board. NRC Report 230, National Research Council Committee on Aviation Medicine, Washington DC, 1943.

38. De Haven H. Relationship of injuries to structure in survivable aircraft accidents. NRC Report 440, National Research Council, Washington DC, 1945.

39. De Haven H (1946) Research on crash injuries. JAMA 131(6):524.

40. De Haven H. The rare occurrence of internal abdominal injury from safety belts or other causes in serious aircraft accidents. N.R.C.

Crash Injury Research, Cornell University Medical College, New York, NY, 1947.

41. De Haven H, Hasbrook AH. Use and effectiveness of shoulder harnesses in surplus military aircraft flown by civilian pilots. AFTR No. 6461, United States Air Force, Wright Patterson Air Force Base, Dayton, Ohio, 1951a.

42. De Haven H. Crash injury research: semi-annual progress report. Cornell University Medical College, NY, 1951b.

43. De Haven H. Current safety considerations in the design of passenger seats for transport aircraft. Cornell University Medical College, New York, NY, 1952a.

44. De Haven H. Accident survival-airplane and passenger car. Society of Automotive Engineers, Detroit, MI, 1952b.

45. De Haven H. Development of crash survival design in personal, executive and agricultural aircraft. Cornell University Medical College, NY, 1953.

46. De Haven H, Tourin B, Macri S. Aircraft safety belts: their injury effect on the human body. Crash Injury Research, Cornell University Medical College, New York, NY, 1953.

47. De Haven H. Beginnings of crash injury research. 13th Stapp Car Crash Conference. Society of Automotive Engineers, Warrendale, PA, 1969.

48. Dille JR, Harraway A. Index to FAA office of aviation medicine reports, 1961 through 1980. FAA-AM-81-1, Federal Aviation Administration, Washington DC, 1981.

49. Domzalski L. Crashworthy military passenger seat development. Eighteenth Annual Symposium of the Survival and Flight Equipment Association. SAFE, Canoga Park, CA, pp 209–215, 1981.

50. DuBois EF (1952) Safety belts are not dangerous. Br Med J 2:685–686.

51. Eiband AM, Simpkinson SH, Black DO. Accelerations and passenger harness loads measured in full scale light airplane crashes. NACA TN 2991, NACA Lewis Flight Propulsion Laboratory, Cleveland, OH, 1953.

52. Eiband AM. Human tolerance to rapidly applied accelerations: a summary of the literature. NASA Lewis Research Center, Cleveland, OH, 1959.

53. Fasanella EL, Alfaro-Bou E. NASA general aviation crashworthiness seat development. SAE 790591, Society of Automotive Engineers, Warrendale, PA, 1979.

54. Follis RH Jr. Memorandum to the AAF Air Surgeon: Geohegan inertia lock for shoulder harness. Hq AAF Flight Control Command, Winston-Salem, NC, 1943.

55. Foret-Bruno JY, Hartemann P, Thomas C, Payon A, Tarriere C, Got C, Patel A. Correlations between thoracic lesions & force values measured at the shoulder of 92 belted occupants involved in real accidents. SAE 780892, Society of Automotive Engineers, Warrendale, PA, 1978.

56. Fox RG. Relative risk, the true measure of safety. 28th Corporate Safety Seminar. Flight Safety Foundation, Arlington, VA, 1983.

57. Fox RG. Realistic civil helicopter crash safety, B-86-SE-24-H000. Meeting on Crashworthiness Design of Rotorcraft. Georgia Institute of Technology, Atlanta, GA, 1986.

58. Fryer DI. Aircraft passenger-seat design and crash survival. FPRC 1055, Flying Personnel Research Committee, Air Ministry, London, 1958.

59. Fulton JF. Measures for increasing safety of flying personnel in crashes: a memorandum to the committee on aviation medicine. NRC Committee on Aviation Medicine Report No. 34, National Research Council, Washington DC, 1941.

60. Geertz A. Limits and special problems in the use of seat catapults. Air Documents Division, Wright Field, OH, 1944.

61. Gilson JG, Stewart WK, Pekarek Z. Prevention of injury in aircraft crashes. Report No. 556, Flying Personnel Research Committee, Air Ministry, London, 1943.

62. Hasbrook AH. Design of passenger "tie-down". AvCir-44-0-66, Aviation Crash Injury Research of Cornell University, Flushing, NY, 1956.

63. Hasbrook AH, Garner JD, Snow CC. Evacuation pattern analysis of a survivable commercial aircraft crash. FAA-AM-62-9, Federal Aviation Agency, Washington DC, 1962.

64. Hass G. An analysis of relations between force, aircraft structure and injuries to personnel involved in aircraft accidents with recommendations for safer principles in design of certain types of aircraft. Report No. 1, Project No. 187, The School of Aviation Medicine, Randolph Field, Texas, 1943.

65. Holbrook HA. Civil Aviation Medicine in the Bureaucracy. Banner Publishing Company, Bethesda, MD, 1974.

66. Kubokawa CC (1974) The NASA Ames integral passenger seat concept. SAFE J 4(4):18–23.

67. NTSB. Safety report-general aviation crash-worthiness project: phase one. NTSB/SR-83/01, National Transportation Safety Board, Washington DC, 1983.

68. NTSB. Safety report—general aviation crashworthiness project: phase two—impact severity and potential injury prevention in general aviation accidents. NTSB/SR-85/01, National Transportation Safety Board, Washington DC, 1985a.

69. NTSB. Safety report—general aviation crash-worthiness project: phase three—acceleration loads and velocity changes of survivable general aviation accidents. NTSB/SR-85/02, National Transportation Safety Board, Washington DC, 1985b.

70. Olcott JW. Proposal on enhanced crash tolerance. Proposal No. 518, V.2, pp. 263–268, Regulatory Review Program, Part 23, Federal Aviation Administration, Washington DC, 1984.

71. Parks DL, Twigg DW. Attendant restraint system technical evaluation and guidelines. Boeing Document D6-44779TN-0, The Boeing Company, Seattle, WA, 1978.

72. Perrone N, Saczalski K. A survey of current government sponsored research & Development programs in vehicle crashworthiness in related biomechanics areas. Office of Naval Research, Washington DC, 1973.

73. Pinkel II, Rosenberg EG. Seat design for crash worthiness. NACA TN 3777, NACA Lewis Flight Propulsion Laboratory, Cleveland, OH, 1956.

74. Pinkel II. A proposed criterion for the selection of forward and rearward-facing seats. ASME Paper No. 59-AV-28, American Society of Mechanical Engineers, New York, 1959.

75. Preston GM, Preman GJ. Accelerations in transport airplane crashes. NACA TN 4158, NACA Lewis Flight Propulsion Laboratory, Cleveland, OH, 1958.

76. Rathgeber RK, Parker PE. Preliminary design research for the caravan 1 crew seat. SAE 850856, Society of Automotive Engineers, Warrendale, PA, 1985.

77. Reed WH, Robertson SH, Weinberg LWT, Tyndall LH. Full scale dynamic crash test of a Douglas DC-7 aircraft. FAA-ADS-37, Federal Aviation Agency Aircraft Development Service, Washington DC, 1965a.

78. Reed WH, Robertson SH, Weinberg LWT, Tyndall LH. Full scale dynamic crash test of a Lockheed Constellation model 1649 aircraft. Federal Aviation Agency Aircraft Development Service, Washington DC, 1965b.

79. Reilly MJ. Crashworthy troop seat investigation. USAAMRDL-TR-74-93, U.S. Army Air Mobility Research and Development Laboratory, Ft. Eustis, VA, 1974.

80. Reilly MJ. Crashworthy troop seat testing program. USAAMRDL-TR-77-13, U.S. Army Research and Technology Laboratories, Ft. Eustis, VA, 1977.

81. Singley GT III. Test and evaluation of improved aircrew restraint systems. USAAVRADCOM-TR-81-D-27, U.S. Army Research and Technology Laboratories, Ft. Eustis, VA, 1981.

81a. Siahaya O, Jarrett W, Iteffield T. A retrofit crash protection installation in two models of general aviation airplanes, SAE 871008 Society of Automotive Engineers, Warrendale, PA, April 1987.

82. Snyder RG. A case of survival of extreme vertical impact in seated position. FAA-AM-62-19, Federal Aviation Agency, Washington DC, 1962.

83. Snyder RG. Human survivability of extreme impacts in free fall. FAA-AM-63-15, Federal Aviation Agency, Washington DC, 1963.

84. Snyder RG. Survival of high velocity free falls in water. FAA-AM-65-12, Federal Aviation Agency, Washington DC, 1965.

85. Snyder RG, Snow CC, Crosby WM, Fineg J, Chandler R. Impact injury to the pregnant female and fetus in lap belt restraint. FAA-AM-68-24, Federal Aviation Administration, Washington DC, 1968.

86. Snyder RG, Crosby WM, Snow CC, Young JW, Hanson P. Seat belt injuries in impact. FAA-AM-69-5, Federal Aviation Administration, Washington DC, 1969a.

87. Snyder RG, Snow CC, Young JW, Crosby WM, Price GT. Pathology of trauma attributed to restraint systems in crash impacts. FAA-AM-69-3, Federal Aviation Administration, Washington DC, 1969b.

88. Snyder RG, Young JW, Snow CC. Experimental impact protection with advanced restraint systems: preliminary tests with air bag and inertia reel/inverted-y yoke torso harness. FAA-AM-69-4, Federal Aviation Administration, Washington DC, 1969.

89. Stapp JP. Tolerance to abrupt deceleration. Chapter 14. In *Collected Papers on*

Aviation Medicine. AGARDograph No. 6, Butterworths Scientific Publications, London, 1955.

90. Swearingen JJ. Design and construction of crash dummy for testing shoulder harness and Safety Belts, Civil Aeronautics Administration, Washington DC, 1951.

91. Swearingen JJ, Morrow DJ. Motions of the head and trunk allowed by safety belt restraint during impact. Project No. 53-204, Civil Aeronautic Administration, Washington DC, 1956.

92. Swearingen JJ, McFadden ER, Garner JD, Blethrow JG (1960) Human voluntary tolerance to vertical impact. Aerospace Medicine 31:989–998.

93. Teare D (1951) Post-mortem examinations on air-crash victims. Br Med J 707–708.

94. Thompson RG, Carden HD, Hayduk RJ. Survey of NASA research on crash dynamics. NASA Technical Paper 2298, Langley Research Center, Hampton, VA, 1984.

95. Trimble EJ. Report on the accident to Boeing 737–400 G-OBME near Kegworth, Leicestershire on 8 January 1989. Aircraft Accident Report 4/90, HMSO, London, 1990.

96. Underhill B, McCullough B. An energy absorbing seat design for light aircraft. SAE 720322, Society of Automotive Engineers, New York, 1972.

97. Villard HS. *Contact!* Bonanza Books, New York, 1968.

98. Watson-Jones R. Fractures of the spine sustained by RAF pilots and the relationship of these injuries to the Sutton harness, parachute harness, and other equipment. Report No. 274, Flying Personnel Research Committee, Air Ministry, London, 1941.

99. Watts DT, Mendelson ES, Kornfield AT. Human tolerance to accelerations applied from seat to head during ejection seat tests. TED No. NAM 25605, Report No. 1, Naval Air Material Center, 1947.

100. Weaver ER. Report of the static and dynamic tests of the Fokker C2-A cabin floor, seat and safety belt. Report A.D.M. 1046, Airplane Branch, Air Corps Material Division, Dayton, Ohio, 1929.

101. Weber Aircraft. (1986) Weber aircraft seat survives 16g forces in structural test. Aviation Week and Space Technology, pp 38–39, January 6, 1986.

102. Webster JL Sr, McGrew JA, Shook WH. Results of the AIA/ATA/FAA dynamic seat testing program. SAE 881375, Society of Automotive Engineers, Warrendale, PA, 1988.

103. Weick FE, Hansen JR. *From the ground up.* Smithsonian Institution Press, Washington and London, 1988.

8
Occupant Restraint Systems

Rolf Eppinger

Introduction

The purpose of an effective transportation system is to convey goods or passengers efficiently, rapidly, and safely from one place to another. While the goods or passengers are being transported, they will naturally acquire a velocity relative to the ground. It should be obvious to everyone that the velocity associated with this transportation process is in and of itself not hazardous to life or limb. This is evidenced by the wide range of velocities that are currently safely experienced by millions and millions of travelers each day, from those who experience a few miles per hour on a bicycle to those who experience over a thousand miles per hour when traveling by air. However, it should be also obvious that there are circumstances (crashes) that exist within the same diverse transportation process that are very hazardous to humans. This is readily evidenced by the fact that over the last 10 years, the annual fatality toll in the United States associated with motor vehicle crashes alone has exceeded 35,000 deaths per year.

A comparative examination of crash events that have and have not proven hazardous to humans has revealed that risk can be generally associated with how much and how fast the human must lose the velocity acquired in the transportation process. That is, risk is simultaneously proportional to the total velocity change and inversely proportional to the time over which the velocity change is accomplished. These examinations have also re-vealed that, as the means by which a specific velocity change is accomplished are altered, a considerable variation in the human risk is also observed.

This realization has led researchers and engineers to combine their knowledge of the physical principles that govern the motion of bodies in space, their knowledge of structures and conditions under which they fail, and their knowledge of human anatomy and injury mechanisms to study these hazardous conditions and to create specialized devices, generically known as occupant restraints, which exploit this knowledge to mitigate the hazardous effects of crash events.

The purpose of this chapter is (1) to provide a general, but not rigorous, statement and discussion of some of the fundamental laws and concepts that govern the motion of bodies in space; (2) to apply these general principles to the transportation process to provide a mechanistic understanding of the structured interplay between forces, motions, and time when governed by these laws of motion and of how specific conditions can become either hazardous or benign in automotive crashes; (3) to introduce a series of maxims, based on the laws of motion and human anatomical and structural failure considerations, that further clarify the characteristics of well-designed and performing occupant restraints; and lastly, (4) to provide examples of how current automotive occupant-restraint technology has applied these maxims to the benefit of the occupant.

Basic Laws and Concepts of Motion

Knowledge of the three basic notions ascribed to Newton, commonly referred to as Newton's laws of motion, together with the concepts of work, energy, and the law of conservation of energy will provide a respectable basis upon which to understand, from a mechanistic viewpoint, the regulation of bodies under the influence of forces and the operation of automotive restraint systems.

Newton's first law states the somewhat obvious but fundamental observation that a body at rest will remain at rest while a body in motion remains in motion unless acted upon by an external force. A force is defined, in a rather circuitous manner, as the cause or agent that alters the motion of an object and represents as a single entity the cumulative effect of the millions of molecular interactions that occur between two bodies. There are two types of forces that can be applied to objects: body forces, which operate from a distance, such as gravity and magnetism, and traction forces, which are forces applied to the surfaces of bodies. Forces have two characteristics: magnitude, i.e., how large or intense they are, and direction. They can be imagined and are often graphically represented as arrows where the arrow's length represents the magnitude of the force, and the arrow's direction, which is direction in which the force acts or pushes on an object.

Newton's second law defines the relationship between the force applied to the body to initiate its change of motion, the length of time that the force is applied, the magnitude of velocity change the body experiences, and the body's mass. The law states that if a force, F, is applied to a body for a period of time, DT, the body will experience a change in velocity, DV, equal to:

$$DV = (F * DT)/M$$

where M is the mass of the body. An alternative, but possibly more familiar form is:

$$F = M * A$$

where A is the acceleration of the body and equal to DV/DT.

The third law states another fundamental but obvious observation that for every force there is an equal and opposite force or reaction. This law can be easily visualized if one considers two bodies contacting and pushing against each other. If the body on the left is examined in isolation, the force of interaction, F, at the contact surface between the two bodies can be seen to be pushing the body to the left. Likewise, if the body on the right is also examined in isolation, it also has a force of magnitude F pushing on it but in the opposite direction, i.e., to the right.

To further develop the concepts that govern motion, two more definitions must first be presented. They are: Energy—which is the capacity for doing work and overcoming resistance, and Work—which is the transference of energy from one body to another. In mechanical systems, a force does work on a body provided that the point where the force is applied has a component of displacement in the direction of the force. The work done, or energy transferred to or from the body, is then equal to the magnitude of the force times the distance over which it acts. This acquired energy manifests itself either as energy associated with the motion of the body, called kinetic energy, or as energy stored within the body, commonly called potential energy. The energy associated with the motion of the body can be readily calculated knowing its mass and velocity. It is:

$$KE = (M * V^2)/2$$

where again M is the mass of the body and V is its velocity.

The final concept that ties everything together is the law of the conservation of energy, from which it can be argued that Newton's laws of motion can be developed. It states that the total amount of energy within a control volume remains constant unless energy is either transmitted into or out of the control volume. When considering, as we are, mechanical systems, the transmitted energy is equal to the work done by forces at the surface of the control

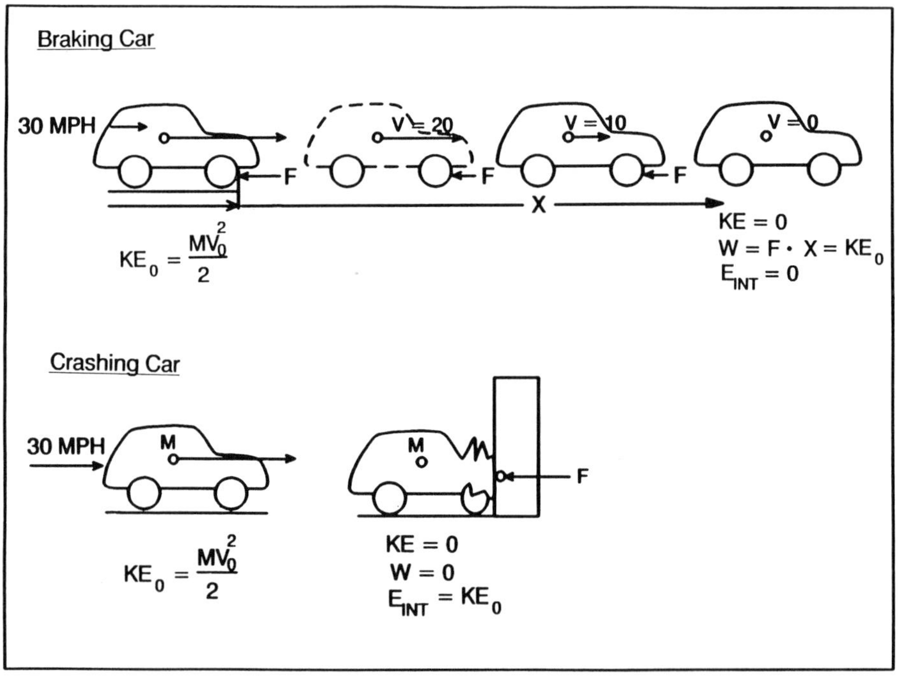

FIGURE 8.1. Comparison of work done and energy absorbed.

volume and is equal to the force times the distance over which it acts.

Application of Concepts to Transportation Process

To put these basic laws and concepts in the context of a transportation system, one can see that Newton's first law implies that anything that participates in the transportation process must be acted upon by forces, both to first acquire the velocity to move from one place to the next, and to stop, once arriving there. Newton's second law states that the velocity acquired by any participant, either positive or negative, is proportional to the product of the applied force and the duration for which it is applied and inversely proportional to the mass of the participant. This obviously begins to explain how certain conditions could become very hazardous to individuals. That is, if for some reason the time available to accomplish a particular velocity change was physically limited to a very short duration rather than a longer one, the second law requires that a very large force must be generated to accomplish the necessary velocity change.

Up to this point, it was implicitly suggested that the bodies under the influence of forces were nondeformable. However, in the case of the real transportation process, all participants (the vehicle, the goods, and the passengers) are actually deformable structures. This capacity to deform, however, does not invalidate the laws of motion or the other concepts previously presented but does introduce an interesting aspect to the concept of energy. The following example, illustrated in Fig. 8.1 and contrasting the two situations, will demonstrate the effect of deformability.

Two identical cars, each initially traveling at 30 mph and possessing the same kinetic energy, decrease their velocity to zero, but by different processes. The first will apply its brakes, generate a force at the tire/road interface that acts on the vehicle, and reduces its velocity to zero. These tire forces will move along with the vehicle, performing negative work, that is, removing kinetic energy, until the vehicle stops. The other vehicle collides with a rigid, immovable barrier, rapidly loses all of its

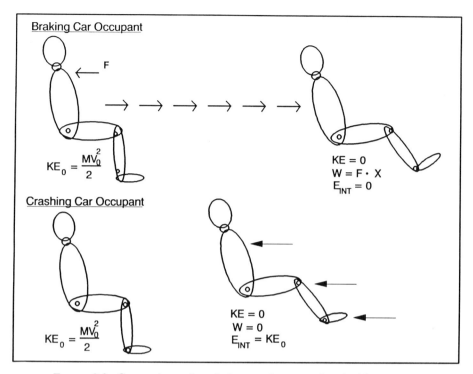

FIGURE 8.2. Comparison of work done and energy absorbed by occupant.

velocity relative to the ground, and, therefore, also all of its kinetic energy. In both cases, the product of the force times the time duration of application will be identical. There are, however, several differences. First, while the product $F * DT$ is the same (as the second law demands), the car that is braking experiences a small force for a long time while the crashing car experiences a large force for a short time. Second, while the point of application of the braking force translates with respect to the ground, performs work, and removes energy from the car, the force at the barrier that arrests the motion of the second car does not move and, therefore, does not transfer any energy away from the car. Since the total energy of the crashing car must be conserved if it is not transmitted away, the kinetic energy is transformed into other forms of energy and remains within the body. This energy is then absorbed by the crushing of the front of the car.

Similar processes occur to the occupants within each of the two cars (Fig. 8.2). The occupant of the braking car will have a variety of small forces acting on him during the braking process such as seat friction force, foot toe-board force, and hands-to-steering-wheel force, which will slow him down with the vehicle and extract his kinetic energy away from his body as these force application points translate over the ground. The unrestrained occupant of the crashing car, however, experiences an event much like the vehicle he is in. That is, because his crashing car stops so quickly, he continues to move forward at his initial velocity within the compartment with little velocity attenuation and strikes interior surfaces that are now not moving. Because these surfaces have already lost all of their velocity with respect to the ground and are very stiff, the forces that these surfaces apply to the occupant to change his velocity to zero are very large, do not translate over the ground, and, therefore, do not extract any energy. Again, because the occupant's kinetic energy is eliminated and none was extracted by forces doing work, the kinetic energy must be trans-

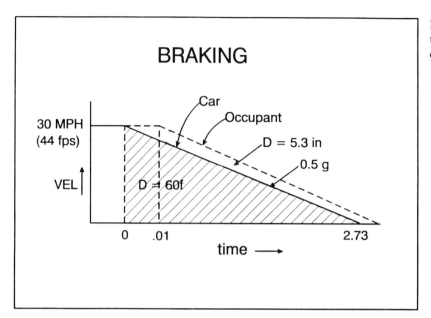

FIGURE 8.3. Velocity-time diagram of braking car and occupant.

formed to other forms of energy and remain within his body. It is this transformed kinetic energy that causes injuries.

The introduction of an occupant restraint into this latter example will significantly modify the sequence of events that occur to the occupant. To examine and illustrate the differences between the above two situations, i.e., the unrestrained occupant in a braking car and a crashing car, and a restrained occupant in a crashing car, the concept of a velocity-time diagram will be introduced. In these diagrams, the velocity of each object over the ground is plotted with respect to time, and differences between the various scenarios discussed above are easily illustrated. In addition, many other parameters are also discernible from this diagram. First, the acceleration of any object is directly related to the slope or steepness of the velocity-time curve at any time T. Also, the displacement of any object over the ground is represented by the area under its velocity-time curve and the relative displacement between any two objects is the area that exists between their corresponding velocity-time curves.

In Fig. 8.3, the first example of the braking car is illustrated. Here, the initial velocity of the car is 30 mph and the brakes are applied at $T = 0$. The braking force is of such an amplitude that the car loses 16.1 ft per second of

velocity per second (this is called a one-half g deceleration rate) and comes to rest 2.73s later. During this deceleration period, the vehicle translates 60 ft over the ground. This is represented by the area under the velocity-time curve between time $T = 0$ and $T = 2.73$ s. If the various forces acting on the occupant through the seat, floor pan, etc., are instantaneously applied, the occupant will also reduce his velocity in the same manner as does the vehicle. However, if the same forces were applied but their onset was delayed by 0.010s, the occupant's change in velocity would be as shown in the figure. His displacement over the ground would be represented by the area under his velocity curve and is now 60 ft, 5.3 inches rather than the 60 ft of the previous example. Since the car still translates the same distance over the ground, the delay of force application has caused the occupant to travel 5.3 inches inside of the compartment. This is represented by the area between his velocity curve and that of the car in the figure.

Figure 8.4 represents the velocity curves of the crashing vehicle and its unrestrained occupant. Here, because the vehicle is crashing into the rigid barrier, we shall assume that the front of the vehicle crushes 24 inches and allow the compartment to translate that amount over the ground. The velocity of the compartment is

FIGURE 8.4. Velocity-
time diagram of crashing
car and unrestrained
occupant

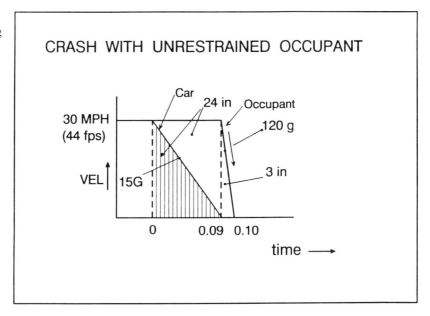

shown in the figure. Again, as before, the area under the vehicle's velocity curve represents the distance it travels over the ground while stopping and is 24 inches. If the occupant is unrestrained and no forces are applied to him, he will continue on after the initiation of the crash at his initial velocity of 30 mph, as required by the first law, until he contacts the instrument panel. If the panel is 24 inches in front of him, he will arrive at the panel just as the vehicle has come to rest and have translated 48 inches with respect to the ground. If the deflection of his body allows only an additional 3 inches of motion, he will come to rest 11 ms later while decelerating at $120g$.

Figure 8.5 shows velocity-time curve of the same crashing car but now with a restrained occupant in it. If we assume the restraint cannot apply any force to the occupant until he has translated 6 inches within the compartment,

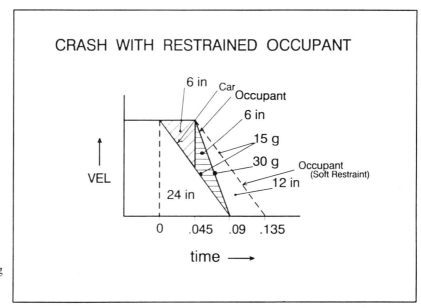

FIGURE 8.5. Velocity-
time diagram of crashing
car and restrained
driver.

the velocity-time diagram shows he will continue at his initial velocity of 30 mph for an additional 0.045 s. Then, if sufficient force is applied to make him lose his velocity in the next 0.045 s, i.e., decelerate at 30g, he will come to rest at the same time as does the vehicle. During this period of restraint, he will translate another 6 inches within the compartment. His total displacement over the ground is then 36 inches, which is comprised of 24 inches of vehicle crush and 12 inches of relative motion within the compartment. Also, because the time to lose the occupant's initial velocity has been increased fourfold, Newton's second law shows that the magnitude of the forces applied to the restrained occupant were reduced to one-fourth the magnitude of the forces applied to the unrestrained occupant.

If, as in the previous example, the instrument panel is initially 24 inches in front of the occupant, he will have, because he only translated 12 inches in the compartment, missed the panel by 12 inches. If one were to modify the applied restraint forces such that the occupant utilizes the entire 24 inches of interior distance to arrest his motion, then his velocity-time curve will be as shown by the dashed line in Fig. 8.5. This indicates that the time to lose his velocity can be extended from 45 to 90 ms. The second law then indicates that the restraint forces will also be one-half as large as in the latter case and one-eighth of the hypothetical unrestrained case.

Maxims for Good Occupant Restraint Performance and Design

The basic concepts discussed above that establish in time the relationships between forces, motions, and energy of bodies can be combined with considerations of general structural failure mechanisms, human anatomy, and human injury mechanisms to suggest certain maxims that should be considered and applied in the design of restraint systems to optimize their safety performance.

These maxims are:

- Maximize the time over which restraint forces are applied.
  Reason: Minimizes the magnitude of the applied forces.
- Maximize the distance that the point of force application on the body moves over the ground.
  Reason: Maximizes the amount of kinetic energy extracted from the body and minimizes energy that must be stored in the body.
- Apply as great a restraint force a possible as soon as possible during the crash event.
  Reason: Maximizes kinetic energy extracted because body translates more over the ground during early phase of crash—thus work and energy extraction are the greatest.
- Minimize body articulations, local deformations and rate of deformations, and local inertial accelerations during the restraint event.
  Reason: Many tissue failure mechanisms are either totally or partially related to either one or more of these parameters.
- Distribute forces over greatest possible area.
  Reason: Structures generally deform less with distributed loads and therefore deformation-based hazards are reduced. Reduces local surface pressures applied to a body region that have also been related to structural failure.
- Apply restraint forces to bony anatomy of the femur, pelvis, upper thorax, shoulder, and head while minimizing loads to compliant anatomical areas.
  Reason: The bony structures of the anatomy are capable of carrying the greatest loads with minimal deflection and least injury, thereby allowing application of most efficient restraint forces without exposing underlying soft tissues to injury-producing conditions. Soft tissues are not capable of sustaining large loads; therefore, if necessary restraint loads are applied, injurious situations are easily created.

Relationship of Occupant Current Restraint Designs to Maxims

There are currently two automotive occupant restraint systems that have achieved a significant level of application and sophistication in restraining occupants and reducing fatalities and mitigating injuries. The most ubiquitous of these is obviously the seat-belt system since it has been a mandatory device on all vehicles produced in the United States since 1966. Currently, the majority of belt systems in service are manual devices requiring an action by the user to be placed in operational position. With the revision of Federal Motor Vehicle Safety Standard No. 208, issued in 1986, which requires passive restraints, that is, restraints that do not require an active action on the part of the user to place in operational position, a number of automatic seat-belt systems have been developed and introduced into the vehicle fleet. Additionally, there has been an increasing trend for manufacturers to install air-bag systems to comply with the passive requirements of FMVSS 208 and to augment them with manual seat-belt systems.

While both types of restraint systems, that is, air bags and seat belts, are finding large application, the mechanics of their operation differ significantly. Current belt systems apply their restraint forces to both the torso and the pelvis to accomplish the needed velocity change while air-bag systems apply their restraint forces to the upper torso and head with some other device, such as a knee bolster, providing forces to restrain the lower portion of the body. With a belt system that lies on the surface of the body, two conditions must prevail in order for it to apply a restraining force to the body. They are: (1) the belt must have a tensile load within it, and (2) the belt must change direction while in contact with the body. Figure 8.6 illustrates this point. On the left of this figure, a belt that has 1,000 pounds

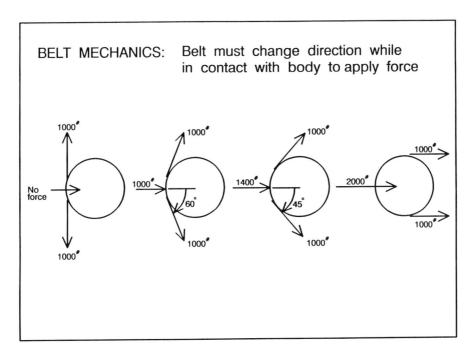

FIGURE 8.6. Applied belt force vs. belt wrap angle.

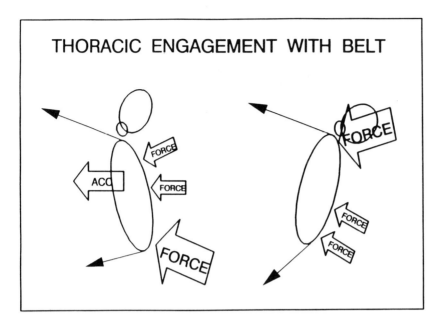

FIGURE 8.7. Applied belt force/geometric engagement examples.

of tension within it touches the body at one point and remains straight. In this position the belt applies no horizontal force to the body. If, as the subsequent illustrations to the right show, the change in direction of the belt while in contact with the body increases, the force applied to the body also increases. Therefore, if one wishes to have a belt system apply restraint forces to selected areas of the anatomy, as recommended in one of the maxims, one must have the belt change direction in those areas. Conversely, if a belt system is applying loads to a portion of the anatomy where a load is not desired, its geometry must be somehow adjusted so that it no longer changes direction in that area.

This concept is illustrated in Fig. 8.7, where two different torso-belt configurations are shown. The occupant on the left, because of his particular translation within the vehicle compartment, has acquired an orientation such that the belt exhibits a greater change in direction in the lower abdominal area than at the shoulders. Therefore, greater forces are being applied in the area than at the shoulders. With the occupant on the right, where the pelvic translation was less and the shoulder translation was more, a more advantageous belt geometry is developed which, as one of the maxims suggests, loads the shoulder area and minimally loads the abdominal area.

An air-bag system, because it has a positive internal pressure, can exert a distributed force on any body that distorts its free surface regardless of the penetrating object's geometry. This characteristic allows the air bag, as another of the maxims suggests, to distribute forces over a large area of the body. Additionally, because the air bag comes into position only after the crash is initiated, it can assume a geometry that can be tailored to apply restraint forces to body areas other than the thorax, such as the head (Fig. 8.8), which then satisfies another maxim that suggests that articulations of the body should be minimized.

With regard to the other maxims presented previously, each restraint addresses and applies them to varying degrees. With respect to the first maxim, which suggests that time over which restraint forces are applied be maximized, the belt system, because it is in place prior to the crash, has the greatest potential to comply with it. However, because of the retraction features that must have large amounts of webbing within the belt system, the time before significant restraint forces can be achieved is not always optimal. This difficulty

FIGURE 8.8. Force
distribution
characteristic of air bag.

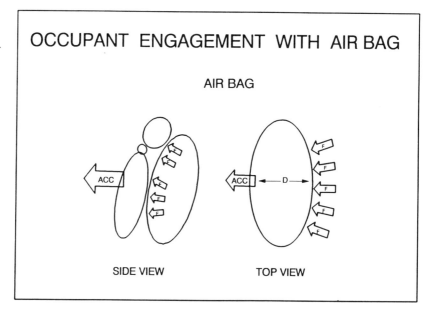

is somewhat alleviated by crash-sensitive pretensioning devices that rapidly remove slack. The air-bag system, because it is not in its operational position before the crash, must devote time after the initiation of the crash to first decide if the crash is of significant intensity to warrant deployment and then to perform the deployment process itself. Because deployment rates are also limited due to special considerations brought about by alternative positions and sizes of the occupant, further reductions of deployment times are difficult to achieve.

Since the time to initiate effective restraint forces is determined by other considerations, the best way for systems to maximize the distance the restraint force moves over the ground, the second maxim, is to allow the occupant to translate within the compartment. The belt system accomplishes this by tailoring the elasticity of the belt webbing or by incorporating a force-limiting device that maximizes internal displacement. These techniques, however, cannot allow the torso to translate to full advantage because the unrestrained head translates forward of the torso and consumes much of the available stroking space. The air-bag system accomplishes additional within-compartment translation by venting the bag so

that it is deflating while still restraining the occupant and also by allowing the steering column to stroke after a predetermined force is achieved. Because the head is restrained by the air bag and remains in a more upright position than in a belt system, more translation distance is available for the occupant without developing concerns about head impacts. The achievement of within-compartment translation in either restraint requires a strict compromise and a total knowledge of the crash conditions the restraint must handle because, if a design allows much or all of the translation space consumed at low crash intensities, it will allow too much translation in high-intensity crashes, involve the occupant in other impacts with interior structures, and have reduced safety effectiveness.

Over the years, a variety of techniques have been devised, developed, and applied to both belt and air-bag restraint systems to improve their safety performance. A listing of some of these techniques together with a short description of each technique's operational principle and objective is given in Table 8.1. Here too, it can be seen that each of these enhancements has as its origin and operation one or more of the maxims for good restraint design.

TABLE 8.1. Restraint performance enhancers.

Belt systems
- Pretensioner—A device, activated by a sensor detecting the onset of the crash, which retracts belts rapidly, removing any slack and coupling the occupant to the vehicle structure sooner than a standard belt system would

  Effect: Maximizes time and distance over which belt forces are applied, applies greater restraint forces earlier in the crash event, and therefore affords greater energy extraction
- Variable stiffness seat cushion—A cushion that is stiffer at the front edge than toward the rear by the seat back

  Effect: Prevents the pelvis from moving down while being restrained by a lap-belt system, thus maintaining correct belt geometry to ensure the belt remains on the bony pelvis and does not slip up and over the pelvis into the soft abdomen and cause injuries
- Force-limiting belt webbing—Seat-belt webbing designed to stretch at a predetermined level

  Effect: Limits the maximum force applied to the body and allows the body to translate more within the occupant compartment as well as over the ground, thus extracting a greater amount of the initial kinetic energy
- Retracting steering system—A steering system designed to move forward within the compartment as the front of the car crushes during an impact

  Effect: Provides a greater translation distance within the compartment for the driver using a safety-belt system, thus increasing the energy extraction potential with reduced force
- Face or head air bags—A small volume air bag mounted on the steering wheel to apply forces to and control the head motions of a three-point belt-restrained driver

  Effect: Provides distributed restraint loads to the head and minimizes head articulations during crash while using a torso belt
- Inflating belts—A torso belt system, which, upon sensing the initiation of a crash, inflates to large-diameter cylinder

  Effect: Increases the contact area between the belt and the thorax as well as removing slack for the system and coupling the occupant to the vehicle earlier in the crash sequence
- Web lockers—A device that clamps the torso belt and prevents it from unwrapping from its take-up spool or reel

  Effect: Prevents torso belt from becoming longer and allowing the occupant to translate within the compartment without substantial restraint forces being applied to him

Air-bag systems
- Dual inflation levels—Air-bag systems that, depending on the logic provided, are either crash sensitive and/ or occupant sensitive, will inflate with different rates and/or volumes of gas depending on the intensity of the crash and/or the size or proximity of occupant to the inflation module

  Effect: Crash or size-sensitive systems modulate the forces applied to the occupant according to need (greater forces in higher-intensity crashes or for

TABLE 8.1. *Continued*

  heavier occupants) thus allowing optimal stroke within compartment. Proximity-sensitive systems reduce inflation rate when occupant near module to prevent unnecessarily high forces being applied
- Dual air bags—An air bag within an air bag where the inflator directly inflates the inner bag and then vents the gases into the outer bag to inflate it

  Effect: Allows the small-volume inner bag to inflate rapidly and apply forces earlier in the crash event with the subsequent large outer bag adding area and force capability later in the crash event
- Precrash sensing (anticipatory)—Means by which an imminent crash is sensed prior to the actual initiation of the crash and restraint operations are begun

  Effect: Allows the restraint system to initiate its application of forces earlier in the crash event by either pretensioning-belt systems or initiating inflation of air bag sooner
- Stroking columns—Specifically designed column support structure that deforms in a specified direction while applying a controlled force

  Effect: Allows the occupant to have greater stroke within the compartment, thus extending the time over which he accomplishes the necessary velocity change and extracting more of his kinetic energy
- Air bag/seat-belt combination—Safety system designed to exploit advantages of both restraint systems

  Effect: Employs the best operational characteristics of both restraint concepts to provide optimal restraint for the occupant

Summary

While the examples and discussions given above have been restricted to only illustrate and explain the performance of occupant restraints in frontal crashes, occupant restraints must operate over a wide variety of crash directions and conditions that exist in today's automotive crash environment. Since the ultimate performance of a restraint system is dependent on its integration into the vehicle structure and that structure's performance characteristics during a crash, even identical restraint systems in different vehicles can have vastly different performance envelopes. It is obvious that their individual performance can only be judged by a detailed analysis of each complete crash event as it affects the human occupant and his biomechanical limits for each of the particular crash types being considered. Since the laws of motion remain the same in all directions; since the risk to the human may have different thresholds for different directions but remains associated with the magnitude of velocity change, how rapidly that change in velocity is accomplished, and the means by which the velocity change is accomplished; the maxims espoused and discussed above, because they are also based on first principles, can be considered universal in their application and can be used to discern why a particular restraint is a poor performer, as well as to suggest potential strategies and modifications to improve performance regardless of the crash direction.

9
Biomechanics of Bone

Steven Goldstein, Elizabeth Frankenburg, and Janet Kuhn

Introduction

The composition and structural integrity of the human skeleton have uniquely evolved, reflecting its need to balance four major functions: protection of vital organs, mechanical support and locomotion, mineral homeostasis, and hematopoiesis. During the past century numerous investigators have carefully attempted to document the mechanical and architectural properties of bone. These studies have provided insight into potential mechanisms of bone remodeling and also contributed to the assessment of fracture risk under normal, aging, or disease conditions.

The mechanical properties of bone, like any structure, are dependent on the material properties of its constituents and the way in which those constituents are arranged. Unlike classical engineering materials, it is highly anisotropic, nonlinear, and viscoelastic and has the ability to alter its structure as a function of mechanical and/or physiologic demand. It is not possible to provide universal constants to characterize the properties of bone or to easily predict its behavior in response to a given set of boundary conditions. It is clear, therefore, that a fundamental understanding of the factors that contribute to bone integrity and response is critical for an appropriate assessment of its ability to withstand the demands of specific activities.

The purpose of this chapter is to review some of the current perspectives on the mechanical and remodeling characteristics of bone.

While the review is not exhaustive, it is hoped that it will provide a framework from which many applications can be assessed. The chapter is organized in a format that parallels the hierarchical order of bone structure and mechanical properties. It summarizes the current understanding of structure/function relationships in bone, the results of experimental measures of bone mechanical properties, and suggested directions for future research.

Bone Structure

General Anatomy/Composition and Microstructure of Bone

Two major types of bone are found in the human body: trabecular and cortical bone. While the chemical, molecular, and cellular components of both types are similar, the organization of these constituents, at both an ultrastructural and a microstructural level, reflect significant differences in their mechanical and metabolic activities.[68,113] While all bone tissue generally consists of cells encased within a two-phase extracellular matrix, the microstructural classifications result from variations in the architecture of the extracellular matrix. The two phases of the matrix include an organic phase composed primarily of collagen type I and a variety of glycosaminoglycans while the inorganic phase or mineral phase is composed of primarily calcium phosphate crystals (hydroxyapatite). Three primary cell lines comprise the metabolic machinery of bone, including the osteoblasts or bone-forming cells; the osteocytes, which become encased within the extracellular matrix and function to maintain bone; and the osteoclasts, which function to resorb bone.

The tissue that comprises both cortical and trabecular bone can be classified into three general microstructural types: woven bone, primary bone, and secondary bone. Woven bone is characterized by randomly oriented collagen fibers, producing a structurally disorganized matrix. The construction of the loosely packed collagen fibers results in a large porosity and the appearance of a reduced density. However, woven bone can become highly mineralized very rapidly. It is the only bone type that can be synthesized in regions where no bone previously existed. Woven bone is expressed in the course of fracture or damage repair since it has the advantage of being quickly deposited and mineralized. As a consequence, however, it has substantially reduced mechanical properties when compared to more highly ordered bone. Woven bone also has an extremely high cell density, enabling it to proliferate quite rapidly. Clearly, it represents an efficient and effective mineralized tissue for repairing damage that results from trauma or pathologic disorders.[40,90,113,155]

The second classification of the microstructural types is primary bone. Primary bone forms on existing surfaces of either cartilage or bone and is arranged in lamellar sheets. In cortical bone, the lamellae are concentrically arranged around a blood vessel, forming a characteristic subunit referred to as a primary osteon. This highly organized structure exhibits excellent mechanical properties.[52,58,68,113]

In the human skeleton, secondary osteonal bone is the primary constituent of the adult cortices. Through a cellularly directed process of resorption and formation, primary bone is remodeled to secondary bone.[68,69,113] The formation of these secondary osteons is detailed in Fig. 9.1. It has been proposed that the incentive to form this osteonal structure

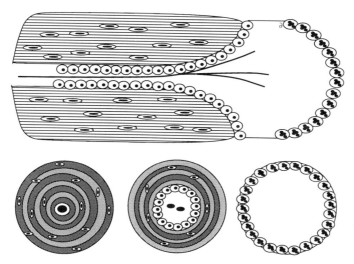

FIGURE 9.1. Remodeling of cortical bone is schematically illustrated. After activation, the large multinucleated osteoclasts resorb the existing bone as denoted by the characteristic cutting cone. The next stage is denoted as reversal when the surface of the bone is prepared for the initiation of osteoblastic expression of unmineralized bone matrix. Once the osteoid is laid down, mineralization follows until both the formation front and mineralization front reach completion and a secondary osteon is formed. Note that the bone is laid down in a lamellar structure surrounding the invaginating blood vessel forming the haversian canal. Osteoblasts that have been surrounded by the matrix that they expressed become the ostecytes incorporated within the tissue lamellae. The osteocytes maintain contact with the haversian canal as well as with each other through canaliculi as described in the text.

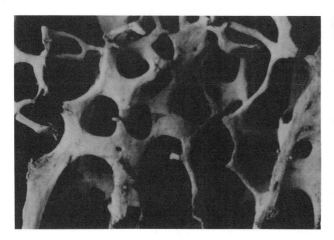 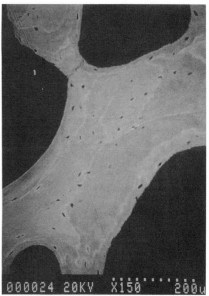

FIGURE 9.2. Trabecular bone at the continuum level is composed of plates, rods, or struts forming a complex anisotropic architecture. Remodeling in trabecular bone occurs on surfaces. As can be recognized from the magnified view of a cross section of an individual trabeculae (on the right), remodeling occurs in discrete packets. These packets can be differentiated from each other by subtle differences in gray scale and are separated by the cement line.

stems from a need to provide nutrients to the interstitial bone (the remnants of preexisting osteons) and is a means for increased resistance to fracture crack propagation and potential failure under cyclic loading.[18,54]

In contrast to cortical bone, trabecular bone is composed of only interstitial lamellae and remodeling occurs on surfaces within discrete regions designated as trabecular packets. The complex three-dimensional latticelike structure of trabecular bone results in a very large surface-to-volume ratio. This increased surface area of bone tissue exposed to marrow provides greater potential for the exchange of minerals through the process of remodeling.[128] In addition, the architecture of trabecular bone provides an effective energy-absorbing structure to attenuate the large loads transmitted across the joints (Fig. 9.2).[28,86]

Cortical Bone Architecture

As described earlier, the most important structural subunit within cortical bone in the human skeleton is the secondary osteon. Each osteon represents a series of concentric lamellae surrounding a central vascular channel (haversian canal). Osteocytes reside within the lamellae surrounding the haversian canal and each osteon is bounded from extraosteonal bone matrix by a 1–5-μm-thick cement line.[113] Typical osteons range in size from 200 to 300 μm in diameter, although it has been reported that these dimensions vary with age.[53,91] Interconnecting vascular channels known as Volkmann's canals complete the distributed vascular network. The osteocytes access nutrients locally through canaliculi that allow the cell processes to directly communicate to either the surface of the bone or the vascular canals (Fig. 9.3).[46]

Variations in the mechanical properties of cortical bone can be significantly influenced by the number, orientation, and size of the osteons.[14,47,33,62,63,66,134] Similarly, the structure of individual lamellae that comprise the concentric "sheaths" of the osteons has been reported to vary in orientation, thereby in-

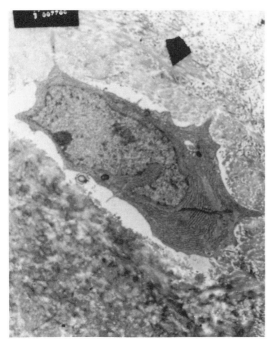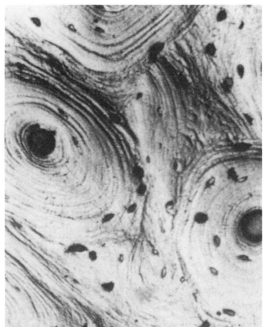

FIGURE 9.3. Magnified view of osteonal bone is demonstrated. Note that the individual osteons are separated from one another and the interstitial lamellae by cement lines. The highly ordered structure of the bone is assumed to be regulated by the mechanical environment to which it is habitually subjected. The osteocytes (on the right) that are embedded within the lamellar structure have cell processes that extend through the canaliculi and form gap junctions with cell processes from the flat lining cells on the surface of the bone. It has been hypothesized that in addition to providing nutrition from the haversian canal to the ostecytes, the processes may also provide direct communication, acting as a distributed sensing mechanism for detecting mechanical or metabolic stimuli.

fluencing the mechanical behavior even at this level of the composite structure.[111,131,148] As a result of these potential architectural variations, all of which are mediated by the remodeling processes, cortical bone can be optimally constructed to satisfy very local demands. For example, in most long-bone diaphyses, the osteons are arranged longitudinally along the long axis of the bone, thereby providing greater mechanical stability and resistance to the dominant bending, torsional, and compressive loads that result from physiologic function. It can be seen, therefore, that careful analysis of bone microarchitecture provides tremendous insight into the mechanical environment that governed the tissue's construction. Similarly, this histologic knowledge coupled with quantifiable boundary conditions may enable the prediction of the mode of failure within the bone.

Trabecular Bone Architecture

Trabecular bone is a highly anisotropic structure composed of a large number of interconnected rods, plates, or beams. Trabecular bone is dominant in the metaphyses of the appendicular skeleton, where it absorbs and dissipates energy transmitted across the diarthrodial joints. In the axial skeleton it is a dominant constituent of the vertebral bodies. The increased porosity of trabecular bone (greater than 30%) contributes to its significantly increased rate of turnover relative to cortical bone. As a result, it is much more susceptible to the morphologic alterations that accompany advancing age, metabolic diseases, and other pathologic processes.[122,129]

Galileo was likely one of the first investigators to note the existence of a relationship between the architecture of the skeleton and the function for which it is designed.[72] Observations of the German anatomists and engineers in the late 1800s, however, described a formalized relationship between trabecular bone architecture and functional loading. These scientists recognized a correlation between the patterns of trabecular alignment and the estimated principal stress directions incurred during normal function in long bones. This relationship is known as Wolff's law.[50,138,151,158] The underlying principles of Wolff's law propose that bone, in particular trabecular bone, is optimally designed. While these concepts have been generally accepted for many years, the mathematical laws relating bone architecture to specific mechanical stresses or strains or their underlying structural optimization objectives remain unknown. While the original tenet of Wolff's law related macroscopic features and stress conditions, it is now believed that mechanical stresses influence bone adaptation and maintenance at the cellular level and that there exist specific relationships between mechanical stimulation and genetic expression mediated by connective-tissue cells.[12,96,137] It is therefore assumed that the microarchitecture of both cortical bone and trabecular bone is significantly influenced by the mechanical stresses associated with normal physiologic function.

Most of the earlier work in quantifying the architecture of trabecular bone can be found in a summary provided by Hayes and Snyder.[86] Primarily using stereologic-based algorithms, measures of bone volume fraction, trabecular-plate thickness, separation and number, connectivity, and anisotropy have been described.[48,64,83,100,126,156] Depending on anatomic location, typical bone volume fractions from 10% to 40% have been reported. Trabecular plate thickness may vary from 100 to 200 μm. The structural anisotropy or orientation of trabecular bone also varies with location, being nearly isotropic in regions such as the center of the femoral head, while highly oriented in the vertebral bodies.[79] The incentive behind recent analyses has been to make direct correlative relationships between architectural and material constants for trabecular bone volumes.

In all of the studies described above the term "trabecular bone" refers to a continuum volume (typically greater than 5 mm per side) suitable for mechanical testing. A few studies have investigated the architecture of the individual trabeculae or struts that make up the volumes. As noted earlier, the individual trabeculae are composed of parallel lamellae organized within discrete remodeled regions known as trabecular packets. In trabecular tissue, the boundary between successive packets is defined as the cement line. Although the importance or contribution of microstructural features (number of lamellae, lamellar thickness, packet volume, cell number) to the mechanical properties is currently unknown, they clearly contribute to its composite properties and the observed patterns of failure.

Repair, Remodeling, and Adaptation

The metabolic activity of bone tissue maintains a supply of mineral for many physiologic functions. As a result, the turnover of bone provides the opportunity for both provision of mineral homeostasis and optimal reformatting of the reconstituted bone under changing mechanical stimulation.

The process by which the bone remodels involves precisely controlled functions of osteoblasts, osteoclasts, and their associated activation factors and cofactors. The remodeling is reported to occur in discrete localized regions and the group of cells participating in this process has been termed the bone multicellular unit (BMU).[68,113,128] Remodeling proceeds through a sequence of activation, resorption, and formation during which one quantum of bone is exchanged. It has been proposed that bone turnover by way of this remodeling process prevents the accumulation of microdamage and maintains access to relatively low-mineral-density bone necessary for maintaining mineral homeostasis.[68,113,128] Parfitt has further differentiated the quantum theory of bone remodeling to include five steps: quiescence, activation, resorption, reversal, and formation.[128] The rationale for extending the theory of remodeling is supported by a need to elucidate the specific function of this complex set of cell-directed processes.

It has been proposed by several investigators that the mechanical stresses associated with normal function tend to suppress the rate of bone remodeling, thereby generally maintaining the bone's inherent mechanical integrity. During habitual underloading the rate and number of sites of remodeling are significantly increased, thereby increasing the potential for significant loss of bone (greater resorption than formation).[67,68,113] Many controlling mechanisms have been proposed, including stress-generated potentials, direct physical stimulation of the associated cells, hydrostatic pressure within the extracellular fluids under load, fatigue damage, and alterations in cell membrane diffusion due to direct loads or fluid flow.[18,113] It can easily be recognized that any interruption in the normal process of bone turnover or maintenance can initiate a cascade of events resulting in loss of bone mass and integrity.

Bone modeling, which is defined as activation and formation without resorption, is typically seen to occur under two conditions: during a process of growth and development and during repair or a fracture-healing processes. Modeling has been characterized by deposition of woven bone that is later remodeled into secondary bone. While modeling is rarely observed in the adult skeleton other than during fracture healing, it can be induced by irritation of the periosteum or surgical manipulation such as insertion of an orthopedic implant.

As noted earlier, the adaptation of bone (modeling or remodeling) is significantly influenced by mechanical stresses or strains. A large number of investigations have attempted to characterize the mechanical conditions that effect bone adaptation using either experimental or analytical techniques.[a] Data suggest that factors such as strain rate, stress or strain magnitude, and direction influence bone adaptation, but the relative importance of these loading characteristics is unknown. It is clear that continuing research is necessary to elucidate the role of these factors.

Additional factors that influence the adaptation of bone are alterations in the metabolic or biochemical environment surrounding the bone. Perhaps one of the most significant factors effecting the adaptation of bone is age.[b] The aging process is associated with specific alterations in the size, geometry, and microstructural features of bone. In cortical bone the diameter and number of osteons varies with age and in trabecular bone a generalized decrease in connectivity and overall trabecular mass is observed during advancing age. In general, all humans begin to lose bone mass after the age of approximately 35 as a result of a physiologic inability to maintain a positive bone balance. The exact causes of age-related bone loss are unknown but are likely related to alterations in availability of factors or cofactors associated with the remodeling processes or perhaps specific changes in the cell's ability to sense mechanical stimuli or to express normal matrix. Despite the propensity for loss of bone during the aging process, the mechanical adaptation mechanisms remain partially intact as reflected in the observations of geometric alterations in bone with age such as increases in diaphyseal diameter, expansion of joint surfaces, and the preservation of vertical trabeculae within vertebral bodies.[c]

Finally, it is important to note that a variety of disease conditions including postmenopausal osteoporosis, rheumatoid arthritis, Paget's disease, and many other conditions significantly affect the amount and distribution of bone and potentially the adaptational mechanisms of the skeleton. In addition, treatment protocols including the use of corticosteroids, chemotherapeutic agents, and others significantly affect the quality and amount of bone in patients being treated. Assessing the mechanical integrity of the skeleton therefore

---

[a] See refs. 18, 34, 35, 36, 37, 41, 49, 70, 74, 77, 78, 84, 85, 87, 88, 96, 103, 105, 106, 110, 137, 139, 145, and 159.

[b] See refs. 3, 13, 20, 68, 98, 113, 120, 122, 123, 126, 129, and 152.

[c] See refs. 3, 13, 20, 68, 73, 98, 113, 120, 122, 123, 126, 129, and 152.

involves the analysis of many factors and conditions.

Details regarding the remodeling, modeling, or adaptational properties of bone, the biologic mechanisms controlling these processes, and the effects of age and common diseases can be found in refs. 68, 69, and 113.

Mechanical Properties of Bone

In this section the mechanical properties of both cortical bone and trabecular bone will be summarized. It is important to note that bone is a nonlinear, viscoelastic, anisotropic, inhomogeneous material, and therefore, unlike typical engineering materials, the properties cannot be simply described by two independent material constants. Instead the properties are dependent on the physiologic condition of the bone, the histologic and architectural features, and the loading conditions to which it is subjected. The data in this section, taken from the vast literature of experimental bone studies, serve as a guideline for understanding the mechanical behavior of bone.

Storage and Preservation of Bone

The mechanical properties of bone can vary significantly depending on the conditions of dissection, storage, and mechanical testing. While it would be optimal to perform biomechanical tests immediately after dissection, issues of practicality necessitate the storage of bone tissue for later careful preparation and testing.

The appropriate method of bone preservation must consider the behavior of its constituents, including collagen, mineral, and water. Early experimental studies reported that drying, embalming, or fixation in various solutions can significantly alter these constituents and influence the mechanical properties of bone.[117,143] As a result of these studies, the most commonly accepted method of preservation involves freezing specimens. Specifically, bone is dissected as soon as possible after death of the donor, wrapped in towels or moistened with normal saline or

physiologic Ringer's solution, and stored in sealed bags at -20 to $-30°C$. Leaving the surrounding periosteum, muscle, and skin intact may help to preserve the moisture content within the bone during long-term storage in the freezer. Data have been less clear concerning the length of time bone may be stored in the freezer. Clearly, excessive drying or freezer "burn" should be avoided.

Cortical Bone Properties

Methods of Testing

As noted, the anisotropic, inhomogeneous properties of bone complicate the accurate assessment of its mechanical behavior. The general approach to the mechanical testing of cortical bone, therefore, has assumed isotropy, transverse isotropy, or orthotropy with mechanical testing in multiple directions and careful documentation of the anatomic location of specimens.

In order to calculate the nine independent elastic coefficients of an orthotropic material (the most frequent assumption for cortical bone), many mechanical tests must be conducted.[8,135] These include tensile and compressive tests in each of the three mutually perpendicular material directions, three torsional tests for shear moduli, and strain measurements for calculation of Poisson's ratios. Implicit in this test method is knowledge of the axes of material symmetry. For diaphyseal bone, these axes are generally directed parallel to the long axis of the diaphysis, circumferential to its cross section, and radial from the longitudinal midline. In order to reduce errors associated with misalignment with material axes it is recommended that specimens of interest be analyzed histologically in an effort to determine the structural orientation of osteons and interstitial lamellae.[92] Further characterization of the anisotropic material properties may be possible with more extensive testing and structural analysis.

A large number of standards have been published by the American Society for Testing of Materials (ASTM) for testing in compression, tension, bending, shear, and torsion.[2] However, when applied to bone, the required size of specimens and difficulties associated with machining specimens to interface with standard grips often make it difficult to comply with the standards precisely. Typical "standards" for cortical bone testing are represented in the work of Reilly et al.[134] These standards pertain to test specimen shape and dimension, machining precautions, compliance of the testing apparatus, methods of load and deformation measurement, and test parameters such as the humidity and temperature of the test and load or displacement rate. The test apparatus compliance should be at least two orders of magnitude less than the test specimen or corrections to the cross-head-displacement measurement are required. Alternatively, localized displacement transducers such as extensometers or optical strain measures can be used.

The specific mode of testing (i.e., tension, compression, bending, shear, torsion) and the test parameters depend on the hypothesis being evaluated. However, typical test parameters include moistened specimens at room or body temperature, and strain rates in the physiologic range of approximately 0.002 to 0.01 pers to simulate normal activities or 0.1 to 1.0 pers to simulate traumatic activities.[25,27,104] Similar to the testing of engineering materials, the critical properties derived from stress–strain curves include elastic modulus, yield strength, ultimate strength, energy absorption, and postyield strain.

Dynamic tests have also been conducted on cortical bone to obtain fatigue and viscoelastic properties.[29,31,38,102,133,150] Due to the limitations of size and shape of available cortical bone specimens it is difficult to comply with standardized methods for fatigue testing used for classic engineering materials. However, since specimen shape, size, and cyclic rate can effect fatigue properties it is important to specify the exact conditions for any fatigue test carried out on cortical bone. Similar to engineering materials, the testing can be applied in fluctuating axial tension, completely reversed axial loading, fluctuating bending, and completely reversed bending. The bending can be accomplished with a rotating beam apparatus in either cantilever or three- or four-point contact. In general, four-point bending is preferred over three-point bending (for monotonic and fatigue testing) due to the more even distribution of stresses that result from the moments generated. Fatigue testing can be accomplished under conditions of constant load or deflection and cyclic frequencies of 2–125 Hz have been reported in the literature.[26,31,101] While the typical presentation of fatigue testing is in the form of SN curve documentation, the reduction in modulus that occurs during fatigue testing of cortical bone has been described recently, providing insight into the mechanisms of failure of bone tissue.[125]

It is important to note the existence of alternative testing techniques, particularly those that are nondestructive. The most important of these is ultrasonic testing, which has been used to a reasonable extent in both cortical and trabecular bone.[7–9] One advantage of ultrasonic testing in comparison to standard materials testing is its ability to calculate several anisotropic properties from specimens without the need for machining complicated shapes. The technique is based on elastic-wave theory, which predicts relationships between stress-wave velocities and anisotropic elastic properties for materials with symmetry of at least orthotropy.[7–9] The important parameters include the density of bone and the velocity of wave propagation. In bone, the most important methods that have been described include pulse transmission, continuous-wave transmission, and pulse-echo techniques.[7–9] Ultrasonic testing is fairly effective for evaluating cortical bone since it is a rather homogeneous nonporous structure. In cancellous bone, its significant porosity makes ultrasonic techniques much more difficult. The use of ultrasonic techniques for evaluating whole bones (in comparison to selected tissue samples) is even more difficult due to the complex geometries and inhomogeneities.[7] As such, most reports in the literature describe only the attenuation and the velocities of the ultrasonic waves. Several investigators have advocated whole-bone evaluation with ultrasonic- or acoustic-wave techniques for the evaluation of healing fractures as well as for the diagnosis of osteopenic disorders.[121,124,130,140]

Elastic Constants

A summary of published data concerning the mechanical properties of cortical bone can be found in Tables 9.1–9.34.

Work on alternative species including bovine and canine reflect both easier access to these materials as well as their use as models for human diseases and conditions. The tremendous variations in properties noted in the tables result from different testing methods, temperature and moisture conditions during testing, and the direction of testing. Within a species as well as within individual bones significant variations have been found reflecting the structural optimization as prescribed by Wolff's law. These variations are due to bone's inherent composite structure: variations in porosity, osteonal orientation, and even cellular density may contribute to its macroscopic behavior.

Viscoelastic Properties

As with all biologic materials, bone is viscoelastic and nonlinear. It has been demonstrated that cortical bone is strain-rate dependent in that it exhibits stiffer and stronger behavior at higher strain rates. Carter and Hayes reported that its ultimate stress and elastic modulus are proportional to strain rate raised to the 0.06 power.[27] Further evidence of bone's viscoelastic behavior was noted in studies designed to characterize creep behavior as well as time-dependent recovery from a deformed state.[29,30,38,133] These variations in properties as a function of strain rate become important in light of the need to predict bone failure under a variety of physiologic and nonphysiologic conditions.

Summary of Macroscopic Properties

The review of the mechanical properties of cortical bone and the details presented in Tables 9.1–9.34 provide data with a macroscopic perspective. At this level cortical bone behaves as a complex composite composed of secondary osteons organized in a specific orientation that reflects physiologic function. The in vivo and in vitro mechanical behavior of cortical bone is affected by many factors: these include variations in composition and structure that might accompany remodeling processes and also the characteristics of the loading regime such as load or strain rate, magnitude, direction, or frequency. As a composite material with many hierarchical levels of microstructure, cortical bone mechanical properties will depend on the structural characteristic that dominates at the chosen level of analysis. Therefore, though discussion in this section was limited to a macroscopic perspective, further insight into the behavior of cortical bone can be gained from more microscopic approaches. These will be described later in the chapter.

Trabecular Bone Properties

Methods of Storage, Preparation, and Testing

Trabecular bone has been extensively evaluated in the literature during the past 100 years. Like cortical bone, trabecular bone is a nonlinear, inhomogeneous, viscoelastic, anisotropic material, requiring similar assumptions for isotropic, transversely isotropic, and orthotropic models of its behavior. However, mechanical evaluation of trabecular bone presents an even greater challenge to biomechanists due to its complex three-dimensional cancellous structure: a structure that varies with anatomic location to a much greater degree than the osteonal structure of cortical bone.[76]

The storage and preparation of trabecular bone specimens follows the same procedures as previously outlined for cortical bone: dissection from the donor as soon as possible after death, maintained moist, sealed, and frozen at −20 to −30°C. The difficulties associated with machining trabecular bone specimens as well as designing appropriate clamping fixtures have made compliance with mechanical testing standards extremely difficult.

TABLE 9.1. Femur: whole-bone compressive and torsional properties.

Source	Comments (years)	Compressive breaking load (kg)	Torsional breaking moment (kg/cm)	Ultimate torsional strength (kg/mm²)	Ultimate angle of twist (°)
Yamada (1970)			1,400	4.62	1.5 (est.)
	Male				
	20–39	5,050			
	40–59	4,780			
	60–89	4,290			
	Female				
	20–39	4,190			
	40–59	3,980			
	60–89	3,540			

TABLE 9.2. Femur: whole-bone bending properties.

Author	Comment	Cross-sectional area (mm²)	Bending breaking load (kg)	Bending strength (kg/mm²)	Ultimate deflection (mm)	Elastic modulus (kg/mm²)	Modulus of rigidity (kg/mm²)
Mather (1967)				16			
Yamada (1970)						1,870	$3,107 \times 10^4$
	Male	330					
	Female	260					
	20–39 years		277 ± 11	21.2 ± 0.8	12.3 ± 0.34		
	40–49 years		252 ± 5	19.9 ± 0.4	11.4 ± 0.30		
	50–59 years		240 ± 9	19.0 ± 0.4	10.6 ± 0.23		
	60–69 years		238 ± 6	18.1 ± 0.5	10.2 ± 0.16		
	70–89 years		218 ± 11	16.5 ± 0.9	9.6 ± 0.44		
	Adult average		250	19.3	11.1		

TABLE 9.3. Tibia: whole-bone compressive and torsional properties.

Source	Comments	Compressive breaking load (kg)	Torsional breaking moment (kg/cm)	Ultimate torsional strength (kg/mm²)	Ultimate angle of twist (°)
Yamada (1970)			1,000	4.43	3.4
	Midsection				
	Male	3,660			
	Female	2,820			

TABLE 9.4. Tibia: whole-bone bending properties.

Author	Comment	Cross-sectional area (mm²)	Bending breaking load (kg)	Bending strength (kg/mm²)	Ultimate deflection (mm)	Elastic modulus (kg/mm²)	Modulus of rigidity (kg/mm²)
Yamada (1970)						1,220	$2,189 \times 10^4$
	Male	240					
	Female	180					
	20–39 years		296 ± 11	21.7 ± 0.4	10.0 ± 0.42		
	40–49 years		257 ± 11	20.9 ± 0.4	9.2 ± 0.33		
	50–59 years		248 ± 5	20.0 ± 0.4	8.6 ± 0.37		
	60–69 years		244 ± 9	19.2 ± 0.3	8.4 ± 0.21		
	70–89 years		234 ± 9	17.1 ± 0.4	7.8 ± 0.25		
	Adult average		262	20.1	9.0		

TABLE 9.5. Fibula: whole-bone compressive and torsional properties.

Source	Comments	Compressive breaking load (kg)	Torsional breaking moment (kg/cm)	Ultimate torsional strength (kg/mm²)	Ultimate angle of twist (°)
Yamada (1970)			116	4.01	35.7
	Midsection				
	Male	860			
	Female	590			
	Distal 4/5				
	Male	890			
	Female	610			

TABLE 9.6. Fibula: whole-bone bending properties.

Author	Comment	Cross-sectional area (mm²)	Bending breaking load (kg)	Bending strength (kg/mm²)	Ultimate deflection (mm)	Elastic modulus (kg/mm²)	Modulus of rigidity (kg/mm²)
Yamada (1970)						1,260	159×10^4
	Male	70					
	Female	50					
	20–39 years		45 ± 2	22.0 ± 0.7	16.2 ± 0.56		
	40–49 years		41 ± 4	20.6 ± 0.9	14.6 ± 0.48		
	50–59 years		40 ± 3	19.8 ± 0.4	13.9 ± 0.39		
	60–69 years		38 ± 2	18.9 ± 0.4	13.3 ± 0.32		
	70–89 years		34 ± 2	17.5 ± 0.4	11.8 ± 0.47		
	Adult average		40	20.1	14.3		

TABLE 9.7. Humerus: whole-bone compressive and torsional properties.

Source	Comments	Compressive breaking load (kg)	Torsional breaking moment (kg/cm)	Ultimate torsional strength (kg/mm²)	Ultimate angle of twist (°)
Yamada (1970)			606	4.35	5.9
	Midsection				
	Male	2,580			
	Female	2,100			
	Distal 4/5				
	Male	2,840			
	Female	2,310			

TABLE 9.8. Humerus: whole-bone bending properties.

Author	Comment	Cross-sectional area (mm²)	Bending breaking load (kg)	Bending strength (kg/mm²)	Ultimate deflection (mm)	Elastic modulus (kg/mm²)	Modulus of rigidity (kg/mm²)
Yamada (1970)						1,020	832×10^4
	Male	200					
	Female	160					
	20–39 years		151 ± 12	21.5 ± 0.5	10.0 ± 0.15		
	40–49 years		142 ± 10	19.5 ± 0.4	9.4 ± 0.28		
	50–59 years		131 ± 10	19.0 ± 0.5	8.3 ± 0.26		
	60–69 years		125 ± 9	18.2 ± 0.3	7.7 ± 0.21		
	70–89 years		115 ± 8	16.4 ± 0.6	7.3 ± 0.34		
	Adult average		136	19.3	8.8		

TABLE 9.9. Radius: whole-bone compressive and torsional properties.

Source	Comments	Compressive breaking load (kg)	Torsional breaking moment (kg/cm)	Ultimate torsional strength (kg/mm^2)	Ultimate angle of twist ($°$)
Yamada (1970)			208	4.95	15.4
	Midsection				
	Male	950			
	Female	780			
	Distal 4/5				
	Male	980			
	Female	800			

TABLE 9.10. Radius: whole-bone bending properties.

Author	Comment	Cross-sectional area (mm^2)	Bending breaking load (kg)	Bending strength (kg/mm^2)	Ultimate deflection (mm)	Elastic modulus (kg/mm^2)	Modulus of rigidity (kg/mm^2)
Yamada (1970)						1,620	140×10^4
	Male	80					
	Female	70					
	20–39 years		60 ± 7	23.2 ± 0.6	10.4 ± 0.24		
	40–49 years		54 ± 4	21.9 ± 0.6	9.6 ± 0.24		
	50–59 years		53 ± 8	21.0 ± 0.3	8.9 ± 0.49		
	60–69 years		49 ± 4	20.1 ± 0.3	8.3 ± 0.22		
	70–89 years		44 ± 3	18.5 ± 0.4	8.0 ± 0.25		
	Adult average		53	21.3	9.3		

TABLE 9.11. Ulna: whole-bone compressive and torsional properties.

Source	Comments	Compressive breaking load (kg)	Torsional breaking moment (kg/cm)	Ultimate torsional strength (kg/mm^2)	Ultimate angle of twist ($°$)
Yamada (1970)			190	4.55	15.2
	Midsection				
	Male	1,140			
	Female	850			

TABLE 9.12. Ulna: whole-bone bending properties.

Author	Comment	Cross-sectional area (mm^2)	Bending breaking load (kg)	Bending strength (kg/mm^2)	Ultimate deflection (mm)	Elastic modulus (kg/mm^2)	Modulus of rigidity (kg/mm^2)
Yamada (1970)						1,570	191×10^4
	Male	90					
	Female	70					
	20–39 years		72 ± 5	23.0 ± 0.5	11.1 ± 0.13		
	40–49 years		64 ± 8	21.6 ± 0.5	10.1 ± 0.31		
	50–59 years		62 ± 6	21.1 ± 0.4	9.2 ± 0.42		
	60–69 years		60 ± 4	20.3 ± 0.8	8.4 ± 0.24		
	70–89 years		56 ± 4	18.7 ± 0.9	8.1 ± 0.46		
	Adult average		64	21.3	9.4		

TABLE 9.13. Femur: cortical-bone tensile properties.

Author	Comment	Yield stress (MPa)	Ultimate stress (MPa)	Percent elongation	Modulus of elasticity (MPa)
Burstein et al. (1972)					14,100
Burstein et al. (1973)	Longitudinal		151 ± 18		17,425
	Transverse				12,700
Burstein et al. (1976)	20–29 years	120	140	3.4	17,000
	30–39 years	120	136	3.2	17,600
	40–49 years	121	139	3.0	17,700
	50–59 years	111	131	2.8	16,600
	60–69 years	112	129	2.5	17,100
	70–79 years	111	129	2.5	16,300
	80–89 years	104	120	2.4	15,600
Evans & Lebow (1951)	*Wet*				
	Proximal $\frac{1}{3}$		77	1.246	13,507
	Middle $\frac{1}{3}$		83	1.274	14,540
	Distal $\frac{1}{3}$		81	1.154	14,265
	Anterior		78	1.198	14,609
	Posterior		80	1.056	14,334
	Medial		80	1.353	13,851
	Lateral		84	1.335	13,989
	Dry				
	Proximal $\frac{1}{3}$		104	0.670	17,159
	Middle $\frac{1}{3}$		111	0.666	19,020
	Distal $\frac{1}{3}$		104	0.670	17,986
	Anterior		99	0.545	17,193
	Posterior		108	0.687	17,228
	Medial		110	0.722	18,055
	Lateral		111	0.691	18,579
Ko (1953)	Longitudinal		122 ± 1.1		17,300
Reilly & Burstein (1975)	Longitudinal		133		17,400
	Transverse		51		12,700
Sedlin & Hirsch (1966)	Longitudinal		86.5		6,260
Yamada (1970)	Wet		122	1.41	17,259
	Dry		151	1.24	20,201
	10–19		113	1.48	
	20–29		123	1.44	
	30–39		120	1.38	
	40–49		112	1.31	
	50–59		93	1.28	
	60–69		86	1.26	
	70–79		86	1.26	

Specimen size and shape are important parameters for valid mechanical tests. Rectangular or cylindrical specimens are usually used for compression, tension, or shear testing. Cubic specimens allow mechanical tests in three directions and provide data for orthotropic descriptions of the mechanical properties. The specimen size must be sufficiently small to avoid structural inhomogeneities but large enough to satisfy the continuum assumption.[16,82] Further, the dimensions of the specimen and the characteristics of the specimen–load-head interface can produce nonuniform strain fields, which in turn affect the calculation of strain-dependent measures such as elastic modulus. Careful analysis of the effect of end conditions and of specimen dimensions can be found in the literature.[16,76,108,109]

Properties measured from experimentally derived stress–strain curves depend on several factors. Recent work by Linde and Hvid in 1989 has suggested that preconditioning of the specimen prior to property determinations is critical in order to enhance the repeatability of the measured characteristics. Like cortical bone, trabecular bone is also load- or stain-rate sensitive; however, evaluation of the effect of load rate has shown that the marrow content within the trabeculated structure provides a viscous stiffening effect at only very high strain

TABLE 9.14. Femur: cortical-bone compressive properties.

Author	Comment	Breaking load (kg)	Ultimate stress (MPa)	Percent contraction	Modulus of elasticity (MPa)
Burstein et al. (1976)	20–29 years		209		18,100
	30–39 years		209		18,600
	40–49 years		200		18,700
	50–59 years		192		18,200
	60–69 years		179		15,900
	70–79 years		190		18,000
	80–89 years		180		15,400
Carothers et al. (1949)	Preserved				26,700
Kimura (1952)					10,400
McElhaney (1970)			140		
Reilly & Burstein (1975)	Longitudinal		193		18,200
	Transverse		133		11,700
Yamada (1970)	(*Midshaft, longitudinal*)				
	Male				
	20–39	5,050			
	40–59	4,780			
	60–89	4,290			
	Female				
	20–39	4,190			
	40–59	3,980			
	60–89	3,540			
	20–29		167	1.9	
	30–39		167	1.8	
	40–49		161	1.8	
	50–59		155	1.8	
	60–69		145	1.8	
Yokoo (1952)			159		

TABLE 9.15. Femur: cortical-bone bending properties.

Author	Comment	Bending strength (MPa)	Ultimate specific deflection (%)	Modulus of rupture (MPa)	Young's modulus (MPa)
Sedlin (1965)		164		181	15,800
Sedlin and Hirsch (1966)		181		176	15,500
Tsuda (1957)		157			
Yamada (1970)	10–19 years	151	8.6		
	20–29 years	174	7.5		
	30–39 years	174	6.6		
	40–49 years	162	6.2		
	50–59 years	154	6.2		
	60–69 years	139	5.3		
	70–79 years	139	5.3		

TABLE 9.16. Femur: cortical-bone torsion properties.

Author	Comment	Utimate torsional strength (MPa)	Ultimate distortion (%)	Shear modulus (GPa)
Reilly & Burstein (1975)		68		3.28
Yamada (1970)	20–29 years	57.0	2.8	3.43
	30–39 years	57.0	2.8	3.43
	40–49 years	52.7	2.5	3.14
	50–59 years	52.7	2.5	3.14
	60–69 years	48.6	2.7	2.94
	70–79 years	48.6	2.7	2.94
	80–89 years	48.6	2.7	—

TABLE 9.17. Femur: cortical-bone shear properties.

Author	Shearing strength (MPa)	Ultimate displacement (mm)
Yamada (1970)	82.37	0.60

TABLE 9.18. Femur: cortical-bone hardness properties.

Author	Comment	Rockwell hardness	Brinell hardness	Vickers hardness (transverse)	Vickers hardness (tangential)
Evans & Lebow (1951)	$\frac{1}{8}''$ diam. steel ball, 45-kg load, 10 seconds				
	Wet				
	Proximal $\frac{1}{3}$	13.2			
	Middle $\frac{1}{3}$	17.3			
	Distal $\frac{1}{3}$	14.2			
	Anterior quad.	15.4			
	Posterior quad.	19.8			
	Medial quad.	14.6			
	Lateral quad.	14.0			
	Dry				
	Proximal $\frac{1}{3}$	22.1			
	Middle $\frac{1}{3}$	26.7			
	Distal $\frac{1}{3}$	24.3			
	Anterior quad.	21.7			
	Posterior quad.	23.1			
	Medial quad.	27.2			
	Lateral quad.	22.4			
Yamada (1970)	*Wet*				
	20–29 years	49	27		
	30–39 years	45	26		
	40–49 years	43	25		
	50–59 years	39	24		
	60–69 years	34	23		
	70–79 years	32	22		
	Dry				
	10–19 years	60	30		
	20–29 years	66	33		
	30–39 years	64	32		
	40–49 years	62	31		
	50–59 years	58	29		
	60–69 years	54	28		
	70–79 years	54	28		
	Surface				
	20–29			24.9	21.5
	30–39			25.7	22.3
	40–49			25.1	21.8
	50–59			25.1	21.4
	60–69			24.7	21.5
	70–79			25.2	21.9
	80–89			25.2	21.9
	Middle				
	20–29			27.9	24.7
	30–39			28.1	24.7
	40–49			28.2	24.8
	50–59			28.2	24.9
	60–69			27.5	24.4
	70–79			27.8	24.6
	80–89			27.8	24.6

TABLE 9.19. Tibia: cortical-bone tensile properties.

Author	Comment	Yield stress (MPa)	Ultimate stress (MPa)	Percent elongation	Modulus of elasticity (MPa)
Burstein et al. (1976)	20–29 years	126	161	4.0	18,900
	30–39 years	129	154	3.9	27,000
	40–49 years	140	170	2.9	28,800
	50–59 years	133	164	3.1	23,100
	60–69 years	124	147	2.7	19,900
	70–79 years	120	145	2.7	19,900
	80–89 years	131	156	2.3	29,200
Dempster & Coleman (1960)	Longitudinal		95.3		
	Transverse		9.9		
Melick & Miller (1966)	*Longitudinal*				
	>60 years		138		
	<60 years		119		
Vincentelli & Grigorov (1985)	Primary bone		162.43	2.58	19,726
	Haversian bone		133.10	2.17	18,014
	>75% Primary bone		161.23	2.66	19,411
	<25% Primary bone		129.53	2.18	17,595
Yamada (1970)	Wet		140.23	1.50	18,044
	Dry		170.63	1.29	20,593

TABLE 9.20. Tibia: cortical bone compressive properties.

Author	Comment	Ultimate stress (MPa)	Modulus of elasticity (MPa)
Burstein et al. (1976)	30–39 years	213	35,300
	40–49 years	204	30,600
	50–59 years	192	24,500
	60–69 years	183	25,100
	70–79 years	183	26,700
	80–89 years	197	25,900
Carothers et al. (1949)	Preserved		28,400

TABLE 9.21. Tibia: cortical-bone bending properties.

Author	Comment	Modulus of rupture (MPa)
Dempster & Coleman (1960)	Along grain	18,926
	Across grain	3,236

TABLE 9.22. Tibia: cortical-bone shear properties.

Author	Shearing strength (MPa)	Ultimate displacement (mm)
Yamada (1970)	80.41	0.66

TABLE 9.23. Fibula: cortical-bone tensile properties.

Author	Comment	Ultimate stress (MPa)	Percent elongation	Modulus of elasticity (MPa)
Ko (1953)	Longitudinal	146		
Yamada (1970)	Wet	146.11	1.59	18.534
	Dry	175.53	1.38	21,084

TABLE 9.24. Fibula: cortical-bone shear properties.

Author	Shearing strength (MPa)	Ultimate displacement (mm)
Yamada (1970)	80.41	0.69

TABLE 9.25. Humerus: cortical-bone tensile properties.

Author	Comment	Ultimate stress (MPa)	Percent elongation	Modulus of elasticity (MPa)
Yamada (1970)	Wet	122.58	1.43	17,161
	Dry	154.94	1.28	20,005

TABLE 9.26. Humerus: cortical-bone shear properties.

Author	Shearing strength (MPa)	Ultimate displacement (mm)
Yamada (1970)	73.55	0.64

TABLE 9.27. Radius: cortical-bone tensile properties.

Author	Comment	Ultimate stress (MPa)	Percent elongation	Modulus of elasticity (MPa)
Yamada (1970)	Wet	149.06	1.50	18,534
	Dry	176.52	1.31	21,378

TABLE 9.28. Radius: cortical-bone shear properties.

Author	Shearing strength (MPa)	Ultimate displacement (mm)
Yamada (1970)	70.61	0.68

TABLE 9.29. Ulna: cortical-bone tensile properties.

Author	Comment	Ultimate stress (MPa)	Percent elongation	Modulus of elasticity (MPa)
Yamada (1970)	Wet	148.08	1.49	18,436
	Dry	177.50	1.30	21,182

rates.[27,76] Lastly, as with cortical bone studies, other test parameters such as test apparatus compliance and test environment (humidity and temperature) must be known or controlled. Ultrasonic techniques have also been applied to the study of trabecular bone mechanics and have offered the advantage of being able to determine a more complete set of anisotropic constants nondestructively.[7,9]

Elastic and Ultimate Properties

As noted in Tables 9.1–9.34, a huge variation in measured moduli and strengths has been reported throughout the literature. These variations have been attributed to differences in testing methods as well as significant variations in the trabecular architectures associated with anatomic location, age, and testing direction. As noted earlier in this chapter, the architecture and mechanical properties of trabecular bone reflect the structural optimization assumptions contained within Wolff's law. Variations as high as two orders of magnitude have been found within individual methaphyses, further exemplifying both the difficulties in assessing trabecular bone properties and that bone's critical dependence on density and architectural configuration.

TABLE 9.30. Ulna: cortical-bone shear properties.

Author	Shearing strength (MPa)	Ultimate displacement (mm)
Yamada (1970)	81.39	0.71

TABLE 9.31. Proximal femur: trabecular-bone compressive properties.

Author	Comment	Breaking load (kg)	Ultimate strength (MPa)	Modulus of elasticity (MPa)
Brown & Ferguson (1980)	9.5-mm length			344.7
	5-mm cubes		120–310	
Ciarell et al. (1986, 1991)	10-mm length		2.1–16.2	58–2,248
	8-mm cubes			49–572
Evans & King (1961)	2.5 × 0.79-cm prisms		0.21–14.82	
Hardinge (1949)	0.25-inch diam., 0.25-inch length	47.6–173		
Martens et al. (1983)	8-mm diameter		0.45–15.6	1,000–9,800
Schoenfeld et al. (1974)	0.79-cm cubes			20.68–965
	4.8-mm diameter		0.15–13.5	

TABLE 9.32. Dstal femur: trabecular–bone compressive properties.

Author	Comment	Ultimate strength (MPa)	Modulus of elasticity (MPa)
Behrens et al. (1974)	5-mm slab	2.25–66.2	
Ciarelli et al. (1986, 1991)	8-mm length		58.8–2,942
	8-mm cubes	18.6 (0.56%)	7.6–800
Ducheyne et al. (1977)	5-mm diameter	0.98–22.5	
Pugh et al. (1973)	9.5-mm diameter 5-mm length		413–1516

TABLE 9.33. Proximal tibia: trabecular-bone compressive properties.

Author	Comment	Ultimate strength (MPa)	Compression at rupture (%)	Modulus of elasticity (MPa)
Behrens et al. (1974)	5-mm slab	1.8–63.6		
Carter & Hayes (1977)	10.3-mm diameter 5-mm length	1.5–45		1.4–79
Ciarell et al. (1986, 1991)	8-mm cubes	0.52–11	5–552	
Goldstein et al. (1983)	7-mm diameter	1–13		8–457
Hvid & Hansen (1985)	10-mm length 5-mm slabs	13.8–116.4		4–430
Lindahl (1976)	14 mm 9 mm			
	Male	3.9	13.4	34.6
	Female	2.2	11.6	23.1
Linde & Hvid (1989)	No constraint			113–853
Williams & Lewis (1982)	5–6-mm cubes	1.5–6.7		10–500

TABLE 9.34. Vertebral bodies: trabecular-bone compressive properties.

Author	Comment	Ultimate strength (MPa)	Ultimate percentage contraction (%)	Modulus of elasticity (MPa)	Shear modulus (MPa)
Ashman et al. (1986)	5-mm diameter 10–15-mm length			158–378	58–89
Bartley et al. (1966)	Lumbar region	2.9			
Galante et al. (1970)	7-, 10-mm diameter	0.39–5.98			
Keller et al. (1987)	1-cm cubes			15–30	
Lindahl (1976)	$10 \times 9 \times 14$ mm Male	4.6	9.5	55.6	
	Female	2.7	9.0	35.1	
McElhaney et al. (1970)	10-mm length	4.13		151.7	
Rockoff et al. (1969)	Lumbar region	0.69–6.9			
Struhl et al. (1987)	8- & 6-mm cubes	0.06–15		10–428	
Weaver & Chalmers (1966)	1-cm cube	0.34–7.72			
Yamada (1970)	40–49 years	1.86	2.5	88.2	
	60–69 years	1.37	2.4	68.6	

The majority of studies have been performed in compression. Far fewer studies have attempted to characterize the tensile and shear properties of trabecular bone. As noted above, its complex latticelike structure has necessitated unusual testing protocols and fixture designs. The use of wedge grips and incorporation of cement in specimen ends have been reported in studies designed to determine the tensile properties of trabecular bone. Care must be taken to ensure that these gripping methods do not significantly alter the inherent properties being measured. Shear properties have been evaluated primarily from cylindrical specimens interposed between sliding plates (Tables 9.1–9.34).

Effects of Physical Properties on Bone Mechanical Properties

Careful review of the tabulated properties of both cortical and trabecular bone from the literature reveal dramatic variations in nearly all properties reported. While there have been significant deviations in the testing methods and the environmental conditions, perhaps the most important factors associated with explaining the variance in properties relates to physical measures of density and architecture of the tested specimens. Driven by the desire to find noninvasive methods of assessing bone properties, nearly all studies have included measures of bone mass or mineralization.

In general, investigators have found significant relationships between the mechanical properties of bone and its bone mineral content, ash weight density, or apparent density.[15,16,30,51] Since the variations in properties of cortical bone are small in comparison to trabecular bone and the variations in bone properties that occur with age or disease affect primarily trabecular bone, most densitometry studies have concentrated on trabecular bone. As noted in the literature, both nonlinear power functions and linear functions have been reported for the relationship between trabecular bone mechanical properties and its apparent density.[76] The results of these in vitro studies suggest that architectural parameters are as important as measures of bone density in explaining trabecular bone's mechanical behavior.

The noninvasive techniques for determining bone mineral density have included single photonabsorptiometry (SPA), dual photon-absorptiometry (DPA), quantitative computed tomography (QCT), and more recently dual-energy x-ray absorptiometry (DXA). All these methods except for QCT are two-dimensionally based and therefore provide a summation of density information for the entire three-dimensional object projected onto a two-dimensional image. Computed tomography provides a three-dimensional description and allows for information on volumetric density distributions. While all of these measures have been relatively successful in providing estimates of mechanical integrity, evaluation of these modalities continues because controversy remains concerning their specificity and sensitivity. More recent developments have included the use of ultrasonography and magnetic resonance imaging for the same general purpose. The readers are referred to the vast literature describing the usefulness of these techniques and their limitations.[d]

Microscopic (Tissue) Properties of Bone

As noted throughout the chapter, bone mechanical properties are dependent on the characteristics of its composite structure, the dominating features of which change with each level of magnification. Therefore, the mechanical properties must be considered with respect to this hierarchy of microstructure. Consistent with this perspective has been a series of studies that have been designed to investigate the microscopic mechanical properties of both cortical and trabecular bone. As discussed earlier, the incentive is provided by the need to better characterize the mechanisms of failure in bone as well as the mechanisms of adaptation or repair.

In cortical bone, several investigators including Amprino, Ascenzi, Bonucci, Frasca, and others have provided unique information regarding the properties of bone at the level of the individual osteons.[1,4–6,65,154] Moduli ranging from approximately 4 to 13 GPa have been reported. Some of the variance can be explained by differences in the ultrastructure and degree of mineralization of osteons. Until recently, few investigators had measured the properties of trabecular tissue at this scale. More recent analytical and experimental studies suggest that the properties of trabecular tissue are significantly lower than cortical tissue in the range of approximately 1–10 GPa with an average of approximately 3–4.[38,39,99,119] These differences may also relate to the ultrastructural features of bone such as lamellar thickness or number, collagen fiber orientations, and lacunar size and number, the features that essentially dominate the next level of hierarchical structure.

Finally, Choi et al. have reported some of the first data concerning the fatigue behavior of bone tissue at the microscopic level.[38] The authors suggest that differences in the observed mechanisms of failure of cortical and trabecular tissue may be explained in part by differences in their ultrastructure.

Future Work

This chapter has emphasized the need to establish structure–function relationships in bone but has also posed numerous questions that remain unanswered. If the future demands better methods to predict fracture risk, or monitor remodeling, more accurate noninvasive measures of bone properties must be developed. Such an endeavor requires continued advances in technology and theory. As the analysis of bone progresses through the hierarchy of structure, eventually, predictions of its behavior near or within the cells will be reached. The future thus calls for parallel advances in the study of the molecular behavior of bone and concurrently, the development of analytical techniques to incorporate these complex microstructural and ultrastructural features into mechanical models.

[d] See refs. 15, 22, 23, 44, 45, 56, 59, 80, 115, 116, and 152.

References

1. Amprino R (1958) Investigations on some physical properties of bone issue. Acta Ancet 34:161–186.
2. *Annual book of ASTM standards*. American Society for Testing of Materials. Philadelphia PA, 1978.
3. Arnold JS (1973) Amount and quality of trabecular bone in osteoporotic vertebral fractures. Clin Endocrin Metab 2(22):221–238.
4. Ascenzi A, Bonucci E (1964) The ultimate tensile strength of single osteons. Acta Anat 58:160–183.
5. Ascenzi A, Benvenlti A (1985) Mechanical hystresis loops from single osteons: technical devices and preliminary results. J Biomech 18:391–398.
6. Ascenzi A, Bonucci E (1967) The tensile properties of single osteons. Anat Rec 158:375–386.
7. Ashman RB, Rho JY (1988) Elastic modulus of trabecular bone material. J Biomech 21(3):177–181.
8. Ashman RB, Cowin SC, Van Buskirk WC, Rice JC (1984) A continuous wave technique for the measurement of the elastic properties of cortical bone. J Biomech 17(5):349–361.
9. Ashman RB, Turner CH, Cowin SC. *Ultrasonic technique for the measurement of the structural elastic modulus of cancellous bone*. Transactions of the Orthopedic Research Society, p 43, 1986.
10. Bartley MH, Arnold JS, Haslam RK, Jee WSS (1966) The relationship of bone strength and bone quantity in health, disease, and aging. J Gerontol 21:517.
11. Behrens JC, Walker PS, Shoji H (1974) Variation in strength and structure of cancellous bone at the knee. J Biomech 7:201–207.
12. Binderman I, Zor U, Kaye AM, Shimshoni Z, Harell A, Somjen D (1988) The transduction of mechanical force into biochemical events in bone cells may involve activation of phospholipase A_2. Calcified Tissue Int 42:261–266.
13. Birkenhager-Frenkel DH, Courpron P, Hupscher EA, Clermonts E, Coutinho MF, Schmitz PIM, Meunier PJ (1988) Age-related changes in cancellous bone structure. Bone and Mineral 4:197–216.
14. Black J, Mattson R, Korostoff E (1974) Haversion osteons; size, distribution, internal structure, and orientation. J Biomed Mat Res 8:299–319.
15. Brassow F, Crone-Munzebrock W, Weh L, Kranz R, Egger-Storeder G (1982) Correlations between breaking load and CT absorption values of vertebral bodies. Eur J Radio 2:99–101.
16. Brown TD, Ferguson AB (1980) Mechanical property distribution in the cancellous bone of the human proximal femur. Acta Orthop Scand 51:429–437.
17. Buckley MJ, Banes AJ, Levin LG, Sumpio BE, Sato M, Jordan R, Gilbert J, Link GW, TranSonTay R (1988) Osteoblasts increase their rate of division and align in response to cyclic mechanical tension *in vitro*. Bone and Mineral 4:225–236.
18. Burr DR, Martin RB, Schaffler MB, Radin EL (1985) Bone remodeling in response to *in vivo* fatigue microdamage. J Biomech 18(3):189–200.
19. Burstein AH, Currey JD, Frankel VH, Reilly DT (1972) The ultimate properties of bone tissue: the effects of yielding. J Biomech 5:34–44.
20. Burstein AH, Reilly DT, Martens M (1976) Aging of bone tissue: mechanical properties. J Bone Joint Surg 58(A):82.
21. Burstein AH, Reilly DT, Frankel VH. Failure characteristics of bone and bone tissue. In Kenedi RM (ed) *Perspectives in biomedical engineering*. University Park Press, Baltimore, 1973.
22. Cann CE, Genant HK, Kolb FO, Ettinger E (1985) Quantitative computed tomography for prediction of vertebral fracture risk. Bone 6:1–7.
23. Cann CE, Genant HK (1980) Precise measurement of vertebral mineral content using computed tomography. J Comput Assist Topmogr 4(4):493–500.
24. Carothers CO, Smith FC, Calabrisi P. The elasticity and strength of some long bones of the human body. Naval Med Research Inst, Project NM, 001, 056.0213, 1949.
25. Carter DR, Spengler DM (1978) Mechanical properties and composition of cortical bone. Clin Orthop Rel Res 135 Sept: 192–217.
26. Carter DR, Caler WE, Spengler DM, Frankel VH (1981) Uniaxial fatigue of human cortical bone—the influence of tissue physical characteristics. J Biomech 14:461.
27. Carter DR, Hayes WC (1977) The compressive behavior of bone as a two-phase porous structure. J Bone Joint Surg 59A:954–962.

28. Carter DR, Fyhrie DP, Whalen WT (1987) Trabecular bone density and loading history: regulation of connective tissue biology by mechanical energy. J Biomech 20(8):785–794.

29. Carter DR, Hayes WC, Schurmann DJ (1976) Fatigue life of compact bone—II. Effects of microstructure and density. J Biomech 9:211–218.

30. Carter DR, Hayes WC (1976) Bone compressive strength: the influence of density and strain rate. Science 194:1174–1176.

31. Carter DR, Hayes WC (1977) Compact bone fatigue damage I. residual strength and stiffness. J Biomechanics 10:325.

32. Carter DR, Hayes WC (1977) The compressive behavior of bone as a two-phase porous structure. J Bone Joint Surg 59A(7):954–962.

33. Carter DR, Spengler DM (1978) Mechanical properties and composition of cortical bone. Clin Orthop Relat Res 135:192–217.

34. Carter DR (1987) Mechanical loading history and skeletal biology. J Biomech 20(11):1095–1109.

35. Chamay A, Tschantz P (1972) Mechanical influences in bone remodeling. experimental research on Wolff's law. J Biomech 5:173–180.

36. Cheal EJ, Hayes WC, Leuzinger RA, Nunamaker DM. *A model for trabecular bone remodeling around an implant.* Trans Orthop Res Sco, p 376, 1985.

37. Cheal EJ, Snyder BD, Nunamker DM, Hayes WC (1987) Trabecular bone remodeling around smooth and porous implants in an equine patellar model. J Biomech 20(11):1121–1134.

38. Choi K, Goldstein SA (1992) A Comparison of the Fatigue Behavior of Human Trabecular and Cortical Bone Tissue. J Biomech 25(12):1371–1381.

39. Choi K, Kuhn JL, Ciarelli MJ, Goldstein SA (1990) The elastic moduli of human subchondral, trabecular and cortical bone tissue and the size-dependency of cortical bone modulus. J Biomech 23(11):1103–1113.

40. Christel P, Cerf C, Pilla A (1981) Time evolution of the mechanical properties of the callus of fresh fractures. Annals Biomed Eng 9:383–391.

41. Churches AE, Howlett CR, Waldron KS, Ward GW (1979) The response of living bone to controlled time varying loading: method and preliminary results. J Biomech 12:35–34.

42. Ciarelli MJ, Goldstein SA, Dickie D, Ku JL, Kapper M, Stanley J, Flynn MJ, Matthews LS. Experimental determination of the orthogonal mechanical properties, density, and distribution of human trabecular bone from the major metaphyseal regions utilizing materials testing and computed tomography. Trans Orthop Res Soc, p 42, 1986.

43. Ciarelli MJ, Goldstein SA, Kuhn JL, Cody DD, Brown MB (1991) Evaluation of orthogonal mechanical properties and density of human trabecular bone from the major metaphyseal regions with materials testing and computed tomography. J Orth Res 9:674–682.

44. Cody DD, Flynn MJ, Vickers DS (1989) A technique for measuring regional bone mineral density (rBMD) in human lumbar vertebral bodies. Med Phys 16(5):766–772.

45. Cody DD, Goldstein SA, Flynn MJ, Brown EB (1991) Correlations between vertebral regional bone mineral density (rBMD) and whole bone fracture load. Spine 16(2):146–154.

46. Cooper RR, Milgram JW, Robinson RA (1966) Morphology of the osteon. an electron microscopic study. JBJS 48A:1239–1271.

47. Cowin SC (ed). *Mechanical properties of bone.* ASME Press, New York, 1981.

48. Cowin SC (1985) The relationship between the elasticity tensor and the fabric tensor. Mech Mat 4:137–147.

49. Cowin SC (1986) Wolff's law of trabecular architecture at remodeling equilibrium. J Biomech Eng 108:83–88.

50. Culmann C. Die Graphische Statik, 1. Auflage. Mayer und Zeller, Zurich, 1866.

51. Currey JD (1970) The mechanical properties of bone. Clin Orth Rel Res 73 Nov–Dec: 210–231.

52. Curry JD (1982) Osteons in biomechanics literature. J Biomech 15:717.

53. Curry JD (1964) Some effects of aging in human Haversion systems. J Anat 98:69–75.

54. Curry JD (1989) Strain rate dependence of the mechanical properties of reindeer antler and the cumulative damage model of bone fracture. J Biomech 22:469–476.

55. Dempster WT, Coleman RF (1960) Tensile strength of bone along the grain. J Appl Physiol 16:355–360.

56. Dickie DL. The determination of lumbar vertebral fracture characteristics using computed tomography. PhD Thesis. University of Michigan, 1987.

57. Ducheyne P, Heymans L, Martens M, Aernoudt E, Meester PD, Mulier JC (1977) The mechanical behavior of intracondylar

cancellous bone of the femur at different loading rates. J Biomech 10:747–762.

58. Enlow DH (1962) Functions of the Haversion system. Am J Anat 110:269–282.

59. Eriksson SAV, Isberg BO, Lindgren JU (1989) Prediction of vertebral strength by dual photon absorptiometry and quantitative computed tomography. Calcif Tissue Int 44:243–250.

60. Evans FG, King AL. Regional differences in some physical properties of human spongy bone. In Evans FG (ed) *Biomechanical studies of the musculo-skeletal system.* CC Thomas, Springfield, IL, pp 49–67, 1961.

61. Evans FG, Lebow M (1951) Regional differences in some of the physical properties of the human femur. J Appl Physiol 3:563–572.

62. Evans FG, Vincentelli R (1974) Relations of the compressive properties of human cortical bone to histological structure and calcification. J Biomech 7:1–10.

63. Evans FG (1958) Relations between the microscopic structure and tensile strength of human bone. Acta Anta 35:285–301.

64. Feldkamp LA, Goldstein SA, Parfitt AM, Jesion G, Kleerekoper M (1989) The direct examination of three dimensional bone architecture *in vitro* by computed tomography. J Bone Mineral Res 4:3–11.

65. Frasca P, Jacyna G, Harper R, Katz JL (1981) Strain dependence of dynamic Youngs modulus for human single osteons. J Biomech 14:691–696.

66. Frasca P, Harper RA, Katz JL (1978) Mineral and collagen fiber orientation in human secondary osteons. J Dental Res 57:526–533.

67. Frost HM (1983) A determinant of bone architecture: the minimum effective strain. Clin Orthop Relat Res 175:286–292.

68. Frost HM. *Intermediary organization of the skeleton.* CRC Press, Boca Raton, FL, 1986.

69. Frost HM. *The laws of bone structure.* Charles C Thomas, Springfield, 1964.

70. Fyhrie DP, Carter DR (1986) A unifying principle relating stress to trabecular morphology. J Orthop Res 4:304–317.

71. Galante J, Rostoker W, Ray RD (1970) Physical properties of trabecular bone. Calcif Tissue Res 5:236–246.

72. Galileo G. Discorsi e dimonstrazioni matematiche, intorno a due nuove scienze attentanti alla meccanica ed a muovementi locali. University of Wisconsin Press, 1638. (As cited by Martin and Burr, 1989.)

73. Gallagher JC (1990) The pathogenesis of osteoporosis. Bone and Mineral 9:215–227.

74. Goldstein SA, Matthews LS, Kuhn JL, Hollister SJ (1991) Trabecular bone remodeling: an experimental model. J Biomech 24:Suppl. 1, 135–150.

75. Goldstein SA, Wilson DL, Sonstegard DA, Matthews LS (1983) The mechanical properties of human tibial trabecular bone as a function of metaphyseal location. J Biomech 16:965–969.

76. Goldstein SA (1987) The mechanical properties of trabecular bone: dependence on anatomic location and function. J Biomech 20(11/12):1055–1061.

77. Goldstein SA, Hollister SJ, Kuhn JL, Kikuchi N. The mechanical properties of trabecular bone. In Mow VC, Radcliffe A, Woo SLY (ed) *Biomechanics of diarthrodial joints.* Vol II. Springer-Verlag, 1990.

78. Goodship AE, Lanyon LE, McFie H (1979) Functional adaptation of bone to increased stress. J Bone Joint Surg 61A: 539–546.

79. Goulet RW, Ciarelli MJ, Goldstein SA, Kuhn JL, Feldkamp LA, Kruger D, Viviano D, Champlain F, Matthews LS (1988) The effects of architecture and morphology on the mechanical properties of trabecular bone. Trans Orthop Res Soc, 73.

80. Hansson T, Roos B, Nachemson A. Bone mineral content and ultimate compressive strength of lumbar vertebrae. Spine 5(1): 46–55.

81. Hardinge MG (1949) Determination of the strength of the cancellous bone in the head and neck of the femur. Surgery Gynec Obstet 89: 439–441.

82. Harrigan TP, Jasty M, Mann RW, Harris WH (1988) Limitations of the continuum assumption in cancellous bone. J Biomech 21(4): 269–275.

83. Harrigan TP, Mann RW (1984) Characterization of microstructural anisotropy in orthotropic materials using a second rank tensor. J Mat Sci 19:761–767.

84. Hart RT, Davy DT, Heiple KG (1984) A computational method for stress analysis of adaptive elastic materials with a view towards applications in strain-induced bone remodeling. J Biomech Eng 106:342–350.

85. Hassler CR, Rybicki EF, Simonen FA, Weis EB (1974) Measurements of healing an osteotomy in a rabbit calvarium: the influence of applied compressive stress on collagen synthesis and calcification. J Biomech 7:545–550.

86. Hayes WC, Snyder B (1981) Toward a quantitative formulation of Wolff's law in trabec-

ular bone in mechanical properties of bone. Am Soc Mech Eng 45:43–68.

87. Hert J, Pribylova E, Liskova M (1972) Reaction of bone to mechanical stimuli. Acta Anat 82:218–230.

88. Hollister SJ, Goldstein SA, Jepsen KJ, Goulet RW (1990) Continuum and microstructural stress morphology relationships for trabecular bone subject to controlled implant loads. ORS 15:74.

89. Hvid I, Hansen SL (1985) Trabecular bone strength patterns at the proximal tibial epiphysis. J Orthop Res 3:464–472.

90. Jaffe HL (1929) The structure of bone with particular reference to its fibrillar nature and the relation of function to internal architecture. Arch Surg 19:24–52.

91. Jowsey J (1966) Studies of Haversion systems in man and some animals. J Anat 100:857–864.

92. Katz JL, Yoon HS (1974) The structure and anisotropic mechanical properties of bone. IEEE Trans Biomed Eng 31:12.

93. Keller TS, Hansson TH, Panjabi MM, Spengler DM (1987) Regional variations in the compressive properties of lumbar trabeculae. Trans Orthop Res Soc 378.

94. Kimmell PL. (1984) Radiologic methods to evaluate bone mineral content (1984) Ann Intern Med 100:908.

95. Kimura H (1952) Tension test upon the compact substance in the long bones of cattle extremities. J Kyoto Pref Med Univ 51:365–372.

96. Klein-Nulend J, Veldhuijzen JP, deLong M, Burger EH (1987) Increased bone formation and decreased bone resorption in fetal mouse calvaria as a result of intermittent compressive force in vitro. Bone and Mineral 2:441–448.

97. Ko R (1953) The tension test upon the compact substance in the long bones of cattle extremities. J Kyoto Pref Med Univ 53:503–525.

98. Kragstrup J, Melsen F, Mosekilde L (1983) Thickness of bone formed at remodeling sites in normal human ilia trabecular bone: variations with age and sex. Metab Bone Dis Rel Res 5:17–21.

99. Kuhn JL, Goldstein SA, Choi K, London M, Feldkamp LA, Matthews LS (1989) A comparison of the trabecular and cortical tissue moduli from human iliac crests. J Orthop Res 7:874–886.

100. Kuhn JL, Goldstein SA, Feldkamp LA, Goulet RW, Jesion G (1990) Evaluation of a microcomputed tomography system to study trabecular bone. J Orthop Res 8:833–842.

101. Lafferty JF, Raju RUU (1979) The influence of stress frequency on the fatigue strength of cortical bone. J Biomech Eng 101:112.

102. Lakes RS, Katz JL, Sternstein SS. Viscoelastic properties of wet cortical bone I. torsional and braxial studies. J Biomech 12:657–678.

103. Lanyon LE, Goodship AE, Pye CJ, MacFie JH (1982) Mechanically adaptive bone remodeling. J Biomechanics 15(3):141–154.

104. Lanyon LD, Hampson WGJ, Sternstein SS (1975) Bone deformation recorded in vivo from strain gauges attached to the human tibial shaft. Acta Orthop Scand 46:256.

105. Lanyon LE (1974) Experimental support for the trajectorial theory of bone structure. J Bone Joint Surg 56B:160–166.

106. Lanyon LE (1987) Functional strain in bone tissue as an objective and controlling stimulus for adaptive bone remodeling. J Biomech 20(11/12):1083–1094.

107. Lindahl O (1976) Mechanical properties of dried defatted spongy bone. Acta Orthop Scand 47:11–19.

108. Linde F, Hvid I (1987) The effect of constraint on the mechanical behavior of trabecular bone specimens. J Biomech 22(5):485–490.

109. Linde F, Hvid I, Pongsoipetch B (1989) Energy absorptive properties of human trabecular bone specimens during axial compression. J Orth Res, 7:432–439.

110. Liskova M, Hert J (1971) Reaction of bone to mechanical stimuli. Part 2: periosteal and endosteal reaction of tibial diaphysis in rabbit to intermittent loading. Folia Morphol 19:301–317.

111. Maj G, Toajari E (1937) A resistenza meccanica del tessuto osseo lamellare compatto inisurata in varie direzioni. Boll Social Biol Sper 12:83–86.

112. Martens M, VanAudekercke R, Delport P, DeMeester P, Muelier JC (1983) The mechanical characteristics of cancellous bone at the upper femoral region. J Biomech 16:971–983.

113. Martin RB, Burr DB. Structure function and adaptation of compact bone. Raven Press, New York, 1989.

114. Mather BS (1967) The symmetry of the mechanical properties of the human femur. J Surg Res 7:222.

115. McBroom RJ, Hayes WC, Edwards WT, Goldberg RP, White AA (1985) Prediction of vertebral body compressive fracture using

computed tomography. J Bone Joint Surg 67A(8):1206–1213.

116. McCubbrey DA, Cody DD, Kuhn JL, Flynn MJ, Goldstein SA (1990) Static and fatigue failure properties of thoracic and lumbar vertebral bodies and their relation to regional density. Trans Orthop Res Soc 15:178.

117. McElhaney JH, Fogle JL, Melvin JW, Haynes RR, Roberts VL, Alem NM (1970) Mechanical properties of cranial bone. J Biomech 3:495–511.

118. Melick RA, Miller DR (1966) Variations of tensile strength of human cortical bone with age. Clon Sci 30:243–248.

119. Mente PL, Lewis JL (1989) Experimental method for the measurement of the elastic modulus of trabecular bone tissue. J Orth Res 7:456–461.

120. Meunier P, Courpron P, Edouard C, Bernard J, Bringuier J, Vignon G (1973) Physiologic senile involution and pathological rarefaction of bone: quantitative and comparative histologic data. Clin Endocrinol Metab 2:239–256.

121. Miller AT, Porter RW. The prediction of fracture of the proximal femur by broadband ultrasonic attenuation. Sixth International Workshop on Bone and Soft Tissue Densitometry. Buxton, England, p 83, 1987.

122. Mosekilde L, Mosekilde L (1990) Sex differences in age-related changes in vertebral body size, density and biomechanical competence in normal individual. Bone 11:67–73.

123. Mosekilde L (1989) Sex differences in age-related loss of vertebral trabecular bone mass and structure—biomechanical consequences. Bone 10:425–432.

124. Nicoll JJ, Collier A, Dougall N, Nuki G, Tothill P. Comparison of bone mineral measurements in the Os calcis using SPA and broadband ultrasonic attenuation. Sixth International Workshop on Bone and Soft Tissue Densitometry. Buxton, England, p 82, 1987.

125. Parfitt AM, Mathews CHE, Villanueva AR, Kleerekoper M, Frame B, Rao DS (1983) Relationships between surface, volume, and thickness of iliac trabecular bone in aging and in osteoporosis. J Clin Invest 72:1396.

126. Parfitt AM (1984) Age-related structural changes in trabecular and cortical bone: cellular mechanisms and biomechanical consequences. Calcif Tissue Int 36:S123–S128.

127. Parfitt AM (1984) The cellular basis of bone remodeling: the quantum concept reexamined in light of recent advances in cell biology of bone. Calcif Tissue Int 36:L5123–5128.

128. Parfitt AM (1987) Trabecular bone architecture in the pathogenesis and prevention of fracture. Am J Med 82(SIB):68–72.

129. Pattin CA, Carter DR, Caler WE (1990) Cortical bone Modulus reduction in tensile and compressive fatigue. Trans ORS 15:50.

130. Petley GW, Hames TK, Cooper C, Langton CM, Cawley MID. The application of broadband ultrasound attenuation to the assessment of osteoporosis. Sixth International Workshop on Bone and Soft Tissue Densitormetry. Buxton, England, p 81, 1987.

131. Portigliatti-Barbos M, Bianco P, Ascenzi A (1983) Distribution of osteonic and interstitial components in the human femoral shaft with reference to structure, calcification, and mechanical properties. Acta Anat 115:J178–186.

132. Portigliatti-Barbos M, Bianco P, Ascenzi A, Boyde A (1984) Collagen orientation in compact bone II. Distribution of lamellae in the whole of the human femoral shaft with reference to its mechanical properties. Metabolic Bone Disease and Related Research 5:309–315.

133. Pugh JW, Rose RM, Radin EL (1973) Elastic and viscoelastic properties of trabecular bone: dependence on structure. J Biomech 6:475–485.

134. Reilly DT, Burstein AH (1975) The elastic and ultimate properties of compact bone tissue. J Biomech 8:395–405.

135. Reilly DT, Burstein AH (1974) Review article: the mechanical properties of cortical bone. J Bone Joint Surg 56A(5):1001–1022.

136. Rockoff SD, Sweet E, Bleustein J (1969) The relative contribution of trabecular and cortical bone to the strength of human lumbar vertebrae. Calc Tiss Res 3:163.

137. Rodan GA, Thomas M, Alan H (1975) A quantitative method for the application of compressive forces to bone in tissue culture. Calcified Tissue Res 18:125–131.

138. Roux W Gesamelte Abhandlungen uber der Entwicklungsmechanik der Organisman. W Engelmann, Leipzig, 1895.

139. Rubin CT, Lanyon LE (1984) Regulation of bone formation by applied dynamic loads. J Bone Joint Surg 66A:397–402.

140. Saha S, Shafkey R (1987) Relationship between ultrasonic and mechanical properties of cancellous bone from human distal tibia. ASME Biomechanics Symposium AMD 84: 105–107.

141. Schoenfeld CM, Lautenschlager EP, Meyer PR, Jr (1974) Mechanical properties of human

cancellous bone in the femoral head. Med Biol Eng 12:313–317.

142. Sedlin ED, Hirsch C (1966) Factors affecting the determination of the physical properties of femoral cortical bone. Acta Orthop Scandinavica 37:29–48.

143. Sedlin ED A theological model for cortical bone. In *a study of the physical properties of human femoral samples*. Acta Orthop Scandinavica, Supplementum 83, 1965.

144. Seireg A, Kempke W (1969) Behavior of *in vivo* bone under cyclic loading. J Biomech 2:455–461.

145. Skerry TM, Pitensky L, Chayen J, Lanyon LE (1987) Strain memory in bone tissue: is proteoglycan-based persistence of strain history a cue for the control of adaptive bone remodeling? Trans Orthop Res Soc 75.

146. Smith JW, Walmsley R (1959) Factors affecting the elasticity of bone. J Anat 93(4):October.

147. Struhl S, Goldstein SA, Dickie DL, Flynn MJ, Matthews LS The distribution of mechanical properties of trabecular bone within vertebral bodies and iliac crest: correlation with computed tomography density. Trans Orthop Res Soc, p 262, 1987.

148. Toajari E (1938) Resistenza meccanica ed elasticita del tessuto osseo studiata in rappor to alla minuta struttwa. Monit Zool Ital 48:148–154.

149. Tsuda K (1957) Studies on the bending test and impulsive bending test on human compact bone. J Kyoto Pref Med Univ 61:1001–1025.

150. Vincentelli R, Grigorov M (1985) The effect of haversian remodeling on the tensile properties of human cortical bone. J Biomechanics 18(3):201–207.

151. vonMeyer GH (1867) Die Architektur der Spongiosa. Arch Anat Physiol Wissenhaftliche

Med (Reichert und Dubois-Reymonds Archiv) 34:615–628.

152. Weaver JK, Chalmers J (1966) Cancellous bone: its strength and changes with aging and an evaluation of some methods for measuring its mineral content. J Bone Joint Surg 48A:289–298.

153. Weaver JK, Chalmers J (1966) Cancellous bone: its strength and changes with aging and an evaluation of some methods for measuring its mineral content. J Bone Joint Surg 48A(2):289–299.

154. Weaver JK (1966) The microscopic hardness of bone. JBJS 48A:273–288.

155. White AA, Panjabi MM, Southwick WO (1977) The four biomechanical stages of healing. JBJS 59A:188–192.

156. Whitehouse WJ (1974) The quantitative morphology of anisotropic trabecular bone. J Micros 101:153–168.

157. Williams JL, Lewis JL (1982) Properties and an anisotropic model of cancellous bone from the proximal tibial epiphysis. J Biomech Eng 104:50–56.

158. Wolff J. Das Gaesetz der Transformation der Knochen. A Hirchwild, Berlin, 1892.

159. Woo SLY, Kuei SC, Amiel D, Gomex MA, Hayes WC, White FG, Akeson WH (1981) The effect of prolonged physical training on the properties of long bone: a study of Wolff's law. J Bone Joint Surg 63A:780–787.

160. Yamada H *Strength of biological materials*. In Evans FG (ed), Williams and Wilkins, Baltimore, 1970.

161. Yokoo S (1952) The compression test upon the diaphysis and the compact substance of the long bones of human extremities. J Kyoto Pref Med Univ 51:291–313.

10
Biomechanics of Soft Tissues

Roger C. Haut

Introduction

The human body is composed of four primary groups of tissues: (1) epithelial tissues are characterized by having cells closely joined one to another and found on free surfaces of the body; (2) muscle tissues are characterized by the high degree of contractility of their cells or fibers—their primary function is to move the skeleton; (3) nervous tissues are composed of cells specialized in the properties of irritability and conductility; and (4) connective tissues are those in which the cells are separated by large amounts of extracellular materials.

Tissues are combined in the body to form organs. Organs are defined as structures composed of two or more tissues integrated in such a manner as to perform certain functions. The heart, for example, has its chambers lined with a special epithelium, its walls are primarily muscle, and there are connective tissues present in numerous forms.

Connective tissues represent wide-ranging types, both in their variety and distribution. They are all characterized, however, by large amounts of extracellular material. Their functions are as varied as the tissues themselves. These tissues bind, support, and protect the human body and its vital organs. Structural integrity and therefore function of vital organs is affected when connective tissue surrounding them is damaged. Connective tissues give us the strength to resist mechanical stresses and a recognizable shape that persists in the face of these forces.[1] The connective tissues can be classified by their extracellular constituents. Connective tissue proper is subdivided into loose, dense, and regular. Loose connective tissue is widely distributed. For example, it is found in the walls of blood vessels, surrounding muscles as fascia, and in the lung parenchyma. Dense connective tissues contain essentially the same elements as loose connective tissue, but there are fewer cells. This type of tissue is found in skin and in many parts of the urinary ducts, digestive organs, and blood vessels. The stromas and capsules of the internal organs, e.g., kidney and liver, are dense connective tissues responsible for maintaining the structural integrity of organs against mechanical forces. Other body components, having primarily mechanical functions, are composed almost exclusively of connective tissue with few cells. The main function of a tendon, for example, is to transmit a tensile force between muscle and bone. Ligaments provide mechanical stability to joints and limit excessive motions across joint surfaces. These functions are carried out by the parallel arrangement of the extracellular components.

The connective tissues of our body are, in fact, complex fiber-reinforced composite materials. The mechanical properties of soft connective tissues depend mainly on the properties and organization of collagen fibers in association with elastin fibers. The fibers are embedded in a hydrated matrix of proteoglycans. The constitution of each particular connective tissue is specially tuned to perform a certain function. The function of a tendon is to transmit large tensile forces precisely to bone—via a muscle. Collagen fibers are primarily responsible for this action. A blood vessel wall, on the other hand, has to distend in response to a pulse wave and subsequently recoil in order to contribute to the propulsion of blood. This function is achieved by the intricate interaction of collagen and elastin fibers. Skin is a soft connective tissue that supports internal organs and protects the body from abrasions, blunt impact, cutting, and penetration while at the same time allowing considerable mobility. These functions are performed by an intricate three-dimensional network of collagen and elastin fibers embedded in a gelatinous matrix. Ligaments provide mechanical stability to joints. These functions are carried out by the parallel arrangement of collagen and elastin fibers. The articular surfaces of body joints are covered with a 1–5 mm dense layer of connective tissue, called articular cartilage. The primary functions of the cartilage are (1) to spread loads across joints and in so doing to minimize contact stress, and (2) to allow relative movement of the opposing surfaces with minimum friction and wear. These functions are performed by connective tissue that has an intricate network of collagen fibers embedded in a large concentration of matrix proteoglycans.

Impact trauma to the body can cause excessive distortions of connective tissues, leading to organ dysfunction. Many studies on the mechanical strength of connective tissues implicate the collagen fiber network.

Collagen

Collagen molecules are synthesized by fibrobastic cells as large precursors (procollagen), which are then secreted and cleaved extracellularly to become collagen.[2] More than a dozen different types of collagen have been isolated.[3] The best-defined (types I–V) clearly represent unique amino acid sequences. The most common collagen is type I. This molecule consists of three polypeptide chains, each coiled in a left-handed helix[3] with approximately 100 amino acids. The three α chains are combined in a right-handed triple helix that gives the collagen molecule a rodlike shape (Fig. 10.1). The length of the molecule is about 280 nm, and its diameter is about 1.5 nm.[3,4] Almost two-thirds of the collagen molecule consists of three amino acids; glycine (33%), proline (15%), and hydroxyproline (15%).[5] Every third amino acid in each α chain is glycine, and this repetitive sequence is essential for the proper formation of the triple helix. Glycine enhances the stability of the molecule by forming hydrogen bonds among the three chains of the superhelix. Hydroxyproline and proline form hydrogen bonds, or hydrogen bonded water bridges, between specific groups on the chains. Type III collagen is thought to be an immature form of type I because of its high concentration in young and healing connective tissues.[3] Type II collagen is unique to cartilage. Type IV collagen is generally found in basement membranes, in vascular tissues, and in skin. Type V is found in basement membranes as well as in cartilage and bone.

Soon after being expressed into the extracellular space, collagen molecules are arranged in a quaternary structure. This structure, in which each molecule overlaps the other, is responsible for the banding observed in the electron microscope (Fig. 10.1). Cross-links are formed between molecules and are essential to the aggregation at the fibril level. The cross-links derive mainly from four lysine and hydroxylysine residues—one at each end of the helical region and one in each telopeptide region.[6] It is the cross-linked character of the collagen fibrils that gives strength to connective tissues. The readers are referred to Nimni[3] for a detailed description of the inter- and intrachain cross-links in collagen. The degree of covalent cross-linking in collagen is altered during maturation.[7] Dietary lathyrogens can inhibit cross-linking by inhibiting the action of an enzyme, lysyl oxidase. Some understanding in the role of covalent cross-linking on mechanical strength has been gained with lathyritic agents.[8,9] The function of intramolecular cross-links is quite obscure, but intermolecular cross-links are essential to the strength of collagen.

The mechanical properties of collagen are often determined in experiments on tendon

Amino acid sequence

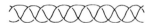

Triple helix of amino acid chains

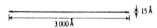

Tropocollagen molecule

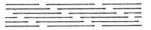

Quarter stagger arrangement of molecules

Banded pattern resulting from overlap and hole zones

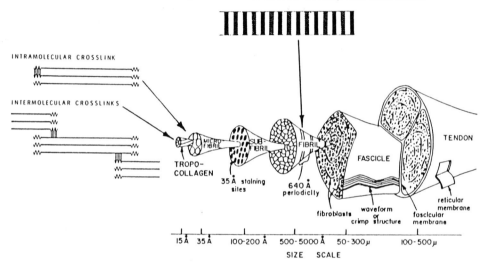

FIGURE 10.1. Schematic representation of the molecular arrangement of collagen in the fiber bundle of rat tail tendon. (From Haut.[8])

and ligaments, where collagen appears as parallel oriented fibrils.[10] The tail tendon of rat (RTT) is an excellent source of pure collagen. The hierarchial organization of collagen in this tendon is well understood (Fig. 10.1). The tensile response of a collagen fiber at low strain (Fig. 10.2) is associated with straightening of crimped collagen fibrils[11,12] and their shear interaction with the hydrated matrix.[13] Kastelic et al.[14] show that the crimp angle in individual collagen fibrils varies radially across the fiber bundle, leading to a sequential uncrimping of fibrils with deformation. Sub-

sequent to the "toe" response, the tensile stress–strain curve is made up of a linear region followed by yield and failure regions. Deformation of RTT up to 2–3% strain has been found reversible with no mechanical damage.[11] The linear region is thought to be due to elastic deformation of collagen fibrils.[15] The modulus of the linear range depends on age.[8] At 1 month of age the modulus is approximately 400 MPa, and it increases to approximately 600 MPa at 4 months of age. The "computed" modulus depends on the length of specimen being tested.[16]

FIGURE 10.2. The static, tensile responses of collagen fiber bundles from the rat-tail tendon at various stages of development. (From Haut.[8])

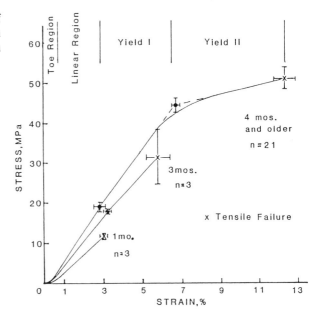

Above approximately 4% strain, permanent damage has been observed in the collagen fiber with a reduction of its tensile modulus and irreversible disruption of the crimp waveform of its fibrils.[11,15] Kastelic and Baer[17] have examined the mechanism of tensile yielding and failure of RTT collagen fibers by using electron microscopy and small-angle x-ray diffraction (SAX). A slight broadening of the SAX pattern and signs of limited intrafibrillar slip are observed when the tendon is deformed into the first yield region. More significant damage is observed when the collagen fiber is deformed in the second yield region. At fracture the fiber seems to separate into filaments averaging 10 μm in diameter.[18]

It appears that resistance to intrafibrillar slip in the collagen fiber starts with maturation concurrent with the appearance of "yield" behavior. The resistance increases with age, as does the apparent modulus of the "yield" region. When exposed to dietary lathrogens, resistance of collagen to intrafibrillar slip is compromised.[8] The tensile strength of collagen from RTT varies from approximately 50 MPa to 100 MPa, depending on the degree of maturation.[8] Failure strains increase from approximately 11% to 18% for the mature fiber. Failure strain increases with age.[7,8]

Betsch and Baer[10] document decreasing failure strains with age.

Viscoelastic behavior of tendon collagen is thought to be due to a shear interaction with the matrix of proteoglycans during collagen fibril uncrimping.[13] Studies also show that tensile strength and failure strain for collagen significantly depend on strain rate.[19] Tensile strength and failure strain are approximately 108 MPa and 18%, respectively, at 720%/sec compared to 61 MPa and 14.7% at 3.6%/sec.[19] The matrix of proteoglycans has been implicated in providing some degree of structural integrity at high strain rates. The sensitivity of each parameter to strain rate is greater in immature collagen, suggesting some dependency on the degree of crosslinking and the content of matrix proteoglycans.

Elastin

Elastin is another major protein of connective tissues. Collagen is the principal protein of white connective tissue, while elastin predominates in yellow tissue. It is normally present at significant levels in tissues such as blood vessels, lungs, and skin. The collagen content of human achilles tendon is about

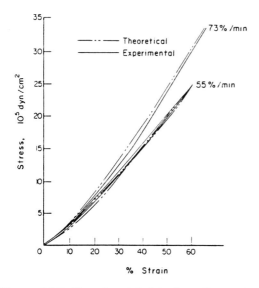

FIGURE 10.3. Experimental data from ligamentum nuchae showing nearly linear tensile response and minimal time dependency. (From Jenkins and Little.[22])

20 times that of elastin, while in yellow ligamentum nuchae the elastin content is about five times that of collagen. Like collagen, glycine accounts for about one-third of the total amino acids of elastin. The contents of proline and hydroxyproline are much lower in elastin than in collagen. The fundamental polypeptide chain in elastin is tropoelastin.[20] Assembly of multiple tropoelastin molecules gives elastin its characteristic elastic properties. Critical in the assembly is the formation of cross-links between tropoelastin molecules. Allysine residues react nonenzymatically with lysine residues for the characteristic cross-link.[21] Each chain forms a fibrillar structure composed of alternating segments of cross-linked regions and structures termed "oiled coils," which may be stretched from 2–2.5 times the length of relaxed molecules.

It is recognized that elastin provides elasticity to connective tissues, but its exact role is not well understood. While the mechanical properties of collagen are typically estimated from those of rat-tail tendon, no such pure form exists for elastin. Human and bovine aorta and bovine ligamentum nuchae are the most common sources of elastin fibers. Aortas

contain approximately 40% elastin by dry weight, while ligamentum nuchae contain 78 to 83% elastin.[22] The load-elongation curve for ligamentum nuchae yields a modulus of 0.3 MPa for elastin.[23,24] Carton et al.[25] conducted experiments on individual elastin fibers after dissection from the ligamentum nuchae of the ox. They found a linear tension–strain curve to approximately 120% strain. Hass[26] reports a modulus of 3 MPa for elastin. Jenkins and Little[22] used formic acid to remove collagen from bovine ligamentum nuchae and showed that the stress–strain curve of elastin is essentially linear and displayed minimal time dependency (Fig. 10.3). Minns and Steven[27] conducted tensile experiments at five stages in the development of fetal bovine ligamentum nuchae. Strips tested to failure suggest that the strain at failure decreases from approximately 280% to 220% at birth. The tensile stress at failure remained constant until birth at approximately 1.4 MPa. Mature elastin fibers can be strained to approximatly 130% at 10 MPa before failure.[25]

Matrix of Proteoglycans

Proteoglycan aggregates are composed of three molecular species: proteoglycan subunits, hyaluronic acid, and link protein[28] (Fig. 10.4). In its formation each component appears separately in the matrix. Proteoglycan subunits noncovalently bind to a single hyaluronate chain. Link protein is then incorporated and appears to stabilize the bond between proteoglycan subunits and hyaluronate. The proteoglycan subunit consists of chondroitin sulfate, keratin sulfate, and possibly dermatin sulfate covalently attached to the protein core. These glycosaminoglycans are linear polymers of sugar residues with a disaccharide repeating unit. Chondroitin sulfate, for example, is composed of 40–60 repeating units, is 20,000–30,000 in molecular weight, and ranges in length from about 40 to 60 nm. The hyaluronic acid chains that form the filamentous backbone of proteoglycan aggregates vary greatly in size, ranging from 200,000 to over two million in molecular weight and from 50 to over 5,000 nm

FIGURE 10.4. Model of a cartilage proteoglycan aggregate, showing the backbone of hyaluronic acid, proteoglycan, subunits and link proteins. (From Rosenberg.[28])

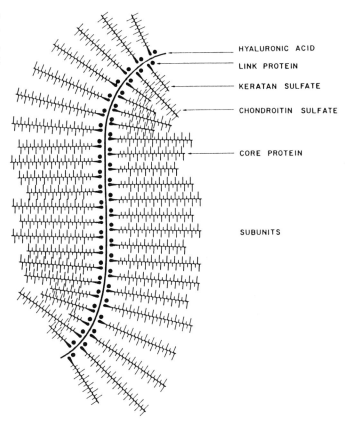

HYALURONIC ACID

LINK PROTEIN

KERATAN SULFATE

CHONDROITIN SULFATE

CORE PROTEIN

SUBUNITS

in length. A proteoglycan subunit may have 100 chondroitin sulfate chains attached to a protein core 200,000 in molecular weight and 200 nm in length. The proteoglycan subunit can be 2 to 3 million in molecular weight. A proteoglycan aggregate containing 100 such proteoglycan subunits would be over 200 million in molecular weight. In tissues like cartilage, the proteoglycan aggregates are effectively immobilized within a fibrous network.[29] In addition, they are hydrophilic because glycosaminoglycan molecules contain a high density of negatively charged groups, which gives rise to imbalance in the concentration of freely diffusible electrolytes.

Proteoglycans also seem to play a major biological role in structure of collagen. Collagen fibrillogenesis, in vivo, may be controlled by a feedback system whereby the stress history on fibroblastic cells determines the synthesis of specific glycosaminoglycans.[30] The importance of two common sulfate-containing glycos-

aminoglycans is evident from in vitro studies. These have shown that in the presence of chondroitin sulfate fine fibrils are formed, while in dermatin sulfate fibrillogenesis is retarded and relatively large fibrils are formed.[31,32] Connective tissues that require high tensile strength usually contain large-diameter collagen fibrils, while those whose primary function is low-load creep resistance have a larger proportion of small-diameter fibrils.[30] In tendon there is clear evidence of specific interactions between collagen and the matrix of proteoglycans, whereas interactions in cartilage are probably less specific, involving entrapment and excluded volumes.[33]

The role played by the matrix of proteoglycans in the mechanical properties of connective tissue is not presently well understood. More is known about the influence of this component in determining the mechanical properties of articular cartilage in compression. This will be discussed later. The matrix comprises only a small fraction of most connective tissues. This noncollagenous component appears partly responsible for the cohesion of tendon fibers.[34] Proteoglycan-based filaments are shown attached to collagen at specific polar locations and interconnecting collagen fibrils.[35] The matrix component is thought to provide a viscous lubrication between individual fibrils of collagen.[34,36,37] Viscoelastic properties, like creep and relaxation, have been associated with the interaction of collagen with the surrounding matrix.[38] The matrix in RTT has been modeled as viscoelastic with a time-dependent shear modulus.[15] The modulus of the matrix at 3 months of age is approximately 0.1 MPa, and is found to increase 15-fold at maturity. The complex shear modulus of purified solutions of proteoglycan monomers and aggregates is approximately 0.01 MPa at concentrations similar to that in cartilage.[39] The shear viscosity is dependent on concentration and shear rate, being approximately 1.0 Pa · s at typical concentrations. Using viscometric flow measurements on high concentrations of purified proteoglycan solutions, Zhu and Mow[40] find that proteoglycan macromolecules interact with each other to form structural networks with significant mechanical strength. The forces of interaction arise from mechanical entanglements of neighboring molecules, electrostatic interactions amongst charge groups, and frictional effects from one molecule sliding over another.

Tensile failure studies suggest that the matrix may help stabilize the collagen fibril, especially at high rates of loading.[8,19,41,42] On the other hand, enzymatic digestion studies indicate that the sensitivity of tissue strength to strain rate is not directly related to the content of matrix proteoglycans.[43]

Ligaments and Tendons

Ligaments and tendons are dense connective tissues known as parallel-fibered collagenous tissues. The roles of ligaments, which connect bone to bone, are to augment the mechanical stability of joints, to guide joint motion, and to prevent excessive motion. The function of tendon is to attach muscle to bone and transmit tensile loads, thereby producing joint motion. Like other connective tissues, tendons and ligaments consist of only a few cells (fibroblasts) and an abundant extracellular matrix. The content of collagen is slightly higher in tendons than ligaments.[44] The content of elastin varies between ligaments, depending on function. While ligaments from the knee, for example, contain small amounts of elastin, spinal ligaments typically contain greater amounts of elastin.[45] While the ratio of collagen to elastin is 1:2 in ligamentum flavum,[46] the interspinous ligament is predominantly collagen.[45] These differences in constitution and organization of collagen and elastin in various spinal ligaments are reflected in their obviously different mechanical properties (Fig. 10.5).

The nonlinear, stiffening response of ligaments is due to the structural responses of collagen and elastin in the matrix of proteoglycans. Bundles of collagen measuring approximately 20 μm in width have a characteristic crimp that varies between ligaments depending on their particular function.[47] Elastin fibers appear straight and always in close association with collagen.[45] Numerous structural-based models have been proposed for soft connective tissues to deal with the uncrimping of collagen during tensile stretch.[48–52] Tensile studies on bone-ligament-bone preparations have shown non-uniform strain patterns with large strains existing near insertions into bone.[53,54] This has lead to structural-based models in which crimp angles in collagen vary down the length of the ligament.[55] During quasi-static tensile deformation, the 20 μm wide bundles of crimped collagen sequentially straighten and bear load.[47] In general, the current concept is that elastin fibers bear load first because they appear to be initially straight in ligaments. Assuming that the crimp angles in collagen are normally distributed,[56] tensile loads in the early "toe" region are due to tensile deformation of elastin fibers and the straightened collagen fibers (Fig. 10.6).

Belkoff and Haut[57] recently modeled the uncrimping of collagen fibers in human patella tendons (PT), based on the model of Lanir,[5] to study the effects of irradiation sterilization

FIGURE 10.5. Tensile responses of selected spinal ligaments showing differences between the posterior longitudinal ligament—primarily collagen—and the ligament flavum—primarily elastin. (From Panjabi et al.[167])

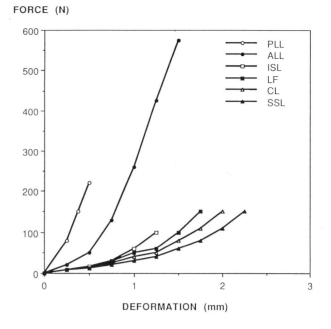

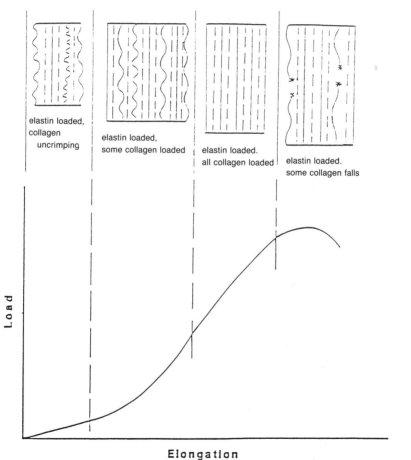

FIGURE 10.6. Schematic drawing to illustrate the micromechanics of ligament deformation during tensile stretch.

According to the model analysis 50% of the collagen fiber bundles are straighten by approximately 5% strain. The tensile modulus of the collagen network ranges from 350 to 400 MPa for donors aged 18 to 63 years. The tensile modulus of the human PT varies between investigators, being 288 ± 18 MPa[58] and 415 ± 31 MPa.[59] The tensile modulus of human digitorus tendons is approximately 600 MPa.[60] Little change has been found in the tensile properties of tendons with age.[60-62] A decrease in the extractability of collagen with pepsin, however, has been correlated with an increase in tensile modulus of the PT.[62]

The tensile properties of ligaments significantly depend on age. The modulus of the human anterior cruciate ligament (ACL) is 111 ± 26 MPa for young specimens (16–26 years), decreasing continuously to 65 ± 24 MPa for older specimens (48–86 years).[63] The structural stiffness of the human ACL decreases continuously with age.[64] Biochemical analyses indicate that these age-related changes correlate with a decrease in collagen synthesis and reducible cross-links in collagen.[65] Immobilization causes a marked decrease in the modulus of ligaments, while exercise has a more limited positive effect.[66] The tangent modulus of the human ligamentum flavum decreases from approximately 100 to 2 MPa with age.[46] This value of tensile modulus reflects a significantly greater content of elastin in the spinal ligament than in the ACL or PT.

When isolated collagen fibers are loaded, damage is reported at strains above approximately 4%.[11] However, for whole ligaments and tendons the linear response can extend above 20% (Fig. 10.7).

Studies, however, have shown that failure of some fine collagen fibers can go undetected in macroscopic tests. Scanning electron micrographs of ligaments stretched into the linear region show ruptured collagen fibers at loads one-half the maximum.[67,68] Near the end of the linear region force reductions represent signs of sequential failure of a few greatly stretched bundles. Tensile failure of bundles gradually progresses until ultimate load is reached. Throughout this process the ligament may visually appear intact until complete

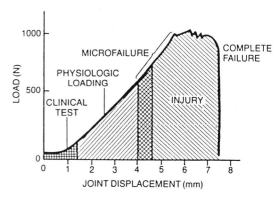

FIGURE 10.7. Tensile curve representing the regions correlating with clinical findings: (1) load imposed during drawer test; (2) range of physiological activity; and (3) partial and complete rupture. (From Nordin and Frankel.[2])

separation ensues. Fiber bundles appear to fail at different points along the length of the ligament, producing the classic "mop-end" appearance.[63]

Measurement of the gross tensile-failure properties of ligaments is often influenced by bone fracture near insertions. With advanced age[63] or immobilization[69] the mechanism of failure in bone-ligament-bone preparations is by avulsion of adjacent bone. For young specimens aged 16–26 years, the tensile strength and failure strain for the human ACL is 37.8 ± 9.3 MPa and 44.3 ± 8.5%, respectively.[63] In a structural sense the ultimate load is 1,725 ± 269 N. More recently Woo et al.[64] documented that for young specimens (22–35 years), the ultimate load is 2,160 ± 157 N and dependent on orientation of the knee preparation with respect to normal anatomy. The tensile failure properties of different knee ligaments also vary.[70] The tensile failure properties of the human PT are 29.1 ± 2.4 MPa at 30.8 ± 3.1% strain,[58] 53.9 ± 2.7 MPa[59] or 39.9 ± 15.8 MPa and 19 ± 8%.[71] Tensile failure properties for the human ligamentum flavum are significantly different than those of the PT tendon, for example, being 10 MPa at 70% strain for young adults and 2 MPa at 30% strain for older adults.[72] The differences in magnitude for the tensile strength of this spinal ligament compared to knee ligaments or tendons are likely due to the relative contents of collagen and elastin.

Few studies have directly addressed the influence of strain rate on the tensile failure properties of ligaments and tendons. Bone-ligament-bone preparations fail more often in the ligament substance, rather than by avulsion, as the loading rate increases.[73,74] While the shape of the stress–strain curve is not significantly altered by strain rate, tensile strength and ultimate strain are increased 20–30% over a 1,000-fold change in strain rate.[75] While the tensile strength of ligaments varies slightly with strain rate, failure strain does not appear dependent.[76]

Skin

Skin is the largest single organ in the body (16% of the human adult weight). It consists of the epidermis with its outer characteristic surface contours and the dermis, which contains collagen, elastin, cells, blood, lymph vessels, nerve endings, hair and hair follicles, and glands together with their associated ducts. All are embedded in the matrix of proteoglycans and glycoproteins. The mechanical and barrier functions of the epidermis stem primarily from the stratum corneum, which is an outer layer of horny keratinized cells.[77] The predominant components of the dermis are collagen fibers in the matrix of proteoglycans. Collagen accounts for 60–80% of the dry weight of the skin depending on age, sex, and site on the body.[78] The collagen (primarily type I, with lesser amounts of type III) appears as a three-dimensional network of wavy or coiled fibers. In the upper (papillary) layer of the dermis collagen fibers are fine.[79] This layer is mainly concerned with connecting the reticular dermis to the epidermis. The deep, reticular dermis contains densely packed fibers running parallel to the surface of the skin[80,81] with some fibers running between the planes, presumably to prevent interplanar shearing.[82] The fibers within the planes also appear to be oriented in a preferred direction.[83] Skin is normally under tension in vivo. This tension (expressed as force per unit length) varies from

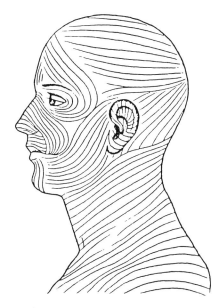

FIGURE 10.8. Schematic showing the lines of skin cleavage—Langer's lines. (From Peterson et al.[90])

0 to 20 N/m depending on site, direction, and body posture.[84] This concept was originally investigated by Langer.[85] The lines drawn by Langer, referred to as cleavage lines, are thought to parallel collagen fibers on the surface of skin (Fig. 10.8).[86–88]

Skin provides the outermost covering of the body and its strength plays a role in lacerative trauma. Observations from accidental injuries as well as experiments with laboratory instruments indicate that skin fails more often in a tensile manner than from a shear or cutting action, even when struck by relatively sharp metal edges or structures.[89] Tensile failure also plays an important role in the lacerative resistance of skin to grazing or glancing blows, such as when the head hits the roof pillar[90] or windshield[91] during an automotive collision. The analyses of Gadd et al.[89] have been generalized and critical shear stresses have been computed for laceration of skin.[92] The severity of lacerative trauma depends on the applied load, the lacerative resistance of skin, and the geometrical shape of the impacting surface.[93]

There exists a great degree of variability in the properties of the skin, depending on

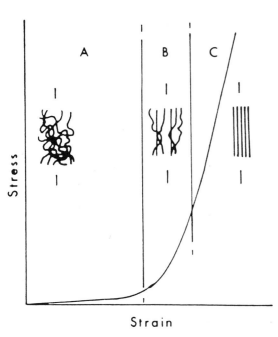

FIGURE 10.9. Schematic showing the relationship between collagen fiber morphology and the mechanical response curve in tension. (From Daly.[101])

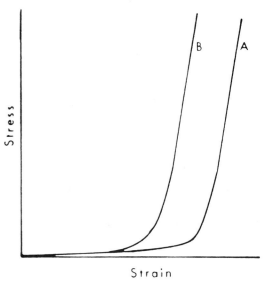

FIGURE 10.10. Effect of specimen orientation on the tensile response of skin. A = specimen taken parallel to craniocaudal axis; B = specimen taken perpendicular to the craniocaudal axis. (From Daly.[101])

species, age, exposure, hydration, obesity, disease, and biological difference between individuals. The basic tensile response of skin is nonlinear stiffening (Fig. 10.9). The first region displays a low modulus response. Some investigators suggest elastin is being deformed in region A.[56,94] Others suggest the tensile response in this region is due to a few straight collagen fibers bearing load.[95] The primary role of elastin, which seems to parallel collagen, may be to restore collagen to its prestretch, crimped configuration.[96] The initial modulus of skin is 0.1–2 MPa.[97,98] In region B collagen fibers are being sequentially straightened and bear load.[80,99] In region C collagen fibers are primarily aligned and the tensile response approaches that of tendon.[100]

As expected from the anisotropy noticed in skin under normal in vivo tension (as evidenced by Langer's lines), there is a difference in the response curves obtained from specimens taken from different sites and different orientations on the body (Fig. 10.10). Test specimens whose orientation primarily parallel the cleavage lines recruit the collagen fiber

network at lower levels of strain.[83,101] Typical values of tensile modulus for normal skin on the human tibia are 22 MPa along Langer lines and 6 MPa across the lines.[103] For skin over the sternum the tensile modulus varies from 20 to 80 MPa from birth to 25 years.[103] Correspondingly, over the thigh the tensile modulus varies from 1 to 5 MPa.

Statistically, lacerative facial injuries parallel the Langer lines in traffic-accident investigations.[93] The resistance of skin to cut across Langer lines is greater than that to cut along the lines. The tensile strength of skin has typical values in the range of 2.5–16 MPa.[104] It varies with site,[105] is higher in the main fiber direction,[106] and is believed to increase with age.[104,107] The tensile strength and failure strain of skin for an average adult are 7.7 MPa and 78%, respectively.[72] Both parameters decrease with age. The tensile strength and failure strain of skin over the sternum are approximately 20 MPa and 40–70%, respectively.[103] No direction effects are documented. Over the thigh area the tensile strength and failure strain are documented to be 1–5 MPa and 40–70%, respectively. Recent studies have shown that the failure strain of rat skin varies with orientation and age.[108] While failure strains perpendicular to skin tension lines decrease with animal age, parallel to these lines the strain at failure increases with age. This parallels with age-related changes in the tensile failure strains of collagen fibers.[19]

The tensile strength of skin also depends on the rate of elongation or strain. Vogel[109] showed that in rat dermis it increases with the logarithm of strain rate. Gadd et al.[89] showed that the tensile strength and failure strain of aged human facial skin increases from 7–14 MPa to 11–20 MPa and from 30–67% to 42–62%, respectively, or approximately 150% over three orders of strain rate. Similar changes have been found in the sensitivity of tensile strength with strain rate in rat,[108] but the failure strain was not found to be dependent on rate of loading. Haut[108] further showed that the sensitivity of tensile strength to strain rate decreased with age and correlated with the content of matrix proteoglycans in the skin. The results parallel with a decrease in the degree of stress relaxation with age and the content of tissue proteoglycans.[109] These results are consistent with the notion that movement of fluid in the hydrated matrix plays an important role in the strain-rate-sensitive responses of connective tissues.[110]

Vascular Tissues

Various clinical investigative teams associate ruptures or tears of major blood vessels with death in 30–45% of automobile fatalities.[111] Crush injury during soft-tissue trauma can also adversely affect blood supply and increase susceptibility of surrounding tissue to infection.[112]

Arteries are blood vessels with a great range of diameters. The human proximal aorta, for example, has a diameter approximately 2.5 cm, while the small arteries—the arterioles—are about 60 μm in diameter. The arterial wall has three layers: the intima, the media, and the adventitia. The innermost component of the intima is a layer of endothelial cells that offer little resistance to internal pressure. The intima

is separated from the media by an internal elastic membrane composed of elastin. The media, which is responsible for most of the strength and elasticity of the arterial wall, is composed largely of collagen. The adventitia is a thin layer of loose connective tissue largely composed of collagen. The walls of veins are thinner, more supple, and less elastic than those of arteries. While most authors distinguish three layers in the walls of veins, these layers are frequently indistinct. The intima contains endothelial cells and is bounded by a network of elastic fibers. The media is much thinner than arteries and consists mainly of circular smooth muscle fibers separated by many longitudinal collagenous fibers. The adventitia is usually much thicker than the media and consists of loose connective tissue with thick longitudinal collagenous bundles and an intricate network of elastin. In larger veins like the inferior vena cava, portal, splenic, iliac, and renal veins the adventitia makes up the greater part of the venous wall.

There exists a huge literature on vascular mechanics and the mechanical responses of blood vessels and correlations with the microstructure of their primary constituents: collagen, elastin, and smooth muscle. An excellent, comprehensive review is given by Dobrin.[113] The tensile mechanical response of the arterial wall stiffens exponentially with elongation similar to skin, ligament, and tendon.[114,115] Krafka[24] noted that the tangent modulus of strips of aorta varied from 0.15 to 0.19 MPa. He suggested in the physiological range a loose network of elastin may be responsible. Roach and Burton[116] attempted to separate the contributions of elastin and collagen in the human iliac artery using crude trypsin to degrade the elastin and formic acid to degrade collagen (Fig. 10.11).

They conclude that elastin fibers primarily bear circumferential load at small distensions and that collagen fibers bear circumferential load at large distensions. These descriptions of the correlation between mechanical properties and ultrastructure are consistent with histological studies of artery under pressure.[117] They have shown that under diastolic pressure collagen fibers show no definite pattern or

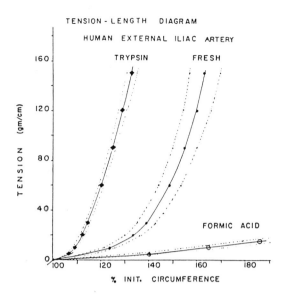

TENSION - LENGTH DIAGRAM

HUMAN EXTERNAL ILIAC ARTERY

FIGURE 10.11. Tensile response of human iliac artery after removal of collagen with formic acid and elastin with trypsin. (From Roach and Burton.[116])

orientation. Above diastolic pressure elastic lamellae appear straight and collagen fibers are circumferentially arranged. They conclude that at physiological pressures the aortic media functions as a two-phase material. At 100 mm Hg the tangent modulus of the thoracic aorta is 0.4–0.8 MPa.[118,119] At 240 mm Hg the tangent modulus varies from 1.2 to 1.6 MPa. These data can be compared with the modulus of elastin[25,23] (0.3–0.9 MPa) and that of collagen (400–600 MPa).[8,11]

The ratio of elastin to collagen in the aortic wall decreases away from the heart, until in the abdominal aorta more collagen exists than elastin.[120] The corresponding tensile responses of circumferential and longitudinal specimens change down the aortic tree.[121] These authors also show that the more distal and smaller arteries relax more and at faster rates, reflecting a change in viscoelastic properties down the aortic tree. No direct correlations, however, have been established between the passive stress–strain properties of arteries and the ratio of collagen to elastin.[122,123] Attempts have been made to describe differences in the tensile-wall mechanics of various vessels with the following simplified equation: $E = W_e E_e +$

$f_c W_c E_c$, where E^e and E^c are the elastic modulus of elastin and collagen fibers, respectively, and W_e and W_c represent the fractional content of these two components. The term f_c had to be included, however, to reflect differences in the recruitment of collagen fibers between arteries.[122] The circumferential tension-elongation response of the human iliac artery stiffens with increasing age,[124] probably due to an increase in the ratio of collagen to elastin.[113] The longitudinal tensile response also shifts with aging, reflecting less influence of elastin fibers (Fig. 10.12).

Tensile modulus of the human iliac artery at 30 years of age varies from 0.01 MPa at zero stretch to 0.7 MPa prior to failure. At 100 mmHg the tensile modulus is 0.5 MPa, and the corresponding longitudinal modulus is approximately 1.7 MPa. These moduli are increased by factors of 2–5 at 80 years of age. Smooth muscle is included as a viscous element in physical models of the active properties of aorta.[125,126]

Fewer experimental data exist on the mechanical properties of veins. The percentage of collagen is typically greater in veins than in arteries, while the percentage of elastin is less.[127] Comparative tests of pulmonary arteries and veins indicate that arteries are more compliant than veins. The mechanical behavior of veins in the longitudinal direction can be regarded as essentially elastic, while that in the circumferential direction is highly viscoelastic.[128] For veins the tensile response curves shift toward the stress axis with increasing age,[127] like for arteries.[124] MacKay et al.[127] state that age-related changes in both arteries and veins are due to alterations in elastin at the molecular and lamellar levels.

The tensile failure properties of vascular tissue have important implications in traumatic injury to the body. The thoracic aorta is the single most significant site of serious vascular injury.[129] Transverse tears of the descending aorta at the isthmus just distal to the left subclavian artery represent the major site of aortic injury. While the mechanisms of aortic rupture are still being debated, both longitudinal and circumferential failure properties appear implicated.[130] Collagen is the primary

FIGURE 10.12. Tension curves for the human iliac artery showing the effect of aging. (From Roach and Burton.[124])

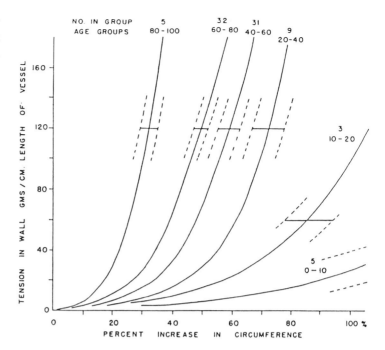

strength-bearing component of the aorta.[131] The circumferential strength of the human ascending, thoracic, and abdominal aorta averages 1.1 MPa, 0.9 MPa, and 1.1 MPa, respectively, across all age groups.[72] The corresponding longitudinal tensile strengths average 0.7 MPa, 0.8 MPa, and 0.8 MPa, respectively. Strengths in both directions decrease with age. The circumferential failure strains are 77%, 71%, and 81%, respectively, and the corresponding longitudinal failure strains are 81%, 56%, and 69%, respectively. More recent experiments on dumbbell-shaped specimens from the human aorta indicate that the longitudinal tensile strength in low-speed experiments varies from approximately 2.7 MPa in the young down to 0.8 MPa in older tissues.[130] The circumferential strengths are slightly higher, but decrease similarly with age. The corresponding failure strains also decrease with age from approximately 179% in young to 129% in aged tissues. Under dynamic strain rates the tensile strength of human thoracic aorta increases, but failure strain does not change with alterations in strain rate.

Questions of the dynamic vs. static strength of veins have recently received attention.

Acute subdural hematoma occurs in approximately 30% of the severely head-injured.[132] The tolerance curve for subdural hematoma has been interpreted in terms of the sensitivity of cerebral bridging veins to strain rate.[133] Their analysis is based on the work of Lowenhielm,[134] in which the ultimate strain for these veins significantly decreases with strain rate. More recent experiments have indicated that while the tensile strength of human subdural bridging veins slightly increases over 3 orders of magnitude change in strain rate, the ultimate stretch ratio is not altered.[135] This is in line with work on human thoracic aorta[130] and on the common carotid artery and jugular vein of the ferret.[136]

Articular Cartilage

Articular cartilage is a connective tissue that lines the contacting surfaces of bones and functions as a bearing material in synovial joints. In order to support the dual functions of managing the transmission of joint loads and providing a bearing surface, the microarchitecture of articular cartilage is unique. Articular

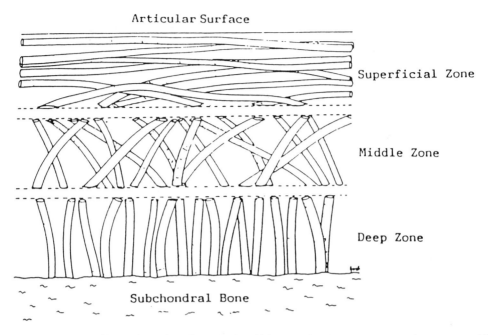

FIGURE 10.13. Collagen fibril orientation through the thickness of articular cartilage. (From Egan.[140])

cartilage is composed of 70–80% aqueous electrolyte and a solid organic matrix of collagen, proteoglycans, glycoproteins, and lipids.[137] The tissue is aneural and avascular and has only a few cells (chondrocytes) that are responsible for synthesizing and maintaining the organic matrix. Although there is some degree of disagreement on the arrangement of collagen in articular cartilage,[138,139] a simplified view has been given (Fig. 10.13).[141] Close to the surface, collagen fibrils run parallel to the surface. This was first demonstrated by Hultkrantz.[141] Below the superficial zone, the fibril alignment becomes progressively more oblique to the articular surface down to the deep zone, where collagen fibers are aligned approximately perpendicular to the cartilage surface and the subchondral bone. Because of its propensity to structure water, the matrix of proteoglycans plays a major role in determining the compressive properties of cartilage. The rigidity and compliance of articular cartilage are due to the osmotic swelling of the proteoglycans against tensile constraint from a network of collagen (type II). The swelling pressure of "normal" articular cartilage is approximately 0.35 MPa.[142] When

stress is applied to articular cartilage there is an instantaneous deformation that changes the shape of the collagen and proteoglycan networks. The instantaneous surface deformation is strongly anisotropic and strongly dependent on the collagen network.[143,144] The proteoglycans secondarily influence the instantaneous response by providing a net pretension in the collagenous network. At the same time fluid within the articular cartilage flows out of the tissue, if the applied stress exceeds the swelling pressure of the tissue.[145] The viscous deformation of cartilage is largely due to fluid flow and is controlled by the osmotic pressure and hydraulic permeability, which both depend on the content of proteoglycans.[142] The long-term "creep" modulus of articular cartilage is dependent on the intrinsic properties of the solid phase.[145] The maintenance of tissue hydration under load can be completely described in terms of a balance between the osmotic pressure of the proteoglycans and the applied pressure.[142,146]

The functional, or biomechanical, properties of articular cartilage are known to depend on exercise, age, and pathology. Immobilization of a joint has been shown to result in a significant, but reversible, loss in proteoglycans and in an increase in the content of water.[147,148] Immobilization thereby causes an increased rate of creep deformation under constant load, decreases the long-term equilibrium modulus, and increases the permeability of joint cartilage.[149] These changes parallel those observed in osteoarthritis[150] and closely parallel those documented in aging.[151] Some distinct differences, however, have been shown between the pathogenesis of osteoarthritis and normal aging.[152] During the course of disease the softened articular cartilage becomes invaded by cells and vessels from the subchondral bone; fraying of the cartilage surface is observed; fissures (fibrillations) penetrate the cartilage; and the cartilage layer is lost and bony sclerosis prevails. The radiographic presence of bone spurs, which limit joint motion, is a definite sign of joint degeneration.[153]

While the onset of degenerative joint disease is not well understood, mechanical insult is suggested to initiate early events similar to those of the disease. While a single insult has been implicated,[154] repeated low-level stresses have also shown degenerative changes.[155] Impact-induced injury to articular cartilage has received little attention. In vitro impacts on human cartilage/bone samples cause radial fissures of the surface extending into the deep zone and death of chondrocytes at contact pressures exceeding 25 MPa, corresponding to 25% strain.[156] These surface fissures orient on the surface parallel to the split lines of Hultkrantz. Repeated impact loading on bovine cartilage-on-bone specimens at 2–12 J of energy suggest microstructural changes in the arrangement of collagen fibrils resembling early osteoarthritic changes.[157] Impact-induced fractures of cartilage in vitro appear oriented 45° to the articular surface and extend to the intermediate zone. Impact experiments onto the patellofemoral joint indicate separation of the cartilage from underlying bone and disruption of the collagen ultrastructure without gross visual damage to the tissue.[158] Subfracture loads on articular cartilage of the patellofemoral joint, in vivo, indicate changes in the zone of calcified cartilage represented by an increase in cellular clones, vascular

invasion, losses in the proteoglycan content, and increases in the content of water without signs of surface damage.[159] These are some of the histological changes observed in early stages of the human disease process.

The function of articular cartilage and its response under impact loading depend on the tensile properties of the tissue. In planes parallel to the surface the tensile mechanical properties of cartilage vary with depth and orientation (Fig. 10.14).[160] In concert with the documented morphology of collagen, the tensile response of surface layers is consistently stiffer and stronger than underlying layers. Tensile stress at failure correlates positively with the content of collagen but not with the content of proteoglycans.[160] Tensile specimens oriented parallel to the split lines of Hultrantz are stiffer and stronger than those oriented perpendicular to these lines. The tensile strength and modulus of the superficial zone increases with age to a maximum of approximately 40 MPa and 220 MPa, respectively, in the third decade, decreasing to 12 MPa and 60 MPa at 90 years of age.[161,162] Similar results have been reported for the bovine model.[163] Recent studies on bovine articular cartilage indicate that proteoglycans act to retard reorganization and alignment of collagen fibers under tensile loading, thereby preventing sudden extension of the collagenous network.[164] The intrinsic tensile modulus of human articular cartilage is typically less than 30 MPa.[165] Tissues from low weight-bearing areas are stiffer than those from high weight-bearing areas, correlating with the collagen/proteoglycan ratio. Osteoarthritic cartilage showing surface fibrillation has a tensile stiffness consistently less than 2 MPa. This is correlated with damage in the network of collagen for diseased tissue.

Summary

Structural integrity of soft connective tissues is essential for the support and protection of the skeleton and major organs of the body. Impact loads can traumatize and damage these tissues, leading to disfigurement and/or dysfunction of

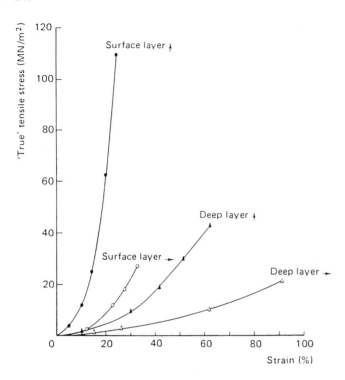

FIGURE 10.14. Tensile experiments on human femoral cartilage cut on the surface and the deep layer in directions parallel and perpendicular to the cleavage lines of Hultkrantz. (From Kempson.[161])

a major organ or joint. We have seen in this chapter that the mechanical properties of soft tissues are dependent on the concentration and arrangement of constituent elements— namely, the fibrous proteins collagen and elastin and the hydrated matrix of proteoglycans. Numerous studies have shown that the strength-bearing properties of connective tissues are associated with collagen. Indeed, a correlation seems evident between the content of collagen in a tissue and its tensile strength (Table 10.1). Yet we have seen that strength, per se, can vary widely depending on the complex organization, physical properties, and concentration of collagen. These data can also be widely divergent due to experimental procedures, species differences, etc. We have seen that the physical strength of collagen varies with age, pathology, etc., reflecting alterations in the degree of covalent cross-linking. Exactly which cross-links perform these functions is currently unknown. We still do not know if the mechanical properties of collagen types I, II, and III are different. In only a few instances can individual fibers be isolated, so analyses with microstructural-based models of these tissues seem essential.

TABLE 10.1. Some tensile strengths and associated biochemical data, based on percentage of weight, for representative soft connective tissues (biochemical data from Woo et al.[166]).

Tissue	Strength (MPa)	% fat-free dry weight		
		Collagen	Elastin	GAGS
Aorta	0.7–1.0[72]	23–35	40–50	2–2.5
Cartilage	5–40[159]	60–65	Trace	10–15
Skin	2–16[105]	65–70	5–10	1.5–2
Ligament	13–38[63]	75–80	<5	2.5–3
Tendon	30[61]–55[59]	75–80	<3	1–1.5

The role played by the matrix of proteoglycans is also largely unknown, except possibly in determining some of the compressive properties of cartilage. Some studies suggest these viscous elements may influence structural integrity at high rates of loading. Since impact trauma occurs at high rates, the role of this matrix component needs further study.

Another area of current and future research deals with the biological functions of modeling and remodeling of soft connective tissues. Do mechanical states of stress help determine the microarchitecture of a soft tissue? What are the mechanisms by which cells are programmed to synthesize specific extracellular constituents? How are these elements arranged in tissues to perform their special functions? While we have certainly witnessed significant advances in our understanding of soft tissues over the past 20 years, many critical questions still need to be answered in future research. Because of the multidisciplinary nature of these questions, we will need the continued cooperation of physical, biological, and clinical scientists.

References

1. Scott J (1986) Molecules that keep you in shape. New Scient 24:49–53.
2. Nordin M, Frankel VH. Biomechanics of tissues and structures of the musculoskeletal system. In Lea, Febringer (ed) *Basic biomechanics of the musculoskeletal system*. Philadelphia, London, 1989.
3. Nimni ME, Harkness RD. Molecular structure and functions of collagen. In Nimni M (ed) *Collagen*. CRC Press, Boca Raton, FL, pp 3–35, 1988.
4. Diamant J, Keller A, Baer E, Litt M, Arridge RGC (1972) Collagen: ultrastructure and its relation to mechanical properties as a function of aging. Proc R Soc Lond B180:293–315.
5. Ramachandran GN. Chemistry of Collagen. In Ramachandran G (ed) *Treatise on collagen*. Academic Press, New York, pp 103–183, 1967.
6. Miller EJ. Collagen chemistry. In Piez KA, Reddi AH (ed) *Extracelluar matrix biochemistry*. Elsevier, New York, pp 41–81, 1984.
7. Vogel HB (1978) Influence of maturation and age on mechanical and biochemical parameters of connective tissue of various organs in the rat. Conn Tiss Res 6:83–94.
8. Haut RC (1985) The effect of a lathyritic diet on the sensitivity of tendon to strain rate. J Biomech Eng 107:166–174. ASME Publishers.
9. Vogel HG (1975) Collagen and mechanical strength in various organs of rats treated with D-penicillamine or aminoacetonitrile. Conn Tiss Res 3:237–244.
10. Betsch DF, Baer E (1980) Structure and mechanical properties of rat tail tendon. Biorheology 17:83–94.
11. Rigby B, Hirai N, Spikes J, Eryring H (1959) The mechanical properties of rat tail tendon. J Gen Physiol 43:265–283.
12. Viidik A (1972) Simultaneous mechanical and light microscopic studies of collagen fibers. Zcshr Anat Entu-gesch 136:204–212.
13. Hooley CJ, Cohen RE (1979) A model for the creep behavior of tendon. Int J Biol Macromol 1:123–132.
14. Kastelic J, Palley I, Baer E (1980) A structural mechanical model for tendon crimping. J Biomech 13:887–893.
15. Torp S, Arridge RC, Armendiades CD, Baer E. Structure property relationships in tendon as a function of age. In *1974 Colston Conf*, pp 197–221, 1974.
16. Haut RC (1986) The influence of specimen length in the tensile failure properties of tendon collagen. J Biomech 19:951–955.
17. Kastelic J, Baer E. Deformation in tendon collagen. In Vincent JFV, Currey JD (ed) *The mechanical properties of biological material*. Cambridge, London, New York, New Rochelle, Melbourne, Sydney, 1980. Cambridge University Press.
18. Yannas IV, Huang C (1972) Fracture of tendon collagen. J Poly Sci A-2(10):577–584.
19. Haut RC (1983) Age dependent influence of strain rate on the tensile failure of rat-tail tendon. ASME J Biomech Eng 105:296–299.
20. Bailey AJ, Etherington DJ. Metabolism of collagen and elastin. In Florkin M, Neuberger A, Van Doren LLM (ed) *Comprehension biochemistry*. Elsevier-North Holland, Amsterdam, 19B:299–460.
21. Gray WR, Sandberg LB, Foster JA (1973) Molecular model of elastin structure and function. Nature 246:461–466.
22. Jenkins R, Little RW (1974) A constitutive equation for parallel-fibred elastic tissue. J Biomech 7:397–402.
23. Hoeve CAJ, Flory PJ (1958) The elastic properties of elastin. J Am Chem Soc 80:6523–6526.
24. Krafka J (1939) Comparative study of the histo-physics of the aorta. Am J Physiol 125(1):1–14.
25. Carton RW, Dainauskas J, Clark JW (1962) Elastic properties of elastic fibers. J Appl Physiol 17:547–551.
26. Hass GM (1942) Elasticity and tensile strength of elastic tissue isolated from the human aorta. Arch Pathol 34:971–981.

27. Minns RS, Steven FS (1976) The tensile properties of developing fetal elastic tissue. J Biomech 9:9–11.

28. Rosenberg LC. Proteoglycans, Chapter 6. In Owen R, Goodfellow J, Bollough (ed) *Scientific foundations of orthopaedics and traumatology*. WB Saunders, Philadelphia, Toronto, pp 36–42, 1980.

29. Lanir Y (1987) Biorheology and fluid flux in swelling tissues. I. Biocomponent theory for small deformations, including concentration effects. Biorheology 24:173–187.

30. Parry DAD, Craig AS. Growth and development of collagen fibrils in connective tissue. In Ruggeri A, Motta PM (ed) *Ultrastructure of the connective tissue matrix*. Martinus Nijhoff, Boston, pp 34–64, 1984.

31. Wood GC (1960) The formation of fibrils from collagen solutons. Effect of chondroitin sulphate and some other naturally occurring polyanions on the rate of formation. Biochem J 75:605–612.

32. Wood GC (1964) The precipitation of collagen fibrils from solution. Int Rev Conn Tiss Res 2:1–31.

33. Scott JE, Orford CR, Hughes EW (1981) Proteoglycan-collagen arrangements in developing rat tail tendon. An electron-microscopical and biochemical investigation. Biochem J 195:573–581.

34. Partington FR, Wood GC (1963) The role of non-collagen components in the mechanical behavior of tendon fibres. Biochim et Biophy Acta 69:485–495.

35. Myers DB, Highton TC, Rayns DG (1973) Ruthenium red-positive filaments interconnecting collagen fibrils. J Ultrastruct Res 42:87–92.

36. Parry DAD, Barnes GRG, Craig AS (1978) A comparison of the size distribution of collagen fibrils in connective tissues as a function of age and a possible relation between fibril size distribution and mechanical properties. Proc R Soc Lond B 203:305–321.

37. Li JT, Armstrong CG, Mow VC (1983) The effect of strain rate on mechanical properties of articular cartilage in tension. ASME Biomech Symp 56:117–120.

38. Minns RJ, Soden PD, Jackson DS (1973) The role of the fibrous components and ground substance in the mechanical properties of biological tissues: a preliminary investigation. J Biomech 6:153–165.

39. Armstrong CG, Mow VC, Lai WM, Rosenberg LC. *Biorheological properties of proteoglycan macromolecules*. 27th Mtging Orthop Res Soc Las Vegas, Nevada, 1981.

40. Zhu W, Mow VC (1991) A nonlinear viscoelastic constitutive equation for the flow behaviors of concentrated proteoglycan solutions. ASME Biomech Symp AMD-120:247–250.

41. Mason P (1965) Viscoelasticity and structure of keratin and collagen. Kolloid Z 202:139–147.

42. Barenberg SA, Filisko FE, Geil PH (1978) Ultrastructural deformation of collagen. Conn Tiss Res 6:25–35.

43. Haut RC, DeCou JM. The effect of enzymatic removal of glycosaminoglycans on the strength of tendon. ASME, Adv Bioeng, 1984.

44. Amiel D, Frank CB, Harwood FL, Fronek J, Akeson WH (1984) Tendons and ligaments: A mophological and biochemical comparison. J Orthop Res 1(3):257.

45. Yahia LH, Garzon S, Strykowski H, Rivard CH (1990) Ultrastructure of the human interspinous ligament and ligamentum flava. A preliminary study. Spine 15(4):262–268.

46. Nachemson AL, Evans JH (1968) Some mechanical properties of the third human lumbar interlaminar ligament. J Biomech 1:211–220.

47. Amiel D, Billings E, Akeson WH. Ligament structure, chemistry, physiology. In Daniel D et al (ed) *Knee ligament: structure, function, injury and repair*. Raven Press, Ltd., pp 77–91, 1990.

48. Comninou M, Yannas IV (1976) Dependence of stress-strain nonlinearity of connective tissues on the geometry of collagen fibres. J Biomech 9:427–433.

49. Markenscoff X, Yannas IV (1979) On the stress strain relation for skin. J Biomech 12:127–129.

50. Kwan MK, Woo S L-Y (1989) A structural model to describe the nonlinear stress-strain behavior for parallel fibered collagenous tissues. J Biomech Eng 111:361–363.

51. Lanir Y (1978) Structure-strength relations for mammalian tendon. Biophy J 24:541–554.

52. Decraemer WF, Maes MA, Van Huyse VJ, Van Peperstraete P (1980) A nonlinear viscoelastic constitutive equation for soft biological tissues based upon a structural model. J Biomech 13:559–564.

53. Woo S L-Y, Gomez MA, Amiel D, Ritter MA, Gelberman RH, Akeson WH (1981) The effects of exercise on the biomechanical and biochemical properties of swine digital flexor tendons. ASME J Biomech Eng 103:51–56.

54. Zernicke RF, Butler DL, Grood ES, Hefzy MS (1984) Strain topography in human tendons and fascia, ASME J Biomech Eng 106:177–180.

55. Stouffer DC, Butler DL, Hosny D (1985) The relationship between crimp pattern and mechanical response of human patellar tendon-bone. J Biomech Eng 107:158–165.

56. Lanir Y (1979) A structural theory for the homogeneous biaxial stress-strain relationship in flat collagenous tissues. J Biomech 12:423–436.

57. Belkoff SM, Haut RC. A microstructural model used to study the effect of gamma irradiation on tendon allografts. Proc Conf Mtging Orthop Res Soc of USA, Japan, Canada, 1991.

58. Haut RC, Powlison AC (1990) The effects of test environment and cyclic stretching on the failure properties of human patellar tendons. J Orthop Res 8(4):532–540.

59. Butler DL, Grood ES, Noyes FR (1978) Biomechanics of ligaments and tendons. Exer Sport Sci Rev 6:125–181.

60. Hubbard RP, Soutas-Little RW (1984) Mechanical properties of human tendon and their age dependence. J Biomech Eng 106:144–150.

61. Haut RC, Powlison AC, Rutherford GW, kateley JR (1988) Some effects of donor age and sex on the mechanical properties of patellar tendon graft tissues. ASME Adv Bioeng 8:75–78.

62. Haut RC, Lancaster RL, DeCamp CE (1992) Mechanical properties of the canine patellar tendon: some correlations with age and the content of collagen. J Biomech 25(2):163–173.

63. Noyes FR, Grood ES (1976) The strength of the anterior cruciate ligament in humans and rhesus monkey. Age-related and species-related changes. J Bone Joint Surg 58A:1074–1082.

64. Woo S L-Y, Hollis JM, Adams DJ, Lyons RM, Takai S (1991) Tensile properties of the human femur-anterior cruciate ligament-tibia complex: the effects of specimen age and orientation. Am J Sports Med 19(3):217–225.

65. Kuiper SD, Amiel D, Harwood FL, et al (1990) Age related properties of the medial collateral ligament and anterior cruciate ligament. A morphological and biochemical analysis. Trans Orthop Res Soc 15:523.

66. Woo S L-Y, Gomez MA, Woo YK, Akeson WH (1982) Mechanical properties of tendons and ligaments II. the relationship of immobil-ization and exercise on tissue remodeling. Biorheology 19:397–408.

67. Butler DL, Noyes FR, Walz KA, Gibbons MJ. Biomechanics of human knee ligament allograft treatment. Trans 33rd Orthop Res Soc p 128, 1987.

68. Yahia LH, Brunet J, Labelle S, Rivard CH (1990) A scanning electron microscopic study of rabbit ligaments under strain. Matrix 10:58–64.

69. Noyes FR (1977) Functional properties of knee ligaments and alterations induced by immobilization. A correlative biomechanical and histological study in primates. Clin Orthop 123:210–242.

70. Kennedy JC, et al (1976) Tension studies of human knee ligaments. J Bone Joint Surg 58-A(3):350–355.

71. Paulos LE, France EP, et al. Comparative material properties of allograft tissues for ligament replacement: effects of type, age, sterilization and preservation. 33rd Mtging Orthop Res Soc p 129, 1987.

72. Yamada H. *Strength of biological materials*. Evans FG (ed) Williams and Wilkins, Baltimore, MD, pp 226–231, 1970.

73. Noyes FR, De Lucas JL, Torvik PJ (1974) Biomechanics of anterior cruciate ligament failure: an analysis of strain rate sensitivity and mechanisms of failure in primates. J Bone Joint Surg 56A(2):236–253.

74. Crowninshield RH, Pope MH (1976) The strength and failure characteristics of the rat medial collateral ligament. J Trauma 16(2):99–105.

75. Peterson RH, Woo S L-Y (1986) A new methodology to determine the mechanical properties of ligaments at high strain rates. J Biomech Eng 108:365–367.

76. France EP, et al (1987) Failure characteristics of the medial collateral ligament of the knee: effects of high strain rate. Aviation Space and Env Medicine 58:488.

77. Wilkes GL, Nguyen A, Wildnauer R (1973) Structure-property relations of human and neonatal rat stratum corneum—I. Thermal stability of the crystalline lipid structure as studied by x-ray diffraction and differential thermal analysis. Biophys Acta 304:267–275.

78. Hult AM, Goltz RW (1965) The measurement of elastin in human skin and its quantity in relation to age. J Invest Dermatol 44:408–412.

79. Brown IA (1973) A scanning electron microscope study of the effects of uniaxial tension on human skin. Br J Dermatol 89:383–393.

80. Finlay B (1969) Scanning electron microscopy of the human dermis under uniaxial strain. Bio-Med Eng 4:322–327.
81. Lavker RM, Zheng P, Gang D (1987) Aged skin: a study by light, transmission electron, and scanning electron microscopy. J Invest Dermatol 88(3):445–515.
82. Millington PF, Gibson T, Evans JH, Barbenel JC. Structural and mechanical aspects of connective tissue. In Kenedi RM (ed) Advances in biomedical engineering. Academic Press, New York, pp 189–248, 1971.
83. Ridge MD, Wright V (1966) The directional effect of skin—a bioengineering study of skin with particular reference to Langer's lines. J Invest Dermatol 46:341–346.
84. Dick JC (1951) Tension and resistance to stretching of human skin and other membranes. J Physiol 112:102–113.
85. Langer K (1861) Zur anatomia und physiologie der haut. I. uber die spaltbarkeit der cutis. SB der Acad in Wien 44:19–46.
86. Gibson T, Stark H, Evans JH (1969) Directional variation in extensibility of human skin in-vivo. J Biomech 2:201–204.
87. Flint MH. The biological basis of Langer's lines. In Longacre JJ, Thomas CC (ed) *The ultrastructure of collagen.* Springfield, IL, 1973.
88. Pierard G, Lapiere CM (1987) Microanatomy of the dermis in relation to relaxed skin tension lines and Langer's lines. Am J Dermatol 9(3): 219–224.
89. Gadd CW et al. Strength of skin and its measurement. ASME Transactions, 65-WA/HUF-8, 1965.
90. Peterson FJ, Lange WMA, Gadd CW. Tear and tensile strength of human skin under static and dynamic loading. ASME Trans, 72-WA/BHF-6, 1972.
91. Mackay GM, Smith CA (1983) Facial injuries from windshields. Am Assoc Auto Med 27: 129–140.
92. Careless CM, Mackay GM (1982) Skin tissue cuttability and its relation to laceration severity indices. Int IRCOBI Conf Biomech Impacts 7:195–206.
93. Leung YC, Lopat E, Fayor A, et al. Lacerative properties of the human skin during impact. 3rd IRCOBI Conf, pp 399–411, 1977.
94. Alexander, H, Cook T. Variations with age in the mechanical properties of human skin in vivo. In *Bedsore biomechanics.* Macmillan, London, pp 109–117, 1976.
95. Daly CH, Odland GF (1979) Age-related changes in the mechanical properties of human skin. J Invest Dermatol 73:84–87.
96. Oxlund H, Manschot J, Viidik A (1988) The role of elastin in the mechanical properties of skin. J Biomech 21:213–218.
97. Wijn PEF. The alinear viscoelastic properties of human skin in vivo for small deformations. PhD Thesis. Kathieke Universiteit, Nijmegen, 1980.
98. Jagtman B. Clinical investigation of skin elasticity. MD Thesis. Katholieke Universiteit Nijmegen, The Netherlands, 1983.
99. Gibson T, Kenedi RM, Craik JE (1965) The mobile microarchitecture of dermal collagen: A bioengineering study. Br J Surg 52:764–770.
100. Dunn MG, Silver FH (1983) Viscoelastic behavior of human connective tissues: relative contribution of viscous and elastic components. Conn Tiss Res 12:59–70.
101. Daly CH (1982) Biomechanical properties of dermis. J Invest Dermatol 79:17–20.
102. Manschot JFM, Brakkee AJM (1986) The measurement and modeling of the mechanical properties of human skin in vivo—II, the model. J Biomech 19(7):517–521.
103. Holzmann H, Korting GW, Kobert D, Vogel HG (1971) Mechanical properties of skin in relation to age and sex. Orchin Fur Klinische and Experimentelle Dermatologic 239:355.
104. Rollhauser H (1950) Die zugfestigkeit der menschlichen haut; Genenbaurs morphol. Jahrb 90:249–261.
105. Fazekas IG, Kosa F, Basch A (1968) On the tensile strength of skin in various body areas. Deutsch Z Ges Gerich Med 64:62–68.
106. Jansen LH, Rottier PB (1958) Some mechanical properties of human abdominal skin measured on excised strips. Dermatologica 117:65–83.
107. Fry P, Harkness MLR, Harkness RD (1964) Mechanical properties of the collagenous framework of skin in rats of different ages. Am J Physiol 206:1425–1429.
108. Haut RC (1989) The effects of orientation and location on the strength of dorsal rat skin in high and low speed tensile failure experiments. J Biomech Eng 111:136–140.
109. Vogel HG (1972) Influence of age, treatment with corticosteroids and strain rate on mechanical properties of rat skin. Biochim Biophys Acta 286:79–83.
110. Li JT, Armstrong CG, Mow VC. The effect of strain rate on mechanical properties of

articular cartilage in tension. ASME, Biomech Symp, pp 117–120, 1983.

111. Mulligan GW, et al. An introduction to the understanding of blunt chest trauma. *The human thorax-anatomy, injury and biomechanics.* Society of Auto Eng, Warrendale, PA, p 67, 1976.

112. Cardany CR, Rodeheaver G, Thacker J, Edgerton MT, Edlich RF (1976) The crush injury: A high risk wound. JACEP 5(12):965–970.

113. Dobrin PB (1978) Mechanical properties of arteries. Physiol Rev 58(2):397–460.

114. Fung YC, Fronek K, Patitucci P (1979) Pseudoelasticity of arteries and the choice of its mathematical expression. J Physiol Soc 237(5):H620–H631.

115. Demiray H, Vito RP (1976) Large deformation analysis of soft biomaterial. Int J Eng Sci 14:789–793.

116. Roach MR, Burton AC (1957) The reason for the shape of the distensibility curves of arteries. Can J Biochem Physiol 35:681–690.

117. Wolinsky H, Glagov S (1964) Structural basis for the static mechanical properties of the aortic media. Circ Res 14:400–413.

118. Bergel DH (1961) The static elastic properties of the arterial wall. J Physiol 156:445–457.

119. Gozna ER, Marble AE, Shaw AJ, Winter DA (1973) Mechanical properties of the ascending thoracic aorta of man. Cardiovascular Res 7:261–265.

120. Wolinsky H, Glagov S (1967) A lamellar unit of aortic medial structure and function in mammals. Circ Res 20:90–111.

121. Tanaka TT, Fung YC (1974) Elastic and inelastic properties of the canine aorta and their variation along the aortic tree. J Biomech 7:357–370.

122. Cox RH (1979) Regional, species, and age related variations in the mechanical properties of arteries. Biorheology 16:85–94.

123. Hayashi K, Nagasawa S, et al (1980) Mechanical properties of human cerebral arteries. Biorheology 17:211–218.

124. Roach MR, Burton AC (1959) The effect of age on the elasticity of human illiac arteries. Can J Biochem Physiol 37:557–569.

125. Apter JT (1964) Mathematical development of a physical model of some visco-elastic properties of the aorta. Bull Math Biophy 26:367–388.

126. Apter JT (1967) Correlation of visco-elatic properties with microscopic structure of large arteries: IV. thermal responses of collagen, elastin, smooth muscle, adn intact arteries. Circ Res 21:901–918.

127. Mackay EH, Banks J, Sykes B, Lee G (1978) Structural basis for the changing physical properties of human pulmonary vessels with age. Thorax 33:335–344.

128. Hasegawa M (1983) Rheological properties and wall structures of large veins. Biorheology 20:531–545.

129. Viano DC, Culver CC, Haut RC, et al. Bolster impacts to the knee and tibia of human cadavers and a part 572 dummy. Soc Auto Eng Trans 780–896, 1978.

130. Mohan D, Melvin JW (1982) Failure properties of passive human aortic tissue. I-uniaxial tension tests. J Biomech 15(11):887–902.

131. Hoffman AS, Park JB (1977) Sequential enzymolysis of human aorta and resultant stress-strain behavior. Biomat Med Dev Art Org 5(2):121–145.

132. Gennarelli TA, Spielman GM, et al (1982) Influence of the type of intracranial lesion on outcome from severe head injury. J Neurosurg 56:26–32.

133. Gennarelli RA, Thibault LE (1982) Biomechanics of acute subdural hematoma. J Trauma 22:680–686.

134. Lowenhielm P (1974) Dynamic properties of the parasagittal bridging veins. Z Rechtsmedizin 74:55–62.

135. Lee M-C, Haut RC (1989) Insensitivity of tensile failure properties of human bridging veins to strain rate: implications in biomechanics of subdural hematoma. J Biomech 22(6/7):537–542.

136. Lee M-C, Haut RC. Strain rate effects on tensile failure properties of the human parasagittal bridging vein and the common carotid artery and jugular veins of ferrets. ASME, Adv Bioeng, pp 111–112, 1985.

137. Muir IHM. The chemistry of the groud substance of joint cartilage. In Sokoloff L (ed) *The joints and synovial fluid II.* Academic Press, New York, pp 27–94, 1987.

138. Broom ND (1986) The collagenous architecture of articular cartilage—a synthesis of ultrastructure and mechanical function. J Rheumatol 13:142–152.

139. Benninghoff A (1925) Form und ban der glenkknorpel in ihren beziehungen zur funktion. II der aufbau des gelenkknorpels in seinen beziehungen zur funktion. Zietschrift

fur Zellforschung und Mikroskopischen Anatomie 2:783–862.

140. Egan JM (1988) A constitutive study of the age-dependent mechanical behavior of deep articular cartilage: model construction and simulated failure. Clin Biomech 3:204–214.

141. Hultkrantz W (1898) Uber die spaltrichtungen der gelenkkorpel. Verh Anat Ges 12:248.

142. Maroudas A, Bannon C (1981) Measurement of swelling pressure in cartilage and comparison with the osmotic pressure of constituent proteoglycans. Biorheology 18:619–632.

143. Mizrahi J, Maroudas A, Lanir Y, Ziv I, Webber TJ (1986) The "instantaneous" deformation of cartilage: effects of collagen fiber orientation and osmotic stress. Biorheology 23:311–330.

144. Jurvelin J, et al (1988) Biomechanical properties of the canine knee articular cartilage as related to matrix proteoglycans and collagen. Eng Med 17(4):157–162.

145. Mow VC, Kuir SC, Lai WM et al (1980) Biphasic creep and stress relaxation of articular cartilage in compression: theory and experiments. J Biomech Eng 102:74–85.

146. Lanir Y (1987) Biorheology and fluid flux in swelling tissues. II. Analysis of unconfined compressive response of transversly isotropic cartilage disc. Biorheology 24:187–205.

147. Behrens F, Kraft E, Oegema TR (1989) Biochemical changes in articular cartilage after joint immobilization by casting or external fixation. J Orthop Res 7:335–343.

148. Troyer H (1975) The effect of short-term immobilization on the rabbit knee joint cartilage. Clin Orthop Rel Res 105:249–257.

149. Jurvelin J, et al (1989) Partial restoration of immobilization-induced softening of canine articular cartilage after remobilization of the knee (stifle) joint. J Orthop Res 7:352–358.

150. Hamerman D (1989) The biology of osteoarthritis. NEJM 320:1322–1330.

151. Armstong CG, Mow VC (1982) Variations in the intrinsic mechanical properties of human articular cartilage with age, degeneration, and water content. J Bone Joint Surg 64-A:88–94.

152. Brandt KD, Fife RS (1986) Ageing in the pathogenesis of osteoarthritis. Clin Rheum Dis 12(1):117–130.

153. Altman R, et al (1986) Development of criteria for the classification and reporting of osteoarthritis: classification of osteoarthritis of the knee. Arth Rheum 29(8):1039–1049.

154. Insall J, Falvo KA, Wise DW (1976) Chondromalacia patellae: a prospective study. J Bone Joint Surg 58:1–8.

155. Simon SR, Radin EL, Paul IL, Rose RM (1972) The response of joints to impact loading—II In vivo behavior of subchondral bone. J Biomech 5:267–272.

156. Repo RU, Finlay, JB (1977) Survival of articular cartilage after known impact. J Bone Joint Surg 60A:1068–1075.

157. Silyn-Roberts H, Broom ND (1990) Fracture behaviour of cartilage-on-bone in response to repeated impact loading. Conn Tiss Res 24:143–156.

158. Armstrong CG, Schoonbeck J, et al Characterization of impact-induced microtrauma to articular cartilage. ASME Adv Bioenging, pp 153–156, 1980.

159. Donohue JM, et al (1973) The effects of indirect blunt trauma on adult canine articular cartilage. J Bone Joint Surg 65-A:948–957.

160. Kempson JE. Mechanical properties of articular cartilage. In Freeman MAR (ed) Articular cartilage. Grune and Stratton, New York, pp 171–227, 1973.

161. Kempson GE. Mechanical properties of articular cartilage. In Freeman MAR (ed) Adult articular cartilage 2nd ed. Pitman Medical Publishers, Kent, England, pp 333–414, 1979.

162. Kempson GE (1982) Relationship between the tensile properties of articular cartilage from the human knee and age. Ann Rheum Dis 41:508–511.

163. Woo S L-Y, et al (1976) Measurements of the nonhomogeneous directional properties of articular cartilage in tension. J Biomech 9:785–791.

164. Schmidt MB, Mow VC, et al (1990) Effects of proteoglycan extraction on the tensile behavior of articular cartilage. J Orthop Res 8:353–363.

165. Akizuki S, Mow VC, et al (1986) Tensile properties of human knee joint cartilage: II. influence of ionic conditions, weight bearing, and fibrillation on the tensile modulus. J Orthop Res 4:379–392.

166. Woo SLY, Gomez MA, Akeson WH. Mechanical behaviors of soft tissues: measurements, modifications, injuries and treatment. In Nahum AM, Melvin J (ed) The biomechanics of trauma. Appleton Crofts, Norwalk, CT, pp 107–133, 1985.

167. Panjabi M, Jorneus L, Greenstein G (1984) Physical properties of lumbar spine ligaments. Trans Orthop Res Soc 9:112.

11
Skull and Facial Bone Trauma: Experimental Aspects

Douglas "L" Allsop

Introduction

Trauma, "a body injury produced by sudden force,"[1] is something that man has had to confront from the beginning of time. Skull and facial trauma has long been a part of war and warring. Early biblical references, such as to David and Goliath,[2] and accounts of early man illustrate the severe effects caused by a substantial blow to the head. While interpersonal violence still accounts for a significant portion of head trauma, the invention, development, and use of motor vehicles provides a medium through which a majority of skull and facial trauma occur.[3] The leading causes of facial fracture trauma are illustrated in Fig. 11.1.

Vehicular accidents and their associated injuries, while not a personal everyday occurrence, occur frequently enough to have an impact on the lives of most. Analysis of the Crashworthiness Data Systems' data (CDS) for 1988 and 1989, shown in Fig. 11.2, suggests that head and facial injuries account for nearly 40% of all vehicular injuries.

Other studies also indicate that a very high percentage of motor vehicle injuries are associated with the head and face. Backaitis and Dalmotas found that 36% of unrestrained driver injuries and 45% of unrestrained passenger injuries were head or facial injuries. Similarly, while the severity of injury was reduced, 39% of restrained driver injuries and 9% of restrained passenger injuries were to the head or face.[4] Thirty percent of restrained frontal occupants were found to have sustained head or facial injuries in a study performed by Cesari et al.[5] When analyzed with the Multiple Injury Priority Rating (MIPR), Viano et al.[6] found that injuries to the head and face accounted for 53% of the total.

Analysis of head and facial injuries, based on the Abbreviated Injury Scale (AIS), as shown in Fig. 11.3, indicates that many are AIS level-1-type injuries. These are minor injuries according to the AIS severity code and include laceration to the lips (no matter how extensive); laceration to the eyelid; nose fracture; and all lacerations not into subcutaneous tissue regardless of length, or into subcutaneous tissue less than or equal to 5 cm in length.[7] While certainly not life-threatening, these facial injuries, as well as more severe head and facial injuries, are often disfiguring and/or disabling, with long-term physical and emotional effects.

Use of Research Data

In 1973, William A. Lange, M.D., suggested: "The importance of designing the automobile interior with emphasis on protecting the human anatomy above the shoulders is recognized when the statistics are studied and the frequency of injuries is noted. Facial injuries with their subsequent disfigurements, functional impairments, and psychological implications make them especially important."[8]

The purpose of obtaining biomechanical data on the face and skull (as far as the automobile designer is concerned) is to provide a

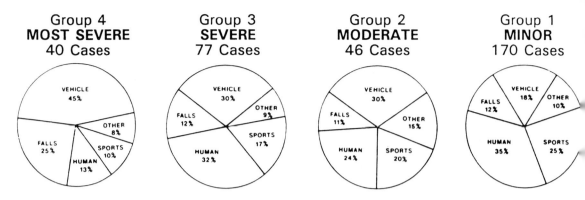

Human refers to interpersonal violence and other refers to other and unknown.

FIGURE 11.1. Distribution of facial fracture causes. (Reprinted with permission, T.A. Karlson, "The Incidence of Hospital-Treated Facial Injuries from Vehicles," *The Journal of Trauma*, Volume #22, Issue #4, Page 305, by Williams & Wilkins, 1982.)

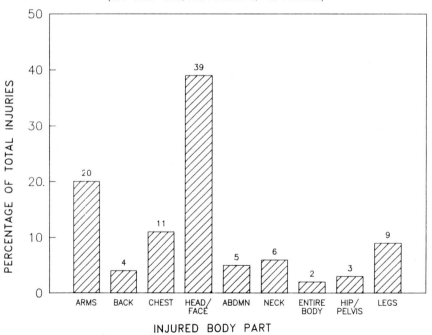

FIGURE 11.2. Automotive vehicle injury distribution by body regions.

basis for the design engineer to evaluate the injury potential associated with various design options. Feedback is provided through vehicle testing, and in order to provide meaningful feedback, test devices based on biomechanical data must be used. Stones from a riverbed may have the size and shape of chicken eggs; however, erroneous results would be obtained,

FIGURE 11.3. Injury severity: head and face compared to all body regions.

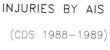

INJURIES BY AIS

(CDS 1988–1989)

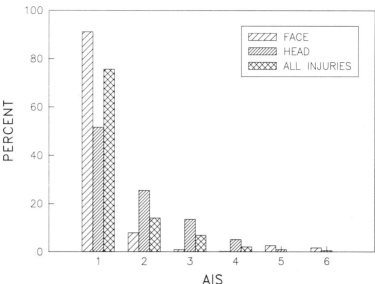

and ineffective products would be the result, if these were used to design and test egg cartons. Geometric similarity may exist, but an obvious difference in fracture characteristics of the test device (the stone) and the actual subject (the egg) exists, making the test device unsuitable as a tool in the design process.

For obvious reasons, humans and human cadavers cannot be used routinely in crash testing; because of this, a "test device" is required.

Early anthropomorphic test dummies (ATDs), i.e., test dummies with humanlike attributes, can be characterized in a manner similar to the stone and the egg. The early test dummies were similar to humans in geometry, but the response of the head, chest, legs, etc., to forces, accelerations, impulses, and the like was not necessarily similar to the response of the human.

One reason was that the response of the human, for the most part, was undocumented. During the last 30 years much effort and money have been spent to define the response characteristics and tolerances of the human. In parallel, the ability of the ATD to accurately model human response has improved as

knowledge and technology have allowed. ATDs in turn were and are being used in efforts to design and build automobiles which are safer than their predecessors.

Early ATD heads were similar to the human in geometry only. Many improvements were made during the 1970s by General Motors. The Hybrid I head was a modified Sierra design with uniform "skin" density and a triaxial accelerometer at the center of gravity. The Hybrid II was the result of a redesign in 1972 to eliminate mechanical resonances found in the Hybrid I. In 1973 the ATD 502 head was designed, and it is currently used on the Hybrid III dummy.[9] It was the first dummy head based on biomechanical data,[10] matching human cadaver response characteristics of the frontal bone documented by Hodgson and Thomas.[11] Since that time, many efforts have been made using various techniques to construct a dummy head capable of sensing contact force or contact pressure during impact in the facial region.[6,12–18]

While the above-referenced dummy heads employed sophisticated instrumentation, none adequately addressed the issue of biomechanical impact response in the facial region.

This is due in part to the fact that essentially no compliance data existed for the human face until Nyquist et al. in 1986[19] and Allsop et al. in 1988[20] published force-deflection data for the zygomatic and maxillary regions of the human cadaver. Based on these data, Perl et al.[21] designed and constructed a modified Hybrid III dummy head capable of measuring contact forces directly, with force-deflection characteristics similar to the human. Melvin and Shee have also built a modified Hybrid III dummy head that exhibits human bio-mechanical response for distributed as well as concentrated loads.[22] These two new dummy heads, shown in Figs. 11.4 and 11.5, due to their humanlike response characteristics, enable direct comparison between results obtained from vehicle crash tests and bio-medical data, thus permitting a quantitative evaluation of injury potential associated with a particular vehicle component. Benson et al. documented the characteristics of the Hybrid III head during lateral impacts and found them similar to those of the human. They also modified a Hybrid III head to measure contact force directly during side impacts (Fig. 11.6).[23]

The remaining portion of this chapter briefly outlines facial and skull anatomy and associated injury patterns; and describes briefly significant biomechanical studies published to date.

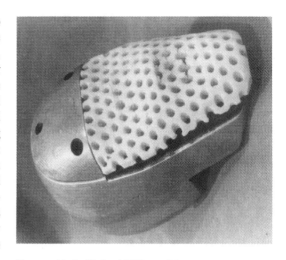

FIGURE 11.4. Volvo/CSE modified Hybrid III head with compliant insert. (Reprinted with permission 1989, Society of Automotive Engineers, Inc.)

Anatomy and Injury Patterns

The face and skull of humans are very complex structures. They consist of many bones fused together and associated suture lines. There is substantial variation between bones with regard to thickness, radius of curvature, etc. Because of this, and other associated factors, there is a great amount of variation in bio-mechanical data. Drawings illustrating head and facial complexity are presented in Figs.

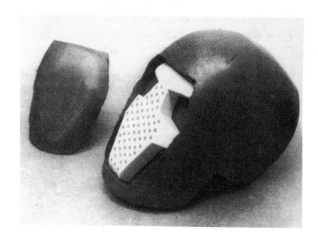

FIGURE 11.5. GM prototype 2 Hybrid III head with the deformable facial element in place and feature-less facial covering. (Reprinted with permission, J.W. Melvin, "Facial Injury Assessment Techniques", *12th ESV*. Volume #1, NHTSA 1989.)

FIGURE 11.6. Volvo/CSE modified Hybrid III head for side impact.

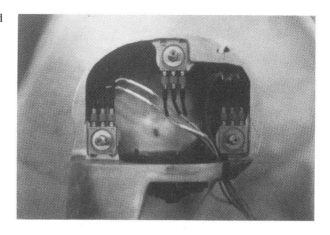

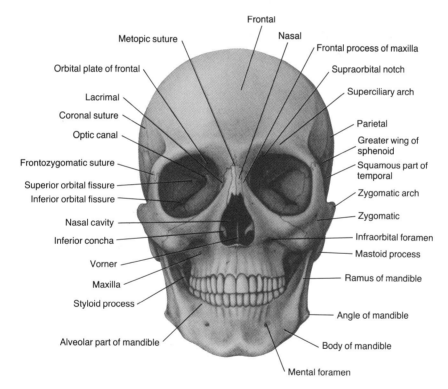

FIGURE 11.7. Skull—anterior view. (Reprinted with permission, R.S. Snell, *Atlas of Clinical Anatomy*, Little, Brown and Company, Inc. Boston, 1978.)

11.7 and 11.8 for frontal and lateral views, respectively. In addition, anatomical axes and planes are outlined in Figs. 11.9 and 11.10.

Pioneering work done by Le Fort,[24] at the turn of the century, mapped typical lines of fracture encountered after facial impact. These lines of fracture are termed Le Fort I, Le Fort II, and Le Fort III fractures. These are illustrated in Figs. 11.11 and 11.12 where the broken line, triangular-dotted line, and the

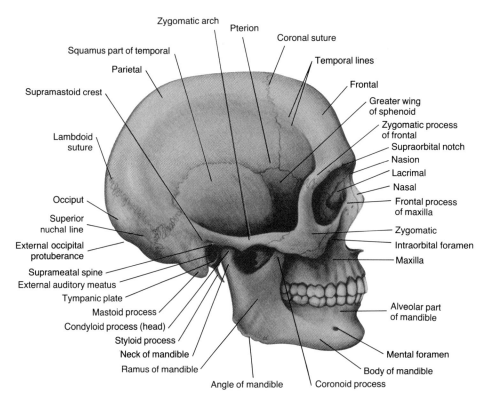

FIGURE 11.8. Skull—lateral view. (Reprinted with permission, R.S. Snell, *Atlas of Clinical Anatomy*, Little, Brown and Company, Inc. Boston, 1978.)

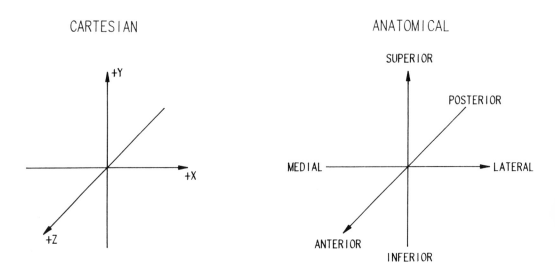

FIGURE 11.9. Anatomical axes.

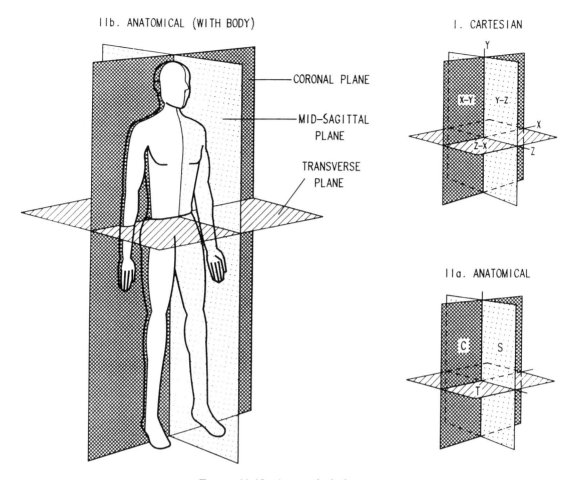

FIGURE 11.10. Anatomical planes.

diagonally-dashed line represent Le Fort I, II, and III fractures, respectively.

Review of Previous Research

Most research dealing with facial injury addresses medical treatment of fractures and lacerations. There has been a small amount of research done to document the force at which facial bones and skulls fracture; however, compliance and stiffness characteristics of the human face and skull during dynamic impact have been, until recently, essentially undocumented. The following sections review facial fracture tolerance and facial bone stiffness. A review of skull tolerance and stiffness is also presented.

Facial Fracture and Facial Stiffness

Facial Fracture

Nearly all facial-impact research, which documents force levels sufficient to fracture the human face, has been conducted by a very few individuals. Schneider summarized the data in 1985.[25] He concluded at that time that usable data came from only three sources; however,

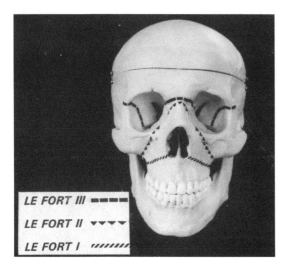

FIGURE 11.11. Le Fort lines of fracture.

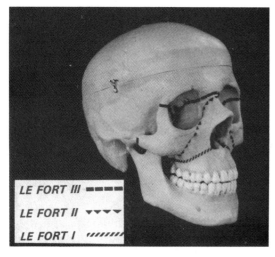

FIGURE 11.12. Le Fort lines of fracture.

since that time, additional significant research work has been conducted.

Hodgson is credited with doing much of the early research dealing with facial fracture. In 1964, he reported on work in which seven cadavers of ages over 60 were impacted with circular impactors ranging in mass from 0.50 to

5.63 kg.[26] The skin was excised from the impact sites at the supraorbital ridge, zygoma, and zygomatic arch, while a 1-inch-thick polyurethane pad was placed on the impactor face. Multiple blows were done at each impact site with impactor mass and velocity varying. Hodgson listed peak force values at impact. Recognizing possible inaccuracies in the data due to his test procedure, he stated:

Since the philosophy of these experiments was to obtain as much information from each cadaver as possible, many blows were struck at each blow location at subfracture impact levels. The data . . . on the strength of the facial bones obtained from these several cadavers should be considered with ⌐the] reservation that they may be on the low side.[26]

1965, Hodgson published additional data that concentrated mainly on the zygoma and again employed the multiple impact technique.[27] Most of the blows were delivered directly to the bone of 15 embalmed cadavers with a circular impactor 2.86 cm in diameter. Impactor mass ranged from 0.50 to 5.63 kg while the velocity varied from 1.3 to 8.7 m/sec. Response differences between embalmed and unembalmed cadavers were addressed; however, no conclusion was presented.

Subsequent work by Hodgson, published in 1967, is deemed more useful because the skin was left intact during impact.[28] Impactors weighing from 0.9 to 7.3 kg were used with a circular face of 6.45 or 33.5 cm². The frontal and mandible bones were impacted in addition to the zygoma. The multiple-blow technique was again used and the number of impacts per site usually was five or six. Accelerometers were mounted on the back of the cylindrical impactor and on the side of the head opposite the impact location. It was suggested that bone fracture could be detected from the shape of the acceleration curve generated by the accelerometer mounted on the impactor. Additionally, it was found that fracture force increased with an increased impactor surface area.

In 1968 Hodgson and Patrick[29] compared the dynamic response of the human head to a simple math model, illustrating that, at certain frequencies, accelerometers placed on the

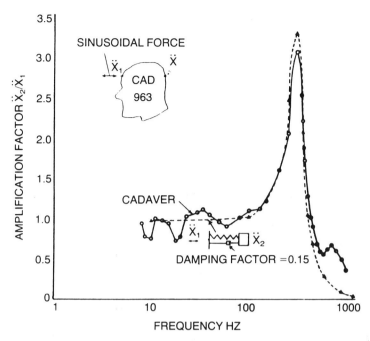

FIGURE 11.13. Occipital acceleration amplification (x_2/x_1) for sinusoidal force input to the frontal bone of the cadaver (silicon-gel-filled cranial cavity) at the first mode frequency (313 Hz), compared to a simple spring mass system having a natural frequency of 313 Hz, damping factor 0.15. (Reprinted with permission 1968, Society of Automotive Engineers, Inc.)

head opposite the impact site give erroneous results (Fig. 11.13).

Swearingen in 1965 reported on research in which instrument panels with head-impact deformation were removed from wrecked vehicles.[30] The medical history for the occupant that made the head print during the accident was used to determine the type and severity of fracture. Undamaged instrument panels from exemplar vehicles were obtained and impacted with a dummy head, recording accelerations, until dents in the accident-vehicle instrument panels were duplicated. It was hypothesized that the forces that caused fracture could be calculated from accelerations observed with dummy heads. However, the results are questionable because the dummy head was much stiffer than the human.

In an additional effort to document the fracture tolerance of the face, Swearingen also conducted 45 impacts to cadavers. Unfortunately, the mass of molded blocks that were fitted to the face where accelerometers were placed was not reported; therefore, conclusions about forces required for fracture cannot be made. In addition, each fracture site was hit multiple times with increased severity until fracture, diminishing the reliability of the data. However, Swearingen did establish that distributing the load over a large surface area significantly increased the force required for facial fracture.

Nahum et al. in 1968 reported on skull and facial impact work in which the frontal bone, the temporoparietal junction, the zygoma, and the mandible were hit.[31] Both embalmed and unembalmed cadavers were used. Each impact site was struck only once and force–time histories were recorded from a load cell that was located on the striking end of a cylindrical impactor. The impactor surface was 6.45 cm^2 in area and was covered with a MetNet crushable nickel pad 0.51 cm thick. Results suggested that clinically significant fractures (more severe than a hairline fracture) occurred at force levels of 1,000 N for the zygomatic area and that the average force at fracture was 1,770 N.

Later work presented in 1972 by Schneider and Nahum[32] augmented prior work by Nahum and presented facial fracture data for the maxilla, mandible in the antersor–posterior (A-P) and lateral directions, and the zygomatic arch. In addition, data on the frontal, temporoparietal, and zygomatic regions were reported. Loadings to the maxilla were at an oblique angle, as were all of the zygoma impacts previously discussed. The impactor was circular with a 6.5 cm² face, covered with MetNet 0.25 cm thick. All experiments were performed with the soft tissue in place, and all fracture data were based on a single impact. The results of this work corroborated the previous work by Nahum, concluding that there was no significant difference between embalmed and unembalmed material, and suggested a minimal fracture force tolerance of 670 N for the maxilla, 1,780 N for the A-P mandible, and 890 N for the lateral mandible. The average force at fracture for these three regions is 1,150 N, 2,840 N, and 1,570 N, respectively.

In 1986 Nyquist et al. reported their efforts to define fracture thresholds for the nasal bone and suborbital ridge. A 2.54-cm-diameter bar, longer than the width of a human head, was attached to the end of 32- and 64-kg cylinders and propelled horizontally into the face at speeds ranging from 2.7 to 7.1 m/sec. Each cadaver was placed upright in a chair so that its suborbital ridge was in line with the minor axis of the bar. The bar was oriented so that it would contact the nasal bone and the bottom of the orbits, roughly simulating contact with a steering wheel during a vehicular crash. Uniaxial accelerometers were placed on the impactor parallel to the path of travel, and on the back of the cadaver head, aligned in the anteroposterior direction. The peak applied force was determined by multiplying the impactor mass by the peak-impactor acceleration values. A threshold value of 3,000 N was suggested to distinguish between nasal fracture and more severe fractures. However, the highest fracture force recorded was from an impact with a specimen in which only the nasal

bone fractured, and the lowest force observed caused a fracture of the nasal bone and transverse fractures of the frontal bone about the nasal notch. These two examples illustrate the great variability encountered in biological testing. This variation was witnessed in all of the referenced research.

Allsop et al., in 1988, presented results of facial impacts to the maxilla, the zygomas just below the suborbital ridge, and the frontal bone just above the supraorbital ridge.[20] They employed a technique in which each specimen was impacted with more than enough energy to cause fracture, with fracture force being detected during the impulse. This was accomplished by employing a 20-mm-diameter rod as the impactor, made up from eight load cells. The load cells had very little mass, which minimized the instrumentation response time, enabling one to determine the point of fracture from the force–time history of the impact. An example of this is shown in Fig. 11.14. Initially the force builds along a relatively smooth path, but at fracture (approximately 1,700 N and 26 msec) a severe discontinuity is observed.

To ensure correctness of fracture forces taken from force–time histories, acoustic emissions–time data were also recorded. This was accomplished by attaching acoustic sensors to each specimen. These sensors detected acoustic (sound) waves or strain energy, which was released as micro- and macrofractures of the bone occurred. An acoustic emissions–time trace, for the maxillary impact shown in Fig. 11.14, is illustrated in Fig. 11.15 and indicates fracture at just over 26 ms. Force–time and acoustic emissions–time traces for that same impact are plotted on the same time scale in Fig. 11.16. The fracture point becomes obvious when the two sets of corroboratory data are analyzed together.

Forces at fracture ranged from 1,000 N to 1,800 N for the maxilla and 900 N to 2,400 N for the zygomas. An observation from this work is that fracture force is often less than the maximum force observed.[33] In each case presented in Fig. 11.17, fracture occurred at a force significantly less than the maximum. No significant correlation between fracture force and mineral content was observed.

FIGURE 11.14. Force/time history. Fracture indicated at 26 msec For Maxillary Impact. (Reprinted with permission 1988, Society of Automotive Engineers, Inc.)

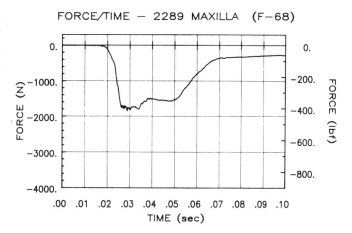

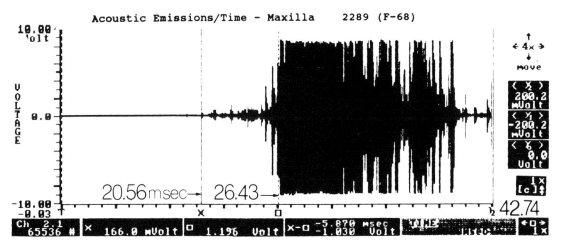

FIGURE 11.15. Acoustic Emissions/Time History. Fracture Indicated at 26 ms. (Reprinted with permission 1988, Society of Automotive Engineers, Inc.)

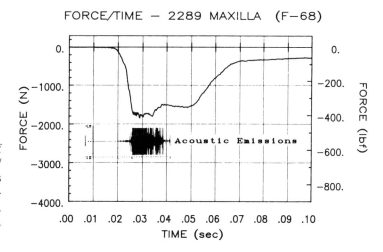

FIGURE 11.16. Comparison of force/time and acoustic emissions/time histories. Both histories indicate fracture at 26 ms. (Reprinted with permission 1988, Society of Automotive Engineers, Inc.)

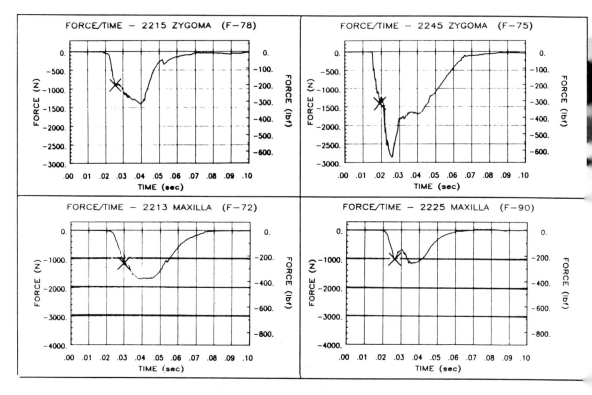

FIGURE 11.17. Force/time curves for facial impacts. Fracture force lower than maximum force. (× indicates fracture.)

Yoganandan et al. in 1988[34] and 1989[35] detailed impacts of the zygoma into two different steering wheels. A standard and an energy-absorbing steering wheel were set at a 30-degree angle and were impacted with 15 cadaver heads. Each head was guided into the steering wheel by a vertical monorail-outrigger system. Forces were measured at the base of the steering-wheel hub. Deflection of the wheel at the impact position was also recorded. A triaxial accelerometer was mounted to the posterior-parietal skull opposite the impact region; however, "the calculated forces based on the system mass and accelerations did not closely predict the measured forces."[35] Impact velocities ranged from 2.01 to 6.93 m/sec, and forces recorded were between 1,499 N and 4,604 N, with a mean value of 2,390 N, in those cases where fractures were observed. It was noted that neither head injury criteria (HIC) nor bone mineral content correlated well with fracture strength.

In 1989 facial impacts to the subnasal maxilla and nasion were reported by Welbourne et al.[36] Eight cadavers were impacted with a horizontal steel bar 25 mm in diameter, roughly approximating the cross section of a steering-wheel rim. The setup was very similar to that of Nyquist, with the cadaver sitting upright being impacted by a T-shaped bar moving in the horizontal plane. The impactor mass was 17 kg, and impact speeds varied from 1.8 to 14 m/sec.

In the subnasal region of the maxilla, maximum forces between 516 N and 1,362 N were observed. Unfortunately, only one fracture occurred, and this was at a maximum force of 788 N. The conclusion drawn from this series of tests was that impact energy was not a good indicator of fracture probability in this region.

Impacts into the nasion caused fracture in five out of seven cases. Maximum force at fracture ranged from 1,875 to 3,760 N. The

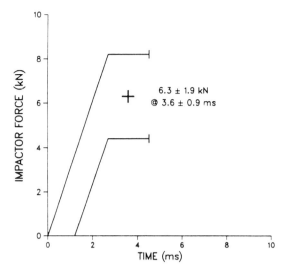

FIGURE 11.18. Preliminary force-time response corridor at 6.7/ms for full-face rigid impact to five cadaver subjects with only nasal bone fractures. (Reprinted with permission, J.W. Melvin, "Facial Injury Assessment Techniques," *12th ESV*, Volume #1, NHTSA 1989.)

minimum force caused a simple nasal fracture, while more severe fractures, including complete craniofacial disjunction (Le Fort III), were observed at higher levels.

Melvin and Shee listed preliminary results of impacts to five cadavers with a 15.2-cm-diameter flat plate.[22] Nasal fractures occurred; however, no significant facial fractures were observed even with a high average force of 6.3 kN and an impact speed of 6.7 m/sec. They suggested a force–time response corridor based on these data (Fig. 11.18) which was used as one of the design criteria for their deformable Hybrid III face.

A summary of facial fracture data, along with references to the author, are presented in Table 11.1.

Facial Stiffness

Research documenting stiffness characteristics of the human face is limited to three studies. The earliest efforts to document the compliance of the human skull were performed by Hodgson, Nakamura, and Talwalker in 1964.[26] Force-deflection characteristics of the zygoma and zygomatic arch were measured; however, the maximum deflection reported was less than 0.025 cm. These tests were conducted by applying force directly to the bone with the soft tissue removed. Deflection was measured by strain gauges attached to a cantilever strip, mounted on a stud, which was screwed to the skull. Because of the very small range of deflections measured, these data are of little value in dummy face design.

TABLE 11.1. Fracture force of facial bones.

| Bone | Force | | Sample size | Impactor area (cm²) | Author (reference) |
	Range (N)	Mean			
Mandible					
Midsymphysis	1,890–4,110	2,840	6	6.5	Schneider (32)
Lateral	818–2,600	1,570	6	25.8	Schneider (32)
Maxilla	623–1,980	1,150	11	6.5	Schneider (32)
Maxilla	1,100–1,800	1,350	6	20-mm-dia bar	Allsop (20)
Maxilla	788	788	1	25-mm-dia bar	Welbourne (36)
Zygoma	970–2,850	1,680	6	6.5	Schneider (32)
Zygoma	910–3,470	1,770	18	6.5	Nahum (31)
Zygoma[a]	1,120–1,660	1,360	4	6.5	Hodgson (28)
Zygoma[a]	1,600–3,360	2,320	6	33.2	Hodgson (28)
Zygomas[b]	2,010–3,890	3,065	4	25-mm-dia bar	Nyquist (19)
Zygomas[b]	900–2,400	1,740	8	20-mm-dia bar	Allsop (20)
Zygoma	1,499–4,604	2,390	13	approx 25-mm-dia bar (steering wheel)	Yoganandan (34)
Nasion	1,875–3,760	2,630	5	25-mm-dia bar	Welbourne (36)
Full face[c]	—	>6,300	5	181.0	Melvin (41)

[a] Multiple impacts prior to fracture.
[b] Both zygomas below suborbital ridges.
[c] Greater than 6,300 N for fractures other than nasal.

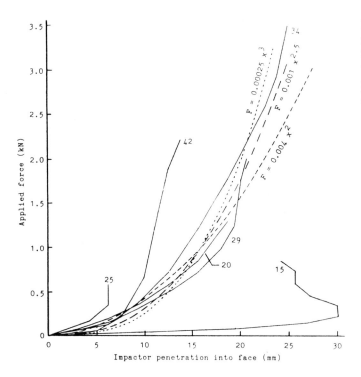

FIGURE 11.19. Force vs. penetration for tests 15, 20, 25, 29, 34, 42. Best fit: force (kN) = (0.001) (penetration mm).$^{2.5}$ (Reprinted with permission 1986, Society of Automotive Engineers, Inc.)

Recent work previously cited by Nyquist et al. presented force-deflection characteristics of the nasal bone and the suborbital ridge. The instrumentation consisted of accelerometers mounted on a cylindrical impactor and to the back of the cadaver's head. A high-speed movie camera was also used. Cross-plotting force–time data and double-integrated acceleration data to generate force-deflection histories proved difficult due to poor quality of the derived deflection data and due to time synchronization problems. Noise problems were encountered with the acceleration traces, making double integration unreliable, and admittedly, the precision of penetration data from the high-speed films was limited. However, a concave upward curve representing facial stiffness characteristics was suggested, with force in Newtons being equal to deflection in millimeters raised to the 2.5 power. This curve, along with stiffness curves for six cadavers, is shown in Fig. 11.19.

As previously cited, Allsop et al. documented the deflection characteristics for several facial impacts by fixing the specimen and measuring the displacement of the rigid impactor during the impact. The displacement–time curves were cross-plotted with their corresponding force–time curves to generate force–displacement curves. Fig. 11.20 displays curves for maxillary impacts, and Fig. 11.21 displays force–displacement data for zygomatic impacts. The mean stiffness for these regions is 120 N/mm for the maxilla and 150 N/mm for the zygomas.

Skull Fracture and Skull Stiffness

Several studies have been conducted in which bones of the skull have been impacted. Some were done with the intent of documenting the response of the brain to frontal or lateral accelerations[37–40] and others with the intent of documenting fracture characteristics of the bones of the skull. This section will give a brief description of studies published on skull fracture, followed by a review of the severely limited data on skull stiffness.

Skull Fracture

Of research conducted on fracture strength of the skull, some has been with full cadaver

FIGURE 11.20. Force/deflection histories for maxillary impacts. (Reprinted with permission 1988, Society of Automotive Engineers, Inc.)

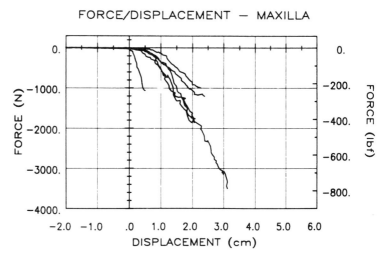

FIGURE 11.21. Force/deflection histories for zygomatic impacts. (Reprinted with permission 1988, Society of Automotive Engineers, Inc.)

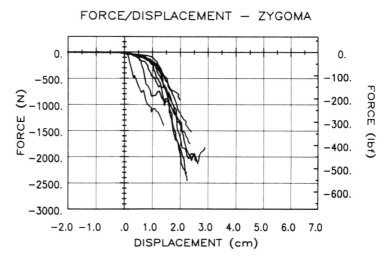

heads and some has been with only portions of the skull or with dry skulls. While quantitative data from research with dry skulls or skull portions is not directly comparable to the human, some quanlitative observations can be made.

In 1969 Melvin et al.[41] presented results of impact studies on skull caps. Three different small-area impactors were used to strike the frontal and parietal areas of the skull. Major conclusions from this work suggest that embalming has little or no effect on the fracture characteristics of the skull and that fracture force is directly related to the thickness of the skull at the point of impact. For example, the

parietal region always fractured at a lower force than the frontal bone (and was thinner than the frontal bone) except in one case in which both bones fractured at approximately the same level. In that case it was observed that the bones had nearly the same thickness. Characteristically, the left and right parietal bones on the same skull cap fractured at approximately the same force, except in those cases in which significant differences in bone thickness were present.

Research by Ono et al.[42] consisted of filling dry skulls with gelatin, covering them with clay, inserting them inside a Hybrid II vinyl skin, and impacting them multiple times from various drop heights. Observation from this study indicate the temporal region fractures at a lower force than the frontal or occipital zones.

The earliest single-impact quantitative data on skull impacts come from Nahum et al.[31] The instrumentation, previously described, employed a 25.4-mm-diameter flat, circular impactor. Eighteen frontal bone fractures were recorded with an average force of 4,930 N and a range of 2,670 to 8,850 N. The average force level for 18 fractures of the temporoparietal region was somewhat lower at 3,490 N. Fracture forces ranged from 2,215 N to 5,930 N. In addition to the fracture data, a minimum tolerance value for the frontal and temporoparietal regions of 4,000 N and 2,000 N was suggested. Nahum concluded that embalming, the impact rate of onset, and pulse duration were not critical factors and had minimal effect on fracture force.

Schneider and Nahum[32] later augmented the above work. Essentially the same instrumentation was used, and fracture studies of the frontal bone, temporoparietal region, and zygomatic arch were conducted. The average fracture force for the zygomatic arch was 1,450 N and ranged from 930 N to 1,930 N. Average fracture for the temporoparietal region occurred at 3,630 N, ranging from 2,110 to 5,200 N. The frontal bone fractured at a significantly higher level of 5,780 N on the average, with a low of 4,140 N and a high of 9,880 N. This study corroborated the previous conclusion by Nahum that embalming and pulse duration do not have a significant effect on fracture force. Additionally, it pointed out that female skulls as a group tend to fracture at lower values than male skulls.

In 1971 and 1973,[46,47] Hodgson and Thomas published results of research on the relationship between impact surface curvature and skull fracture. Impact surfaces included flat plates, cylindrical "bars" ranging in diameter from 3.2 mm to 25.4 mm, and hemispherical shapes with radii from 76 mm to 420 mm. In addition, the impactor stiffness varied from rigid to 60 durometer. Eighty cadavers were tested, and most received multiple impacts before fractures were observed. However, some impacts caused fracture on the first hit. Among these peak force ranged from 4,310 N to 8,990 N for frontal impacts and 2,670 N to 4,450 N for blows to the left frontal boss. No significant relationship between impact surface curvature and fracture force was observed.

The remaining data on frontal-bone fracture characteristics was completed by Allsop in 1988.[20] The instrumentation used was previously described, the impactor was a 20-mm-diameter bar made up from eight load cells. As with fracture of the facial bones, acoustic emissions were used to verify the fracture force. Thirteen cadaver heads were impacted with a resulting average fracture force of 4,780 N. The minimum force to cause fracture was 2,200 N and the maximum was 8,600 N.

Research presented in 1991 by Allsop augmented data on fracture characteristics of the temporoparietal region of the human cadaver.[43] Two impactors were used: one was a flat circular disk 25.4 mm in diameter with a mass of 10.2 kg; the other was a flat rectangular plate approximately 5 cm by 10 cm with a mass of 12 kg. This plate was actually made from eight small load cells 5 cm by 1.2 cm each.

Impacts with the flat disk were to the temporoparietal region, while the rectangular flat plate contacted somewhat higher on the head in the parietal region. Each reported impact was conducted with more than enough energy to ensure fracture, and fracture was detected from the force–time and acoustic emissions–time curves as previously described. Fracture force for the circular disk ranged from 2,500 to 10,000 N and averaged 5,200 N. For the rectangular flat plate the average force at fracture was 12,500 N, with a range of 5,800 N to 17,000 N. It was determined in this study that mineral content did not significantly affect fracture force.

The only data found for dynamic superior-inferior impacts to the head consisted of a 9.9-kg padded impactor loading a supine cadaver at 6.8–10.2 m/sec.[44] No skull fractures were observed; however, it was established that cervical fractures began at 5,700 N.

A summary of the skull fracture data, along with references to the author, is presented in Table 11.2.

TABLE 11.2. Fracture force of the skull.

Bone	Force Range (N)	Mean	Sample size	Impactor area (cm²)	Author (reference)
Frontal	2,670–8,850	4,930	18	6.45	Nahum (31)
Frontal	4,140–9,880	5,780	13	6.45	Schneider (32)
Frontal	2,200–8,600	4,780	13	20-mm-dia bar	Allsop (20)
Frontal	5,920–7,340	6,370	4	6.4-mm-dia bar	Hodgson (47)
Frontal	8,760–8,990	8,880	2	25.4-mm-dia bar (sagittal)[a]	Hodgson (47)
Frontal	N/A	6,550	1	50.8-mm-dia bar (90 durometer, sagittal)[a]	Hodgson (47)
Frontal	N/A	6,810	1	203-mm-radius hemisphere	Hodgson (46)
Frontal	4,310–5,070	4,690	2	76-mm-radius hemisphere	Hodgson (46)
Frontal	N/A	5,120	1	50.4-mm-dia bar (sagittal)[a]	Hodgson (46)
Left frontal boss	2,670–4,450	3,560	2	25.4-mm-dia bar	Hodgson (46)
Temporoparietal	2,215–5,930	3,490	18	6.45	Nahum (31)
Temporoparietal	2,110–5,200	3,630	14	6.45	Schneider (32)
Temporoparietal	2,500–10,000	5,200	20	5.07	Allsop (43)
Parietal	5,800–17,000	12,500	11	50	Allsop (43)
Zygomatic arch	930–1,930	1,450	11	6.45	Schneider (32)

[a] Major axis of bar parallel to sagittal plane.

FIGURE 11.22. Force/deflection histories for frontal impacts. (Reprinted with permission 1988, Society of Automotive Engineers, Inc.)

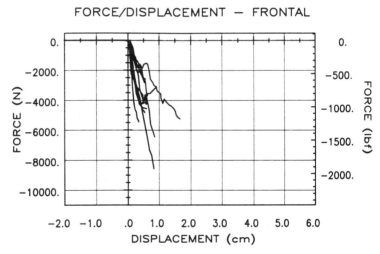

Skull Stiffness

Stiffness of the frontal bone was determined by Allsop et al.[20] in exactly the same manner described for the zygomas and maxilla. Results of 13 frontal impacts, hit with a 20-mm-diameter rod, are shown in Fig. 11.22. An average of the stiffnesses yields a value of approximately 1,000 N/mm.

Later research by Allsop et al.[43] (previously described) computed stiffness values from lateral impacts in a similar manner to that of the frontal bone. Stiffness curves for each of the temporoparietal impacts with the 25.4-mm-diameter circular plate impactor are presented in Fig. 11.23. The average for the 20 cadavers tested is 1,800 N/mm. Stiffness curves for parietal region, impacted by the 5 by 10-cm flat plate, are shown in Fig. 11.24. The average stiffness is 4,200 N/mm.

A summary of the facial and skull stiffness data is presented in Table 11.3.

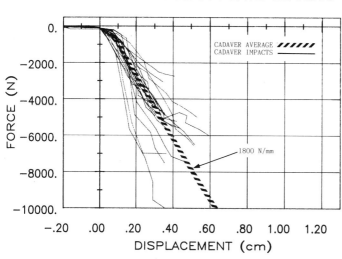

FIGURE 11.23. Force/deflection histories for impacts to the temporoparietal region. (Reprinted with permission 1991, Society of Automotive Engineers, Inc.)

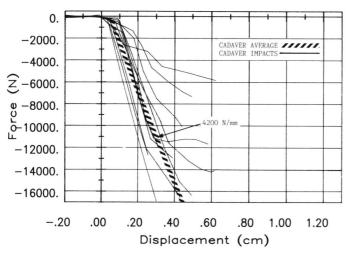

FIGURE 11.24. Force/deflection Histories for impacts to the parietal region. (Reprinted with permission 1991, Society of Automotive Engineers, Inc.)

TABLE 11.3. Stiffness of the face and skull.

| Bone | Stiffness (N/mm) | | Sample size | Impactor area (cm^2) | Author (reference) |
	Range	Mean			
Maxilla	80–180	120	6	20-mm-dia bar	Allsop (20)
Zygoma	Force (N) = [displacement (mm)]$^{2.5}$		6	25-mm-dia bar	Nyquist (19)
Zygoma	90–230	150	8	20-mm-dia bar	Allsop (20)
Frontal	400–2,200	1,000	13	20-mm-dia bar	Allsop (20)
Temporoparietal	700–4,760	1,800	20	6.45	Allsop (43)
Parietal	1,600–6,430	4,200	11	50	Allsop (43)

Conclusions

Research conducted in the last 5 years has helped document fracture and stiffness characteristics of the face and skull. Much of the new data, particularly those documenting stiffness characteristics, have been employed in the design and construction of new, truly anthropomorphic, ATD heads. However, a quick review of Tables 11.1–11.3 illustrates that the total number of specimens tested is still small, and that, coupled with the variation in impactor size, advanced specimen age, diversity of test procedures, and differences in data interpretation techniques, meaningful statistical analysis is made difficult. The many factors affecting fracture and stiffness should be carefully considered when employing the data presented herein.

While a meaningful statistical analysis is not yet possible, some trends have been observed and are listed below:

1. Embalming has little effect on fracture characteristics of skull and facial bones.[31,32,41]
2. Mineral content does not significantly affect fracture characteristics.[20,34,35,43]
3. Pulse duration, within limits normally encountered in occupant–vehicle interaction, does not substantially affect fracture force.[31,32]
4. Rate of onset and strain rate, within limits normally encountered in occupant–vehicle interaction, do not significantly affect fracture force.[6,31]
5. Initial fracture may occur at levels less than the maximum force recorded.[33,45]
6. Fracture force is significantly affected by skull bone thickness.[41]
7. Fracture force is significantly affected by impactor area.[28,30,43]

The data presented in this chapter provide a basis for quantitative analysis; however, it is hoped that future research into skull and facial bone fracture will be undertaken to augment and corroborate that which has been conducted in years past. Additionally, it is felt that new technology and creative application of new instrumentation can increase the quantity and quality of data gathered from each of the difficult-to-obtain test specimens.

References

1. *Random House Dictionary*, Random House, New York, 1978.
2. Old Testament, I Samuel 17:49.
3. Karlson TA (1982) The incidence of hospital-treated facial injuries from vehicles. Trauma 22(4).
4. Backaitis SH, Dalmotas DJ. Injury patterns and injury sources of unrestrained and three point belt restrained car occupants in injury producing frontal collisions. *29th AAAM*, p 365, October 7–9, 1985.
5. Cesari D, Ramet M, Welbourne E. Experimental evaluation of human facial tolerance to injuries. 1989 IRCOBI, Stockholm, Sweden, September 13–15, 1989.
6. Viano DC, Melvin JW, McCleary JD, Madeira RG, Shee TR. Measurement of head dynamics and facial contact forces in the Hybrid III dummy. *30th Stapp*, #861891, SAE P-189, p 269, October 27–29, 1986.
7. *The abbreviated injury scale*. American Association for Automotive Medicine, 1980 revision.
8. Lange WA. Facial Injury, Biomechanics and its applications to automotive design. *Society of Automotive Engineers P-49*, Warrendale, PA, January 1973.
9. Foster JK, Kortge JO, Wolanin MJ. Hybrid III—a biomechanically-based crash test dummy. *21st Stapp*, #770938, p 973, October 19–21, 1977.
10. Hubbard RP, McLeod DG. Definition and development of a crash dummy head. *18th Stapp*, #741193, p 599, December 4–5, 1974.
11. Hodgson VR, Thomas LM. Comparison of head acceleration injury indices in cadaver skull fracture. *15th Stapp*, #710854, Coronado, CA, November 17–19, 1971.
12. Grosch L, Katz E, Kassing L, Marwitz H, Zeidler F. New measurement methods to assess the improved protection potential of airbag systems. In *Restraint technologies: front seat occupant protection*. #870333, SP-690, p 161, February 1987.
13. Newman JA, Gallup BM. Biofidelity improvements to the Hybrid III headform. *28th Stapp*, #841659, p 87, November 6–7, 1984.
14. Warner CY, Niven J. A prototype load-sensing dummy faceform test device for facial injury

hazard assessment. *23rd AAAM*, p 67, October 3–6, 1979.

15. Moulton JR, Warner CY, Mellander H. Design, development and testing of a load-sensing crash dummy face. In *advances in belt restraint systems: design, performance and usage*. SAE #840397, pp 271–277, February 27–March 2, 1984.

16. Warner CY, Wille MG, Brown SR, Nilsson S, Mellander H. A load sensing face form for automotive collision crash dummy instrumentation. In *passenger comfort, convenience and safety: test tools and procedures*. #860197, p 85, February 24–28, 1986.

17. Warner CY, Allsop DL, and Wille MG. *Surface pressure sensors and ATD application SBIR final report*. DOT DTRS-57-86-C-00100, April 1987.

18. Nilsson S, Planath I. Facial injury occurrence in traffic accidents and its detection by a load sensing face. *11th ESV Conference*, p 613, May 12, 1987.

19. Nyquist GW, Cavanaugh JM, Goldberg SJ, King AI. Facial impact tolerance and response. *30th Stapp*, #861896, SAE P-189, p 379, October 1986.

20. Allsop DL, Warner CY, Wille MG, Schneider DC, Nahum AM. Facial impact response—a comparison of the Hybrid III dummy and human cadaver. *32nd Stapp*, #881719, p 139, October 17–19, 1988.

21. Perl TR, Nilsson S, Planath I, Wille MG. Deformable load sensing Hybrid III face. *33rd Stapp*, #892427, p 29, October 4, 1989.

22. Melvin JW, Shee TR. Facial injury assessment techniques. *12th ESV*, Vol 1, May 29–June 1, 1989.

23. Benson BR, Perl TR, Smith GC, Planath I. Lateral load-sensing Hybrid III head. *35th Stapp*, San Diego, CA, November 18–20, 1991.

24. Le Fort R. Etude experimentale sur les fractures de la machoire superieure. Rev Chir 1901(23):208,360,479.

25. Schneider DC. Biomechanics of facial bone injury: experimental aspects. *In the biomechanics of trauma*. p 281, Norwalk, Connecticut, 1985.

26. Hodgson VR, Nakamura GS, Talwalker RK. Response of the facial structure to impact. *8th Stapp*, p 229, October 21–23, 1964.

27. Hodgson VR, Lange WA, Talwalker RK. Injury to the facial bones. *9th Stapp*, p 144, October 20–21, 1965.

28. Hodgson VR (1967) Tolerance of the facial bones to impact, *American Journal of Anatomy* 120:113–122.

29. Hodgson VR, Patrick LM. Dynamic response of the human cadaver head compared to a simple mathematical model. *12th Stapp*, #680784, p 280, October 22–23, 1968.

30. Swearingen JJ. Tolerances of the human face to crash impact. Office of Aviation Medicine, Federal Aviation Agency, June 1965.

31. Nahum AM, Gatts JD, Gadd CW, Danforth JP. Impact tolerance of the skull and face. *12th Stapp*, #680785, p 302, October 22–23, 1968.

32. Schneider DC, Nahum AM. Impact studies of facial bones and skull. *16th Stapp*, #720965, p 186, November 8–10, 1972.

33. Allsop DL. Human facial fracture and compliance. PhD Dissertation. Department of Mechanical Engineering, Brigham Young University, December 1989.

34. Yoganandan N, Pintar F, Sances A, Myklebust J, Schmaltz D. Steering wheel induced facial trauma. *32nd Stapp*, #881712, p 45, October 1988.

35. Yoganandan N, Sances A, Pintar F, Harris G, Larson S. Three-dimensional computerized tomography analysis of steering wheel. Dept Neurosurgery, Medical College of Wisconsin. Paper presented at *12th ESV*, #89-4A-W-020, Gothenberg, Sweden, May 29, 1989.

36. Welbourne ER, Ramet M, Zarebski M. A comparison of human facial fracture tolerance with the performance of a surrogate test device. *12th ESV*, #89-4A-0-004, Gothenberg, Sweden, May 1989.

37. Nahum AM, Ward CC, Raasch FO, Adams S, Schneider DC. Experimental studies of side impact to the human head. *24th Stapp*, #801301, Troy, MI, October 15–17, 1980.

38. Nahum AM, Ward CC, Schneider DC, Raasch FO, Adams S. A study of impacts to the lateral protected and unprotected head. *25th Stapp*, #811006, San Francisco, CA, September 28–30, 1981.

39. Stalnaker RL, Roberts VL, McElhaney JH. Side impact tolerance to blunt trauma. *17th Stapp*, #730979, Oklahoma City, OK, November 12–13, 1973.

40. Got C, Patel A, Fayon A, Tarriere CH, Walfisch G. Results of experimental head impacts on cadavers: the various data obtained and their relations to some measured physical parameters. *22nd Stapp*, #780887, October 24–26, 1978.

41. Melvin JW, Fuller PM, Daniel RP, Pavliscak GM. Human head and knee tolerance to localized impacts. SAE #690477, May 19–23, 1969.

42. Ono K, Kikuchi A, Kobayashi H, Nakamura N. Human head tolerances to sagittal and lateral impacts—estimation deduced from experimental head injury using subhuman primates and human cadavers skulls. In *Head injury prevention past and present research*. Wayne State University, Department of Neurosurgery, Detroit, MI, December 4, 1985.

43. Allsop DL, Perl TR, Warner CY. Force/deflection and fracture characteristics of the temporo-parietal region of the human head. *35th Stapp*, San Diego, CA, November 18–20, 1991.

44. Culver R, Bender M, Melvin JW. Mechanisms, tolerances and responses obtained under dynamic superior-inferior head impact. Ann Arbor, MI: Highway Safety Research Institute, University of Michigan, UM-HSRI-78-21, PB 229-292, May 1978.

45. McClellan SB, Warner CY, Allsop DL, Perl TR. Compliance of the human cadaver head in the temporal-parietal region. Internal publication, Collision Safety Engineering, Orem, UT, December 1990.

46. Hodgson VR, Thomas LM. Breaking strength of the human skull vs. impact surface curvature. Wayne State University School of Medicine Department of Neurosurgery, Final report, contract No. FH-11-7609, June 1971.

47. Hodgson VR, Thomas LM. Breaking strength of the human skull vs. Impact surface curvature. Detroit: Wayne State University School of Medicine. NHTSA DOT-H-S-801-002. PB 233 041. November 1973.

12
Brain Injury Biomechanics

John W. Melvin, James W. Lighthall, and Kazunari Ueno

Introduction

The brain may be the organ most critical to protect from trauma, because anatomic injuries to its structures are currently non-reversible, and consequences of injury can be devastating. The experimental study of brain-injury mechanisms is unparalleled, because effects of trauma to the organs responsible for control and function of the body are the objects of the study. Injury of the central nervous system results not only from local primary effects, but from effects on physiologic homeostasis that may lead to secondary injury. The brain controls the flow of information, including autonomic control as well as sensory perception and motor function. The brain is the source of intentional actions, and it functions in time to store, retrieve, and process information. The state of self-awareness or consciousness is the highest level of brain function in man.

This chapter addresses the current state of knowledge in the biomechanics of brain injury. It is organized to provide a summary of head and brain anatomy and of clinical head-injury issues, followed by sections on experimental brain-injury models and bio-mechanical mechanisms of brain-injury and head-injury criteria. It closes with of discussion of future research directions in brain-injury biomechanics.

Anatomy of the Head

This section is a brief summary of head anatomy, starting with the scalp and skull, followed by more detailed descriptions of the structures internal to the skull. It is intended to provide a basic description for use in the following sections of the chapter. More complete descriptions can be found in standard anatomy texts.

Scalp

The scalp is 5 to 7 mm (0.20 to 0.28 inches) thick and consists of three layers: the hair-bearing skin (cutaneous layer), a subcutaneous connective-tissue layer, and a muscle and fascial layer. Beneath the scalp there is a loose connective-tissue layer plus the fibrous membrane that covers bone (periosteum). The thickness, firmness, and mobility of the outer three layers of scalp as well as the rounded contour of the cranium function as protective features. When a traction force is applied to the scalp, its outer three layers move together as one.

Skull

The skull is the most complex structure of the skeleton. This bony network is neatly molded around and fitted to the brain, eyes, ears, nose, and teeth. The thickness of the skull varies between 4 and 7 mm (0.16 and 0.28 inches) to snugly accommodate and provide protection to these components. The skull is composed of eight bones that form the brain case, 14 bones that form the face, as well the teeth. Excluding the face, the cranial vault is formed by the ethmoid, sphenoid, frontal, two temporal, two parietal, and occipital bones. The inner surface of the cranial vault is concave and relatively smooth. The base of the braincase is an irregular plate of bone containing depressions and ridges plus small holes (foramen) for arteries, veins, and nerves, as well as the large hole (the foramen magnum) that is the transition area between the spinal cord and the brainstem.

Meninges

Three membranes known as the meninges protect and support the brain and spinal cord. One function of the meninges is to isolate the brain and spinal cord from the surrounding bones. The meninges consist primarily of connective tissue, and they also form part of the walls of blood vessels and the sheaths of nerves as they enter the brain and as they emerge from the skull.

The meninges consists of three layers: the dura mater, the arachnoid, and the pia mater. The dura mater is a tough, fibrous membrane that surrounds the spinal cord and, in the skull, is divided into two layers. The outer cranial, or periosteal layer, lines the inner bony surface of the calvarium. The inner layer, or meningeal layer, covers the brain. In the braincase, the two layers of dura mater are fused except where they separate to form venous sinuses, which drain blood from the brain. Folds of the meningeal layer form the falx cerebri, which projects into the longitudinal fissure between the right and left cerebral hemispheres; and the tentorium cerebelli, a shelf on which the posterior cerebral hemispheres are supported.

The arachnoid mater is a delicate spiderweb-like membrane that occupies the narrow subdural space. The pia mater is a thin membrane of fine connective tissue invested with numerous small blood vessels. It is separated from the arachnoid by the subarachnoid space. The pia mater covers the surface of the brain, dipping well into its fissures.

The subarachnoid space and the ventricles of the brain are filled with a colorless fluid (cerebrospinal fluid, or CSF), which provides some nutrients for the brain and cushions the brain from mechanical shock. Cerebrospinal fluid is formed in the lateral and third ventricles by the choroid plexus and passes via the cerebral aqueduct into the fourth ventricle. From this site the fluid circulates in the subarachnoid spaces surrounding both the brain and the spinal cord. The majority of the CSF is passively returned to the venous system via the arachnoid villi. The specific gravity of cerebrospinal fluid is about 1.008 in the adult, which is approximately that of blood plasma. About 140 ml of CSF constantly circulates and surrounds the brain on all sides, so it serves as a buffer and helps to support the brain's weight. Since the subarachnoid space of the brain is directly continuous with that of the spinal cord, the spinal cord is suspended in a tube of CSF. For normal movement, a shrinkage or expansion of the brain is quickly balanced by an increase or decrease of CSF.

Central Nervous System

The central nervous system (CNS) consists of the brain and the spinal cord. At a microscopic level, the CNS is primarily a network of neurons and supportive tissue functionally arranged into areas that are gray or white in color. Gray matter is composed primarily of nerve-cell bodies concentrated in locations on the surface of the brain and deep within the brain; white matter is composed of myelinated nerve-cell processes (axons) that largely form tracts to connect parts of the central nervous system to each other.

The brain can be divided structurally and functionally into five parts: cerebrum, cerebellum, midbrain, pons and medulla oblongata. In addition, it has 4 ventricles (CSF cisterns with exits), 3 membranes (meninges), 2 glands (pituitary and pineal), 12 pairs of cranial nerves, and the cranial arteries and veins. The average length of the brain is about 165 mm (6.5 inches), and its greatest transverse diameter is about 140 mm (5.5 inches). Because of size differences, its average weight is 1.36 kg

(3.0 pounds) for the male and a little less for the female. The specific gravity of the brain averages 1.036, and it is gelatinous in consistency. The brain constitutes 98% of the weight of the central nervous system and represents about 2% of the weight of the body.

Cerebrum

The cerebrum makes up seven-eighths of the brain and is divided into right and left cerebral hemispheres. These are incompletely separated by a deep midline cleft called the longitudinal cerebral fissure. The falx cerebelli process projects downward into this fissure. Beneath the longitudinal cerebral fissure, the two cerebral hemispheres are connected by a mass of white matter called the corpus callosum. Within each cerebral hemisphere is a cistern for cerebrospinal fluid called the lateral ventricle. The surface of the each hemisphere is composed of gray matter and referred to as the cerebral cortex. In man, the cerebral cortex is arranged in a series of folds or convolutions. The ridge of the fold is referred to as a gyrus whereas the valley of the fold is called a sulcus. Each cerebral hemisphere is further subdivided into four lobes by fissures, each lobe being named by its association to the nearest cranial bone. Thus, the four lobes are the frontal, parietal, temporal, and occipital lobes.

The interior of each cerebral hemisphere is composed of white matter arranged in tracts that serve to connect one part of a cerebral hemisphere with another, to connect the cerebral hemispheres to each other, and to connect the cerebral hemispheres to the other parts of the central nervous system. In addition, within these interior areas of white matter are concentrations of gray matter called nuclei.

Midbrain

The midbrain connects the cerebral hemispheres above to the pons below. Anteriorly the midbrain is composed of two stalks that consist of fibers passing to and from the cerebral hemispheres above. The midbrain also contains gray matter nuclei. Within the midbrain is a narrow canal, the cerebral aqueduct, that connects to the third ventricle above and the fourth ventricle below.

Pons

The pons lies below the midbrain, in front of the cerebellum, and above the medulla oblongata. It is composed of white matter nerve fibers connecting the cerebellar hemispheres. Lying deep within its white matter are areas of gray matter that are nuclei for some of the cranial nerves.

Medulla Oblongata

The medulla oblongata appears continuous with the pons above and the spinal cord below. In the lower part of the medulla oblongata, motor fibers cross from one side to the other so that fibers from the right cerebral cortex pass to the left side of the body. Some sensory fibers passing upward toward the cerebral cortex also cross from one side to the other in the medulla oblongata. The medulla oblongata also contains areas of gray matter within its white matter. These are nuclei for cranial nerves and relay stations for sensory fibers passing upward from the spinal cord.

Cerebellum

The cerebellum lies behind the pons and the medulla oblongata. Its two hemispheres are joined at the midline by a narrow, striplike structure called the vermis. The outer cortex of the cerebellar hemispheres is gray matter; the inner cortex is white matter. The outer surface of the cerebellum forms into narrow folds separated by deep fissures. Nerve fibers enter the cerebellum in three pairs of stalks that connect the cerebellar hemispheres to the midbrain, pons, and medulla oblongata.

Traumatic Brain Injury from Clinical Experience

Introduction

Data complied by the Department of Health and Human Services (1989) indicate that someone receives a head injury every 15 seconds in the United States. This places the total number of injuries at over two million per year with half a million severe enough to require hospital admission. This study further indicates that 75,000–100,000 die each year as a result of traumatic brain injury, and it is the leading cause of death and disability in children and young adults.

Types of Brain Injuries

Clinically brain injuries can be classified in two broad categories: diffuse injuries and focal injuries. The diffuse injuries consist of brain swelling, concussion, and diffuse axonal injury (DAI). The focal injuries consist of epidural hematomas (EDH), subdural hematomas (SDH), intracerebral hematomas (ICH), and contusions (coup and contrecoup). Studies (Gennarelli 1981; Tarriere 1981; Chapon et al. 1983) have attempted to describe the incidence and sequelae of the above brain injuries. The results of these studies vary somewhat, however, mainly due to the criterion of selection of the patients in the studies. For example, the patients in the Chapon et al. study were all critically injured with immediate unconsciousness without a lucid interval after accidents involving automobiles (occupants and pedestrian) and two-wheelers. Only 7% of their sample contained injuries from falls and sports. Gennarelli's study contained 48% patients whose injuries were due to falls and assaults while the other 52% were from automobile accidents (occupants and pedestrians). Gennarelli's data indicate the average injury was serious to severe. This difference in the population considered may explain the different results in the two series, since Gennarelli's study shows a marked difference in the type of brain injuries sustained by automobile accident victims as compared to assault and fall victims. In this study, it was found that, three out of four automobile/ pedestrian brain injuries were of the diffuse type, and one out of four were of the focal type. The assault and fall victims had one out of four diffuse injuries and three out of four focal injuries.

Gennarelli's study points out that acute subdural hematoma and diffuse axonal injury were the two most important causes of death. These two lesions together accounted for more head injury deaths than all other lesions combined. The injuries most often associated with a good or moderate recovery were cerebral concussion and cortical contusion.

Diffuse Injuries

Diffuse brain injuries form a spectrum of injuries ranging from mild concussion to diffuse white matter injuries. In the mildest forms, there is mainly physiological disruption of brain function and, at the most severe end, physiological and anatomical disruptions of the brain occur.

Mild concussion does not involve loss of consciousness. Confusion, disorientation, and a brief duration of posttraumatic and retrograde amnesia may be present. This is the most common form of diffuse brain injury, it is completely reversible, and due to its mildness it may not be brought to medical attention. According to Scott (1981), minor concussions form approximately 10% of all minor-to-serious injuries involving the brain, skull, and spinal column.

The classical cerebral concussion involves immediate loss of consciousness following injury. Clinically, the loss of consciousness should be less than 24 hours and is reversible. Posttraumatic and retrograde amnesia is present, and the duration of amnesia is a good indicator of the severity of concussion. Thirty-six percent of these cases involve no lesions of the brain. The remainder may be associated with cortical contusions (10%), vault fracture (10%), basilar fracture (7%), depressed fracture (3%), and multiple lesions (36%) (Gennarelli 1982). Hence, the clinical outcome of patients with this type of symptom depends on the associated brain injuries. In general, 95% of the patients have good recovery at the end of 1 month. Close to 2% of the patients might have severe deficit, and 2% might have moderate deficit (Gennarelli 1982).

The injury considered to be the transition between pure physiological dysfunction of the brain to anatomical disruption of the brain generally involves immediate loss of consciousness lasting for over 24 hours. This injury is also called diffuse brain injury. It involves occasional decerebrate posturing, amnesia lasting for days, mild-to-moderate memory deficit, and mild motor deficits. At the end of 1 month, only 21% of these cases have good recovery. Fifty percent of the cases end up with moderate to severe deficits, 21% of the cases have vegetative survival, and 7% are fatal (Gennarelli 1982). The incidence of diffuse injury among severely injured patients is 13% (Gennarelli 1982) to 22% (Chapon et al. 1983).

Diffuse axonal injury (DAI) is associated with mechanical disruption of many axons in the cerebral hemispheres and subcortical white matter. Axonal disruptions extend below the midbrain and into the brainstem to a variable degree (Gennarelli 1982). These are differentiated from the less-severe diffuse injuries by the presence and persistence of abnormal brainstem signs. Microscopic examination of the brain discloses axonal tearing throughout the white matter of both cerebral hemispheres. It also involves degeneration of long white-matter tracts extending into the brainstem. High-resolution CT scans may show small hemorrhages of the corpus callosum, superior cerebellar peduncle, or periventricular region. These hemorrhages are quite small and may often be missed on CT scans.

Diffuse axonal injury involves immediate loss of consciousness lasting for days to weeks. Decerebrate posturing, with severe memory and motor deficits, is present. Posttraumatic amnesia may last for weeks. At the end of 1 month, 55% of the patients are likely to have died, 3% might have vegetative survival, and 9% would have severe deficit (Gennarelli 1982).

Brain swelling, or an increase in intravascular blood within the brain, may be superimposed on diffuse brain injuries, adding to the effects of the primary injury by increased intracranial pressure (Gennarelli 1982). Penn and Clasen (1982) report from 4% to 16% of all head-injured patients and 28% of pediatric head-injured patients have brain swelling. Tarriere (1981) has reported the incidence of

edema in 21% of CT-scanned head-injured subjects. It should be noted that in general brain swelling and edema are not the same but are often used interchangeably in the literature. Cerebral edema is a special situation in which the brain substance is expanded because of an increase in tissue fluid (Penn and Clasen 1982). The course of treatment for the two may be different. According to Penn and Clasen (1982), the mortality rate due to brain swelling among adults is 33–50% and 6% in children.

Focal Injuries

Acute subdural hematoma (ASDH) has three sources: direct lacerations of cortical veins and arteries by penetrating wounds, large-contusion bleeding into the subdural space, and tearing of veins that bridge the subdural space as they travel from the brain's surface to the various dural sinuses. The last mechanism is the most common in the production of ASDH (Gennarelli and Thibault 1982). Gennarelli and Thibault report a high incidence (30%) of ASDH among severely head-injured patients, with a 60% mortality rate. From various earlier studies, Cooper (1982a) reports the incidence rates of ASDH to be between 5% and 13% of all severe head injuries. According to Cooper, acute subdural hematomas generally coexist with severe injury to the cerebral parenchyma, leading to poorer outcome when compared to chronic subdural and extradural hematomas that generally do not coexist with injuries to the cerebral parenchyma. The mortality rate in most studies is greater than 30% and greater than 50% in some.

Extradural hematoma (EDH) is an infrequently occurring sequel to head trauma (0.2–6%). It occurs as a result of trauma to the skull and the underlying meningeal vessels and is not due to brain injury (Cooper 1982a). Usually skull fracture is found, but EDH may occur in the absence of fracture. From 50% to 68% of the patients have no significant intracranial pathology (Cooper 1982a). The remainder of the patients may have subdural hematoma and cerebral contusions associated with the EDH. These associated lesions influence the outcome of the EDH. The mortality rate from various studies ranges from 15% to 43%. This rate is greatly influenced by age, presence of intradural lesions, the time from injury to the appearance of symptoms, level of consciousness, and neurological deficit (Cooper 1982a).

Cerebral contusion is the most frequently found lesion following head injury. It consists of heterogeneous areas of necrosis, pulping, infarction, hemorrhage, and edema. Some studies have shown the occurrence of contusions in 89% of the brains examined postmortem (Cooper 1982a). CT-scan studies have shown incidence rates from 21% to 40%. A recent CT-scan study by Tarriele (1981) shows an incidence of 31% for contusions alone and 55% associated with other lesions. In contrast, Gennarelli's study (1982) shows an incidence of contusions in only 13% of the patients studied.

Contusions generally occur at the site of impact (coup contusions) and at remote sites from the impact (contrecoup contusions). The contrecoup lesions are more significant than the coup lesions (Cooper 1982a). They occur predominantly at the frontal and temporal poles, which are impacted against the irregular bony floor of the frontal and middle fossae. Contusions of the corpus callosum and basal ganglia have also been reported (Cooper 1982a). Contusions are most often multiple and are frequently associated with other lesions (cerebral hemorrhage, SDH, and EDH). Contusions are frequently associated with skull fracture (60–80%). In some cases they appear to be more severe when a fracture is present than when it is absent (Cooper 1982a). Mortality from contusions is reported to range from 25% to 60% (Cooper 1982a). Adults over 50 years of age fare worse than children. Patients in coma have a generally poor outcome.

Intracerebral hematomas (ICH) are well-defined homogeneous collections of blood within the cerebral parenchyma and can be distinguished from hemorrhagic contusions (mixture of blood and contused and edematous cerebral parenchyma) by CT scans. They are most commonly caused by sudden acceleration/deceleration of the head. Other causes are penetrating wounds and blows to the head producing depressed fractures below which ICH develop. Hemorrhages begin superficially and extend deeply into the white matter. In one-third of the cases they extend as far as the lateral ventricle. Some cases of the hematomas extending into the corpus callosum and the brainstem have been reported (Cooper 1982a).

According to Cooper, the incidence of ICH has been underestimated in the past. With the advent of the CT scan, better estimates are now available. Recent studies show the incidence to be between 4% and 23%. Gennarelli (1982) shows an incidence rate of 4%. Chapon et al. (1983) show an incidence rate of 8% in severely injured patients.

Depending on the study, the mortality for traumatic ICH has been as high as 72% and as low as 6%. The outcome is affected considerably by the presence or absence of consciousness of the patient (Cooper 1982a).

Skull Fractures

Clinically the presence or absence of linear skull fracture does not have much significance for the course of brain injury, although the subject is still controversial. This controversy continues because some studies show that, when dangerous complications develop after an initial mild injury, they are associated with skull fracture (Jennett 1976). According to Cooper (1982b), failure to detect fractures would have little effect on the management of the patient. Cooper further cites a study in which half the patients with extradural hematomas had skull fracture and half did not. Another study showed the occurrence of subdural hematomas in twice the number of patients without skull fracture as in those with skull fractures.

Gennarelli (1980) found the incidence of fracture to be similar across all severities of brain injuries in 434 patients. There was a slight tendency for the severity of fracture to increase as the severity of brain injuries increased. However, this tendency was not statistically significant. Similar conclusions were drawn by Chapon et al. (1983). Cooper (1982b) states that there is no consistent correlation between simple linear skull fractures and neural injury. Comminuted skull fractures result from severe impacts and are likely to be associated with neural injury. Cooper further states that clinically depressed fractures are significant where bone fragments are depressed to a depth greater than the thickness of the skull.

The incidence of depressed skull fracture is 20 per 1,000,000 persons per year, with an associated mortality rate of 11% related more to the central nervous system (CNS) injury than the depression itself. From 5% to 7% have coexisting, intracranial hematoma and 12% have involvement of an underlying venous sinus (Cooper 1982b).

Clinically, basal skull fractures are significant because the dura may be torn adjacent to the fracture site, placing the CNS in contact with the contaminated paranasal sinuses. The patient will be predisposed to meningitis (Landesmann and Cooper 1982).

The incidence of basal fracture is estimated to be between 3.5% and 24%. Part of the reason for such variation in estimates is that it is hard to see basal fractures during clinical examination. Further, they are difficult to visualize radiographically.

Experimental Brain-Injury Models

Mechanical injury to the brain can occur by a variety of mechanisms. General categories include (1) direct contusion of the brain from skull deformation or fracture; (2) brain contusion from movement against rough interior surfaces of the skull; (3) reduced blood flow due to infarction or pressure; (4) indirect (contrecoup) contusion of the brain opposite the side of the impact; (5) tissue stresses produced by motion of the brain hemispheres relative to the skull and each other; and (6) subdural hematoma produced by rupture of bridging vessels between the brain and dura mater. The latter three mechanisms are hypothesized to be involved in both impact and nonimpact (intertial acceleration) head injury (Ommaya 1985).

Regardless of the experimental-outcome variable to be studied by the neurotraumatologist, the model chosen by the researcher will produce the injury by mimicking one or more of the mechanisms described earlier. Experimental models of brain injury have used different techniques and a variety of species, with the common objective to develop a reproducible model of trauma that exhibits anatomical, physiological, and functional responses similar to those described clinically. Despite these efforts, there is not a single "ideal" experimental injury model; rather the goals and objectives of the research must dictate what is required of the model.

To this end there exist a variety of models. However, there is no entirely satisfactory experimental model that succeeds in producing the complete spectrum of brain injury seen clinically and yet is sufficiently well controlled and quantifiable to be a useful model for experimental studies. Experimental injury models that can be characterized biomechanically are required for physical and analytical modeling of tissue deformation. These modeling efforts will be useful for correlation of experimental results and injury response with human-injury initiation and response. Assuming that neural and vascular tissues are injured by induced local stresses and strains, the technique used to load or deform the neural tissue at the contact surface is unimportant if the pattern of injury seen is comparable to that observed in clinical brain injury. One can argue that since the structural changes, such as contusion, hemorrhage, or axonal injury, are distributed in patterns similar to those observed clinically, the local mechanics of the injury at a tissue level are comparable even if the gross-level input is different (Lighthall et al. 1989a, 1990).

This section will review specific experimental models of brain injury developed to study biomechanical and physiological mechanisms of clinical CNS trauma. The experimental brain injury models will be divided into three general categories: (1) head impact; (2) head acceleration; and (3) direct brain deformation.

Examples will be reviewed and discussed for each model category. Finally, the use, value, and appropriate validation of physical and analytical models will be discussed in relation to development of predictive criteria for functional neural injury in humans.

The section focuses on experimental models of nonpenetrating mechanical brain injury and will discuss the appropriateness and applications of these models for investigation of injury biomechanics, pathophysiology, and histopathology.

Method Development

The development and evolution of any experimental model of traumatic neural injury depends in part on the investigator's objectives. Differing scientific objectives and goals may result in different, but equally appropriate, models. A goal of injury prevention through improved understanding of injury biomechanics poses somewhat different constraints and requirements for the design of the model than, for example, testing efficacy of pharmacologic interventions on specific physiologic aspects of the injury response. However, all models must mimic to some extent the mechanical mechanisms of brain trauma observed in real world trauma to assure comparability of mechanisms. Despite differing experimental objectives, there are certain requirements that are common to any successful experimental model for traumatic brain injury: (1) The mechanical input used to produce the injury must be controlled, reproducible and quantifiable; (2) The resultant injury must be reproducible and quantifiable and produce functional deficit and neuropathology that emulate human brain injury; (3) The injury outcome, whether specified in anatomical, physiological, or behavioral terms must cover a range of injury severities; (4) The level of mechanical input used to produce the injury should be predictive of the outcome severity.

The primary objective for any experimental model of brain injury is to create specific pathophysiologic outcomes in a reproducible manner. The importance of reproducible,

intermediate-severity injury levels should be emphasized, because valuable data are likely to be found at transition- or threshold-level regions. Whether one is evaluating the relationship of injury biomechanics to outcome severity or the efficacy of a particular treatment regimen, the range of outcome modification due to altered mechanical input or treatment is likely to be greater at the intermediate-severity level than at either supramaximal or trivial injury-severity levels.

Although the mechanical input to the brain mimics, at least in part, the biomechanics of human trauma, some simplifications are helpful and indeed necessary to enable interpretation of mechanisms of injury at a tissue level. For example, direct brain deformation reproduces only some of the dynamics of closed head-impact trauma, but can be characterized biomechanically. Provided that the injury technique is designed to be relevant to hypothesized biomechanics and pathophysiology of clinical injury, the critical factor becomes the production of functional and anatomic sequelae comparable to those observed in human neurologic injury.

A simplified model, once characterized biomechanically and physiologically, can be combined with analytic and physical models of the neural, vascular, and skeletal structures to define injury-tolerance criteria at the tissue level. A reproducible, well-defined mechanical input simplifies to a degree the interpretation of the pathophysiologic, biomechanical, and biochemical mechanisms of the resultant injury.

Models of Brain Injury

Head-Impact Models

Nonpenetrating head-impact models can be grouped according to whether the resulting head motion is constrained to a single plane or whether the head is allowed to move freely in an unconstrained manner. These two types of head impact models were first studied in primates and later in non-primate species. Controlled nonpenetrating head impact was pioneered by Denny-Brown and Russell in primates (Denny-Brown 1945; Denny-Brown and Russell 1941).

In early experiments performed by these researchers, the head motion resulting from the impact to the head was unconstrained. Their experiments laid the groundwork for the use of controlled impact to the unrestrained head as a common experimental technique because it was observed that when the head was fixed, cerebral concussion was less likely to result. The neurological and physiological indicators of injury produced by direct impact to the head were evaluated in fully anesthetized animals. Since a surgical plane of anesthesia is required to assure absence of discomfort to the animal during the experimental impact procedures, immediate assessment of the injury severity is limited to brainstem reflexes and systemic physiologic changes.

Gurdjian and associates used an impact piston with a 1-kg mass to strike the head of anesthetized primates at a predetermined location on the skull. Physiologic parameters, impact force, and head acceleration were monitored in an effort to determine thresholds for concussion and coma, coup and contrecoup contusions, and relative brain motions (Gurdjian et al. 1954, 1966; Hodgson et al. 1969). Later experiments performed by Ommaya and others used a molded protective skull cap to prevent fracture. Slight variations of this technique have been used to evaluate changes in intracranial pressure, behavior, systemic physiology, cerebral metabolism and histopathology following impact injury to the primate head (Ommaya 1966; Folz and Schmidt 1956; Ommaya et al. 1966; McCullough et al. 1971; Lewis and McLaurin 1972; Martins and Doyle 1977; Ommaya et al. 1971).

Head motion in these primate studies was constrained only by the neck, resulting in complex and poorly characterized three-dimensional head movement. Severity was determined by selection of impactor velocity, impactor mass, interface material, and impactor contact area. However, like human brain injury the potential injury mechanisms

remained complex. While a wide range of biomechanical responses exhibiting clinical relevance were likely produced, including local skull deformation, development of pressure gradients within the brain tissue, and relative motion between the brain and skull, because of the dynamics of the resultant head movement it was not technically feasible to quantify or separate the various biomechanical components of the injury event for more detailed analysis of injury mechanisms. Although some studies attempted to evaluate the effects of rotational and translational head acceleration separately, careful biomechanical analysis of the experiments found that impact to the unrestrained head always produced both rotational and translational acceleration.

The various direct head-impact methods are successful at producing either fatality or short-duration unconsciousness but generally suffer from a high degree of variability in the response. This variability may result from a lack of control over the precise conditions of the impact, an absence of control of head dynamic response, and inconsistent impactor-skull interface parameters. As a result, the expected variability due to biological differences is confounded by mechanical variability of the injury event, necessitating a large number of experiments to obtain a representative sample of pathophysiologic response. In addition, the uncontrolled injury biomechanics make analysis of brain-injury biomechanics or testing of therapeutic efficacy difficult at best.

A number of studies have therefore constrained, at least partially, the head motion during and after impact in an effort to increase the reproducibility of injury outcome (Langfitt et al. 1966; Gosch et al. 1970; Shatsky et al. 1974). Full constraint was not obtained, but the head motion was typically confined to a single plane. An analysis of the pathophysiology and relation of impact biomechanics to outcome in these studies indicates that the partial control of head motion does not represent a significant improvement over the gradation and reproducibility of impact to the unconstrained head.

Closed head impact has been applied to nonprimates, including rat and cat, with limited success (Beckman and Bean 1970;

Bakay et al. 1977; Hall 1985; Bean and Beckman 1969; Tornheim et al. 1976, 1979, 1981, 1983). Similar to early experiments involving primates, biomechanical interpretation of the test results was initially impeded by the unpredictable head movement resulting from the impact. This was due in part to unspecified level of head support or restraint. As a result, biomechanical analysis of head and brain dynamics following head impact was inconsistent.

Head-impact studies performed in cats, using a captive bolt pistol to deliver the impact, have been most extensively developed by Tornheim et al. (Tornheim et al. 1976, 1979, 1981, 1983). Oblique impacts delivered to the coronal suture cause a reproducible contusion with associated edema and skull fracture. The captive-bolt head-impact model has been used successfully to test efficacy of antiedema drugs. Subsequent experiments have used an oblique lateral impact, with the head resting on a collapsible hex-cell support (Tornheim et al. 1979, 1983). This model is useful for studies of cerebral contusion and resultant edema, though reliable gradation of impact severity is still needed.

In general, whole head impact has not been successful at producing clinically relevant brain injury in the rat. In most cases, early attempts using direct head impact to the rat resulted in either no identifiable injury or immediate convulsions associated with apnea. This finding highlights a common problem shared by early whole head-impact models in subprimates, particularly the rat. That problem is the inability to produce a graded, reproducible range of injury outcomes by varying the biomechanical parameters of the impact. In some rat impact models high-level input parameters resulted in either fatality or a brief period of unconsciousness, usually measured by absence of the righting reflex (Bakay et al. 1977; Ommaya et al. 1971; Govons et al. 1972; Nilsson et al. 1978; Bergen and Beckman 1975).

Skull fracture commonly occurs at impact-severity levels insufficient to produce prolonged coma in the rat; moreover, the occurrence of skull fracture is generally not well correlated

with injury severity. Convulsive activity, a common result of direct head impact in the rat, may affect overall outcome and must be considered in interpretation of cerebral metabolic, neurophysiologic and electroencephalographic changes which follow injury. The histopathological evidence of neural injury is typically restricted to the lower brainstem in contrast to findings in human brain injury. Finally, the injury response curve is extremely steep; only a slight change in impact parameters is needed to produce an injury spectrum from minor to fatal.

Recently Goldman and collaborators have reported results obtained using a newly developed closed head-impact model of mild to moderate head injury in the rat (Goldman et al. 1991). Moderate concussion in this model is characterized by 4–10 minutes of unconsciousness in the absence of skull fractures or brain contusions. This new experimental brain-injury model utilizes a pendulum to deliver a controlled impact to the intact skull. The skull and maxilla rest on an energy absorbing rubber mat to reduce the likelihood of a skull fracture. The pendulum impact surface incorporates a load cell that enables measurement of the amplitude and duration of force produced by the impact. This model reproducibly produces brain swelling accompanied by increases in intracranial pressure lasting more than 3 days postinjury. Significant morphologic changes include edema and neuronal death.

The model developed by Goldman is significant and unique in producing a reproducible range of mild- to moderate-severity injury based on pendulum stroke, impact load, and animal body weight, in the absence of skull fracture. Repeatability of experimental outcome is dependent on brain mass and is affected by skull strength. A key step in the success of this model was development of an impact force/body-weight nomogram that compensates for differences in skull strength over the body-weight range (330–430 g) so that similar cerebrovascular responses are achieved in animals at the extremes of body weight. Well-controlled animal husbandry conditions are critical for the reproducibility achieved by these investigators. Goldman reported variances in estimates of regional cerebral permeability that were well within the range encountered in other studies (Rapoport 1980). Physiologic and morphologic changes parallel many aspects of human head trauma, particularly elevation of intracranial pressure. These observations suggest this may be a useful and relatively inexpensive tool for investigating the mechanisms and therapeutics of brain trauma, and especially edema and elevated intracranial pressure.

Head Acceleration Models

Various head acceleration models have been developed, some of which tightly control the motions of the head and others of which allow free head motion. Free head acceleration is attained through an abrupt deceleration of a moving frame to which the rest of the body is firmly affixed. This produces a whiplash head motion and can result in concussion (Ommaya and Hirsch 1966; Ommaya et al. 1973). These studies have been performed in large nonhuman primates since the anatomic relationships between brain, brainstem, and spinal cord are most similar to man, as is the ratio of brain mass to head mass.

In any whole head acceleration model it is the geometry and mass distribution that will determine the brain dynamics and resultant injury. A significant difference between the head-impact and head-acceleration models is the relative absence of skull fracture in the acceleration models; however, in real situations the range of induced accelerations that produce injury experimentally is only achieved in man when head impact occurs.

Since unconstrained head dynamics make analysis of the injury biomechanics difficult and contribute to outcome variability, the majority of studies using head acceleration techniques have employed some type of helmet and linkage to control the head motions (Gennarelli et al. 1982; Unterharnscheidt 1982). Such a system controls the path direction, path length, and duration of acceleration so that the head motion is comparable between

experiments with a comparable input. In addition, controlling the path of head movement during acceleration reduces the incidence of skull fracture and local skull deformation, which are common occurrences in impact techniques.

The most extensive series of experiments studying acceleration induced brain injury was initiated by Ommaya and Gennarelli and concluded by Gennarelli and Thibault. The investigators were able to produce graded anatomic and functional injury severities, including prolonged traumatic unconsciousness (>30 minutes) in nonhuman primates (Gennarelli et al. 1982). This series of experiments built upon earlier head-acceleration studies that had indicated that loss of consciousness was more readily produced by high levels of angular acceleration than high levels of translational acceleration (Unterharnscheidt 1969; Ommaya and Gennarelli 1974; Gennarelli and Thibault 1983). Consequently, a device and control linkage was designed to allow high levels of angular acceleration to be delivered to the primate head without skull fracture (Gennarelli et al. 1982).

The technique used a pneumatic thrust column, helmet, and pivoting linkage to apply $60°$ of angular rotation within $11-22\,\mathrm{ms}$, attaining peak angular accelerations of $1-2 \times 10^5$ radians/sec^2. The acceleration pulse was biphasic, with a relatively long, ramp like acceleration phase followed by an abrupt deceleration phase, with injury presumed to occur during the deceleration phase. In addition to prolonged traumatic coma, these animals exhibited diffuse axonal injury in the subcortical white matter, comparable to pathology observed in clinical brain injury (Gennarelli et al. 1982; Adams and Doyle 1984). Histopathological evaluation of the brains shows a high degree of comparability to clinical brain injury pathology, substantiating the relevance of the technique (Adams et al. 1985, 1986, 1989). The spectrum of injury obtainable using this technique ranges from mild, subconcussive brain injury with only sparse histologic evidence of axonal damage, through prolonged (hours to days) traumatic coma with extensive axonal injury throughout the white matter and brainstem, to immediately fatal injury.

Biomechanical analysis has been partially successful in relating the magnitude of acceleration input to the severity of injury outcome in this model, although interpretation is confounded by the two-phase acceleration— deceleration pulse, which results in nearly comparable acceleration and deceleration force peaks and the potential for neural and vascular injury during either or both pulses. Nevertheless, the need to use nonhuman primates for the technique (because of geometrical considerations) slows the progress of research since it is not possible to perform the large number of experiments necessary to fully use the experimental power of the technique. The injury device is also complex and very costly to duplicate. It requires collaboration of medical scientists and biomechanical engineers for implementation and meaningful data interpretation. Finally, due to the biphasic acceleration—deceleration pulse, conclusions regarding the biomechanics and timing of neural and vascular tissue injury must be drawn cautiously.

Nelson and his colleagues developed a controlled nonimpact head acceleration model in the cat, using repetitive accelerations (Nelson et al. 1979, 1982; Barron et al. 1980). Repeated acceleration/deceleration is delivered at 1,200–1,400 oscillations/minute and combined with induced posttraumatic hypoxia or ischemia. Injury severities were categorized into three outcomes: immediate fatality, delayed mortality, and extended coma. Although clinical brain injury may involve a period of hypoxia or relative cerebral ischemia, the biomechanics of brain neural and vascular tissue response to rapid repetitive accelerations is unknown. The outcomes observed, however, are clearly relevant to clinical brain injury. This technique induces a consistent range of injury, with a reproducible percentage distribution in each of the three outcome categories, but does not allow prediction of the injury severity that is likely to result from a specific exposure. Hence, testing for efficacy of pharmacologic intervention is limited to observations regarding changes in the percent

immediate fatality, delayed mortality, and prolonged coma, requiring larger sample sizes and impairing interpretation on a mechanistic basis.

Direct Brain Deformation Models

Nonpenetrating focal deformation of cortical tissue has been employed as an alternative to head-impact and induced-acceleration models of brain injury. From a theoretical point of view, since brain tissue is injured by the induced stresses and pressures within the cerebrum and brainstem, if a direct cortical deformation results in the same pattern of intracerebral forces within the brain as that resulting from an acceleration or impact model, then the injuries induced are directly comparable.

The extent to which this can be successfully achieved remains an open question; however, since the functional changes and histopathology are in many aspects comparable to clinical brain injury, these models have become widely used. Further, since the brain deformation is under direct experimental control, it is unnecessary to restrict studies to primate species on the basis of brain geometry, as has sometimes been required for clinical relevance in head-impact or acceleration techniques. Theoretically, direct brain-deformation models should allow better control over the mechanics of the injury input and therefore pose some potential advantages for biomechanical analysis of the injury event and relation of brain-tissue deformation to injury outcome. However, these advantages remain potential since in almost every instance, little or no analysis of the brain-tissue deformation has been performed.

Early experimental work produced a direct focal cortical compression using either weight-drop devices or gas-pressure jets (Feeney et al. 1981; Meyer 1956; Gurdjian 1954). Although different mechanical inputs were used to produce cortical deformation, each model type displayed both localized cortical contusions and distributed cerebral metabolic effects (Dail et al. 1981). In both models the pathologic changes in neural and vascular elements were predominantly observed in the impact region. For this reason direct focal cortical compression is a useful model in studies in which a desired histopathological outcome is cortical contusion, and for testing the efficacy of therapies aimed at reducing cortical contusion size. However, widespread diffuse injuries of clinical relevance are not produced, nor are long-term function consequences of importance to clinical brain injury. From a mechanistic viewpoint this may be due to damping of the mechanical input by the dura and cortical tissue, effectively preventing propagation of the input throughout the remainder of the brain. The absence of biomechanical data on brain deformations in these injury models prevents any further conclusions.

Currently the fluid percussion method is the most widely accepted direct brain-deformation technique for producing experimental brain trauma, including reactive axonal injury, in subprimate species such as cat and rat (Clifton et al. 1989; Dixon et al. 1987, 1988; Hayes et al. 1987; McIntosh et al. 1987, 1989; Povlishock et al. 1978, 1983; Stalhammar et al. 1987; Sullivan et al. 1976). In this technique, a brief fluid pressure pulse is applied to the dural surface of the brain through a craniotomy. The procedure has been applied to both cats and rats to generate a range of brain injury from mild to severe (Sullivan et al. 1976; Povlishock et al. 1978, 1983; Dixon et al. 1987, 1988; Lewelt et al. 1980). The pressure pulse is delivered via a fluid column to the intact dura of the brain and results in functional changes accompanied by subcortical axonal damage and brainstem pathology. By increasing or decreasing the magnitude of the pulse pressure (1.0–4.0 atm, with relatively constant duration of 20 ms), a graded, reproducible range of injury severities can be produced.

The fluid-percussion technique reproduces some of the features associated with moderate head injury in man, characterized clinically by transient unconsciousness with prolonged alteration of mental status, a low incidence of hematomas, and prolonged neuropsychological deficits (Clifton et al. 1989; Rimel et al. 1982). A key aspect of human head injury that is not reproduced in midline fluid percussion is the cortical contusion; this likely reflects the distributed nature of cortical loading in the technique. Recently, McIntosh and colleagues have shown that the fluid percussion technique applied through a lateral craniotomy produces cortical contusion, a histological endpoint previously unreported using this technique (Cortez et al. 1989; McIntosh et al. 1989).

While the fluid percussion technique may be suitable for studying the physiology and pharmacology of moderate-severity head injury, it is not well suited for the study of the biomechanics of trauma. Experimental evidence taken from high-speed radiographic movies of the fluid-percussion event demonstrate a consistent, though complex, movement of fluid within the cranial cavity in the rat (Dixon et al. 1988; Lighthall et al. 1989). Identical experiments performed in the ferret showed a consistent, though less complex, wave pattern of fluid flow in the epidural space; however, the pattern observed was completely different from that observed in the rat. This would indicate that the pattern of cerebral deformation resulting from fluid percussion is species dependent (Lighthall and Dixon, unpublished observation). The interaction of the fluid pulse with the cranial contents does not lend itself to accurate biomechanical analysis of tissue deformations that produce the injury.

Although the mechanics of the fluid-percussion injury model have been investigated, they are not yet well defined, and are arguably different from closed head injury in man. However, the pathophysiologic changes offer a reasonable model in which to study mechanisms for brainstem injury and secondary cerebrometabolic abnormalities. The ability to produce graded brainstem and subcortical axonal injury continues to make the fluid-percussion technique a useful model for those aspects of clinical brain injury.

A direct cortical-impact model developed by our laboratory allows independent control of brain contact velocity and level of brain deformation. This technique was originally developed to study spinal-cord injury (Anderson 1982) and later modified to be used for experimental brain-injury research (Lighthall 1988). Initially characterized in the laboratory ferret, the cortical impact model has now been applied with success to the rat (Dixon et al. 1991). The controlled impact is delivered using a stroke-constrained pneumatic impactor. The impact device and impact procedures have been described elsewhere (Lighthall 1988). Briefly stated, the device consists of a stroke-constrained stainless-steel pneumatic cylinder with a 5.0 cm stroke. The cylinder is mounted in a vertical position on a crossbar that can be adjusted in the vertical axis. Impact velocity can be adjusted between 0.5 and 10 m/sec by varying the air pressure driving the pneumatic cylinder. Depth of impact is controlled by vertical adjustment of the crossbar that holds the cylinder.

Results from our laboratory indicate that cortical impact produces acute vascular and neuronal pathology that is similar to observations in currently accepted experimental models and, most importantly, in clinical brain injury. Controlled impacts using the pneumatic impactor produce a range of injury severities that are a function of contact velocity, level of deformation, and site of impact. This model is unique in its ability to produce graded cortical contusion, subcortical injury and, in high-severity impacts, brainstem contusion. Impacts performed at 4.3 m/sec or 8.0 m/sec, with $\simeq$ 10% compression (2.5 mm), produce extensive axonal injury at 3 and 7 days postinjury using both velocity/compression combinations (Lighthall et al. 1990). Regions displaying axonal injury were the subcortical white matter, internal capsule, thalamic relay nuclei, midbrain, pons, and medulla. Axonal injury was also evident in the white matter of the cerebellar folia and the region of the deep cerebellar nuclei.

Because diffuse axonal injury was observed, this would imply, based on clinical and experimental observation, that rapid mechanical deformation of the brain can produce behavioral suppression and/or functional changes similar to coma. Behavioral assessment showed functional coma lasting up to 36 hours following 8.0 m/sec impacts, with impaired movement and control of the extremities over

the duration of the postinjury monitoring time. The spectrum of anatomic injury and systemic physiologic responses closely resembled aspects of closed head injury seen clinically.

This procedure complements and improves upon existing techniques by allowing independent control of contact velocity and level of deformation of the brain to facilitate biomechanical and analytic modeling of brain trauma. Graded cortical contusions and subcortical injury are produced by precisely controlled brain deformations, thereby allowing questions to be addressed regarding the influence of contact velocity and level of deformation on the anatomic and functional severity of brain injury.

These cortical impact experiments confirm that direct brain deformation models of experimental injury can produce many aspects of traumatic brain injury in humans and can be used to investigate mechanisms of axonal damage and prolonged behavioral suppression.

Biomechanical Mechanisms of Brain Injury and Injury Criteria

Introduction

Impact injury to the brain can be caused by forces applied to the head and by the resulting abrupt motions imparted to the head. These forces can either be external to the body and act directly on the head and/or internal to the body and act on the head through the head/neck junction. Forces transmitted to the head from the neck are a combination of muscle forces and cervical spinal forces. In the case of involuntary loading due to impact, these forces are the result of external loads applied to other body regions, such as vehicle restraint forces applied to the torso, and are sometimes referred to as forces due to "whiplash".

Application of external forces to the head can result in local injury to the scalp, bones of the skull and/or brain tissue due to the effects of concentrated load. In the case of the brain, local injury at the site of impact can occur due to penetration of the skull by the striking surface or due to local deflection of the skull without skull fracture. Externally applied head impact forces can also deform the skull globally, which can cause pressure and deformation gradients throughout the brain.

Motions of the head associated with impacts to the head and torso quite often result in severe accelerations and large attendant velocity changes which, typically, are both translational and rotational in nature. Such abrupt motions result in inertial or body forces being developed in the brain tissue that in turn result in stresses and deformations throughout the brain. Thus, the state of deformation of the tissue in a region of the brain in a head undergoing impact loading will depend on (1) its location relative to the point of force application, (2) the nature of the distribution of the force, and (3) the nature of the motion of the head due to the forces acting on the head. In addition, abrupt head motion can also result in relative motion of the brain or parts of the brain with respect to the skull. Such relative motions can deform brain tissue due to impingement upon irregular skull surfaces or interaction with meningeal membranes and can stretch the connecting blood vessels between the surface of the brain and the skull. Finally, one last mechanism of deformation of brain tissue is that of local stretching of the brainstem and spinal cord due to motions produced at the head/neck junction. This motion can occur as a result of either head impact or head motion due to torso loading.

If the magnitudes of the deformations and stresses induced in the tissues by any of the above mechanisms are sufficiently great, the tissues will fail, either in the physiological or the mechanical sense, and injury will occur. It is evident from the above discussion that there are many possible combinations of loading conditions that could result in injury to the tissues of the head. Because of the multiplicity of conditions, the history of head injury biomechanics has produced a wide variety of proposed mechanical factors that have been presented as being responsible for producing injury. Ideally, a biomechanical understanding of brain injury mechanisms requires a description of the mechanical states that occur in the tissue during an impact and of the resulting

dysfunction in the physiological processes at the tissue level. The resulting tissue stresses and strains must be related to the dysfunction in order to develop truly predictive injury criteria. It is our view that this is best done through finite element modeling of the brain response to impact.

The sections that follow discuss the major studies that have addressed one or another aspect of brain injury biomechanics and their associated attempts at developing biomechanical injury criteria. It should be noted that the resulting injury criteria are all based on mechanical inputs to the head, rather than the more desirable mechanical responses of the brain itself.

Early Studies

The earliest studies of the biomechanical factors associated with brain injury were those of Scott (1940), Denny-Brown and Russell (1941), Holbourn (1943), Walker et al. (1944), Gurdjian and Lissner (1944), and Pudenz and Sheldon (1946). The early studies with experimental animals were severely limited by the lack of suitable dynamic measurement methods available for characterizing the impact severity and the responses such as intracranial pressure. Holbourn did no actual experiments on animals but, rather, used simple photoelastic models of the head to demonstrate his theories. He hypothesized that translational acceleration of the head would not produce significant deformations in the brain due to the incompressible nature of confined brain tissue. He thus concluded that shearing deformations, which produce no volume change, caused by rotational acceleration could develop the shear strains throughout the brain required to produce the diffuse effects needed for concussive brain injuries. Gurdjian and Lissner, on the other hand, attributed intracranial damage to deformation of the skull and changes in intracranial pressure brought about by skull deformation and acceleration of the head due to a blow to the head. Later, Gurdjian et al. (1955) also recognized that movement of the brain relative to the skull and resulting injuries can be caused by head rotation.

Rotational Brain-Injury Studies

Holbourn's hypothesis, that rotational acceleration is the primary means by which diffuse brain injury is produced, makes no differentiation between direct impact and indirect loading in terms of the outcome if the rotational acceleration levels are the same in both exposures. This led some subsequent researchers to explore the concept in experiments with monkeys in which abrupt rotational motion was imparted without direct impact loading to the head. Ommaya et al. (1966) demonstrated that abrupt rotation with impact could affect sensory responses in the monkey and that a cervical collar that reduced the rotational acceleration in occipital impacts also raised the impact severity needed to reach the threshold for concussion. This work demonstrated that the angular accelerations necessary to produce concussion by direct impact were approximately half those needed by indirect or inertial loading and, thus, did not support Holbourn's hypothesis. Ommaya and Hirsch (1971) subsequently revised the rotational theory to state that "Approximately 50 per cent of the potential for brain injury during impact to the unprotected movable head is directly proportional to the amount of head rotation . . . the remaining potential for brain injury will be directly proportional to the contact phenomena of impact (e.g., skull distortion)." The authors reported on experimental head impact and whiplash injury studies with three different sizes of subhuman primate species in support of their hypothesis. The data from the experiments were compared with values predicted from scaling considerations based on dimensional analysis. The authors predicted that a level of head rotational acceleration during whiplash in excess of 1,800 rad/sec^2 would have a 50% probability of resulting in cerebral concussion in man.

Gennarelli, Thibault, and co-workers, in a series of studies, continued the investigation into the relative roles of translational and rotational accelerations in causing brain in-

juries by using experimental devices that could produce large translational and rotational head accelerations independently and without deforming the skull of subhuman primate subjects. The nature of the test apparatus produced an acceleration followed by a deceleration since it employed a limited stroke motion. While such a start-stop motion is typical of angular motions due to impact, it is not typical of translational motions in which an initial velocity is usually involved. In an early study using these techniques, the effects of translational and angular acceleration on the brain were studied using squirrel monkeys (Ommaya and Gennarelli 1974). Two groups of animals were subjected to similar acceleration loading. The first group received translational accelerations and the second group received angular accelerations in a 45 degree arc about a center of rotation in the cervical spine. The physiological and pathological results were quite different in each of the groups. Pure translation did not produce diffuse injury although focal lesions were produced. It was only when rotation was added to translation that diffuse injury types were seen. At the highest acceleration exposures, it was impossible to induce a cerebral concussion in animals subjected to pure translational acceleration, while the combination of angular acceleration and translational acceleration easily produced concussion for the same tangential acceleration exposure level measured at the top of the head.

Later studies in this series reported by Abel et al. (1978) and Gennarelli and Thibault (1982) applied accelerations in the sagittal plane by subjecting the heads of rhesus monkeys to controlled rotation about a lateral axis in the lower cervical spine. The Abel et al. study focused on the production of subdural hematomas and expressed the results of these tests in terms of a translational component, tangential acceleration, which is the product of the initial angular acceleration and the radius of curvature of the applied motion. The test results were plotted as functions of the two parameters with maximum tangential acceleration shown as a series of lines of constant magnitude. The line denoting a maximum tangential acceleration of 714G was found to be the apparent boundary separating those cases in which subdural hematoma occurred from those in which it did not.

In the later study, Gennarelli and Thibault chose to use the angular deceleration phase of the enforced motion, rather than the initial acceleration phase, as the mechanical parameter with which to relate to the occurrence of brain injuries. They plotted the test results as functions of the peak angular deceleration and the associated pulse duration of the stopping phase of the motion. They found the occurrence of cerebral concussion to generally follow a decreasing angular deceleration level as pulse duration increased. Diffuse brain injuries occurred at higher levels of angular deceleration and generally followed the same trend as that for concussion. Plotting the subdural hematoma data on the same graph produced the unusual result that the magnitude of the angular deceleration necessary to produce subdural hematoma increased for increasing pulse duration. They attributed this effect to rate sensitivity of the failure strength of the bridging veins.

Lee and Haut (1989) have shown that the bridging veins are not rate sensitive, however. Lee et al. (1987) used a two-dimensional finite element model representation of the rhesus monkey brain to simulate these experiments to better understand the mechanisms of traumatic subdural hematoma and to estimate its threshold of occurrence in the rhesus monkey. The brain was treated as an isotropic homogeneous elastic material with and without structural damping and the skull was treated as a rigid shell. The complete acceleration and deceleration time history of the enforced motion was applied to the model. During both phases of the motion, high shear strains occurred at the vertex where the parasagittal veins are located.

The conclusions of the model analysis indicated that subdural hematoma may have occurred during the acceleration phase in the primate experiments. Because the experiments used a fixed total angle of rotation, the relationship between maximum angular acceleration and its pulse duration is fixed. Thus, if the angular deceleration and its pulse duration

were increased in the experiments, the initial angular acceleration would also be very high and its pulse duration would, conversely, be shortened. This finding may explain the apparent anomaly of the Gennarelli and Thibault analysis of the subdural hematoma data and supports the Abel et al. analysis using the initial acceleration data. Lee et al. were able to replot the experimental data as a function of both tangential and angular accelerations to show their combined effect on bridging vein deformation and estimate tolerance thresholds for subdural hematoma in the rhesus monkey as a linear combination of both types of acceleration.

Further analysis of the injuries produced in the rhesus monkey experiments led Gennarelli et al. (1982, 1987) to conclude that the extent of axonal injury, duration of coma, and outcome of this type of experimental injury correlate better with coronal (lateral)-plane rotational impacts rather than sagittal (frontal)-plane rotational impacts. In an effort to understand the implications of the injury data in terms of estimating equivalent exposures for the human, they duplicated the lateral rotation tests using physical models of skull–brain structures of the baboon and human. The skulls were prepared as coronal hemisections that allowed visual determination of shear deformations in a silicone gel simulation of brain material (Margulies et al. 1990). The falx cerebri membrane was simulated in both models. Since no measurement of brain biomechanical response, such as pressure or displacement within the head, was made in any of the experimental animals, there was no direct way to verify the reality of the response of the physical animal model. Instead, the authors chose to compare the overall deformation pattern with the pattern of diffuse axonal injury found in the animals. This method allowed them to estimate an empirically derived value of approximately 10% for critical shear strain associated with the onset of severe diffuse axonal injury in primates. This estimate of critical shear strain was then used to determine a corresponding coronal plane rotational acceleration value for the human head model. This resulted in an estimate of 16,000 rad/sec² rotational acceleration for the threshold of severe diffuse axonal injury in man.

The above study indicates the difficulty in developing comprehensive injury-prediction criteria for functional brain injury. As noted above, the lack of biomechanical measurement in the experimental animal brains during the test required estimations of brain responses through completely separate physical-model tests. The very high level of angular and translational accelerations necessary to produce closed head injury in the small brains of animals makes such measurements difficult. Additionally, the shapes of the brains of animals typically used for brain-injury studies make them more resistant to impact injury and also make it very difficult to scale the results to man, since structural scaling laws assume geometric similitude (Ueno et al. 1989).

Translational Motion Studies

The early emphasis on skull deformations and intracranial pressure gradients as sources of brain injury led Gurdjian, Lissner, and their co-workers to focus their brain injury studies on direct blows to the head and the resulting translational accelerations associated with such blows. In impact experiments in which blows were delivered to the fixed or free heads of dogs, Gurdjian et al. (1966) demonstrated that cellular damage in the upper spinal cord occurred as frequently with the head fixed as with the head free to move. They attributed the damage to shear stresses at the craniospinal junction as a result of pressure gradients in the brain. These researchers used an indirect approach to study human concussion by impact testing embalmed cadaver heads. The rationale for using a nonphysiological test subject was based on the clinical observation that concussion is present in 80% of patients with simple linear skull fractures. Even though most concussions do not involve skull fractures, the easily observed occurrence of a skull fracture was felt to be an endpoint that could be studied in the cadaver. Thus, by impacting the foreheads of embalmed cadaver heads against rigid surfaces at different impact energies, it would

be possible to determine the levels of head acceleration associated with the onset of linear skull fractures. By extension, then, the results could be used to infer the onset of concussion for the case of rigid head impacts to the front of the head. The translational head acceleration in the anterior–posterior direction was measured in the tests with a uniaxial accelerometer attached to the back of the skull of the cadaver.

This work was summarized in terms of acceleration level and impulse duration by Lissner et al. (1960). The relationship between acceleration level and impulse duration was presented by a series of six data points that indicated a decreasing tolerable level of acceleration as duration increased. This relationship became known as the Wayne State Tolerance Curve (WSTC), for the affiliation of the researchers, and has become the foundation upon which most currently accepted indexes of head injury tolerance are based. The original data only covered a duration range of 1–6 ms and, of course, only addressed the production of linear skull fractures in embalmed cadaver heads. The curve was later extended to durations above 6 ms with comparative animal and cadaver impact data and with human volunteer restraint system sled test data. The volunteer information consisted of whole body deceleration without head impact at very long (100 ms and greater) durations. The WSTC was subsequently used by Gadd (1961) to develop the weighted impulse criterion that eventually became the Gadd Severity Index (GSI) (Gadd 1966). In 1972, the National Highway Traffic Safety Administration proposed a modification of the GSI that has become known as the Head Injury Criterion (HIC) currently used to assess head injury potential in automobile crash test dummies. It is based on the resultant translational acceleration rather than the frontal axis acceleration of the original WSTC. A complete discussion of the development of the current HIC and its predecessors, the GSI and WSTC, is contained in *SAE Information Report, J885-APR84* (1984).

The WSTC has been criticized on various grounds since its inception. The paucity of data points, questionable instrumentation techniques, lack of documentation regarding the scaling of animal data used in its extension to longer durations, and uncertainty of definition of the acceleration levels have all been questioned. From a biomechanical standpoint the main criticism of the WSTC is that, just like the work of those advocating a rotational acceleration-induced mechanism of brain injury, there has been no direct demonstration of functional brain damage in an experiment in which biomechanical parameters sufficient to determine a failure mechanism in the tissue were measured. The assumption behind the WSTC work is that translational acceleration produces pressure gradients in the region of the brainstem that result in shear-strain-induced injury. The extension of this hypothesis to human brain injury remains to be verified. Ono et al. (1980) conducted an extensive series of experiments with monkeys and demonstrated that cerebral concussion can be produced by impacts that produce pure translational acceleration of the skull. Using additional experiments with cadaver skulls and scaling of the animal data, the authors developed a tolerance curve for the threshold of cerebral concussion in humans. The curve was called the Japan Head Tolerance Curve (JHTC). The difference between the JHTC and the WSTC in the 1–10 ms duration range was shown to be negligible, while minor differences exist in the longer duration region of the curves. The Ono et al. data show that the threshold for human skull fracture is slightly higher than that for cerebral concussion.

In both the above discussions researchers attempted to predict various kinds of brain injury from one specific head impact input parameter, such as rotational or translational acceleration, with little regard for the effects of the other parameter. In the vast majority of head impact situations it can be expected that both rotational and translational accelerations are present and combine to cause the brain responses that produce the injury in the tissue. As discussed at the beginning of this section, the global patterns of stress and deformation in the brain during an impact are complex. Accordingly, comprehensive brain-injury pre-diction will require a complete description of tissue mechanical states throughout the brain for any combination of mechanical inputs. This state of knowledge has yet to be realized and will depend on future research in brain injury and the development of sophisticated analytical models for the prediction of brain mechanical response to impact.

Future Brain-Injury Biomechanics Research

Standardization of experimental protocols dictates and encourages the use of a simple, single, controlled mechanical input to produce a neural injury. Several advantages accrue. If the mechanical input is designed to be quantifiable and graded, then correlations can be made between the tissue deformation parameters, including applied force, the amount of deformation and its time-history, and the resultant pathology and functional changes. Such analysis will ultimately lead to enhanced understanding of the interaction between the physical input, the severity of the physiologic injury response, and the functional outcome.

The restriction to one quantifiable mechanical input variable facilitates biomechanical analysis of experimental CNS injury. Parallel analysis utilizing physical and analytical modeling of tissue deformation then allows correlation to the more complex dynamics of human CNS injury, especially involving the brain, through derivation of tissue biomechanical parameters that produce transient neurological changes, coma, or fatality.

In all cases, physiological responses to the mechanical injury must be considered in the design of the experimental model and must be taken into account when ascribing hypothesized modalities of treatment. In addition, anesthetic interaction with the desired physiological outcome must be considered. While a surgical plane of anesthesia is mandatory during the experimental impact procedures, anesthesia will mask certain aspects of neurological outcome and behavioral assessment. Ethically there is no way to avoid this aspect of experimental CNS trauma research; however, consistent use of specific standardized anesthetic protocols between laboratories using the same experimental technique will enhance comparability of experimental results.

Techniques for producing experimental brain injury are sometimes not compatible with detailed biomechanical analysis required for development of an injury criterion. The cortical-impact technique described here in general has provided the ability to reproducibly generate graded levels of functional-injury severity in order to investigate mechanisms of clinical injury, and to conduct initial evaluations of potential therapeutic interventions. Species differences in brain mass and geometry and the nature of the interaction between the physical and physiological factors dictate first that certain simplifications will add to the usefulness of an experimental model and second that analytical or mathematical methods such as finite element models are necessary to make extrapolations from experimental studies to humans (Ueno et al. 1989). The approach of using a finite element model of the human brain will allow information from impact tests with dummies to be analyzed to predict the potential for brain injury. The method characterizes the brain as a deformable body bounded by the skull. The complete head motion from an impact is enforced on the skull by the accelerations. The contact surface of the skull–brain boundary transfers the motion from the skull to the brain resulting in stresses and strains in the brain tissue. Critical sites of potential injury may be indicated by maximum pressure, stress, strain, or displacement relative to the boundary. These potential injury sites must then be assessed using tissue-level injury criteria that have been validated using anatomical and functional data from experimental physiologic models.

We feel that development of tissue-level injury criteria for the central nervous system can only be achieved by using a three component approach consisting of (1) a simplified, biomechanically characterized physiological model that produces clinically relevant injury; (2) a physical model constructed from material that incorporates geometry, mass, and physical material properties matching the physiological model; and (3) a comprehensive finite- element model of the brain. Analytical modeling of the tissue response leading to injury requires that mechanical input to the tissue be quantifiable and reproducible. Therefore simplification of the input is required in designing a model that can be used to address the mechanics of neural and vascular injury at a tissue level. Validation of analytical finite-element models using experimental data requires correlation of the mechanical responses of the system in terms of pressures, displacements, and local accelerations of the important regions of the brain. We feel this approach will lead to tissue-level injury criteria, which, after physiological and anatomical validation of the analytical model, can be applied to the analysis of neural injury risk for impact and acceleration trauma in humans.

References

Abel JM, Gennarelli TA, Segawa H (1978) Incidence and severity of cerebral concussion in the rhesus monkey following sagittal plane angular acceleration. 22nd Stapp Car Crash Conference, Society of Automotive Engineers 22:35–53.

Adams JH, Doyle D, Ford I, et al (1989) Diffuse axonal injury in head injury: definition, diagnosis and grading. Histopathology 15:49–59.

Adams JH, Doyle D, Graham DI, et al (1986) Gliding contusions in nonmissile head injury in humans. Arch Pathol Lab Med, 10:485–488.

Adams JH, Graham DI, Gennarelli TA (1985) Contemporary neuropathological considerations regarding brain damage in head injury. In Becker DP, Povlishock JT, (eds). *Central nervous system trauma status report*. Sponsored by NIH, NINCDS, pp 143–452.

Adams JH, Doyle DI (1984) Diffuse brain damage in non-missile head injury. In Anthony PP, MacSween RNM (eds). *Recent advances in histopathology*. Churchill Livingstone, Edinburgh, pp 241–257.

Anderson TE (1982) A controlled pneumatic technique for experimental spinal cord contusion. J Neurosci Methods 6:327–333.

Bakay L, Lee JC, Lee GC, Peng JR (1977) Experimental cerebral concussion. Part I: An electron microscopic study. J Neurosurg 47:525–531.

Barron KD, Auen EL, Dentinger MP, Nelson L, Bourke R (1980) Reversible astroglial swelling in a trauma-hypoxia brain injury in cat. J Neuropath Exp Neurol 39:340.

Bean JW, Beckman DL (1969) Centrogenic pulmonary pathology in mechanical head injury. J Appl Physiol 37:807–812.

Beckman DL, Bean JW (1970) Pulmonary pressure-volume changes attending head injury. J Appl Physiol 29:631–636.

Bergren DR, Beckman DL (1975) Pulmonary surface tension and head injury. J Trauma 15:336–338.

Chapon A, Verriest JP, Dedoyan J, Trauchessec R, Artru R (1983) Research on brain vulnerability from real accidents. ISO document No. ISO/TC22SC12/GT6/N139.

Cheng CLY, Povlishock JT (1988) The effect of traumatic brain injury on the visual system: A morphologic characterization of reactive axonal change. J Neurotrauma 5:47–60.

Clifton GL, Lyeth BG, Jenkins LW, et al (1989) Effect of D, α-tocopheryl succinate and polyethylene glycol on performance tests after fluid percussion brain injury. J Neurotrauma 6:71–81.

Cooper PR (1982a) Post-traumatic intracranial mass lesions. Head Injury, pp 185–232. Edited by PR Cooper. Williams and Wilkins, Baltimore/London.

Cooper PR (1982b) Skull fracture and traumatic cerebrospinal fluid fistulas. Head Injury, pp 65–82. Edited by PR Cooper. Williams and Wilkins, Baltimore/London.

Cortez SC, McIntosh TK, Noble LJ (1989) Experimental fluid percussion brain injury: vascular disruption and neuronal and glial alterations. Brain Res 482:271–282.

Dail WG, Feeney DM, Murray HM, Linn RT, Boyeson MG (1981) Responses to cortical injury II: Widespread depression of the activity of an enzyme in cortex remote from a focal injury. Brain Res 211:79–89.

Denny-Brown D, Russell WR (1941) Experimental cerebral concussion. Brain 64:93–164.

Denny-Brown D (1945) Cerebral concussion. Physiol Rev 25:296–325.

Dixon CE, Lyeth BG, Povlishock JT, et al (1987) A fluid percussion model of experimental brain injury in the rat. J Neurosurg 67:110–119.

Dixon CE, Lighthall JW, Anderson TE (1988) Physiologic, histopathologic, and cineradiographic characterization of a new fluid-percussion model of experimental brain injury in the rat. J Neurotrauma 5:91–104.

Dixon CE, Clifton GL, Lighthall JW, Yaghmai AA, Hayes RL (1991) A controlled cortical impact model of traumatic brain injury in the rat. J Neurosci Methods 39:3, pp 253–262.

Feeney DM, Boysen MG, Linn RT, Murray HM, Dail WG (1981) Responses to cortical injury. I. Methodology and local effects of contusions in the Rat. Brain Res 211:67–77.

Folz EL, Schmidt RP (1956) The role of the reticular formation in the coma of head injury. J Neurosurg 13:145–154.

Gadd CW (1961) Criteria for injury potential. Impact Acceleration Stress Symposium, National Research Council publication no. 977. National Academy of Sciences, Washington DC, pp 141–144.

Gadd CW (1966) Use of a weighted impulse criterion for estimating injury hazard. 10th Stapp Car Crash Conference. Society of Automotive Engineers 10, pp 164–174.

Gennarelli TA (1980) Analysis of head injury severity by AIS-80. 24th Annual Conference of the American Association of Automotive Medicine, pp 147–155. AAAM, Morton Grove, Ill.

Gennarelli TA (1981) Mechanistic approach to head injuries: clinical and experimental studies of the important types of injury. Head and neck injury criteria: a consensus workshop, pp 20–25. Edited by AK Ommaya. U.S. department of transportation, national highway traffic safety administration, Washington DC.

Gennarelli TA, Thibault LE (1982) Biomechanics of acute subdural hematoma. J Trauma 22:680–686.

Gennarelli TA, Thibault LE (1983) Experimental production of prolonged traumatic coma in the primate. In Villiani R (eds) Advances in neurotraumatology. Excerpta Medica, Amsterdam, pp 31–33.

Gennarelli TA, Thibault LE (1985) Biological models of head injury. In Becker DP, Povlishock JT (eds) Central nervous system trauma status report. Sponsored by NIH, NINCDS, pp 391–404.

Gennarelli TA, Thibault LE, Adams JH, Graham DI, Thompson CJ, Marcincin RP (1982) Diffuse axonal injury and traumatic coma in the primate. Ann Neurol 12:564–574.

Gennarelli TA, Thibault LE, Tomei G, Wiser R, Graham D, Adams J (1987) Directional dependence of axonal brain injury due to centroidal and non-centroidal acceleration. Society of Automotive Engineers, 31st Stapp Car Crash Conference. Warrendale, PA, 31:49–53.

Goldman H, Hodgson V, Moorehead M, Hazlett J, Murphy S (1991) Cerebrovascular changes in a rat model of moderate closed-head injury. J Neurotrauma 8(2):129–144.

Gosch HH, Gooding E, Schneider RC (1970) The lexan calvarium for the study of cerebral responses to acute trauma. J Trauma 10:370–376.

Govons SR, Govons RB, VanHuss WD, Heusner WW (1972) Brain concussion in the rat. Exp Neurol 34:121–128.

Graham DI, Adams JH, Doyle D (1978) Ischemic brain damage in fatal non-missile head injuries. J Neurol Sci 39:213–234.

Gurdjian ES and Lissner HR (1944) Mechanism of head injury as studied by the cathode ray oscilloscope preliminary report. J Neurosurgery 1:393–399.

Gurdjian ES, Webster JE, Lissner HR (1955) Observations of the mechanism of brain concussion, contusion, and laceration. Surg Gynecol Obstet 101:680–690.

Gurdjian ES, Lissner HR, Webster JE, Latimer FR and Haddad BF (1954) Studies on experimental concussion. Neurology 4:674–681.

Gurdjian ES, Roberts VL, Thomas LM (1966) Tolerance curves of acceleration and intracranial pressure and protective index in experimental head injury. J Trauma 6:600–604.

Hayes RL, Stalhammar D, Povlishock JT, et al (1987) A new model of concussive brain injury in the cat produced by extradural fluid volume loading: II. Physiological and neurophysiological observations. Brain Injury 1:93–112.

Hall E (1985) High-dose glucocorticoid treatment improves neurologic recovery in head-injured mice. J Neurosurg 62:882–887.

Hodgson VR, Thomas LM, Gurdjian ES, Fernando OU, Greenber SW, Chason JL (1969) Advances in understanding of experimental concussion mechanisms. 13th Stapp Car Crash Conf. Society of Automotive Engineers 13:18–37.

Holbourn AHS (1943) Mechanics of head injury. Lancet 2:438–441.

Human tolerance to impact conditions as related to motor vehicle design. Society of Automotive Engineers, Human Injury Criteria Task Force. SAE Handbook Supplement J885–84. Society of Automotive Engineers, Warrendale, PA, 1984.

Interagency Head Injury Task Force report. Department of Health and Human Services, National Institutes of Health, NINDS, pp 1–29, February 1989.

Jennett B (1976) Some medicolegal aspects of the management of acute head injury. British Medical Journal, 1:1383–1385.

Landesman S, Cooper PR (1982) Infectious complications of head injury. Head Injury, pp 343–362. Edited by PR Cooper. Williams and Wilkins, Baltimore/London.

Langfitt TW (1978) Measuring the outcome from head injuries. J Neurosurg 48:673–678.

Langfitt TW, Tannanbaum HM, Kassell NF (1966) The etiology of acute brain swelling following experimental head injury. J Neurosurg 24:47–56.

Lee MC, Melvin JW, Ueno K (1987) Finite element analysis of traumatic subdural hematoma. 31st Stapp Car Crash Conference. Society of Automotive Engineers 31:67–77.

Lee MC, Haut RC (1989) Insensitivity of tensile failure properties of human bridging veins to strain rate: implications in biomechanics of subdural hematoma. J Biomech 22:537–542.

Lewelt W, Jenkins LW, Miller JD (1980) Autoregulation of cerebral blood flow after experimental fluid percussion injury of the brain. J Neurosurg 53:500–511.

Lewis HP, McLaurin RL (1972) Cerebral blood flow and its responsiveness to arterial pCO_2: alterations before and after experimental head injury. Surg Forum 23:413–415.

Lighthall JW (1988) Controlled cortical impact: a new experimental brain injury model. J Neurotrauma 5(1):1–15.

Lighthall JW, Melvin JW, Ueno K (1989) Toward a biomechanical criterion for functional brain injury. Experimental Safety Vehicle Conference. Goteberg, Sweden Paper #89-4a-0-002, pp 2–10.

Lighthall JW, Dixon CE, Anderson TE (1989) Experimental models of brain injury. J Neurotrauma 6:83–99.

Lighthall JW, Goshgarian HG, Pinderski CR (1990) Characterization of axonal injury produced by controlled cortical impact. J Neurotrauma 7(2):65–76.

Lindgren S, Rinder L (1965) Experimental studies in head injury, I: Some factors influencing results of model experiments. Biophysik 3:320–329.

Lissner HR, Lebow M, Evans FG (1960) Experimental studies on the relation between acceleration and intracranial pressure changes in man. Surg Gynecol Obstet 111:329–338.

Lowenhielm P (1974) Dynamic properties of the parasagittal bridging vein. Zeitschrift fur Rechtsmedizin 74:55–62.

Margulies SS, Thibault LE, Gennarelli TA (1990) Physical model simulations of brain injury in the primate. J Biomech 23:823–836.

Martins AN, Doyle TF (1977) Blood flow and oxygen consumption of the focally traumatized monkey. J Neurosurg 47:346–351.

McIntosh TK, Noble L, Andrews B, Faden AI (1987) Traumatic brain injury in the rat: characterization of a midline fluid-percussion model. CNS Trauma 4(2):119–134.

McIntosh TK, Faden AI, Bendall MR, et al (1987) Traumatic brain injury in the rat: Alterations in brain lactate and pH as characterized by $_1$H and $_{31}$P nuclear magnetic resonance. J Neurochem 49:1530–1540.

McIntosh TK, Vink R, Noble L, et al (1989) Traumatic brain injury in the rat: characterization of a lateral fluid-percussion model. Neuroscience 28:233–244.

McCullough D, Nelson KM, Ommaya AK (1971) The acute effects of experimental head injury on the vertebrobasilar circulation: angiographic observations. J Trauma 11:422–428.

Melvin JW Evans FG (1972) A strain energy approach to the mechanics of skull fracture. 15th Stapp Car Crash Conf. Society of Automotive Engineers 15:666–685.

Meyer JS (1956) Studies of cerebral circulation in brain injury, III: Cerebral contusion, laceration and brain stem injury. Electroenceph Clin Neurophysiol 8:107–116.

Millen JE, Glauser FL, Zimmerman M (1980) Physiological effects of controlled concussive brain trauma. J Applied Physiol 49:856–861.

Nelson LR, Auen EL, Bourke RS, Barron KD (1979) A new head injury model for evaluation of treatment modalities, Neurosci Abstr 5:516.

Nelson LR, Auen EL, Bourke RS, et al (1982) A comparison of animal head injury models developed for treatment modality evaluation. In Grossman RG, Gildenber PL (eds) *Head injury: basic and clinical aspects.* Raven Press, New York, pp 117–128.

Nilsson B, Ponten U, Voigt G (1978) Experimental head injury in the rat. Part I: mechanics, pathophysiology, and morphology in an impact acceleration trauma. J Neurosurg 47:241–251.

Ommaya AK. Experimental head injury in the monkey. In Caveness WF, Walker AE (eds) *Head injury conference proceedings*. JB Lippincott, New York, pp 321–342.

Ommaya AK (1985) Biomechanics of head injury: experimental aspects. In Nahum AM, Melvin JW (eds) *The biomechanics of trauma*. Appleton-Century-Crofts, Norwalk, CT, pp 245–269.

Ommaya AK, Corrao P, Letcher FS (1973) Head injury in the chimpanzee. Part 1: biodynamics of traumatic unconsciousness. J Neurosurg 39:167–177.

Ommaya AK, Geller A, Parsons LC (1971) The effects of experimental head injury on one-trial learning in rats. Int J Neurosci 1:371–378.

Ommaya AK, Gennarelli TA (1974) Cerebral concussion and traumatic unconsciousness. Correlation of experimental and clinical observations on blunt head injuries. Brain 97:633–654.

Ommaya AK, Grubb RL, Naumann RA (1971) Coup and contre-coup injury: observations on the mechanics of visible brain injuries in the rhesus monkey. J Neurosurg 35:503–516.

Ommaya AK, Hirsch AE, Flamm ES, Mahone RH (1966) Cerebral concussion in the monkey: an experimental model. Science 153:211–212.

Ommaya AK, Hirsch AE, Martinez JL (1966) The role of whiplash in cerebral concussion. 10th Stapp Car Crash Conference, Society of Automotive Engineers 10:314–324.

Ommaya AK, Hirsch AE (1971) Tolerances for cerebral concussion from head impact and whiplash in primates. J Biomech 4:13–31.

Ono K, Kikuchi A, Nakamura M, Kobayaslli H, Nakamura N (1980) Human head tolerance to sagittal impact reliable estimation deduced from experimental head injury using subhuman primates and human cadaver skulls. 24th Stapp Car Crash Conference. Society of Automotive Engineers 24:101–160.

Parkinson D, West M, Pathiraja T (1978) Concussion: Comparison of humans and rats. Neurosurgery 3(2):176–180.

Penn RD, Clasen RA (1982) Traumatic brain swelling and edema. Head Injury, In PR Cooper (ed) *Head Injury*. Williams and Wilkins, Baltimore/London, pp 233–256.

Povlishock JT, Becker DP, Cheng CLY, et al (1983) Axonal change in minor head injury. J Neuropathol Exp Neurol 42:225–242.

Povlishock JT (1985) The morphopathologic responses to experimental head injuries of varying severity. In Becker DP, Povlishock JT (eds) *Central nervous system trauma status report*. Sponsored by NIH, NINCDS, pp 443–452.

Povlishock JT, Becker DP, Sullivan HG, Miller JD (1978) Vascular permeability alterations to horseradish peroxidase in experimental brain injury. Brain Res 153:223–239.

Pudenz RH, Sheldon CH (1946) The Lucite calvarium—A method for direct observation of the brain. II. Cranial trauma and brain movement. J Neurosurg 3:487–505.

Rapoport SI, Fredericks W, Ohno K, Pettigrew KD (1980) Quantitative aspects of reversible osmotic opening of the blood-brain barrier. Am J Physiol 238:R421–R431.

Rimel RW, Giordani B, Barth JT, et al (1982) Moderate head injury: Completing the clinical spectrum of brain trauma. Neurosurgery 11:344–351.

Rinder L (1969) Concussive response and intra-cranial pressure changes at sudden extradural fluid volume input in rabbits. Acta Physiol Scand 76:352–360.

Scott WW (1940) Physiology of concussion. Arch Neurolog Psychiat 43:270–283.

Scott WE (1981) Epidemiology of head and neck trauma in victims of motor vehicle accidents. *Head and Neck Criteria: A consensus Workshop*, Ommaya AK (ed) U.S. Department of Transportation, National Highway Traffic Safety Administration, Washington DC, pp 3–6.

Shatsky SA, Evans DE, Miller F, Martins AN (1974) High-speed angiography of experimental head injury. J Neurosurg 41:523–530.

Stalhammar D, Galinat BJ, Allen AM, et al (1987) A new model of concussive brain injury in the cat produced by extradural fluid volume loading: I. Biomechanical properties. Brain Injury 1:79–91.

Sullivan HG, Martinez J, Becker DP, Miller JD, Griffith R, Wist AO (1976) Fluid-percussion model of mechanical brain injury in the cat. J Neurosurg 45:520–534.

Tarriere C (1981) Investigation of brain injuries using the C.T. Scanner. In Ommaya AK (ed) *Head and neck injury criteria: a consensus workshop*. U.S. department of transportation, national highway traffic safety administration, Washington DC, pp 39–49.

Thibault LE, Galbraith HA, Thompson CJ, Gennarelli TA (1982) The effects of high strain rate uniaxial extension on the electrophysiology of isolated neural tissue. In Viano DC (ed) *Advances in bioengineering*. ASME, New York.

Tornheim PA, McLaurin RL, Thorpe JF (1976) The edema of cerebral contusion. Surg Neurol 5:171–175.

Tornheim PA, McLaurin RL (1981) Acute changes in regional brain water content following experimental closed head injury. J Neurosurg 55:407–513.

Tornheim PA, Linwicz BH, Hirsch CS, Brown DL, McLaurin RL (1983) Acute responses to blunt head trauma: experimental model and gross pathology. J Neurosurg 59:431–438.

Tornheim PA, McLaurin RL, Sawaya R (1979) Effect of furosemide on experimental traumatic cerebral edema. Neurosurg 4:48–52.

Ueno K, Melvin JW, Lundquist E, Lee MC (1989) Two-Dimensional finite element analysis of human brain impact responses: application of a scaling Law. *In Crashworthiness and Occupant Protection in Transportation Systems*. AMD-Vol 106. The American Society of Mechanical Engineers, New York, pp 123–124.

Unterharnscheidt FJ (1969) Pathomorphology of experimental head injury due to rotational acceleration. Acta Neuropath 12:200–204.

Walker AE, Kollros JJ, Case TJ (1944) The physiological basis of concussion. J Neurosurg 1:103–116.

Ward CC, Nahum A (1979) Correlation between brain injury and intracranial pressure in experimental head impacts. 4th IRCOBI Conference. Goteborg, Sweden, pp 67–74.

13
Biomechanics of Human Trauma: Head Protection

James A. Newman

Introduction

Protection from injury caused by a blow to the head has been of interest since the beginning of recorded time. Injuries to the brain and its container, the skull, and to the outer covering of the head, the scalp, can be inflicted through a variety of mechanisms. Injuries include lacerations, abrasions, fractures, and other forms of tissue disruption. These are nearly always caused by excessive movement[1] of one part of the head relative to another. A scalp laceration is the result of a mechanical action (cutting or tearing) that separates formerly contiguous pieces of scalp. A skull fracture will occur when the skull bone bends more than it is capable of doing without breaking. A brain contusion, for example, is a collection of blood caused by the rupture of blood vessels that have been stretched too much. Separating, bending, and stretching are merely descriptors of somewhat different kinds of movement. To protect against all these kinds of injuries may require a variety of approaches. Basically, however, it comes down to padding and load distribution.

In order to appreciate the influence of the relevant variables, a basic understanding of head injury mechanisms is helpful. In this regard, the reader is referred to the previous chapter. The head injury of most interest is, of course, that to the brain. Brain injury can occur if any part of it is distorted, stretched, or compressed, or if it is torn away from the interior of the skull. An impact to the head can cause the skull to deform and, even if it does not fracture, the underlying brain tissue can be injured as it distorts under the influence of the deforming skull. Even if the skull does not bend, if it is caused to move violently, distortion within the brain will occur. It is the minimization of brain tissue distortion that is the object of head protection.

This chapter examines the basic physics and design considerations related to head protection devices. The principles reviewed apply to padded surfaces as well as to helmets. Protective headgear systems encompass a large number of user and functional variables. These could include penetration resistance, retention, stability, ventilation, aesthetics, etc. Most of these will not be addressed here. The primary emphasis here will be upon impact energy attenuation and the means by which this can be optimized.

The helmet, of course is the most common form of head protection. Worn on the head, its purpose is to reduce the severity or probability of injury, to which the head would otherwise be subjected, caused by an inadvertent[2] impact

---

[1] The deformation of certain parts of the head also constitutes relative movement. "Excessive" movement is meant to imply that there is some limited amount of relative motion below which injury would not occur.

[2] It may be argued that military and some forms of athletic head impacts are purposeful rather than inadvertent. It depends, one would suppose, if one is the giver or receiver of such blows.

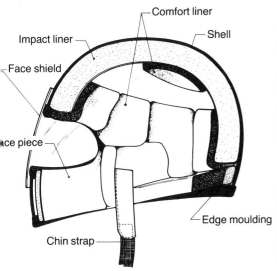

Comfort liner

Impact liner

Face shield

Shell

ce piece

Edge moulding

Chin strap

FIGURE 13.1. Cross section of a typical motorcycle helmet.

o the head. A cross-sectional view of a typical motorcycle helmet is shown in Fig. 13.1. The basic features of all head protection are embodied in the concepts illustrated there.

A helmet, like other forms of head protection, accomplishes its protective function by "cushioning" the blow to the head. As shown in Fig. 13.1, it does this by encasing the head of the wearer in a specialized type of padding. To understand this cushioning process, which has to do with reducing the forces that produce the kinds of movement referred to above, some elementary physics are in order.

Physics of Motion

It is common in discussing head injury mechanisms and the performance of protective devices, to refer to the acceleration of the head. Usually, this is in terms of g's, or gravity units. It is important to recognize that acceleration (expressed in g's or any appropriate unit) is merely a measure of movement. By itself, it tells us nothing about forces, stresses, energy, or any other physical quantity. Only in its relation to other variables does its meaning becomes clear.

There are two basic kinds of motion, both of which can play a role in the head injury process. They are translational and rotational. There is considerable discussion about the relative importance of each kind of motion in head protection. The following review endeavors to clarify the similarities and differences between the two types. The theoretical study of motion, kinematics, applies to any real object, including the human head.

"Translation" means, quite simply, that the object does not rotate. The movement is often simply called linear. The motion may be rectilinear or curvilinear. "Rectilinear" means the body moves in a straight line. The velocity may, however, change as the body moves. "Curvilinear motion" means the body moves on a curved path. In the latter case the body does not rotate but the velocity of the body does change direction.[3] In both cases, the velocity of every point within the body will always be the same. If this were not true, the body would be either deforming or rotating. Figure 13.2 illustrates the two kinds of linear motion.

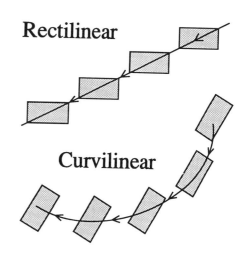

FIGURE 13.2. Rectilinear and curvilinear motion.

[3] A body tends to move in a straight line unless a force acts upon it to cause it to deviate. Hence, curvilinear motion can only occur if forced to occur. In fact, a body moving at constant velocity along a curved path is accelerating (i.e., centripetal or centrifugal acceleration).

"Rotation" means the angular orientation of the body changes. If the rotation is about some fixed point, like the axle of a wheel, the motion is referred to as plane circular motion. In general, the point about which the body will rotate is not fixed to the body and its location may change with time. A body that is rotating is one for which the translational movement of every point within the body, though related, is different. If the body can be considered to be rigid, certain simple, fundamental relations between the linear and angular kinematics exist.

In the case of pure translation, the movement of the whole body can be characterized completely in terms of linear kinematics of *any* point on the body. These kinematic parameters include the familiar displacement x, the velocity v, and linear (or translational) acceleration a. The displacement, velocity, and acceleration vary in time during an impact and there are fundamental relations between each of them. The general relations are of the form:

$$v(t) = \frac{dx(t)}{dt}$$
$$a(t) = \frac{dv(t)}{dt} \qquad (13.1)$$

That is, velocity is numerically equal (exactly) to the instantaneous rate of change of displacement. Similarly, acceleration is the rate of change of velocity. Given the displacement time-history of a point on the body $x(t)$, it is thus possible to determine the changes in velocity and acceleration of that point on the body. Likewise, knowing $a(t)$ is sufficient to completely characterize the velocity and displacement (i.e., the relative movement) of that point. For a body that is deformable, and we can assume that the head is (i.e., some parts can move relative to some other parts), the motion $x(t)$ of different points on the body can be different. In fact they can be different even if the body is considered nondeformable (i.e., rigid). In this case, however, the body must be rotating.

In the case of rotation, the movement of the body can be characterized in terms of the rotational kinematic terms; θ, the angular dis-placement; ω, the angular velocity; and α, the angular acceleration. The relationships between these terms is analogous to the linear equations:

$$\alpha = \frac{d\omega}{dt}$$
$$\omega = \frac{d\theta}{dt} \qquad (13.2)$$

Unlike the case of linear motion, rotational motion is not with respect to a point but rather is a description of the motion of a body. A wheel rotates about its axle. A boxer's head following an uppercut rotates about some undetermined, and moving, center of rotation. In fact, the rotation of a rigid *body* can be fully characterized by the linear motion of *points* within the body without reference to a center of rotation per se. Consider the movement of points A and B on the body shown in Fig. 13.3.

If the body is rigid, the distance between the two points, r, cannot change. That is, the velocity of point B toward A is always zero.[4] If point B moves relative to A at all, it can only move at right angles. If it does, the body is considered to be rotating. The angular velocity is, by definition:

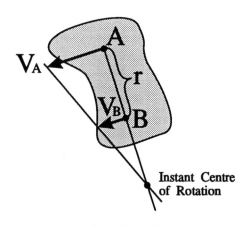

FIGURE 13.3. Free body in motion.

_____

[4] Said differently, point A moves away from point B as fast as point B moves toward it.

$$\omega = \frac{(V_A - V_B)}{r} \qquad (13.3)$$

At any time when the linear velocity difference is not equal to zero, there is a point somewhere in space where the velocity is zero. This point can be located by extrapolation as shown in Fig. 13.3. This point, by definition, is the instant center of rotation. It may be fixed in space (on or off the body itself), as in the case of a wheel on an axle, or it may move if $(V_A - V_B)$ changes.[5]

If $(V_A - V_B)$ is *changing in time*, the body is undergoing angular acceleration. The relationship between these linear velocity changes and the angular acceleration is:

$$\frac{\frac{d}{dt}(V_A - V_B)}{r} = \alpha \qquad (13.4)$$

As stated earlier, head injury comes about principally by the movement of some part of the head relative to another. That is, the head is deformable. Thus, the application of the above rules for rigid body motion must be treated with some caution when applying them to head injury mechanisms. This is important because, as stated earlier, the effectiveness of various forms of head protection will often be described in terms of the acceleration of the head. In order to discuss that, it is appropriate to review some additional physics that have a bearing on these matters.

Dynamics of Impact

A body will accelerate (linearly) when a force F is applied to it. During an impact, acceleration[6] occurs because of the forces generated by the collision of the body with something else. If the body does not deform, the relation between force and acceleration is the well-known expression:

$$F = ma \qquad (13.5)$$

where m is the mass of the body in question.

A rigid body will undergo *angular* acceleration when a torque T is applied to it. During an impact, angular acceleration occurs because a torque is generated. This is usually associated with impacts that have a component that tries to induce rotational motion. The equivalent expression for rotational motion is:

$$T = I\alpha \qquad (13.6)$$

where T is the applied (generated) torque, I the moment of inertia, and α the angular acceleration.

Since torque is a force acting about a lever arm, it is important to note that efforts to reduce force will typically reduce torque. Thus reductions in a will be accompanied by reductions in α.

A head, or any other body of mass m moving at a velocity V, possesses translational kinetic energy defined as follows:

$$KE = \tfrac{1}{2}mV^2 \qquad (13.7)$$

A body in rotation, will possess a rotational kinetic energy defined as follows:

$$RKE = \tfrac{1}{2}I\omega^2 \qquad (13.8)$$

If the head is caused to accelerate (or decelerate) its velocity will change according to the principles of equations 13.1 and 13.2. That is, it will be caused to possess more (or less) energy. This process will be associated with the application (or creation) of a force F in accordance with equations 13.5 and 13.6. The relationships between these variables is not important for the moment. What is important is:

1. The process of energy transfer takes time; and
2. The head is not rigid.

The head can, during the energy transfer process, deform under the influence of the force. It can thus be injured.

It is a fundamental tenet of physics that energy cannot be created or destroyed. When

---

[5] Note that if V_A equals V_B, ω equals zero. That is, translation is rotation about a point infinitely far away.

[6] The term "acceleration" will be used interchangeably with deceleration. In general, acceleration means increasing velocity; deceleration, decreasing.

the kinetic energy of a body changes, that energy is either transferred elsewhere (by changing the velocity of the colliding objects) or is used to do work (i.e., it is used to deform something[7]). The energy of deformation is often considered to be "absorbed." The basic principle of head protection is to reduce the forces that could injure the head by absorbing some of the kinetic energy through the deformation or destruction of something else (i.e., padding, helmet).[8]

If the moving head strikes some object, and that object absorbs some of the kinetic energy of the head, the forces generated in the impact will be less. The extent of this reduction is a function of how much deformation is achieved and the force required to deform the object. The simplest relationship between the forces produced and the space required to absorb the energy is:

$$Fd = \tfrac{1}{2}mV^2 = KE \qquad (13.9)$$

where d is the stopping distance, F is the average force during the impact, and V the change of velocity. Clearly, for a given kinetic energy of the head, the larger the d, the lower the force F.[9] The actual force that will be developed will be a function of the strength, the amount, and the shape of the padding material on the impacted object or in the helmet itself and, of course, the mass, shape, and stiffness of the head.

The simplest type of relationship between crushing force and stopping distance is that of a simple spring:

$$F = kx \qquad (13.10)$$

where k, the proportionality constant, is the stiffness of the spring.[10] Many materials are springlike, though most do not follow the above simple linear relationship (i.e., k is not a constant). Nevertheless, the force generally increases with increasing deformation. Since x changes with time, i.e., $x(t)$, the force also changes with time. Given that force is proportional to acceleration, then acceleration changes with time. The relation between $x(t)$ and $a(t)$ will always be governed by equation 13.1.

Material Considerations

Materials can be classified in two broad categories: plastic and elastic. If the material is plastic, it will not recover from any deformation that occurs during loading. When fully compressed, the velocity of deformation is zero. That is, all of the kinetic energy has been dissipated (absorbed). If the padding material is elastic, it will recover its original shape. As it does so, the force will follow a similar relationship but will decrease as the recovery takes place. In this situation, there is no net energy absorbed and the object will resume its initial velocity (but in the opposite direction). The maximum force developed will not be affected but the time during which the head is loaded will be doubled.

Most real materials are neither perfectly elastic nor perfectly plastic but fall somewhere between. If the duration of loading is a significant concern, materials that are essentially plastic should be used. If the particular application is one where the helmet is to function more than just once (for example as in football), materials that recover their shape and their material properties are to be preferred. The best of all possible material options would be one that deforms plastically, then slowly recovers its shape and its strength, and is able thereby to deal with subsequent impacts.

---

[7] When a car crashes into a rigid barrier for example, the forces generated are used to destroy the front end of the car. The kinetic energy that the car possessed before striking the barrier is numerically equal to the work done on the car.

[8] It may also be appropriate to reduce the *duration* of the force to the extent possible, as injurious effects may be exacerbated if the loading persists for too long. The extent to which this is a significant consideration will be discussed later.

[9] The force generated by impact can never be reduced to zero unless there is an infinite amount of space in which to do it.

---

[10] The torsional analogy is that of an old-fashioned alarm clock spring. The torque required to wind the spring is proportional to the angle through which it is twisted.

The actual force that is produced when a material is crushed depends not only on the extent of crush x, but also on the inherent strength of the material and the size of the area loaded.[11]

The force developed when a helmeted head strikes something, or as the head strikes a padded surface, depends on the crushing characteristics of the material impacted and the amount of it used.[12] These characteristics are defined in terms of material stress–strain relationships.

"Stress" is defined as force per unit area, whereas "strain" is deformation divided by the initial undeformed thickness. The effect of area is quite simple. To compress 1 square inch of material to a certain strain requires the application of a specific force F. To crush twice the area requires twice the force. Hence, the greater the area of padding crushed, the higher is the force developed. Conversely, increasing the initial undeformed thickness of the padding reduces the strain for the same deformation, thereby maintaining a lower force.[13]

Curiously, perhaps at first glance, one of the primary objectives of good helmet design is to maximize the area of padding that can interact with the head during impact. Since higher forces induce higher acceleration and are associated with higher deformations (which in turn are related to higher injury severity), this seems to be something of a contradiction. It is not, for the following reason:

Maximizing the amount of material used in the collision maximizes the kinetic energy absorption, thereby minimizing the transfer of energy to the head. If the "high" force that is developed in this process is less than that necessary to produce injury, then this constitutes effective design. Doing that in practice, however, is another matter. In an accident situation, one cannot always know how much energy is to be dealt with, what the relative velocities are going to be, what are the shapes and stiffness of the things that the head might strike, and so on. Obviously, no known form of head protection can completely protect the wearer against all foreseeable head impacts. To consider these limitations, let's get back to a few basics.

Figure 13.4 illustrates a number of different stress–strain profiles, during the loading phase, for a number of hypothetical materials. Curve A corresponds to the linear spring, curve B to a stress behavior that is unchanging with strain, and curve C to a more realistic stress–strain curve of typical padding material.

For a given area loaded, and a known thickness of padding material, the curves translate directly to force-deformation curves. The area bounded by the curve and the deformation axis is numerically equal to the energy absorbed. It has been suggested that curve B in Fig. 13.4 is the optimum type of material to use for padding. To confirm this, consider the following:

---

[11] It may also depend on the velocity of deformation, being higher when compressed faster. Such materials are called rate sensitive and are often viscoelastic. Most padding materials are not particularly rate sensitive.

[12] It also depends on the stiffness of the head, which, as discussed, is not infinitely high, i.e., rigid. However, for the time being it can be assumed that the stiffness of the skull is so much greater than the padding material that the rigid head assumption is not an unreasonable one. Notwithstanding, it is indeed the deformation of the head that corresponds to injury.

[13] These generalizations are for an essentially flat piece of material being compressed across its thickness over a constant area. When the surface being compressed, or when the impacting object, is not flat, these simple relations will not hold exactly, as, for example, for a helmet or for a head impacting a flat, padded surface.

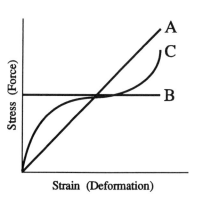

FIGURE 13.4. Hypothetical stress-strain curves.

As a constant area impact is delivered to each of the materials depicted above, the material will begin to deform. Each will continue to deform until all the kinetic energy of the colliding object has been used up. At this point, the deformation will have reached its maximum value. The area under the force-deformation curve will be numerically equal to this energy. As the energy being absorbed increases, the force generated will be governed by the stress–strain (force-deformation) characteristics of the padding material. For material A, the force increases continually as the energy is absorbed. For material B, the force remains constant throughout the deformation process. Initially, material A produces a lower force than does B. If the energy of impact is low, material A will actually generate a lower force than B. As the energy increases, there comes a point at which the forces generated are the same. If even more energy is to be absorbed, the force produced by material A continues to increase, whereas that of B remains low. Hence material B is capable of absorbing more energy, at lower force than material A. If the force, as limited by B, is lower than that which would produce an injury, then it clearly is a better choice than A. Even though at low energy A seems better, when it counts, i.e., when the energy is high, B is better.

Most real materials do not behave like A or B. However, materials whose stress-strain behavior approaches B are better. Though curve C in Fig. 13.4 is typical of a good hypothetical padding material, it will be recalled that most materials recover somewhat following impact. Figure 13.5 illustrates the stress-strain characteristics of several real padding materials during impact. The net energy absorbed is that absorbed during the loading phase *minus* that given back during the recovery phase. One important feature to observe for all these materials is that there is a definite limit to their energy-absorbing capability. They cannot crush more than their original thickness. When a real material is nearly fully crushed, it will become very stiff and the forces then developed become very high. When the material is no longer capable

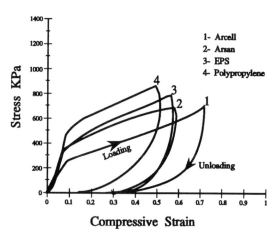

FIGURE 13.5. Stress-strain of padding.

of absorbing additional impact energy, the unabsorbed energy is transferred to the head by accelerating it or deforming it and, potentially, injuring it. Thus, the head can be protected if the following two general conditions are met:

1. The reduction in the kinetic energy of the head during impact (i.e., that absorbed by the padding) is less than that which would completely crush the padding material.
2. Both the area and the depth of the padding crushed are small enough that, for its particular crushing characteristics, the force developed is less than that necessary to produce sufficient relative movement within the head to constitute an injury.

The probability of meeting these criteria increases with:

Increased padding thickness
Increased padding area
Decreased crushing strength of the padding
Uniform crushing strength.

The first two maximize the energy absorbed; the second two minimize the force developed. Given that there is some limit beyond which increasing the padding thickness is impractical, the potential conflict presented by these criteria should be readily apparent.

Helmet Design

Notwithstanding the generality of the above concepts, helmet design is further complicated by the following additional facts:

- A helmet is more or less spherical in shape, not flat.
- The amount of energy that will be delivered in any accident situation can never be forecast with great accuracy.
- The shape, mass, area, and stiffness of the striking object cannot be always anticipated.
- The user of the helmet will have specific needs that will limit the choices of design options.[14]

The object of good helmet design is to insure that, regardless of the characteristics of the striking object, the loading area is sufficiently high that x does not exceed some critical value x_c. Furthermore, the force that is developed must be less than some critical value F_c if injury is to be avoided. The dilemma facing the helmet designer is illustrated in Fig. 13.6. If the helmet is too strong (high stiffness, high crushing strength, high area), the force developed, for a given amount of energy to be

absorbed, can exceed F_c. Conversely, if the helmet is too weak, the deformation will become excessive and, as the helmet deformation approaches its limit, again F will exceed F_c.[15] These two extremes are illustrated in Fig. 13.6. Also illustrated is the force deformation response of a more suitable padding system.

A helmet usually consists of two primary elements. They are the outer shell and an energy absorbing liner.[16]

From a functional point of view, the object of the shell is to provide a hard, strong, outer surface that serves to distribute the impact load over a large area. It also provides a penetration shield against high-speed objects and, in addition, serves to protect both the wearer and the underlying liner of the helmet from abrasion with the impacting surface. In engineering terms, this means that the shell must be:

- rigid, i.e., high stiffness
- tough, i.e., high bulk strength
- hard, i.e., high surface strength.

In addition, it should have a high strength-to-weight ratio and, usually, a smooth[17] exterior finish.

Interior to the shell is the liner of the helmet. It is this element that, through its partial destruction, is largely responsible for absorbing the energy of impact. In order to perform its function effectively, it must deform at force levels below that which would cause head injury.[18] Its strength should be largely insensitive to impact velocity and, to maximize net energy absorption, it should have slow

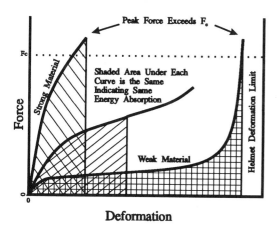

FIGURE 13.6. Effect of padding strength when the same energy is absorbed.

---

[14] Helmets for different applications, e.g., football, hockey, motorcycling, etc., not only look different from each other, but are different for these reasons.

[15] This behavior of the material is frequently referred to as "bottoming out."

[16] Though usually true, some contemporary bicycling helmets have virtually no shell and others, principally military and industrial headgear, have a webbing suspension to manage impact energy rather than padding.

[17] Smoothness is desirable as it will limit the generation of tangential forces. It is these forces that can generate a torque that in turn may produce angular acceleration. Thus smoothness reduces the probability of brain injury that might be associated with angular acceleration of the head.

[18] Or, if at a magnitude for which some minor injury might be expected, for as brief a time as possible.

recovery (rebound) characteristics. These requirements dictate that the liner should:

- have a well-defined, relatively constant low crushing strength
- be relatively strain-rate insensitive
- be essentially plastic in its crushing behavior.

These elements must be fitted together in such a fashion that the entire assembly satisfies the primary functional criteria. The choice of particular materials that meet the above requirements is but one aspect of the decision-making process. In principle, a great number of materials, if properly used, can be made to exhibit the desired properties. Within the constraints imposed by the intended application, however, the choice is somewhat limited.

Material Options

Shell

Common alternatives for this purpose are fiber-reinforced plastics (FRP) (e.g., fiberglass/resin composites) and thermoplastics (the most popular being polycarbonate). There are, however, others whose attractiveness depends on the particular application (e.g., racing, police, military). These include ABS, high-density polyethylene, ABS/polycarbonate alloys, and even metal. Recently, polyaramide fabrics have been found suitable.

The FRP materials can be compression molded, or a hand lay-up process can be used. The former, in conjunction with so-called chopped-strand techniques, produces a relatively homogeneous structure of broken fibers embedded in a plastic matrix. The latter produces a laminated structure that, properly made, is inherently stronger per unit weight in the normal direction for the fabric layers.

The thermoplastic shells are, for large-scale production, cheaper to produce as they can be readily injection-molded. For the same volume of material, they are also lighter than the FRP materials. However, they also tend to be less rigid unless molded with a very high wall-thickness. Furthermore, they are susceptible to stress concentrations set up, for example,

around rivet holes, and in these areas they can be inherently weak.

One final factor is that, relative to FRPs, the thermoplastics can be brittle. This particular behavior may be amplified under certain environmental conditions (e.g., extreme cold). FRPs, on the other hand, tend to crush or delaminate rather than fracture on impact and are far less sensitive to environmental conditions.

Liner

The most widespread materials used for energy-absorbing liners are either semirigid polyurethane foams or expanded polystyrene bead (EPB) foams.

The former is produced by introducing, into a closed mold, two liquid constituents. The resulting exothermic process produces a foaming reaction that, given sufficient time, cures to produce a pliable helmet liner. The resultant properties of the foamed liner are highly dependent on such factors as initial mixture ratio, mold temperature, and curing time, and great care must be exercised to insure consistent physical properties.

The EPB liners are produced by introducing a known amount of pre-expanded polystyrene bead into a closed mold and injecting steam. This causes the individual beads to expand and to adhere to each other. The resulting liner is a relatively stiff homogeneous structure possessing desirable stress-strain properties. The one governing factor that determines the crushing properties of the material is its bulk density and this can be controlled quite accurately.

Both of the above materials are generally considered suitable. Both are relatively inexpensive.

Other materials that have either been used or have been considered include cross-linked polyethylene foams and synthetic rubber-based foams. Even honeycomb structures and inflatable bladders (filled with liquid) have been found to be effective for some situations.

The above-discussed alternatives provide some insight into the considerations regarding material selection and production methods.

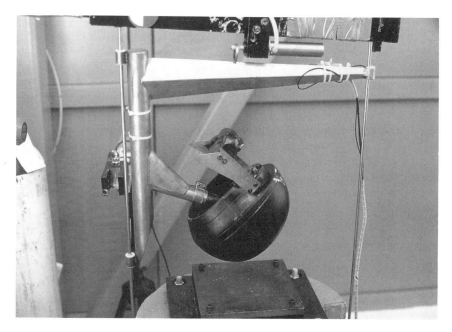

FIGURE 13.7. Typical helmet-impact vertical-drop test setup.

This clearly is only part of the design process as the geometric design itself leaves many areas in which decisions must be made.

In order to insure that reasonable levels of impact protection are maintained regardless of the specific design requirements, performance standards have been developed for different helmet applications.

Helmet Impact Performance Standards

All helmet standards for impact performance are essentially the same in their overall approach. They each entail the following:

- The helmet is placed on an artificial head form in the way it would be worn by a real person. Different standards use different head forms, though all try to model the important features of the human head.
- The helmeted head form is subjected to an impact. The impact typifies the type of blow that could be encountered in the specific application. Energy level, environmental

factors, and impact surface characteristics are considered.[19]
- The linear acceleration $a(t)$ of the head form is monitored throughout the duration of the impact.[20]

A typical helmet impact vertical drop test setup is shown in Fig. 13.7.

In these kinds of tests, the helmeted head form is raised to some predetermined height and released. At the moment of impact, the assembly will have acquired a kinetic energy, proportional to the drop height and its weight.

---

[19] For example: Football helmets will be struck by surfaces that represent the playing surface and other players. Hockey helmets are expected to perform when striking a hard flat surface when cold. Military helmets are to protect against high-speed low-mass fragments. Equestrian helmets are impacted by an object intended to represent a horse's hoof.

[20] Helmet performance standards do not monitor for a helmet's ability to moderate angular acceleration of the test head form. The reason for this is that the helmeted head form is constrained to move in an essentially linear fashion during impact. This feature of the test protocol is usually related to matters of test repeatability and impact site location.

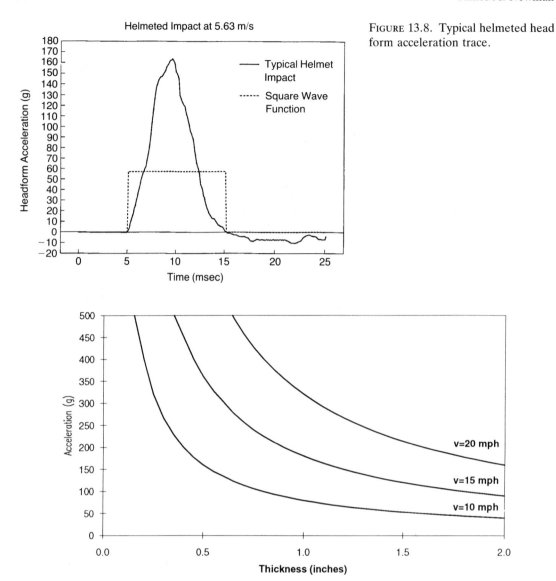

Helmeted Impact at 5.63 m/s

FIGURE 13.8. Typical helmeted head form acceleration trace.

FIGURE 13.9. Minimum acceleration achievable.

This energy will be dissipated during collision with the impact anvil. The downward motion of the head form is arrested by the force that is developed on it during this process. It is this force, changing in time, that causes the head form's velocity to change from its preimpact speed to zero. A typical helmeted head form acceleration trace is shown in Fig. 13.8. Regardless of the particular standard, in order to be considered acceptable the response of the head form must fall within prescribed acceleration limits. Some examples of these

limits and their corresponding impact parameters are given in Table 13.1.

The Future of Head Protection

Improvements in head protection are always going to be limited by the laws of physics. In terms of acceleration, the minimum values achievable for various velocities and padding-liner thickness, are shown in Fig. 13.9. These levels cannot be achieved in practice as they represent theoretical limits. For a given

TABLE 13.1. Descriptions of impact energy attenuation test methods and requirements of selected helmet standards.

Helmet type	Test method	Head form material	Drop assembly weight (lbs)	Impact surface	Impact energy (ft-lbs)	Impact sites	Rejection criteria
Industrial	ANSI Z89.1	Wood or metal	Missile 7.8–8.0	Steel hemisphere	40	Top	F > 1,000 lbs; F_{ave} > 850 lbs
Industrial	ISO 3873	Hardwood or metal	Striker 11–11.2	Hemisphere	37	Top	F > 1,124 lbs; a > 100 g
Industrial	CSA Z94.1–M1977	Not specified	Ball 7.8	Steel ball	40	Top	F > 989 lbs; F_{ave} > 854 lbs
Firefighter's	NFPA	Metal	Head form 11–11.8	Steel flat	69	Front, sides, back	a > 400 g; a > 200 g, t > 3 ms; a > 150 g, t > 5 ms
			Impactor 7.8–8.0		40	Top; Top	a > 150 g; F > 1,000 lbs; F_{ave} > 850 lbs
Police riot	NILECJ 0.0104	Metal	Head form 11–13.2	Steel hemisphere	80	Front, sides, back, top	a > 400 g; a > 200 g, t > 3 ms; a > 150 g, t > 5 ms
Police riot	CAN/CSA Z611–M86	CSA D230 Standard head form sizes E, J, M	Head form	Cylindrical anvil	103; 52	All points above test line	a > 300 g, for 103 ft-lb; a > 200 g, for 52 ft-lb
Hockey	CAN3–Z262.1–M83	Polyurethane head form 4 sizes 6.3, 6.9, 7.4, 7.8	Striker 10	Flat rectangular birch block	20 (3×)	Top, 45° front, side, rear 90° side, rear	F > 1,850 lbs; F_{ave} > 1,500 lbs; T < 45 sec; T > 60 sec
Football	ASTM F717–81 F429–79	Metal	Head form 11	MEP	56 (3×)	Front, side, rear front boss, crown lower rear boss	a > 275 g (1st 3×); a > 300 g (2nd 3×)
Football	NOCSAE	Humanoid	Head form 3 sizes 8.3, 9.8, 11.7	38 shore A durometer rubber	25–35; 33–47; 42–59	Front, side front boss, top rear boss, rear	SI > 1,500
Crash helmets	NILECJ 105	Metal	Head form 11–13.2	Steel flat	80 (1st); 70 (2nd)	front, sides, back, top	a > 400 g; a > 200 g, t > 3 ms; a > 150 g, t > 5 ms
Ballistic helmets	NILECJ 106	Metal	9.9–12.1	Bullets		Front, sides, back	a > 400 g
Motorcycle, auto racing	Snell	Metal	Head form 14.3	Steel flat hemicylinder	103 (1st); 81 (2nd); 103 (3×)	4 sites above test line separated by > 1/6 max circumference	a > 300 g
Motorcycle	ANSI Z90.1	Metal	Head form 11–11.2	Steel flat hemicylinder	88 (1st); 66 (2nd)	4 sites above test line separated by >1/6 max circum	a > 300 g

TABLE 13.1. *Continued*

Helmet type	Test method	Head form material	Drop assembly weight (lbs)	Impact surface	Impact energy (ft-lbs)	Impact sites	Rejection criteria
Motorcycle	DOT 218	Metal	Head form 11–11.2	Steel flat hemicylinder	88 (1st) 66 (2nd)	4 sites above test line separated by >1/6 max circum	a > 400 g a > 200 g, t > 2 ms a > 150 g, t > 4 ms
Motorcycle	CAN3–D230–M85	ISO head form sizes, A, E, J, M	Head form 11–11.3	Steel flat Steel hemicylinder	52 103 37 74	All points above test line	a > 300 g at high energy level a > 200 g at low energy level
Bicycle	ANSI Z90.4	Metal	Head form 10.9–11.1	Steel flat hemicylinder	38.6 38.6	4 sites above test line separated by >1/5 max circum	a > 300 g
Bicycle	Snell	Metal	14.3	Steel flat hemicylinder	100 65	4 sites above test line	a > 300 g
Bicycle	CSA D113.2	ISO head form sizes A, E, J, M		Steel flat, cylinder	80 55	6 sites above test line	a > 200 g a > 250 g a > 250 g
Equestrian	ASTM F1163	ISO head form sizes A, E, J, M	Head form 10.9–11.1	Steel flat, V-anvil	66 46	4 sites above t, line separated by >1/6 max circum	a > 300 g
Equestrian	U.S. Polo Assoc., proposed	Humanoid	Head form 3 sizes 8.3, 9.8, 11.7	Steel hemicylinder 38 Shore A Flat	42–59 42–59 58–70	Front, side, rear top, random	SI > 1,500
Equestrian	Snell	Metal	Head form 14.3	Steel flat hemicylinder	66	4 sides above t, line separated by >1/6 max circum	a > 300 g

Based on McElhaney, J., COPE 1988, October 31–November 2, 1988, Toronto, Canada.

velocity change and liner thickness, the optimum helmet minimizes the acceleration by maximizing the time duration of the impact event. To approach the theoretical limits, some refinements to current design and material technology are possible if not immediately feasible.

The curve in Fig. 13.8 shows a typical acceleration response for a "good" contemporary motorcycle helmet when impacted against a flat, hard surface at a velocity of 5.63 m/sec. This helmet has a liner thickness of approximately 35 mm. The actual velocity change that occurs is the area under the acceleration–time curve. In this case, the velocity change is 7.7 m/sec, i.e., the helmet rebounds at a speed of 2.1 m/sec. Based on the acceleration response, it can be determined that the maximum liner compression was only 21 mm. That is, only 60% of the thickness available was used. Figure 13.8 also shows a hypothetical trace that, for the same impact velocity and using 80% of the available liner thickness, produces the lowest possible acceleration. The challenge for the helmet designer is to change the behavior of the headgear from that shown to, as close as possible, that theoretical limit.[21] To do this requires the following:

Compress all the available padding/liner material to the fullest extent possible (80% compression is a practical upper limit before bottoming).

Minimize the velocity change, i.e., eliminate rebound.

Maximize the onset rate.

Maintain constant acceleration throughout the impact.

Maximize the finishing rate.

Let us consider each of these separately.

A helmet is essentially spherical in shape. An idealized sectional view of a head within a helmet having an infinitely rigid shell and within a helmet having no shell, or a zero stiffness shell, each with a liner of constant

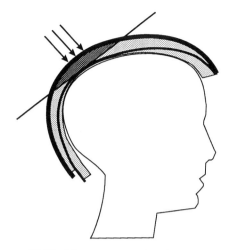

FIGURE 13.10. Liner compression shapes.

thickness, is shown in Fig. 13.10. Also shown is the maximum compression of the liner thickness that could be achieved subject to these geometrical constraints. Notice how much of the liner is not fully used! The liner is compressed to its maximum only at the central region of the deformation. It is apparent that the rigid shell causes more liner to participate in the impact than does the no-shell helmet. This is the basis for the rigid shell concept from the beginning. In terms of maximizing the amount of liner that participates in the impact, however, even the theoretical, infinitely rigid shell seems far from optimal. Two possibilities exist to improve this situation: One is to completely fill the space between the head and the interior of the shell. The other is to cause the shell to somehow conform more closely to the shape of the head as it moves in toward the head. This, as illustrated in the shell-less helmet case, is opposite to the way the shell would want to deform.

Achieving the former might be feasible by custom fitting each helmet to each wearer. Indeed, such has been the practice with certain aircrew helmets. Of course, such a procedure can be expensive and may not be practical for widespread use. How the latter suggestion might be achieved remains something for future consideration.

The next consideration in creating the optimum helmet is to reduce the rebound

---

[21] In undertaking this exercise, it will be recognized that one can never anticipate exactly where on the helmet an impact will occur and of what violence it will be. A helmet must be designed to accommodate a range of possibilities.

velocity to zero. Most usual liner materials are permanently deformed when impacted and recover quite slowly if at all. Hence they produce little rebound velocity. Helmet shells, on the other hand, because they are usually required to be rigid and strong, tend to be fairly elastic (until the loading causes a structural failure of the shell). Thus, after they deform, they bounce back. In doing so, some energy may be transferred back to the head. To minimize this, it is required, then, that the maximum deformation of the helmet assembly during impact also be the final shape at the end of the pulse. How zero rebound could be accomplished with contemporary helmet materials is also a subject for future consideration.

The third desirable feature to minimize head acceleration is to maximize the onset rate. That is, get the force generated by the crushing of the helmet up to the highest acceptable level as fast as possible. As seen in Fig. 13.5, the initial stiffness of a flat, uniform piece of typical padding/liner material, is not very high. If it could be made stiffer, without changing the crushing strength, such a material used in a helmet would produce a higher acceleration onset rate. Similarly, a high stiffness during the recovery phase, would maximize the finishing rate of acceleration.

Maintaining a uniform crushing strength for the padding/liner material has been a challenge for material technology for some time. One of the best examples of this kind of material is metal honeycomb. Unfortunately, it works best when flat and its properties are very unidirectional. Another interesting material is metal foam. Quite stiff up to a point, it then crushes very uniformly. Once crushed it stays that way. Being a foam, its properties are preserved in all three directions. It is, as might be expected, rather heavy and expensive. Another potential candidate material consists of very small hollow glass beads embedded in a resin matrix. Lighter than metal foams it has certain potential that has not yet been fully explored.

In the absence of full contact between the head and the liner material, as in contemporary helmet design, or in the case of the unhelmeted head striking, for example, the interior padded surface of a car, the stiffness of the material should actually decrease with increasing deformation if a constant force/acceleration is to be maintained. This is because the area of padding being deformed increases as the nonflat head penetrates into the essentially flat padded surface. A material with such a reversed stiffness has yet to be invented. Possibly, in the not-too-distant future, some clever combinations of existing materials will be shown to possess such a characteristic.

Discussion

Helmets work. They do so by reducing the force that would be generated when an object strikes the head, or when the head strikes something. This force reduction is accomplished by the conversion of kinetic energy to work of deformation of something other than the head (i.e., the padding). Reducing the force on the head reduces its acceleration and, if well distributed, reduces the likelihood of skull bending. Both mechanisms reduce the likelihood of brain tissue distortion.

Thus, a helmet:

1. Cushions the blow to the head; and
2. Spreads the blow over a larger area.

Notwithstanding the advent of shell-less bicycle helmets, and the provision of very aggressive impact anvils in certain standards (equestrian headgear for example), few standards for protective headgear attempt to measure directly the ability of the device to perform the second function listed above. For impacts with common flat surfaces (such as the roadway), this should not be a problem. Protrusions of one form or another could, however, present some difficulties. In the future, it will be important to develop standard methods to measure load distribution and to set criteria of acceptability.

A second important feature of protective headgear is its relatively unknown capacity to protect against rotationally induced injuries.

Since it is generally acknowledged that rotational movement is more likely to produce brain injury than is translation, and since contemporary helmets have been observed to be generally effective, one must conclude that they are effective in preventing injuries that would be due to rotation. Nevertheless, in the future, it may be important to try to develop standard methods to monitor for head form rotational acceleration and to set appropriate performance criteria.

A final area that needs future consideration is that of the head protection requirements specifically for infants and children. With the increasing emphasis on head protection for children riding bicycles or riding in bicycle carrier seats, it will become more important that children not be merely regarded as scaled-down adults. Their anatomy, anthropometry, and tolerance to brain injury cannot likely be adequately dealt with by extrapolating from adults. Additional research in this area must be conducted.

Acknowledgments. The author would like to thank his colleagues at Biokinetics for their help in preparing the chapter. Special thanks to Tom Gibson and Terry Smith for their technical input and to Jodi McGrath for her extra efforts in preparing the manuscript.

Bibliography

1. Aldman B, Balldin U, Gustafsson H, Nygreen A, Sporrong A, Astrand I. Carbon dioxide retention inside motorcycle helmets. 1981 International IRCOBI Conference on the Biomechanics of Impacts. Salon de Provence, France, September 8–10, 1981.

2. Aldman B, Gustafsson H, Nygren A, Johansson B, Jonasson H, Wersall J. The sound attenuation and the aerodynamically generated noise inside motorcycle helmets. 1981 International IRCOBI Conference on the Biomechanics of Impacts. Salon de Provence, France, September 8–10, 1981.

3. Aldman B, Thorngren L. The protective effect on crash helmets—a study of 96 motorcycle accidents. 1979 International IRCOBI Conference on the Biomechanics of Trauma. Goteborg, Sweden, September 5–7, 1979.

4. Aldman B, Thorngren L, Gustafsson H, Nygren A, Wersall J (1990) Motorcycle and moped accidents—study of the protective effect on crash helmets. International Motorcycle Safety Conference. Vol II. Washington DC.

5. Bishop PJ, Briard DB (1984) Impact performance of bicycle helmets. Can J Applied Sport Sci 9:94–101.

6. Bowman BM, Schneider LW, Rohr PR, Mohan D. Simulation of head neck impact responses for helmeted and unhelmeted motorcyclists. 25th Stapp Car Crash Conference. 811029, San Francisco, California, September 1981.

7. Bunketorp O, Lindstrum L, Peterson L, Orgengren R. Heavy protective helmets and neck injuries—a theoretical and electromyographic study. 1985 International IRCOBI Conference on the Biomechanics of Impacts. Goteborg, Sweden, June 1985.

8. Chamouard F, Walfisch G, Fayon A, Tarriere C. Prototype of lightweight helmet for users of low-speed two-wheeled vehicles, combining satisfactory head protection with characteristics of acceptable design and wearer's comfort. 1984 International IRCOBI Conference on the Biomechanics of Impacts. Delft, The Netherlands, September 1984.

9. Chandler S, Gilchrist A, Mills NJ. Motorcycle helmet load spreading performance for impacts into rigid and deformable objects. 1991 International IRCOBI Conference on the Biomechanics of Impacts. Berlin, Germany, September 11–13, 1991.

10. Chenier TC, Evans L. Motorcyclist fatalities and the repeal of mandatory helmet wearing laws. 29th AAAM Conference. Washington DC, October 7–9, 1985.

11. Colyer MM, Hallam JCF, Hui K, Lewis GDW, Morfey CL, Thorpe JE. User acceptability and economic benefits of hard-Shell Bicycle Helmets—Results of a U.K. Survey. 1986 International IRCOBI Conference on the Biomechanics of Impacts. Zurich, Switzerland, September 1986.

12. Cooter RD, David DJ. Motorcyclist craniofacial injury patterns. International Motorcycle Safety Conference. Vol I. Orlando, Florida, October 31–November 3, pp 3-1–3-13, 1990.

13. Dart OK. Motorcycle helmet effectiveness in louisiana. International Motorcycle Safety Conference. Washington DC, May 18–23, 1980.

14. Dorsch M, et al (1987) Do bicycle safety helmets reduce severity of head injury in real crashes. Accident Analysis and Prevention, 19(3):183–190.

15. Dorsch MM, Woodward AJ, Somers RL. Effect of helmet use in reducing head injury in bicycle accidents. Proceedings 28th AAAM Conference. Denver, Colorado, October 1982.

16. Doyle D, Duffy EM. Protective helmets and cranio-cerebral trauma in motorcycle accidents: a preliminary study. 1990 International IRCOBI Conference on the Biomechanics of Impacts. Bron, (Lyon) France, September 1990.

17. Evans L, Frick MC. Helmet effectiveness in preventing motorcycle driver and passenger fatalities. 31st AAAM Conference. New Orleans, Louisiana, September 28–30, 1987.

18. Fan WRS. A simple, practical method of assessing foam padding materials for head impact protection. Passenger Comfort, Convenience and Safety: Test Tools and Procedures. Detroit, Michigan, SP-174, SAE 860199, February 1986.

19. Gilchrist A, Mills NJ. Improvements in the design and performance of motorcycle helmets. 1987 International IRCOBI Conference on the Biomechanics of Impacts. Birmingham, England, September 1987.

20. Glaister DH (1985) A new standard for protective headgear. 23rd Annual SAFE Symposium. Las Vegas, Nevada.

21. Goodnow RK. Injury severity, medical costs and associated factors for helmeted and unhelmeted motorcyclist crash cases transported to hospitals in Amarillo, Austin, Corpus Christi, and San Antonio, TX. International Motorcycle Safety Conference. Vol 1. Orlando, Florida, October 31–November 3, pp 3-14–3-17, 1990.

22. Grandel J, Schaper D. Impact dynamic, head impact severity and helmet's energy absorption in motorcycle/passenger car accident tests. 1984 International IRCOBI Conference on the Biomechanics of Impacts. Delft, The Netherlands, September 1984.

23. Hirsch AE, Ommaya AK. Protection from brain injury: the relative significance of translational and rotational motions of the head after impact. 14th Stapp Car Crash Conference. Ann Arbor, Michigan, November 1970.

24. Hope PD, Chinn BP. The correlation of damage to crash helmets with injury and the implications for injury tolerance criteria. 1990 International IRCOBI Conference on the Bio-mechanics of Impacts. Bron, (Lyon) France, September 1990.

25. Hurt HH Jr, Ouellet JV, Wagar IJ (1981) Effectiveness of motorcycle safety helmets and protective clothing. 25th Annual Conference of the American Association for Automotive Medicine. San Francisco.

26. Hurt HH, Thom DR. Laboratory tests and accident performance of bicycle safety helmets. 29th AAAM Conference, October 1985.

27. Hurt HH, Thom DR, Fuller PM. Accident performance of motorcycle safety helmets. International Motorcycle Safety Conference. Vol 1. Orlando, FL, October 31–November 3, pp 3-44–3-69, 1990.

28. Kostner H, Stocker UW. Improvement of the protective effects of motorcycle helmets based on a mathematical study. 1988 International IRCOBI Conference on the Biomechanics of Impacts. Bergisch, Gladbach, Germany, September 1988.

29. Kroon PO, Bunketorp O, Romanus B. The protective effect on bicycle helmets—a study of paired samples in a computer-based accident material in Gothenbury, Sweden. 1986 International IRCOBI Conference on the Bio-mechanics of Impacts. Zurich, Switzerland, September 1986.

30. Kruse T, Jorgensen K, Nielsen HV, Nordentoft EL. AIS as a measure of injury related incapacitation time among selected age and sex groups. 1979 International IRCOBI Conference on the Biomechanics of Trauma. Goteborg, Sweden, September 5–7, 1979.

31. Liu WJ. Analysis of motorcycle helmet test data for FMVSS No. 218. International Motorcycle Safety Conference. Washington DC, May 18–23, 1980.

32. Liu WJ. Current status of FMVSS No. 218, Motorcycle Helmets. International Motorcycle Safety Conference. Vol 1. Orlando, Florida, October 31–November 3, pp 3-105–3-126, 1990.

33. McSwain Willey Janke. The impact of re-enactment of the motorcycle helmet law in louisiana. 29th AAAM Conference. Washington DC, October 7–9, 1985.

34. Mills NJ, Gilchrist A. The effectiveness of foams in bicycle and motorcycle helmets. 34th AAAM Conference. Scottsdale, Arizona, October 1990.

35. Mills NJ, Gilchrist A. The effectiveness of foams in bicycle and motorcycle helmets. 34th AAAM Conference. Scottsdale, Arizona, October 1–3, 1990.

36. Mills NJ, Gilchrist A, Rowland FJ. Mathematical modelling of the effectiveness of helmets in head protection. 1988 International IRCOBI Conference on the Biomechanics of Impacts. Gergisch, Gladbach, Germany, September 1988.
37. Mills NJ, Ward RF (1985) The biomechanics of motorcycle helmet retention. International IRCOBI/AAAM Conference on the Biomechanics of Impacts. Goteborg, Sweden.
38. Newman JA (1978) Engineering considerations in the design of protective headgear. 22nd Conference of the American Association for Automotive Medicine. Michigan.
39. Newman JA (1980) Motorcycle helmets—their limits of performance. International Motorcycle Safety Conference. Vol III. Washington DC.
40. Otte D, Jessl P, Suren EG. Impact points and resultant injuries to the head of motorcyclists involved in accidents, with and without crash helmets. 1984 International IRCOBI Conference on the Biomechanics of Impacts. Delft, The Netherlands, September 1984.
41. Pedder JB, Hagues SB, Mackay GM (1982) Head protection for road users with particular reference to helmets for motorcyclists. AGARD Conference No. 322, impact injury caused by linear acceleration: mechanics, prevention and cost. Cologne, Germany.
42. Pedder JB, Newman JA. After helmets—is there anything else?. 1987 International IRCOBI Conference on the Biomechanics of Impacts. Birmingham, England, September 1987.
43. Richards PG (1984) Detachment of crash helmets during motorcycle accidents. Br Med J 288.
44. Rutledge R, Stutts J, Foil B, Oiler D, Meredith W. The association of helmet use with the outcome of motorcycle crash injury when controlling for crash/injury severity. 35th AAAM Conference. Toronto, Canada, October 7–9, 1991.
45. Sarrailhe SR. Do tougher standards lead to better helmets?. 1984 International IRCOBI Conference on the Biomechanics of Impacts. Delft, The Netherlands, September 1984.
46. Schaper D, Russelsheiim AO, Grandel J. Motorcycle collisions with passengers cars–analysis of impact mechanism, kinematics and effectiveness of full-face safety helmets. Field Accidents: Data Collection, Analysis, Methodologies, and Crash Injury Reconstructions. Detroit MI, SP-159, SAE 850094, March 1985.
47. Schuller E, Beier G. Safety helmets shell material and head injury incidence in motorcycle accidents. 1981 International IRCOBI Conference on the Biomechanics of Impacts. Salon de Provence, France, September 8–10, 1981.
48. Stocker U, Loffelholz H. Investigation into the protective effects of helmets on users of powered two-wheelers. 1984 International IRCOBI Conference on the Biomechanics of Impacts. Delft, The Netherlands, September 1984.
49. Thom DR, Hurt HH. Conflicts of contemporary motorcycle safety helmet standards. International Motorcycle Safety Conference. Vol 1. Orlando, Florida, October 31–November 3, pp 3-71–3-86, 1990.
50. Thompson et al (1989) A case-controlled study of the effectiveness of bicycle safety helmets. N Engl J Med 320(21):1361–1367.
51. Vallee H, Hartemann F, Thomas C, Tarriere C, Patel A, Got C. The fracturing of helmet shells. 1984 International IRCOBI Conference on the Biomechanics of Impacts. Delft, The Netherlands, September 1984.
52. Wager IJ, Fisher D, Newman JA. Head protection in racing and road traffic. International Motorcycle Safety Conference. Washington DC, pp 1347–1363, May 1980.
53. Walfisch G, Chamouard F, Fayon A, Tarriere C, Got C, Guillon F, Patel A. Facial protection of motorized two-wheeler riders. New features of a specification for "full-face" helmet. 1984 International IRCOBI Conference on the Biomechanics of Impacts. Delft, The Netherlands, September 1984.
54. Walz FH, Dubas L, Burkart F, Kosik D. Head injuries in moped and bicycle collisions—implications for bicycle helmet design. 1985 International IRCOBI/AAAM Conference on the Biomechanics of Impacts. Goteborg, Sweden, June 1985.
55. Wasserman RC, Waller JA, Monty MJ, Emery AB, Robinson DR (1988) Bicyclists, helmets and head injuries: a rider-based study of helmet use and effectiveness. Am J Pub Health 78(9): 1220–1221.
56. Wasserman RC, Waller Monty MJ, et al. Helmet use and head injury among adolescent bicyclists: a missed opportunity for injury control. 25th Annual Meeting of the Ambulatory Paediatric Association. May 1985.
57. Watson GS, Zador PL, Wilks A (1981) Helmet use, helmet use laws and motorcyclist fatalities. Am J Pub Health 71(3):297–300.

310

James H. McElhaney and Barry S. Myers

58. Weiss BD (1986) Bicycle helmet use by children. Paediatrics 77(5):677–679.
59. Weiss BD (1986) Bicycle helmet use by children: knowledge and behaviour of physicians. Am J Pub Health 76(8):1022–1023.
60. Williams M (1991) The protective performance of bicyclists helmets in accidents. Accident Anal Prevention 23(2/3):119–131.

14
Biomechanical Aspects of Cervical Trauma

James H. McElhaney and Barry S. Myers

Introduction

From a mechanical and structural point of view, the cervical spine is a very complex mechanism. The human neck contains vital neurologic, vascular, and respiratory structures as well as the cervical vertebrae and spinal cord. Although injury statistics generally attribute only 2% to 4% of serious trauma to the neck, any neck injury can have debilitating if not life-threatening consequences. Permanent paralysis is a particularly devastating and costly injury. When it is a consequence of accidental trauma, frequently a young productive member of society is transformed into a totally dependent member. The advent of high-speed land and air transportation has made us increasingly aware of the serious consequences that can result from a structural failure of the neck. Also, as more people pursue leisure-time activities, the potential for serious neck injuries increases. Football, diving, gymnastics, skiing, hang gliding, mountain climbing, and amusement rides are but a few activities that expose the neck to a risk of serious injury. As a result, a variety of devices have evolved that offer a measure of protection to the neck from mechanical trauma. Head and seat restraints, motorcycle and football helmets, energy-absorbing pads and collars, and gymnastic mats are but a few examples of head and neck protective devices. Unfortunately, the design of many of these has proceeded with insufficient biomechanical input because of the lack of relevant data.

This chapter summarizes research aimed at providing some biomechanical responses of the neck in a form that, it is hoped, will be useful in the design of protective systems and in the development of societal strategies to reduce the number of cervical spine injuries. To that end, various biomechanical characteristics of the neck, tolerance criteria, and injury mechanisms are presented. Neck injuries are described and classified. Accidents that involve neck injuries are analyzed. Real-life neck injuries are presented, and laboratory and mathematical simulations discussed.

It should be recognized at the outset that much of the work described here is ongoing, and the results are therefore preliminary and subject to modification as more data is accumulated. Nor is it claimed that this presentation is complete. It is not possible to cover, in a single chapter, all of the important research that has been done on this subject.

Incidence

The National Head and Spinal Cord Injury Survey estimated the occurrence of spinal cord injury with quadriplegia in the United States at 5 per 100,000 or in excess of 10,000 cases each year. Since, with proper medical care, the life span of a quadriplegic is not significantly reduced, an estimate of 200,000 living quadriplegics may be made at an annual maintenance and medical cost of over $2 billion per year. This does not include the loss to society of many productive individuals.

TABLE 14.1. Activity associated with cervical spinal cord injury.

Category	Number	Percent
Auto accident	842	36.7
Fall	365	15.9
Gunshot wound	268	11.7
Shallow water diving	243	10.6
Motorcycle accident	143	6.2
Hit by falling/flying object	124	5.4
Other	61	2.7
Other sports	60	2.6
Football	29	1.3
Pedestrian	29	1.3
Med/surg complication	28	1.2
Bicycle	22	1.0
Other vehicular	19	0.8
Fixed-wing aircraft	7	0.3
Trampoline	15	0.7
Stabbing	9	0.4
Rotating-wing aircraft	7	0.3
Snow skiing	6	0.3
Snowmobile	5	0.2
Waterskiing	4	0.2
Unknown	4	0.2
Boat	2	0.1
Total	2,292	

Reported cases

Data from the National Spinal Cord Injury Data Research Center (NSCIDRC).

While injuries to the cervical spine can result from almost any activity, the literature suggests that automobile and aircraft accidents, sports, and falls are the circumstances most represented (Table 14.1).

The distribution of injuries depends somewhat on the location of the data collection as is evidenced by the comparison of Table 14.1 with the Canadian experience (Table 14.2). However, the general trends are similar.

Automobile and aircraft accidents undoubtedly produce extensive injuries because of the speeds involved and the associated energy that must be dissipated in a crash. According to Huelke et al. (1980), 56% of all spinal cord injuries are the result of highway accidents, with 67% of those involved in highway accidents being vehicle occupants. Pedestrians and motorcyclists were also significantly involved in the injury statistics. Other studies of automobile and highway-related cervical spine injuries include the

papers of Alker et al. (1975), Mertz et al. (1978), Schutt, and Donan (1968), Sims et al. (1976), Thorson (1972), Tonga et al. (1972), Voight and Wilfert (1969), and Yule (1972).

Automobile restraint systems have also been associated with spinal cord injuries. These injuries are frequently described as shearing injuries produced in high-speed crashes with the upper torso belt providing a fulcrum for forced spinal rotation. Authors who discuss the relationship between restraint systems and spinal injury include Burke (1973), Epstein et al. (1978), Gogler and Athanasiadis (1979), Horsch et al. (1979), Marsh et al. (1975), Nyquist et al. (1980), Schmidt et al. (1975), and Taylor et al. (1976). It should be realized, however, that the reduction in injury by restraint systems far exceeds these relatively uncommon injuries.

Sports and leisure activities account for a significant portion of injuries to the cervical spine. In 1978, Shield, Fox, and Stauffer analyzed 10 years of data on 152 cervical spinal

TABLE 14.2. Cause and severity of spinal fractures in Canada (1980–1986).

Cause of injury	Total (N)	Injuries (%)
Motor vehicle accident	768	53
Occupational	221	15
Domestic	203	14
Sporting and recreational	202	14
Other	54	4
Total	1,448	

Adapted from Allan, D.G., Reid, D.C. and Saboe, L. (1988).

TABLE 14.3. Sport activity causing cervical spinal cord damage in 153 individuals.

Activity	Number	Percent
Diving	82	54
Football	16	11
Gymnastics	5	3
Snow skiing	5	3
Surfing	29	19
Track and field	3	2
Trampoline	2	1
Water skiing	7	5
Wrestling	3	2
Total	152	

cord injuries caused by sports participation that were treated at the Rancho Los Amigos Hospital (Table 14.3).

Considerable regional variation in sports-related cervical injury exists primarily due to the degree of participation in the various activities. However, these injuries can be generally classified as resulting from contact sports of which football is the most well known, or from falls and dives from height. The incidence of these injuries in the game of football is described by Torg (1982) using the National Football Injury Register.

The development and use of improved head protection in football resulted in a significant increase in cervical injury in the 1960s. Unfortunately, because of the increased security provided by facial and head protection, players began using the head as a method for tackling other players. Awareness of this problem, and the subsequent use of "heads-up" tackling together with penalizing spearing, have resulted in a significant drop in neck injury in football.

Schneider, in his book on football injuries as well as in his numerous papers, related trauma due to the impingement of the rear of the helmet shell on the neck. Subsequent authors have described the role of the helmet in producing neck injuries and have seriously debated the mechanism proposed by Schneider. These authors, such as Hodgson and Thomas (1980), Mertz et al. (1978) and Virgin (1980), have attempted to verify Schneider's experiments without much success.

Swimming and diving accidents have also been identified as causing significant numbers of fractures and dislocations of the cervical spine. Kewairamani and Taylor (1975) found that 18% of all spinal cord injuries in their series were related to diving accidents. Albrand and Walter (1975) published curves that related depth in feet and the velocity of the head to the height from which a diver dove into the water. McElhaney et al. (1979) also provided experimental data relative to body velocity and the depth of the water. Their series of accidents included not only springboard diving but water slides as well. They suggest that a head velocity of approximately

TABLE 14.4. Spine injuries in specific sports.

Sport	Total injuries	Percent of all sports
Diving	43	21
Snowmobiles*	20	10
Parachute/skydiving	20	10
Equestrian	19	10
Dirt bikes	18	9
All-terrain vehicle	15	7
Toboggan*	11	5
Alpine skiing*	11	5
Ice hockey*	6	3
Rugby	6	3
Bicycle	5	3
Football	4	2
Wrestling	3	1
Mountaineering	3	1
Surfing	3	1
Other	15	7
Total	202	

Adapted from Reid, D.C., Saboe, L. (1989).
* Winter sports: 48 injuries (24%).

10 feet per second with a following body is sufficient to cause compression fractures of the cervical spine, most frequently at the level of C5, the fifth cervical vertebra. As this is equivalent to a vertical drop height of only 19.4 inches, we realize that many activities contain the potential for neck injury. Reid and Saboe (1989) (Table 14.4) provide a proportionate distribution of these injuries in specific sports. Care must be exercised in interpreting data of this type because the incidence is determined more by the number of participants and exposures than by other factors.

Structure and Anatomy

The complete spine is a structure composed of 7 cervical, 12 thoracic, 5 lumbar, 5 sacral, and 4 coccygeal vertebrae. Each vertebra is composed of a cylindrical vertebral body connected to a series of bony elements collectively referred to as the posterior elements. The posterior elements include the pedicles, lamina, spinous and transverse processes, and the superior and inferior facet joint surfaces. This structure is also known as the neural arch. It provides mechanical protection for the spinal

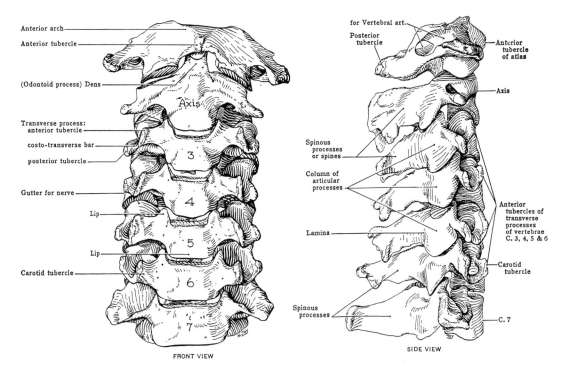

FIGURE 14.1. Cervical vertebrae (from Grant's *Anatomy*).

cord and contributes to the stability and kinematics of the vertebral column.

As noted, the cervical spine is comprised of seven vertebrae forming eight motion segments between the base of the skull and the first thoracic vertebra, T1 (Fig. 14.1). The vertebrae are numbered such that the uppermost vertebra is denoted C1 and the lowermost vertebra is C7. The motion segments are similarly numbered C1 through C8. C1 denotes the articulation of the base of the skull with the first cervical vertebra and C8 denotes the articulation of the C7 vertebra with T1. The cervical spine is divided morphologically and mechanically into two regions, the upper cervical and lower cervical spine.

The lower cervical spine contains vertebrae C3 through C7 and motion segments C3 through C8. The vertebrae are geometrically similar, increasing in absolute size from superior to inferior. The vertebral bodies are connected to one another by a fibrocartilaginous joint, the intervertebral disc (Fig. 14.2). This structure is composed of a central

fluid-like nucleus pulposus bounded by a laminar set of spirally wound fibrous sheets denoted the annulus fibrosus. The anterior surfaces of the vertebral bodies are connected from the sacrum through to the base of skull by the anterior longitudinal ligament. Similarly, the posterior longitudinal ligament connects the posterior surface of the vertebral bodies and forms the anterior surface of the spinal canal. The pedicles run posterolaterally from the posterior of the vertebral bodies and terminate in the pars interarticularis. The pars interarticularis denotes a bony region bounded superiorly by the superior facet surface, inferiorly by the inferior facet surface, laterally by the transverse process, and medially by the spinal canal. Lateral to these elements are the transverse processes, which contain the vertebral artery, the major blood supply for the brainstem, and the posterior portions of the brain. This artery is contained in the foramen transversarium of the transverse process. The lamina project posteromedially from the pars interarticularis and meet at the

FIGURE 14.2. Schematic representation of the ligamentous anatomy of the cervical spine. (From White and Panjabi, 1980c.)

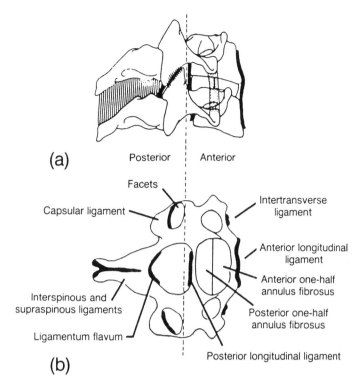

(a)

Posterior | Anterior

Facets

Capsular ligament

Intertransverse ligament

Anterior longitudinal ligament

Anterior one-half annulus fibrosus

Interspinous and supraspinous ligaments

Posterior one-half annulus fibrosus

Ligamentum flavum

Posterior longitudinal ligament

(b)

midline. The lamina form the posterior surface of the spinal canal. Protruding from the midline fusion of the two lamina on each vertebra is the spinous process. The spinous processes are the palpable protuberances on the dorsal surface of the neck and back.

The interspinous and supraspinous ligaments connect the spinous processes of adjacent vertebra. The flaval, yellow, ligaments similarly connect adjacent lamina from the sacrum to the base of the skull. The facet joints are formed by the inferior facet surface of the superior vertebra and the superior facet surface of the inferior vertebra. These are synovial joints, which are wrapped in a capsular ligament. The spinal canal of the vertebrae is the location of the spinal cord. Nerve roots exit between adjacent vertebrae through the intervertebral foramen. This foramen is comprised of the inferior vertebral notch of the superior vertebra and the superior vertebral notch of the inferior vertebra.

The upper cervical spine consists of three bony elements: the occiput (the base of the skull), and the atlas (C1) and the axis (C2),

which produce two joints—the occipitoatlantal joint (C1) and the atlantoaxial joint (C2) (Fig. 14.3). The atlas is a bony ring with enlarged facets on the lateral portions of the ring and no vertebral body. The atlas is divided into the anterior and posterior arches. The anterior arch forms a synovial articulation with the second cervical vertebra, the axis, and the posterior arch provides protection for the spinal column and brainstem.

The axis is composed of a vertebral body and a posterior bony arch, but it has an additional element, the odontoid process (the dens). The odontoid process points superiorly from the C2 vertebral body and its anterior surface articulates with the posterior portion of the anterior arch of the atlas. The lateral portions of the axis contain flattened, enlarged articular facet surfaces, and lateral to these surfaces are the transverse processes.

The occipitoatlantal joint is formed by two bony protuberances on the base of the skull, the occipital condyles, and the atlas. The atlantoaxial joint is composed of three synovial articulations between the atlas and the axis.

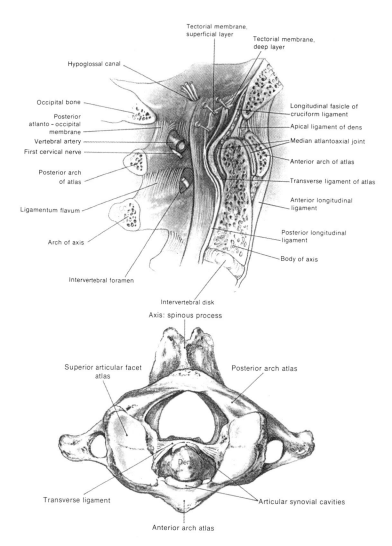

FIGURE 14.3. Anatomy of the first two cervical vertebrae. (From Gehweiler et al., 1980.)

The superior facet surfaces of the axis form two synovial articulations with the inferior facet surfaces of the atlas. The other synovial joint is formed by the articulation of the anterior arch of the atlas with the odontoid process of the axis.

The ligamentous structures of the occipitoatlantoaxial complex include continuations of the lower cervical ligaments and an additional set of structures unique to the upper cervical spine. The transverse ligament is a stout horizontal ligament that connects the medial portions of the C1 lateral masses and constrains the odontoid process posteriorly. The transverse ligament is the horizontal portion of the cruciate ligament. The vertical portion of this ligament attaches to the anterior inferior aspect of the foramen magnum of the base of the skull and the posterior aspect of the C2 vertebral body. The apical ligament is a midline structure that connects the apex of the odontoid to the base of the skull anterior to the cruciate ligament. The alar ligaments originate on the posterior lateral aspect of the odontoid process and ascend laterally to insert directly to the base of the skull. The posterior longitudinal ligament inserts on the base of the skull posterior to the transverse ligament and is named the tectorial membrane. The anterior longitudinal ligament inserts on the base of the skull. The anterior atlantoepistrophical and atlantooccipital ligaments lie posterior to the anterior longitudinal ligament and connect the C2 vertebral body to the atlas and the atlas to the base of the skull, respectively. The lower cervical flaval ligaments insert on the base of the skull and are denoted the posterior atlantooccipital membrane. Finally, the nuchal ligament, which is formed by the midline fusion of the paravertebral muscular fascia, inserts on the occipital protuberance, which is a small bump on the back of the head just above the neck.

Injury Mechanisms and Classifications

Introduction

Because the study of cervical spine trauma has evolved from a wide variety of institutions and sources, several authors have attempted to classify the injuries so that there can be agreement as to what each investigator is referring to as he describes a particular injury. Babcock (1976), in his article in the Archives of Surgery, developed a classification that is complete and should be more widely used. Other classifications of injury have been developed by Melvin et al. (1976), Moffatt et al. (1971), Portnoy et al. (1978), Allen et al. (1982), White and Panjabi (1978c), Dolen (1977), and Harris et al. (1986). The rationale for these classifications has included retrospective reviews of patient data, whole and segmental cadaveric experimentation, and retrospective evaluations of various known injury environments (Allen et al., 1982; McElhaney et al., 1979; Torg, 1982; and Yoganandan et al., 1989a). The following discussion will draw on all three methods in an attempt to bring the advantages of each to our understanding of injury.

Some of the confusion in understanding injury classification schemes has evolved from the nomenclature describing it. For example, flexion of the head may be produced by rotation of the head on the neck, or may be the result of anteroinferior translation of the head

relative to the torso. The confusion is further compounded by the communication differences between the disciplines that study injury. As an example, the term "extension" is properly defined in a clinical setting as a motion that brings the long axis of the distal portion of a joint parallel with the long axis of the proximal portion (Stedman, 1982). In the context of the cervical spine, extension refers to a posteroinferior motion of the head relative to the torso, and is usually associated with rotation of the head and spine. In contrast, in engineering terms, extension refers to the elongation of a member along its long axis, the clinical equivalent of traction (Figs. 14.4 and 14.5).

Injury classification is further complicated by the methods used to determine the mechanism. For example, as the global motion of the head relative to the torso may not be the same as regional motions of the cervical spine, the observation of a flexion motion of the head relative to the torso may actually be concurrent with local (i.e., a single motion segment) extension in the cervical spine and may produce a so-called extension injury. Further, small movements of the impact point or the initial position of the head (less than 1.0 cm) have been shown to change the injury from compression-flexion to compression-extension in various cadaveric studies (McElhaney, 1983a; Myers et al., 1991c; Nusholtz et al., 1983). Thus, the reconstruction of an injury mechanism must be performed with great precision.

In addition, the observed motions of the head may occur after the injury has occurred, and thus not reflect the true injury mechanism, but rather the motions of an unstable spine. In this context, understanding whether the classifications are based on global motions of the head (as in Harris et al., 1986), local deformations of the motion segment (Allen et al., 1982), review of videotaped injuries, careful evaluation of patient data, or cadaveric experimentation is key to an understanding of injury classification.

Thus, in any discussion of injury, it is important to clarify an unambiguous nomenclature and to interpret the results accordingly.

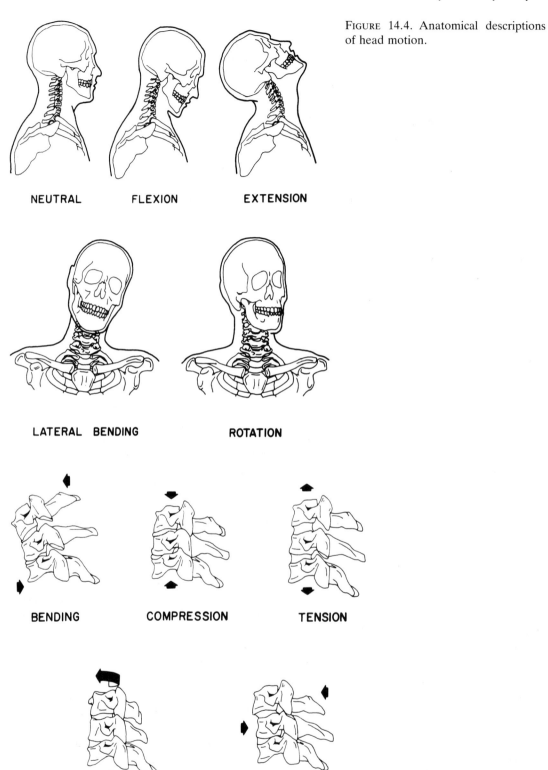

FIGURE 14.4. Anatomical descriptions of head motion.

NEUTRAL   FLEXION   EXTENSION

LATERAL BENDING   ROTATION

BENDING   COMPRESSION   TENSION

TORQUE   SHEAR

FIGURE 14.5. Engineering descriptions of neck loading.

In the following discussion, unless otherwise stated, the nomenclature used will refer to the principal applied loading of the motion segments, and not the observed motions of the head, or the loads on the head required to produce the resultant motion segment loads (the reader is forewarned of the conflicts in nomenclature and proposed mechanisms that this will produce!). The classification system used is summarized in Table 14.5.

Compression, Compression-Flexion, and Compression-Extension

Compression

Purely compressive loading of the cervical spine occurs infrequently due to the complexity

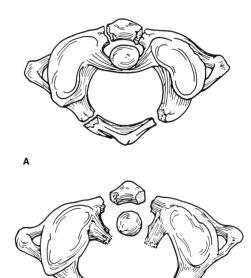

FIGURE 14.6. Jefferson burst fracture of the atlas vertebra. (From Gallie et al., 1989.)

TABLE 14.5. Cervical spine injuries: mechanism of injury.

Compression (vertical compression)
  Jefferson fracure
  Multipart atlas fracture
  Vertebral body compression fracture
  Burst fracture
Compression-flexion
  Vertebral body wedge compression fracture
  Hyperflexion sprain
  Unilateral facet dislocation
  Bilateral facet dislocation
  Teardrop fracture
Compression-extension
  Posterior element fractures
Tension
  Occipitoatlantal dislocation
Tension-extension
  Whiplash
  Anterior longitudinal ligament tears
  Disk rupture
  Horizontal vertebral body fracture
  Hangman's fracture
  Teardrop fracture
Tension-flexion
  Bilateral facet dislocation
Torsion
  Rotary atlantoaxial dislocation
Horizontal shear
  Anterior and posterior atlantoaxial subluxation
  Odontoid fracture
  Transverse ligament rupture
Lateral bending
  Nerve root avulsion
  Transverse process fracture
Other fractures
  Clay shovelers' fracture

of the structure. Notwithstanding, many events may be considered to be predominantly vertical compressive loading. Cadaveric and clinical studies (Allen et al., 1982; McElhaney et al., 1983a; Yoganandan et al., 1989b), have demonstrated that axial displacement of the head can produce both upper and lower cervical compression injuries.

Upper cervical compression injuries consist largely of multipart fractures of the atlas. While these fractures are frequently described as Jefferson fractures, the Jefferson fracture properly refers to a particular four-part fracture of the atlas (Jefferson, 1920) (Fig. 14.6). Fatalities and instability from this group of injuries are common (White and Panjabi, 1978c).

Lower cervical vertebral body compression injuries occur at all vertebral levels from C2 to T1. These lesions may consist of destruction of the cancellous bony centrum with loss of disk height, vertebral end-plate fracture with vertical herniation of the nucleus pulposus into the centrum producing the so-called Schmorl's node, or multipart fractures of the vertebral

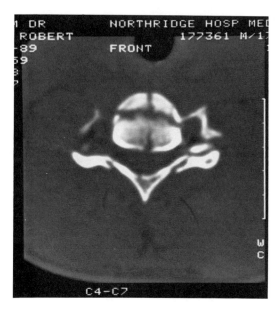

FIGURE 14.7. Cleavage fracture through the body and posterior arch.

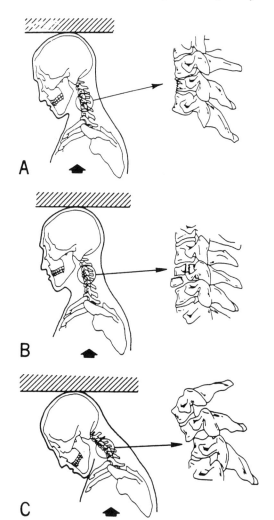

FIGURE 14.8. Flexion-compression injury mechanisms. A. Wedge fractures. B. Burst fracture. C. Anterior dislocation.

body, the latter being referred to as a burst fracture (Figs. 14.7 and 14.8). The most common sites of compression fractures are C4, C5, and C6 (McElhaney et al., 1979). Ligamentous injury is relatively uncommon in pure vertical compression injuries, whereas damage to the facet joints and pars interarticularis can occur, though usually only in association with severe vertebral body injury. The risk of spinal cord injury from these fractures is somewhat variable in the reported literature (approximately 40% to 75%), but tends to increase with the degree of comminution of the vertebral fracture, and with the loss of disk and body height.

Compression-Flexion

Wedge compression fractures of the vertebral bodies are thought to be the result of a combination of a flexion bending moment and compressive loading of the vertebral motion segment resulting in greater compressive stresses and failures in the anterior of the vertebral body (White and Panjabi, 1978c). This type of injury, classified clinically as compression-flexion, may be produced by eccentric compressive loading of the head,

with or without actual head rotation. This has been demonstrated in cadaveric studies by McElhaney et al., (1983a), in which increasing the eccentricity (the effective moment arm of the applied axial load) during an axial displacement of the head produced wedge compression fractures, whereas decreased eccentricity of the applied loading produced compression and burst fractures. Both of these types of fractures were produced in the absence of head rotation. These fractures usually occur in the lower three cervical segments where the flexible cervical spine joins the less flexible thorax, the flexion moments are the angular motion, and the angular motion between vertebrae is the greatest.

A second group of injuries in the lower cervical spine has been classified clinically as both compressive-hyperflexion (Braakman and Penning, 1971), and distractive-flexion (tension-flexion) (Allen et al., 1982, Crowell et al. 1987) The latter term refers to the presence of tensile stresses of the posterior elements, and compressive loading of the vertebral body as a result of a flexion bending moment acting on the motion segment. The former term refers to blows occurring on the posterior portions of the head resulting in flexion of the head and compression of the spine. As discussed below, it would appear that both descriptions are accurate. This group of injuries includes unilateral facet dislocation, bilateral facet dislocation, and the hyperflexion sprain.

Bilateral facet dislocation describes an injury in which the superior vertebral body is displaced anteriorly over its subjacent vertebra. This displacement results in a dislocation of both facet joints with subsequent locking of the surfaces in a tooth-to-tooth fashion secondary to muscle spasm (Fig. 14.9). The lesion is more common in the lowest cervical motion segments; however, it can occur throughout the lower cervical spine (Allen et al., 1982). Unfortunately, this injury results in a significant reduction in the anteroposterior diameter of the neural canal and is therefore usually associated with spinal cord injury. Braakman and Vinken (1967) report permanent partial or complete spinal cord injury in 27 of 35 patients with bilateral dislocations. Experimentally, the lesion has been produced by Bauze and Ardran (1978) and subsequently by Myers et al. (1991c) by applying a compressive axial displacement to cervical spines in which unconstrained posteroanterior displacement was permitted; however, rotation of the head was constrained. Analysis of load cell data from these experiments show that the lower cervical spine was in a state of combined compression and flexion and analysis of local deformations revealed the presence of tensile

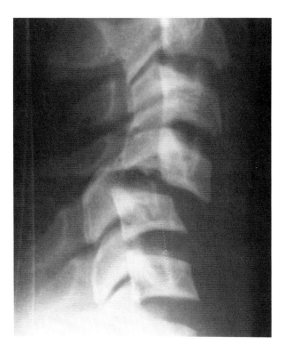

FIGURE 14.9. Bilateral facet dislocation at C4–C5.

strains in the posterior ligaments prior to dislocation. Evaluation and reconstruction of injury case histories suggest that loading of the head occurs more frequently in compression-flexion than in tension-flexion (Yoganandan et al., 1989a); however, it also suggests that both types of loading may produce facet dislocations. Based on this observation it would appear that the primary injury vector is a lower cervical bending moment that is the result of an eccentric load, either tensile or compressive.

Unilateral facet dislocation refers to the anterosuperior displacement of a facet over the facet of the inferior vertebra with subsequent locking in a tooth-to-tooth fashion (see Fig. 14.17). In unilateral dislocation, the dislocation occurs in only one of the two facet joints of a motion segment. The most common sites of this injury are the C5, C6, and C7 interspaces (Braakman and Vinken, 1967). Clinically, the lesion is frequently asymptomatic or associated with radicular pain on the side of the injury (25 of 39 patients). Spinal cord injury is relatively uncommon in this type of injury, occurring in only 5 of 39 patients.

The etiology of this lesion has been the subject of great interest and controversy. Huelke et al. (1980) and Harris et al. (1986) reported that unilateral dislocation was the result of combined flexion and rotation. Gosch et al. (1972) reported that in purely anterior to posterior deceleration sled tests of primates, axial rotation was observed and unilateral facet dislocation produced. Roaf (1960) reported that torsion was required to produce lower cervical ligamentous injury and dislocation and that hyperflexion alone could not produce ligamentous injury. Rogers (1957) and White and Panjabi (1978c) noted that unilateral dislocation resulted from an exaggeration of the normal coupling of lower cervical lateral bending and rotation but did not describe the loads required to produce the injury. Braakman and Vinken (1967) suggested that unilateral facet dislocation was the result of combined flexion and rotation. Torg (1982) stated that the lesion was the result of compression and buckling. Bauze and Ardran (1978) noted that a number of specimens, while being loaded in compression and flexion, suffered unilateral dislocation. Importantly, their apparatus applied no torque to the specimen, and yet, lower cervical rotation was observed prior to unilateral dislocation. Myers et al. (1991b) demonstrated that while unilateral facet dislocation could be produced by direct torsional loading of the lower cervical spine, the lesion could not be the result of torsional loading of the head because of the comparative weakness of the atlantoaxial joint. The authors currently believe that the lesion is produced in a similar mechanism to bilateral facet dislocations with the difference being the result of bending out of the plane of symmetry, or the presence of preexisting facet tropism (structural asymmetry). Facet dislocations are frequently referred to as fracture dislocations in that the apical portions of the facets are typically fractured or abraded during the injury (Harris et al., 1986).

Hyperflexion sprain, is a clinical entity in which the ligamentous structures of the posterior arch are torn or stretched without producing dislocations or fractures of the facet joints. It is thought to be produced by the same mechanism as bilateral facet dislocation, only with a less extensive disruption of the motion segment (Allen et al., 1982). Harris et al. (1986) report 30% to 50% of patients with this diagnosis develop late instability as a result of the ligamentous injury. Allen et al. (1982) note that 2 of 12 patients with this diagnosis had spinal cord syndromes. It has been hypothesized based on this data that hyperflexion sprain may represent a similar degree of injury as the other dislocations, with a spontaneous reduction of the dislocation at the time of injury.

Compression-Extension

Extension injuries are thought to produce both lower and upper cervical injuries. The type of injury produced by extension bending moments (i.e., anterior ligamentous injury versus posterior bony injury) depends largely on the type of loading of the head that produced the extension moment, including anteroposterior shearing force (horizontal shear), a compressive force directed posterior to the occipital condyles (compression-extension), and tensile forces with a line of action anterior to the occipital condyles (tension-extension). Local extension injuries may also occur in the presence of a "flexion" motion of the head relative to the torso. The effect of pure extension moment on cervical injury has not been investigated in a dynamic study as this type of loading is not likely to occur in the accident environment. Extension loading producing structural damage to the lower cervical spine is less common than flexion injuries. The reasons for this may include the increased flexibility of the neck in extension over flexion, which allows the head to move out of the load path of the torso more easily, or a decrease in the incidence of blows to the face as opposed to the crown and posterior of the head.

Compression-extension loading produces fractures of the posterior elements of the cervical spine. This has been observed in both clinical studies and experimental studies on cadaveric specimens (Allen et al., 1982; McElhaney et al., 1983a). These injuries occur throughout the upper and lower cervical spine and appear to be the result of direct bony impingement of the posterior bony elements against each other. The types of injuries produced naturally depend on the relative magnitudes of the compression force and extension bending moments. These include laminar fractures, pedicle fractures, crushing injuries of the pars interarticularis, and fractures of the spinous processes. These fractures can occur in isolation, but are frequently multiple. They may also be associated with neurologic deficit as a result of impingement on the spinal cord by the bony or ligamentous fragments, or as a result of canal compromise from spondylolisthesis of the unstable spine. It has been suggested, but not evaluated experimentally, that the larger the component of compression relative to the extension moment, the greater the likelihood of pars interarticularis fractures over more posterior element fractures (i.e., laminar fractures).

Tension, Tension-Extension, Tension-Flexion

Tension

Pure tensile injury to the human cervical spine appears to be restricted to the upper cervical spine. In particular, tensile loading appears to produce occipitoatlantal distraction, with unilateral or bilateral dislocation of the occipital condyles. This is perhaps the result of the comparatively small size and laxity of the craniocervical ligaments compared to the remainder of the cervical spine. These dislocations tend to produce ligamentous injury without bony fracture and are most frequently lethal due to the associated distraction and subsequent transection of the spinal cord near the brainstem. Montane et al. (1991) report on four cases of occipitoatlantal dislocation resulting from rapid decelerations in motor vehicle accidents in which the victims survived past the immediate event. The prevalence of this type of injury is debated. Because of the nature of the injury and the method of dissection at autopsy, occipitoatlantal dislocations are frequently undetected, and were thus

thought to be uncommon. According to Bucholz and Burkhead (1979), however, the lesion is a relatively common cause of death in motor vehicle accidents. Specifically, it occurred in 9 of 112 automotive fatalities. The authors postulated, based on the presence of submental lacerations, that the injury mechanism is also associated with hyperextension. Yoganandan et al. (1989a) report an association of this injury with passenger ejections during motor vehicle accidents. The other known cause of this injury is high-speed decelerations associated with military aircraft crashes into water, with inertial tensile loading of the neck by the mass of the head and helmet. Estimates based on these events suggest that decelerations must exceed $100g$ to produce the injury in this healthy and muscular population. Notably, other authors have postulated that occipitoatlantal dislocations may be the result of extension, flexion, or shear loading of the head. It is likely that all these types of loading lead to the final common path of tensile loading of the spinal ligaments inserting to the occiput.

Tension-Extension

Tension-extension loading is common and is responsible for a group of injuries including whiplash, hangman's fractures, and structural injury to the anterior column of the spine. Tension-extension loading can occur in three primary ways (Fig. 14.10):

A. Fixation of the head with continued forward displacement of the body. This occurs commonly in unbelted occupants hitting the windshield, and as a result of falls and dives.
B. Inertial loading of the neck following an abrupt forward acceleration of the torso as would occur in a rear-end collision (whiplash mechanism).
C. Forceful loading below the chin directed posterosuperiorly (as in a judicial hanging).

Whiplash injury, while not associated with overt structural injury to the cervical spine or the central nervous system, is both a common and potentially debilitating injury. Unfortunately, this injury has the bad reputation of

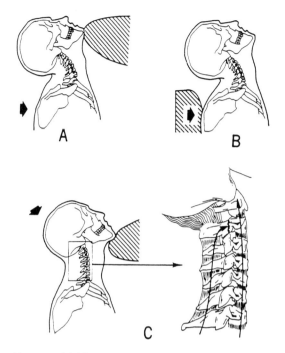

FIGURE 14.10. Tension-extension injury mechanisms.

being associated with unjustified litigation and the expression of psychiatric disorders. It typically occurs as a result of a rear-end collisions in autombles, which may be minor (low g) or major (high g). It is considered a hyperextension injury because of the extension bending moment resulting from inertial loading of the neck by the head. Strictly speaking, this load represents a inertial (D' Alembert) anteroposterior shearing force acting through the center of gravity of the head producing extension bending moments in the cervical spine. Scaled primate data collected by Ommaya and Hirsh (1971) suggest that rotational accelerations of the head as low as 1,800 rad/s^2 may produce these injuries, and that these angular accelerations could occur as a result of linear accelerations of as small as $5g$. The acute symptoms consist of muscle stiffness and neck pain. Conventional radiographs are typically normal or show a straightening of the normal lordotic curve of the cervical spine. While this radiographic finding also represents a normal anatomic variant, Hohl (1974) showed that local changes in lordosis are

associated with a poorer prognosis. The chronic symptoms of the injury include head and neck pain, muscle stiffness and tension, malaise, dysequilibrium, and emotional disturbances, including anxiety and depression. Recent work by Chester (1991) has suggested that patients with chronic whiplash syndrome may be suffering from vestibular dysfunction and injury, and that therapy directed at that organ may be beneficial to patients with chronic whiplash syndrome.

Larger accelerations, in addition to producing whiplash symptoms, may produce disruption of the anterior longitudinal ligament and intervertebral disk, horizontal fractures though the vertebra, and rotational brain injury (Fig. 14.11). Marar (1974) produced anterior longitudinal ligament tears and horizontal vertebral body fracture by manually applying a rearward rotation to the head. The injury has also recently been produced and evaluated more quantitatively by Shea et al. (in press) in which a combination of tension and extension displacements were applied. Concerning the risk of disk rupture versus

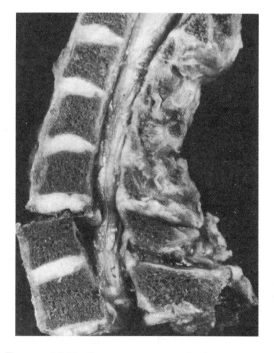

FIGURE 14.11. Severe rupture of the anterior longitudinal ligament and the intervertebral disk with resulting compression of the spinal cord.

vertebral bony injury, experimental data would suggest that victims with low bone mineral density indicative of low ultimate vertebral body strength, but normal ligamentous strength would tend to suffer vertebral fracture over intervertebral disk injury. Marar, based on a review of 45 such injuries, noted that horizontal fracture through the vertebral body was more common than disk lesions however. This, despite the young age and therefore higher bone mineral content of the victims.

Traumatic spondylolisthesis of the axis, or the hangman's fracture, describes a fracture of the pedicles or pars interarticularis of the posterior arch of the second cervical vertebrae. It is thought by most authors to be the result of hyperextension and distraction (tension and rearward rotation of the head), which can result from blows to the face and chin or as its name would suggest, the result of hanging (Braakman and Penning, 1971; Harris et al., 1986; Huelke et al., 1980; White and Panjabi, 1978c).

The mechanism of cord damage resulting from extension injuries has been observed in cadaver studies to be impingement of the spinal cord between the posteriorly displaced vertebral body and the posterior elements (Marar, 1974). The clinical finding of a spinal cord injury in the absence of cervical spine structural injury and in the presence of facial injury by Taylor and Blackwood (1948), prompted interest in extension as a causative agent. Subsequent cadaveric study by Taylor (1951), which combined myelography with manual loading of the head in flexion and extension demonstrated posterior canal defects as seen in the lateral projection myelogram in "forced" hyperextension. These defects were thought to be the result of bulging of the flaval ligaments into the neural canal and were produced without overt structural damage to the spine. The author postulated, based on this observation, that extension could produce this "atraumatic" spinal cord injury. Further evaluation and the recognition of disk bulging during loading reinforced this as a possible mechanism of spinal cord injury (Barnes, 1948; Schneider et al., 1959).

Tension-Flexion

Bilateral facet dislocation, in addition to being the result of compression-flexion loadings has also been observed to be the result of tension-flexion loading in a number of well-documented injuries, and thus should be mentioned in this section. This suggests that the flexion bending moment is the primary basis for the injury, with less importance being placed on the direction of the applied load to the head required to produce the flexion bending moment.

Torsion

Cadaveric studies have shown that torsional loading of the head can produce rotary atlantoaxial dislocation, with or without tearing of the alar ligaments (Goel et al., 1990; Myers et al., 1991b). Other types of atlantoaxial subluxations include unilateral anterior and posterior subluxations as well as bilateral anterior and posterior subluxations. These injuries refer to the dislocation of one or both of the atlas facet surfaces (a lateral mass) on the axis facet joint surface, and are thought to represent combinations of shear and torsion (White and Panjabi, 1978c). As discussed above, torsion has been thought to be a principal mediator of both upper and lower cervical injury and dislocation (Roaf, 1960). Myers et al. showed that the lower cervical spine is stronger in torsion than the atlantoaxial joint, mitigating torsion as a primary mediator of lower cervical injury. The contribution of torsion in predisposing the lower cervical spine to injury from other types of loading (i.e., flexion), while a common belief, is also in question. The authors believe that the absence of development of significant torques at axial rotations of $\pm 67°$ or less from the neutral position reduce the likelihood of torsion contributing to other types of injuries in real-world accidents (Myers et al., 1989a). Rather, that rotation of the head in injury is frequently the result of a coupled motion of an acutely injured and unstable spine as was observed in the primate deceleration studies of Gosch et al. (1972).

Horizontal Shear

Anterior and posterior atlantoaxial sub-luxations are thought to be the result of shear loading (Braakman and Penning, 1971). The injury can produce either transverse ligament rupture or fracture of the odontoid process (Fig. 14.12). These injuries are frequently unstable and are of considerable importance because of the resulting potentially lethal spinal cord impingement that can occur, and the technical difficulty associated with surgical stabilization of the injury. A true traumatic rupture of the transverse ligament is thought by many not to occur, as the ligament is felt to be stronger than the odontoid process (Werne, 1957). More recent experimental work by Fielding et al. (1974), based on shear loads applied directly to the atlas, suggest that the transverse ligament can fail in posteroanterior

shear loading, prior to odontoid fracture indicating that a traumatic transverse ligament injury could occur. However, direct loading of the cervical spine is extremely rare. Thus a definitive experimental study in which transverse ligament injury is produced by direct loading the head, as would occur in the real accident environment, has not been performed to validate the existence of traumatic transverse ligament failures. Atraumatic tearing of the transverse ligament of the axis occurs in patients with preexisting soft tissue laxity or collagen vascular disease (e.g. rheumatoid arthritis). In these patients, the trauma producing the lesion is minor and the injury is described as a "spontaneous" atlantoaxial dislocation.

Odontoid fracture has been classified clinically by Anderson and D'Alonzo (1974) into three groups. Group I includes avulsion

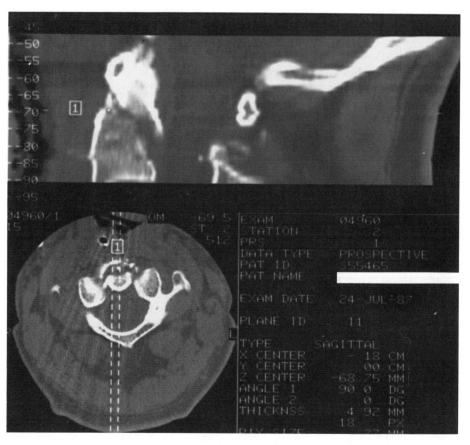

FIGURE 14.12. Type II odontoid fracture seen on axial CT and on midsagittal reconstruction.

fractures of the superiormost tip of the odontoid, group II are fractures through the body of the odontoid, and group III are fractures through the base of the odontoid that extend into the axis vertebral body. Clinically, type I injuries are stable, and type III injuries tend to heal with appropriate immobilization. Type II injuries, however, have a high incidence of nonunion, and surgical repair is recommended. Cadaveric studies of direct shear loading of isolated axis vertebrae by Doherty et al. (1992) suggest that type II fractures tend to be the result of anteroposterior loading, and type III fractures tend to occur in combined antero-posterior and lateral shear loading of the odontoid process. A clinical review of 51 patients with dens fracture by Blockey and Purser (1956) suggested that extreme flexion, extension, or rotation may avulse the odontoid process. They felt that tension in the alar ligaments was responsible for the avulsion. Rogers (1957) presented five cases of undisplaced fractures of the odontoid and suggested the mechanism to be forceful flexion and rotation because of an associated crushing of the superior articular process of C2 on one side. He indicated that posterior fracture dislocation was produced in two cases by forceful hyperextension and in one of these cases "the vertebral arch of the atlas was fractured, evidently by compression against the second cervical vertebra." Anterior fracture dislocation of the dens occurred twice and he suggested that this was produced by a violent shearing force directed anteriorly, the dens being carried forward with the atlas by the transverse ligament. It would appear from these clinical and experimental studies that horizontal shear loading represents the final common pathway of this group of injuries.

Lateral Bending and Lateral Shear

Injuries due to coronal plane motions from lateral bending or lateral shear are considerably less common than those due to loading in the sagittal plane (flexion-extension) (Allen et al., 1982). This is likely due to the relatively lower incidence of lateral loading and the flexibility of the neck in lateral bending.

Experimental studies using whole cadavers in automotive side impact of far-side belted occupants at impact velocities of 50 km/h (30 mph) produced minor injury in only two of seven tests performed (Kallieris and Schmidt, 1990). Lateral bending and lateral shear in combination with other loads are thought to produce the injuries described above with a greater degree of trauma on the side to which the lateral loads are directed (Allen et al., 1982, Harris et al., 1986). Roaf (1963) reported the association of radicular symptoms and bracheal plexus injury with forced lateral bending injury. Lateral shear loading can produce nerve-root avulsion injuries and may also play a role in the type of odontoid fracture produced, as noted above.

Other Fractures

Clay shovelers' fracture is an isolated fracture of the spinous process of the C6, C7, or T1 vertebra (Harris et al., 1986). It is named for its occurrence in people shoveling clay; the clay sticks to the shovel resulting in a whiplash motion of the head with avulsion of the spinous process. Gershon-Cohen et al. (1954) support this finding based on production of the injury in the cadaver following whiplash loading. Harris et al. and others suggest that the lesion is the result of flexion, being produced by tensile loading of the spinous process by the ligamentum nuchae and interspinous and supraspinous ligaments. White and Panjabi (1978c) suggest, however, that the lesion is produced by cyclic muscular loading and not by the action of these ligaments, as the ligaments are of rather limited size and strength. They also suggest, as a rationale for this fatigue mechanism, that clay shovelers were frequently overworked and in poor nutritional status. The lesion has also been thought to occur as a result of direct impingement of one spinous process against another and therefore can also be considered an extension, extension-compression injury. Norton (1962) states that the lesion can also be the result of direct trauma to the spine. Clinically, the lesion is of little significance, as it is associated with neither neurologic deficit nor spinal instability.

Teardrop, or limbus, fractures refer to the bony avulsion of either the anteroinferior or anterosuperior portion of the vertebral body in the lower cervical spine. These fragments were designated as teardrop by Schneiderard Kahn in 1956 '... because of their water droplet appearance in the lateral view on x-ray, and because of the strong emotional component frequently associated with such lesions.'

These fractures can occur in isolation, or in association with ligamentous injury, vertebral burst fractures, and intervertebral disk rupture. The size of the fragment is also highly variable, from as small as a bony chip attached to an avulsed anterior longitudinal ligament, to a large fragment comprising a third of the mass of the vertebral body. Because of the variability of structural injury, a simple relationship between teardrop fractures, spinal stability, and the risk of spinal cord injury does not exist (Torg and Pavlov, 1991). However, the risk for spinal cord injury due to retropulsed bony fragments associated with the presence of a teardrop fracture must always be considered.

An extensive discussion of the etiology of these lesions has occurred over the years based largely, but not exclusively, on subjective evaluation of patient injury data (Babcock, 1976; Barnes, 1948; Braakman and Penning, 1971; Harris et al., 1986; Norton, 1962; Schneider and Kahn, 1956; Torg and Pavlov, 1991; Whitley and Forsyth, 1960). Not surprisingly, then, teardrop fractures have been attributed to nearly every combination of sagittal plane loading including axial compression, compression-flexion, extension-tension, and extension-compression loading of the motion segment. Many authors assert that the anterosuperior teardrop fractures are the result of extension tension (Harris et al., 1986; Whitley and Forsyth, 1960). They also assert that the size of the lesion may also determine the injury mechanism. However, review of the literature reveals a wide variety of mechanisms through which teardrop fractures may be formed, and suggest that the size and geometry of the fragment depends as much on host factors (i.e., local bone strength, ligamentous strength, and the presence of degeneration)

as on the type of applied loading. Thus, generalizations about the injury based solely on the presence of a teardrop fracture are somewhat premature, but when viewed together with other factors may be useful in determining the type of injury produced. The clinical importance of these lesions, therefore, stems from the recognition of their association with other structural injuries and the associated instability and neurologic injury that they can produce.

Activity-Related Injuries and Case Studies

Introduction

Studies of accidents involving serious cervical injuries can provide important information about etiology, injury mechanisms, and human tolerance. The mechanisms of falls and diving accidents are frequently simple enough that many of the parameters can be estimated by calculations or computer-based simulations. Some sports activities, especially football, are videotaped and the body motions involved in the injury are preserved for analysis. Statistical data of automobile injuries is readily available but these accidents are usually too complex for scientific analysis without a great effort.

Many serious neck injuries result in litigation irrespective of the actual responsibility of the defendant because of the tremendous health care costs and loss of income, the great sympathy evoked by a paralyzed person, and the extreme contingency fees afforded the plaintiff's attorney. These litigated injuries usually produce extensive discovery, documentation, accident analysis, and laboratory simulations.

This section describes some of the observations made in the course of investigating serious neck injuries. These investigations generally include:

1. Review of pertinent medical records and x-rays
2. Patient and eyewitness interviews
3. Study of the accident situation

4. Analysis of the impact energies and velocities.

In addition, for those situations where it is felt sufficient information was available, laboratory or mathematical simulations are performed.

Automobile Accidents

Today, automobile accidents are the most common cause of fractures and dislocations of the cervical spine. The impacted structures, force directions, and velocities are extremely varied and result in a wide range of cervical spine injuries. Because of the large numbers involved, it is possible to draw good correlations between the head impact site and the type and level of cervical fracture. Frequently, there are facial or scalp lacerations that can be associated with permanent structural deformations or imprints in the vehicle. However, the vehicle motions and occupant kinematics are usually too complex to allow the detailed analysis required to estimate the impact forces, velocities, and accelerations. Thus, these accidents do not provide much neck tolerance data.

A review of 87 serious neck injuries in automobile and motorcycle accidents (Portnoy, et al., 1971) shows the cervical fracture pattern associated with a head or facial impact site (Table 14.6).

Yoganandan et al. (1989a), in a thorough study of the epidemiology and injury biomechanics of cervical injuries in motor vehicle accidents (MVAs) concluded:

1. Cervical spine injuries from MVAs concentrate in the upper cervical region and around C5–C6 in the lower cervical region.
2. The craniocervical junction and upper regions of the cervical spine (O–C1–C2) are the most common sites of trauma in fatal spinal injury from MVAs.
3. Among survivors with spinal injury from MVAs, the lower cervical spine is a more frequently injured region than the upper cervical spine.
4. A strong association exists between craniofacial injury and serious cervical spine trauma; the overall beneficial role of belt restraint in the reduction of serious cervical spine injuries is most likely due to inhibition of head/face impact with vehicle contact.

Yogandan et al. provided the data shown in Table 14.7 after reviewing 103 automobile accidents with cervical injuries.

Regardless of the circumstance of the accident, in most instances the victim is propelled into head contact with some object. The position of the head and neck, the impact site, the nature of the impacted surface, and the direction of the cervical spine loading

TABLE 14.6. Fracture level—automobile and motorcycle accidents.

Level	Low facial impact extension-tension	High facial impact extension-compression	Head impact flexion-compression
C1	2		
C1–2	9		
C2–3	4		
C2–3–4		2	
C3–4		2	2
C4	1	2	5
C4–5	1	1	6
C4–5–6		3	2
C5		6	12
C5–6		2	7
C5–6–7		1	1
C6		2	7
C6–7			1
C7			
T4–5–6–7			2
Total	17	21	45

TABLE 14.7. Injury score—spinal level.

Spinal level	AIS injury level				
	2	3	4	5	6
C1					1
C2	1	8	1		1
C3		4		1	
C4		4	4	2	
C5	1	5	11	15	
C6		10	9	17	
C7		4	3	2	

determines the resulting cervical fracture. The head and neck is either flexed, neutral, extended, laterally flexed, or rotated, and the cervical spine can be subjected to bending, compression, tension, shear, and/or torque. Impacts about the face and frontal regions tend to produce extension, whereas flexion results from vertex, parietal, or occipital contact. When the impact is off the midline, a lateral flexion and/or torsional component may also be imparted to the head and neck.

Obviously, many combinations of head-neck position, impact site, and cervical spine loading can occur. From a practical standpoint, however, a review of these accidents suggests that in most instances one of the following conditions exists:

1. Head, neck, and torso aligned—cervical spine subjected to compression (compression fractures with possible buckling).
2. Head and neck extended—cervical spine subjected to compression (compression-extension fractures).
3. Head and neck flexed—cervical spine subjected to compression (compression-flexion fractures).
4. Head and neck extended—cervical spine subjected to tension (tension-extension fractures).
5. Lateral loading with axial rotation—(lateral bending).

In a few instances, the head is not impacted and the cervical fracture is the result of direct trauma or impulsive motion of the torso with inertial loading of the neck by the head.

Multiple noncontiguous fractures of cervical spine reported by Spear et al. (1988) also occur in automobile accidents. Why such accidents preferentially injure the lower cervical segments in some, the upper segments in others, and both levels in these cases presumably depends on such factors as the strength and state of the supporting ligaments and muscles and the orientation of the vertebrae at the instant of the injury. In cases of multiple non-contiguous fracture-subluxations of the cervical spine, the trauma must be violent. If one assumes that a fracture-subluxation dissipates the applied traumatic force, the magnitude of the force responsible for multiple non-continuous fracture-subluxations must be very great in order for sufficient force to persist after the first fracture-subluxation to cause a second injury. Alternatively, each injury may be the result of a specific component of the complex traumatic forces.

Illustrative Case Reports

Case 1: (Spear)

A 39-year-old woman sustained an immediate complete motor and sensory quadriplegia at C5 in a motor vehicle accident in which she was the passenger in a vehicle struck broadside on the passenger side. In addition to her spinal injuries, she suffered a closed head injury (GCS 7), facial lacerations, bilateral forearm fractures, and a fractured left acetabulum. Radiographs revealed a burst fracture of the fifth cervical vertebral body with a 25% forward subluxation of C4 on C5, in addition to a fracture of the posterior arch of C1. The cervical spine injuries were managed with initial skeletal traction, followed by a posterior fusion of C3 to C6. The patient's complete sensory and motor paralysis remained unchanged.

Case 2: (Spear)

A 21-year-old man sustained an immediate complete motor and sensory quadriplegia at C7 when he lost control of his car, which struck a tree. Radiographs revealed a 50% forward subluxation of C6 on C7 with fractures through the pedicles of C6. Additionally, there was a type III fracture of the odontoid and a fracture through the anterior arch of C1. The cervical spine injuries were treated with initial skeletal traction, followed by posterior interlaminar and anterior fusion of C5 to C7, with Halo vest immobilization. He improved with some sensory recovery to a complete motor loss with incomplete sensory loss.

Case 3: (Spear)

A 20-year-old intoxicated man sustained an immediate complete motor and sensory loss at C7 when his car overturned in a ditch. Radiographs demonstrated a hangman's fracture in addition to a compression fracture of C7 with a 25% forward subluxation of C6 on C7. His spinal injuries were treated with initial skeletal traction, followed by external immobilization, using a Halo vest and a subsequent anterior decompression and fusion of C6 and C7. He recovered some sensory function.

When a mechanism for a fracture or fracture-dislocation in the cervical spine is sought, the assumption is usually made that there has been loading of the head. However, this may not be the case. In an extensive study, Dr. Donald Huelke identified the "non–head impact" cervical spine injury as occurring more often than previously thought. He reports the following cases.

Case 4: (Huelke)

A 1972 AMC Gremlin two-door coupe was struck in the left side by a 1964 Ford Falcon. Damage was to the driver's door and to the B-pillar immediately behind it. The 17-year-old lap-shoulder–belted male driver (5'7", 157 lb) sustained a dislocation of the atlas from the base of the skull with ligamentous tearing, bruising of the spinal cord, abdominal injuries, and other minor injuries about the body. His fractures of the neck were of a dislocation type; no head contact was indicated by the investigators of this crash.

Case 5: (Huelke)

A 1973 Toyota Corolla four-door turned in the path of a motorcycle. The impact caused the

automobile to roll over onto its right side. The 17-year-old (5'2", 110 lb) lap-shoulder–belted female driver of the Toyota had a fracture of the first cervical vertebra with transection of the medulla, and severe injuries of the pelvis and lower extremities. Also, there were abrasions of the hands and face. This is an example of lateral whiplash injury without any record of head contact.

Motorcycle Accidents

A study of spine injuries in motorcycle accidents by Kupferschmid et al. (1989) reports that of 266 motorcycle accident victims treated at the Allegheny General Hospital, 13 cases of thoracic spine fractures, 4 cases of cervical spine fractures, and 2 cases of lumbar spine fractures were identified. The association of cervical and thoracic injuries (i.e., multiple noncontiguous fractures) is a common finding in motorcycle accidents. This is likely the result of the high kinetic energy of the victim and the kinematics. The typical accident situation associated with this injury involves the victim somersaulting over the handlebars of the motorcycle and landing on his/her head, shoulders, or upper back (Fig. 14.13). Thus, the victim may experience significant impact to the head and the upper thorax.

In many motorcycle accidents, the helmet can provide a unique opportunity to improve our understanding of human tolerance and recreate the injury mechanism. Specifically, in many helmets, a clearly discernible crush area in the Styrofoam helmet liner and a characteristic imprinting of the helmet shell at the point of impact are observed. Since the liner provides a permanent record of the impact pressure on the head, researchers have been studying methods of interpreting it. As an example, compression tests have been made in 10 Exemplar helmets in an attempt to duplicate the liner crush that occurred in an accident. Loads of 1,400 to 1,800 lb were required to approximate the crush patterns. This is a crude first attempt to establish neck tolerance in this way, but the method offers considerable promise. We are currently exploring finite element models of the helmet liner so as to

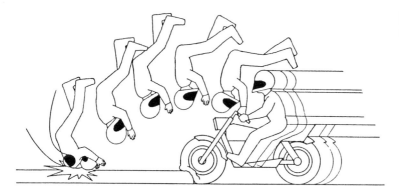

FIGURE 14.13. Motorcycle vaulting accident.

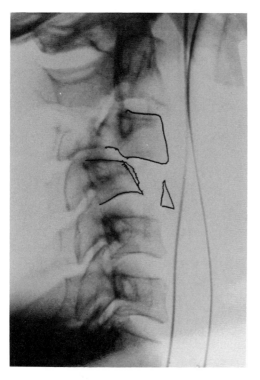

FIGURE 14.14. Severe flexion-compression injury from motorcycle vaulting accident.

better define the sources of error, sensitivity, and accuracy of this method.

Case 6: (McElhaney)

A 27-year-old man riding a motorcycle struck the side of a car at approximately 30 mph. The victim vaulted over the car and tumbled and rolled approximately 50 feet. He was wearing a helmet, suffered no head injury, and was conscious and lucid after the accident. He suffered a 2-cm anterior subluxation of C3 on C4, a mild compression fracture of C4, a significantly displaced teardrop fracture of the anterior margin of C4, which was avulsed about 1 cm forward of the body of C4, and bilateral fractures through the pedicles of C3. In addition, unilateral facet dislocations on the right side of C7, T1, and T2, and a fracture of the lamina of T2 on the left side was observed on x-rays (Fig. 14.14). He survived the accident with a high-level complete spinal cord lesion.

Football

Much of this section is a summary of the writings of Joseph S. Torg and Richard C. Schneider who have studied football-induced head and neck injuries for many years. With the introduction of the modern football helmet, coaches and players assumed head and neck protection, and a new style of blocking and tackling was developed that used the head to spear the opposition. The incidence of serious cervical spine injuries increased dramatically. Torg and Schneider correctly analyzed the cause of this increase and assisted in initiating a rule change prohibiting the use of head-first blocking and tackling. The most common injury mechanism identified by Torg was "axial compression." His analysis showed that this mechanism caused the highest percentage of football cervical fracture and dislocations with and without quadriplegia. From 1971 to 1975, 39% of nonquadriplegic cervical spine injuries and 52% of the quadriplegic injuries were attributed to this mechanism. During the years between 1976 and 1987, 52.5% of the quadriplegic injuries and 49% of the nonquadriplegic cervical spine injuries were caused by the same mechanism. Documentation of axial loading as an important mechanism of injury in the production of catastrophic football cervical spine injuries was obtained by the review of game films of actual injuries. Interestingly, Schneider identified a wide variety of injury mechanisms in his studies. The case studies that follow are quite valuable because they illustrate a number of injury mechanisms, and they are extremely well documented by the game film and medical records.

Case 7: (Schneider)

While carrying the ball, a high school football halfback received a neck injury when two tacklers held his arms at his side as he fell with his neck flexed and his head bent downward. A third opponent struck the group so that the ball carrier fell forward with the neck so completely flexed that both shoulders rested directly on the ground. The halfback had an immediate complete paralysis of all four extremities with a total loss of sensation, for a few minutes after injury, in his lower extremities. Between the time of injury and admission to his community hospital, the patient gradually recovered all motor function and only noted pain and tingling radiating along the inner aspect of his forearms. Five weeks later, a neurosurgical examination revealed some right triceps paresis and weakness of his interosseus muscles. X-rays of the cervical spine demonstrated bilateral facet dislocation of C6 on C7 with marked vertebral subluxation. A fracture of the lateral mass of C7 and possible C6 vertebral fracture was demonstrated.

Comment. This injury occurred in the position of forced cervical flexion and the football player was extremely fortunate not to have transected his cervical spinal cord. Initially, he sustained an acute cervical cord injury and recovered complete function except for a residual C7 nerve root impairment. Flexion

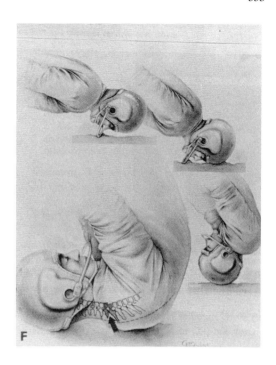

FIGURE 14.15. Melvin's hyperflexion mechanism through the face mask catching in soft ground.

injuries of the cervical spine in football are more frequent than is usually recognized. In Canadian football, Melvin, as in Schneider (1973), has described a similar mechanism of cervical hyperflexion due to the single-bar face guard catching on the ground. With "forced flexion" they sustained fracture-dislocation injuries (Fig. 14.15).

Case 8: (McElhaney)

A 20-year-old college football player attempted to tackle a charging ball carrier. Just prior to this attempt a teammate hit the ball carrier at an angle, causing him to tumble forward (Fig. 14.16). The tackler struck the back of the now upside-down ball carrier with his head, neck, and torso in line. A severe compression-flexion dislocation resulted with complete neurologic deficit below the C4–5 level.

Comment. An analysis of the game film showed a closing velocity between the tackler's head and the ball carrier's back of 14 feet per second. With the axial alignment of the head,

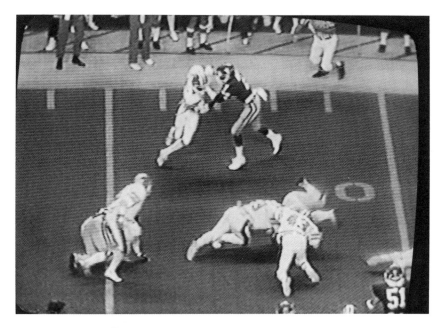

FIGURE 14.16. Flexion-compression injury.

neck, and torso, the stage was set for a catastropic injury. The situation was compounded by a strap placed by the equipment manager between the face mask and shoulder pads to reduce the risk of an extension injury.

Case 9: (McElhaney)

This accident involved a ball carrier who was tackled and lying flat on his back. A late tackler struck the ball carrier's head with his knee, dramatically flexing the neck forward and to the right. The impact was severe enough to disrupt the spinous ligaments and cause a unilateral facet dislocation of C5, with sufficient anterior subluxation to disrupt the spinal cord (Fig. 14.17).

Comment. This injury mechanism is an unusual example of the relatively common knee-to-head injury mechanism (Fig. 14.18). Schneider notes that this injury often occurs on kickoffs and punt returns where fast running and high driving knees are more common. This particular injury is unusual in that complete cord transection occurs in only 12% of unilateral facet dislocations.

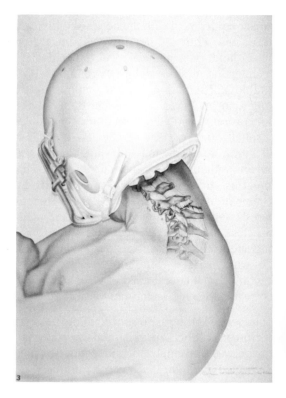

FIGURE 14.17. Off-axis bending due to knee impact with rear of head.

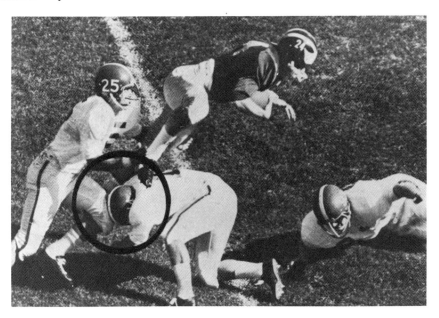

FIGURE 14.18. Football knee-to-head accident.

Gymnastics

Unlike football, where the predominant mechanism of catastrophic cervical spine injuries involves axial compression, gymnastic injuries usually have a much larger flexion component. Many of these injuries present unilateral or bilateral dislocations with no compression of the vertebral body or disk space. This is due to a variety of factors. Gymnasts usually intend to forward roll or somersault on impact. As a result, they tend to tuck their heads at impact, increasing the effective moment arm and flexion moment due to the axial load. In addition, they usually strike their heads on a mat that cushions the axial compression force but provides a pocket, constraining motion of the head. Under these conditions the head is stopped and fixed by the mat and the trampoline, and the torso continues moving, forcing the neck into a serpentine configuration.

No firm conclusions can be drawn from the literature regarding any clearly definable pathology patterns. In 58 cases in which the level of the lesion is determined, however, the distribution is as follows: C-1, 2 cases; C2-3, 1 case; C3-4, no cases; C4-5, 21 cases; C5-6, 31 cases; C6-7, 1 case; and C-7 to T-1, 2 cases. With regard to pathology type, a variety of lesions have been reported: vertebral body compression and burst fractures, facet dislocations and subluxations without fractures, and fracture-dislocations. It appears that irreversible injury to the spinal cord can occur with various injury patterns at any level of the cervical spine, but dislocations at the C4-5 and C5-6 level are most likely (90%).

Case 10: (McElhaney)

This accident involved a university varsity gymnast who somersaulted from a trampoline into a 5-ft pit filled with foam pieces. He suffered a C4-5 dislocation with bilateral locked facets and a complete cord lesion. Experiments with an instrumented volunteer showed torso deceleration of less than 5g when diving into the foam pit in a heads-up attitude (Fig. 14.19).

Case 11: (McElhaney)

A high school boy was participating in an olympic mud diving contest, which involved running on a board and diving into an 18-inch-

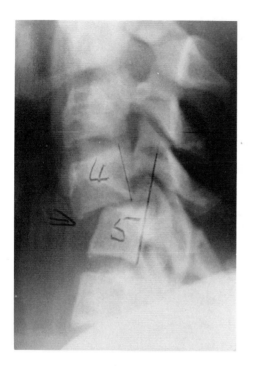

FIGURE 14.19. Severe flexion injury from gymnastic tumbling accident.

deep, specially constructed mud pit. This case is somewhat unique because a photographer took a very clear flash photograph at the instant of impact. The victim had his head flexed with the chin against the sternum. He sustained a C4–5 dislocation and a splitting or bursting of the body of C5 with a complete cord lesion (Fig. 14.20).

Case 12: (McElhaney)

A middle-aged man dove head first on a toy known as a "Slip and Slide." This is a plastic sheet that is spread on the ground and sprinkled with water. Children are encouraged to dive onto this slippery surface and slide on their chest. The victim struck his face with sufficient force to produce a posterior dislocation of C5 on C6 and a central splitting of the body of C6. Witnesses were certain that he did not strike the top of his head. He suffered incomplete sensory and motor loss.

Comment. The rearward dislocation of C5 on C6 is a result of the shearing action of his face against the relatively flat ground and the torso motion. The inability of the head to freely extend is a major factor in this injury. It is not clear, however, what caused the central splitting of the body of C6 as shown in the computed tomography scan. The author has studied two other neck injuries to adult males that occurred on this device.

Diving

A multidisciplinary team led by M. Alexander Gabrielsen, including this author, has studied

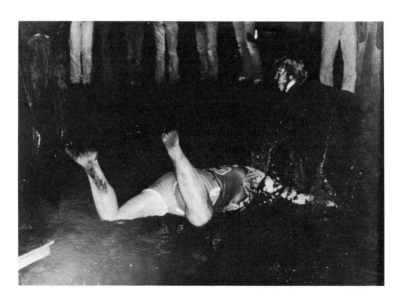

FIGURE 14.20. Mud diving accident.

TABLE 14.8. Level of injury.

Level	Male	Female	Total
C-1	2	1	3
C-1,2	3	0	3
C-2	1	0	1
C-2,3	1	0	1
C-3	1	0	1
C-3,4	6	0	6
C-4	6	0	6
C-4,5	37	4	41
C-5	88	18	106
C-5,6	92	21	113
C-6	17	1	18
C-6,7	26	7	33
C-7	3	0	3
T-1	1	0	1
T-1,2	1	0	1
T-1,3	1	0	1
T-5,6	0	1	1
T-6,7	1	0	1
Some neurological impact	9	2	11
Brain hemorrhage	1	1	2
Fx: Skull	2	1	3
Fx: Jaw	0	1	1
Fx: Shoulder	1	0	1
Total	300	58	358

486 diving injuries. Of this number, 360 occurred in pools and 126 occurred in a natural environment. The pool-related injuries included 76 from dives from springboards, 194 from dives into in-ground pools, and 90 in above-ground pools. The most-frequent site of injury was C-5 and C5–6 with 219 (60.8%) of the injuries occurring at those locations. These injuries were predominantly compression-flexion injuries. Table 14.8 shows the distribution of the injury level.

It is remarkable how few skull fractures and brain injuries occur in diving even though in many of these accidents the head strikes a concrete pool bottom. It is also noteworthy to consider the number of dives made into swimming pools that lead to these injuries. There are approximately seven million swimming pools in the United States. In 1989 the United States Consumer Product Safety Commission summarized the diving problem as follows: Approximately 700 spinal cord diving injuries are estimated to occur in the United States annually as a result of recreational diving into residential pools, public pools, and

other bodies of water. It has been further estimated that there are approximately 200,000 people presently living in the United States who have suffered traumatic spinal cord injury and that diving may account for 9% to 10% of them. The mean life expectancy for these spinal cord injury victims is estimated at 30.2 years.

Spinal cord injuries (SCIs) from all types of sports represent 14.2% of the annual total SCIs (7,900 total survivors). Recreational diving is estimated at 54% to 66% of these, which is nearly twice as much as all other sports combined including football, surfing, gymnastics, skiing, trampoline, horseback riding, etc. The National Swimming Pool Foundation states that 9 out of 10 diving injuries occur in 6 ft of water or less. The conclusion is that only a very small fraction of dives result in a serious cervical injury. However, there are a very great number of dives made each year and therefore a significant number of catastrophic injuries.

Approximately half of diving injuries occur in rivers, lakes, and oceans, according to John S. Young. The distribution of the injury level in these dives shows a similar clustering at the C5 and C5–6 levels (Gabrielson, 1990).

A general observation is that these injuries include fewer compression and more flexion injuries than the in-pool injuries. This is probably related to the much softer bottoms in the natural environment and because many of these injuries were to divers who launched themselves from the water bottom while running on the beach or lake bottom. Estimated depth of water where the victim struck the bottom, was derived from statements of witnesses (Tables 14.9 and 14.10). In 23 (18.3%) of the accidents the impact depth was 2 ft or less. In 107 (84.9%) of the accidents the water was 4 ft deep or less.

Sixty-seven of the diving accidents reported by Gabrielson have been reconstructed by McElhaney et al. (1979) by observing anthropometrically similar volunteers performing the same dives in deeper water. These include shallow water dives from the edge of the pool, springboard dives, and head-first entry from a water slide. Dive kinematics where quantified

TABLE 14.9. Level of injury.

Level	Male	Female	Total
C-1	1	0	1
C-2,3	1	0	1
C-3	1	0	1
C-4	0	2	2
C-4,5	6	0	6
C-5	45	3	48
C-5,6	41	1	42
C-6	4	0	4
C-6,7	11	1	12
C-7	3	0	3
T-1,2	0	1	1
T-3	1	0	1
Some neurological impact	2	1	3
Paraplegia	1	0	1
Total	117	9	126

TABLE 14.10. Number of injuries vs. water depth.

Depth	Number	Depth	Number
0'00"	2	3'01"–3'06"	22
0'06"	1	3'07"–4'00"	15
0'07"–1'00"	1	4'01"–4'06"	11
1'01"–1'06"	11	4'07"–5'00"	3
1'07"–2'00"	8	5'01"–5'06"	1
2'01"–2'06"	17	5'07"–6'00"	3
2'07"–3'00"	30	10'00"	1

using 200 frame/sec film and a grid placed behind the diver (Fig. 14.21). In this way, a lower bound for critical head impact velocity resulting in cervical injury has been developed. Based on these studies, in a clear dive hydro-

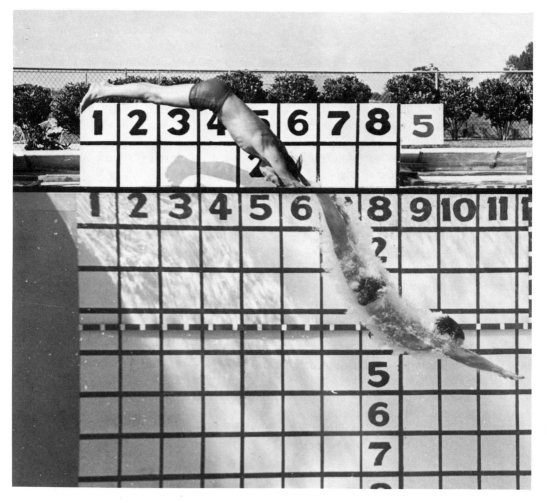

FIGURE 14.21. Diving accident reconstruction.

TABLE 14.11. Head speeds.

Depth (ft)	Head speed (ft/sec)	Depth (ft)	Head speed (ft/sec)
0.5	14.0	4.0	11.2
1.0	14.4	4.5	9.7
1.5	14.9	5.0	8.4
2.0	15.3	5.5	7.2
2.5	15.7	6.0	7.0
3.0	14.3	6.5	6.8
3.5	12.8		

dynamic drag generally does not start to slow the diver's in-water speed to values less than that at water entry until a significant portion of the diver's body is immersed. On the order of one-half to three-fourths of the body must be in the water when executing a clean dive before deceleration commences. Indeed, under the action of gravity, the diver's in-water head speed increases for the first few feet of penetration. Table 14.11 shows the head velocity versus water depth for a typical dive with an entry angle of 45°. In this dive, the diver's maximum in-water speed was not achieved until the top of the head reached a depth of 2.5 ft, or about 42 inches of the diver's body was immersed in the water. The speed of the diver's head was nearly the same as at water entry when about 55 inches of the diver's body was immersed.

For dives from the edge of the pool, fall heights ranged from 116 cm (3.8 ft) to 219 cm (7.2 ft) (Fig. 14.22). Estimated head impact speeds ranged from 3.11 m/sec (10.2 ft/sec) to 6.55 m/sec (21.5 ft/sec). Springboard and platform dives had a wide range of fall heights and water depths; however, impact velocities remained between 3.8 m/sec (12.5 ft/sec) and 8.1 m/sec (26.5 ft/sec). Head-first entry from a water slide has the potential for neck injury when, instead of skimming across the surface, the head and hands are lowered and a snap roll or tumble occurs. Head impact velocities for the snap-roll mode range from 3.57 m/sec (11.7 ft/sec) to 4.94 m/sec (16.2 ft/sec).

It is clear from the number and severity of the accidents presented here that diving or head-first sliding into shallow water is potentially very dangerous and should be actively discouraged. The snap-roll motion

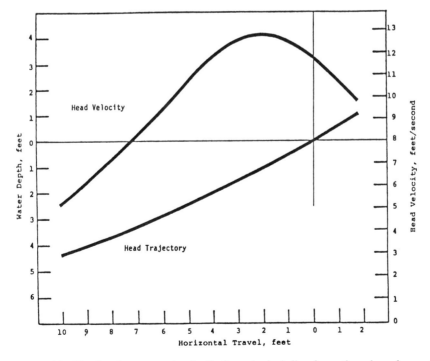

FIGURE 14.22. Head trajectory and velocity for a typical dive from the edge of a pool.

probably occurred in many of these accidents. Keeping the head and hands up and the back arched is critical in shallow water diving.

As noted, the neck injuries observed in diving are amazingly similar. There were only two head injuries, and no facial trauma was reported in the study. In the head-down impacts that probably occurred in the majority of these accidents, the forces were less than that required to cause head trauma but because of the body driving into the neck, catastrophic neck injuries occurred. In the head-up configuration, the face will impact the pool bottom with a glancing blow. Of course, this happens in the swimming pool environment. But the lack of serious, reported head and neck injuries connected with facial impacts indicates that the velocity range associated with diving is less than critical for this extension mode of injury.

The results therefore indicate that flexion-compression injuries can occur with head impacts in a diving mode at velocities greater than 10 ft/sec, where the head is suddenly stopped and the neck must stop the torso.

Experimental Studies

Simulated Injuries with Cadavers

This section reviews a variety of studies in which cervical injuries were caused to occur in whole, unembalmed cadavers. This type of experimental simulation is very valuable in developing head-neck kinematic data with potentially injurious excursions and to measure force and acceleration levels associated with various injury mechanisms.

Nusholtz et al. (1983) performed impacts to the vertex of 12 unembalmed cadavers. A guided 56 kg impactor was used with impact velocities of 4.6 to 5.6 m/sec. The impactor had a padded surface and incorporated a biaxial load cell. Extension-compression cervical injury occurred with the necks buckling in extension or flexion. Head impact loads ranged from 1.8 to 11.1 kN. Nusholtz et al. also performed free-fall drop tests on eight unembalmed cadavers with the initial impact to the crown of the head.

Drop heights that varied from 0.8 to 1.8 m produced extensive cervical and thoracic fractures and dislocations. Head impact forces varied from 3.2 to 10.8 N. Nusholtz et al. drew a variety of conclusions from cadaver tests that are still quite valid:

1. The initial orientation of the spine is a critical factor in influencing the type of response and damage produced. Some of these aspects are:
   A. The degree of involvement of the thoracic spine depends on its initial orientation with respect to the impact axis. Damage can be produced as low as the fourth thoracic vertebra.
   B. The initial cervical spinal orientation can affect the resulting motion of the head. It also influences the relative magnitude and nature of the forces produced by the neck on the head.
   C. The orientation of the spinal elements can have an effect on the type of damage produced. Flexion damage seems to be influenced by a combination of both cervical and thoracic spinal orientation.
2. Descriptive motion of the head relative to the torso is not a good indicator of neck damage. Flexion damage can occur with extension motion, and extension damage can occur with flexion motion.
3. Under high loads (9,000 N), the head response is three-dimensional in nature and must be characterized by translation and rotation.
4. Energy-absorbing materials are effective methods for reducing peak impact force but do not necessarily reduce the amount of energy transferred to the head, neck, and torso or the damage produced in a cadaver model.
5. The complex nature of cervical spine kinematics and damage patterns in crown impact may preclude the determination of a single tolerance criterion such as maximum force.

Alem et al. (1984) conducted two series of impacts to the heads of 19 unembalmed cadavers in the superior-inferior direction.

They used a 10 kg impactor that struck the vertex of the head approximately in line with the spinal axis at speeds between 7 and 11 m/sec. In most of the tests, the impactor was paddled with 5-cm thick Ensolite foam to control the duration of the contact force and to minimize local skull fractures. Compression fractures and tearing of the anterior longitudinal ligaments occurred with impact forces of 3,000 to 6,000 N.

Cheng et al. (1982) tested six unembalmed cadavers by applying a distributed frontal load to the chest through a predeployed driver air-bag system. A sled was used to apply decelerations of 32g to 39g. Severe neck injuries were found in four of the six cadavers. Observed cervical injuries included C1–C2 fracture dislocations, ligament tears, ring fractures, and cord transections.

Lange (1971) performed 15 simulations of frontal collisions with cadavers placed on automobile bucket seats and three-point seat belts. Head accelerations were measured with an instrumented helmet. Sled accelerations varied from 20g to 27g, while torso acceleration varied from 22g to 51g. In 10 of these tests a steering wheel was in front of the cadavers and the head hit the wheel. A variety of neck injuries were observed including fracture of the dens, disk, ligament ruptures, and vertebral body fractures. Another five head-on collisions were simulated without a steering wheel. Chest accelerations ranged from 28g to 47g. More extensive tearing of cervical ligaments was observed with head rotations as large as 123°. Eight cadavers were tested in rear-end simulations with sled accelerations ranging from 19g to 29g and helmet accelerations between 24g and 47g. No head rest was used and extreme hyperextension was observed. Cervical tension-extension injuries were quite varied, ranging from minor to severe.

Yoganandan et al. (1986) conducted a study to evaluate the mechanism of spinal injuries with vertical impact. Sixteen fresh, intact, human male cadavers were suspended head down and dropped vertically from a height of 0.9 to 1.5 m. In 8 of the 16 specimens, the head was restrained to simulate the effect of muscle tone. The head-neck complexes of the specimens were suitably oriented to achieve maximal axial loading of the cervical spine. Head-impact forces ranged from 3,000 N to 7,100 N in the unrestrained and from 9,800 N to 14,700 N in the restrained specimens. There were more upper thoracic and cervical fractures in the restrained compared to the unrestrained cases. High-speed films (16-mm) taken at 1,000 frames/sec revealed that upper thoracic fractures occurred primarily due to the bending of the thoracic spine. Cervical vertebral body damage was observed most commonly when the cadavers remained in contact with the impacting surface without substantial rotation or rebound. This caused the neck to be a major element in stopping the torso motion.

One important factor, not well controlled in all of these studies, is the degree of head fixation. When the head is free to rotate on the condyles, bending of the neck occurs with minimal compression. When head rotation is constrained, bending of the neck is restricted and the system becomes much stiffer. The factors that influence head motion are the stiffness and conformability of the impacting surface and the cadaver head. Another factor that cannot be controlled is the extent to which failure progresses. A certain amount of kinetic energy is available and failures progress until this energy is dissipated. It is these factors as well as lack of muscle action that make interpretation of injury mechanisms from cadaver tests difficult.

Excised Cervical Spinal Properties

Characterization of the mechanical properties of the cervical spine remains a challenge to biomedical engineers. The spine is a segmented structure composed of nonlinear viscoelastic elements and kinematic elements. The motions of the spine are coupled and the local deformations of the various elements produce large strains. Efforts to characterize this complex structure have included *in vivo* range of motion, cadaveric whole spines, motion segments, and isolated spinal ligament studies. Methodologies of evaluation have also

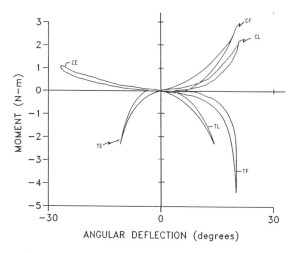

FIGURE 14.23. Cervical spine bending responses.

been highly varied, and include instrumented volunteer decelerations, quasi-static flexibility studies of isolated motion segments, and static and dynamic stiffness of whole spines. Limitations in these methods are numerous and include primarily the method of reporting data. As an example, consider Fig. 14.23 showing the flexion moment–angle relationship for a whole spine in combined bending. Clearly the use of a single value to describe the stiffness/flexibility of this structure is inadequate. Thus, mechanical properties must include the method of derivation in order to be meaningful. The interpretation of mechanical data is made more complex by the realization that with large strains and deformations, the anatomic or material axis deviates significantly from the spatial axis system. Thus, reported values of stiffness must state the formulation used in applying and measuring loads [i.e., Lagrangian (material) or Eulerian (spatial) coordinate systems]. Notwithstanding these limitations, significant contributions to understanding spinal structural properties have been made.

Compression, Compression-Flexion, Compression-Extension

Probably the earliest empirical study of excised spine properties was Messerer's (1880) work on the mechanical properties of the vertebrae.

He reported compressive breaking loads ranging from 1.47 to 2.16 kN (330 to 486 lb) in his extensive compilation on the strength of biological tissues, and he provided data on the static load-deflection properties of the vertebral bodies and discs. Roaf (1960) loaded single cervical spinal units in compression, extension, flexion, lateral flexion, horizontal shear, and rotation. He found that the intact disc, which failed at approximately 7.12 kN (1,600 lb), was more resistant to compression than wet vertebrae, which failed at approximately 6.23 kN (1,400 lb). Selecki and Williams (1970) conducted an extensive study of cadaveric cervical spines loaded with a manually operated hydraulic jack. Unfortunately, they monitored the pressure in the hydraulic line and reported their results in terms of hydraulic pressure without indicating the ram piston diameter. They were able, however, to duplicate several types of clinically observed injuries. White et al. (1975) measured rotation and translation of the upper vertebra as a function of transection of the components in single units of the cervical spine. Liu and Krieger (1978) reported load-deflection responses from axial compression tests on single cervical spinal units. Sances et al. (1982) tested isolated cadaver cervical spines in compression, tension, and shear. A quasi-static compression failure was observed at a load of 645 N (145 lb) and dynamic flexion-compression failures were reported at loads ranging from 1.78 to 4.45 kN (400 to 1,000 lb).

Pintar et al. (1990), in a carefully designed experiment, measured the compression failure loads of seven excised cervical spines separated at the T2–T3 junction and including the bottom half of the skull. Axial compression, compression-flexion, and compression-extension quasi-static failure mechanisms occurred with compressive loads of 1,355 to 3613 N. Compressive deformation to the maximum load point ranged from 9 to 37 mm. Composite before and after lateral views of the specimens were constructed from x-rays to demonstrate failure buckling modes. Pintar et al. continued these studies with six additional specimens. The head was intact and loads were applied through the vertex of the skull. The head was stabilized through a weight and pulley system. High-speed loading rates of 295 to 813 cm/sec were achieved. Compressive failure loads of 1,177 to 6193 N were measured. Failure mechanisms included wedge compressions and burst fractures and were quite similar to those observed clinically. Except for studies by Fielding et al. (1974) Liu and Krieger (1978), Pintar (1986), and Sances et al. (1984), all of these tests were quasi-static and most researchers recorded only the maximum load. Thus, the viscoelastic, rate-dependent, effects that result in higher failure loads and different failure mechanisms (burst fractures vs. simple crushing) have not been well studied.

The results of a study by McElhaney et al. (1983a) on compression tests of whole cervical spines are presented in some detail because it demonstrates the effects of viscoelasticity and initial position on the failure load, injury mechanism, stiffness, and energy to failure measurements in cervical spine testing.

Load relaxation, the decrease in load with constant deformation, is indicative of the prominence of viscoelastic effects. Figure 14.24 shows a typical relaxation test for a human cervical spine. This figure demonstrates the differences in load (approximately 70%) that would be observed between high test rates and quasi-static tests.

In addition, a variable rate of load relaxation was demonstrated. Initially, the load decay was extremely rapid. Thereafter, the load decayed at a much slower rate. This observation renders a standard lumped parameter

viscoelastic model with a single dominant long-term time constant a poor predictor of neck behavior. Instead, a generalized Maxwell-Weichert model must be used since it incorporates an ensemble of associated time constants.

Deformation rate sensitivity of structural stiffness is another measure of viscoelastic effects. Varying load rate by a factor of 500 resulted in a change in stiffness from 1,285 to 2,250 N/cm for a single specimen. This behavior may be characterized by a generalized quasi-linear viscoelastic Maxwell-Weichert model (Fig. 14.25).

In addition to having a significant component of viscoelasticity, the spine also demonstrates a second component of time dependence—preconditioning. Following larger periods (hours) of inactivity, additional fluid is absorbed by the soft tissues of the spine, placing it in a stiffened state called the fully reequilibrated state. Following activity this additional fluid is extruded from the structure and the stiffness of the structure decreases. Eventually, a steady state is reached in which subsequent activity does not produce a change in stiffness. This is the mechanically stabilized or preconditioned state. Defining the cyclic modulus as the peak load over the peak deflection during sinusoidal loading, the cyclic modulus of the mechanically stabilized state ranged from 45% to 55% of the fully reequilibrated state. Given that most individuals are continually active, all structural testing should be performed in the mechanically stabilized state.

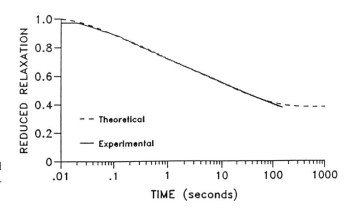

FIGURE 14.24. Experimental and exponential-integral model of relaxation modulus of the cervical spine.

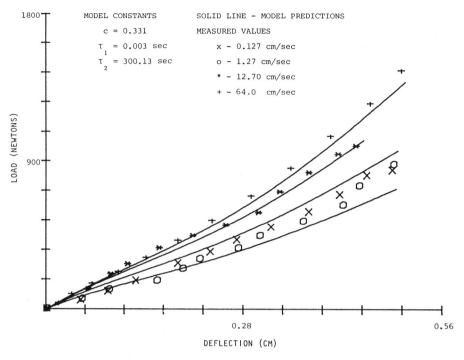

FIGURE 14.25. Rate sensitivity of cervical spine in compression.

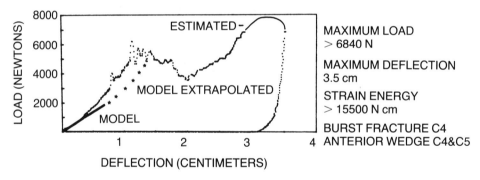

FIGURE 14.26. Compression load vs. deflection of human cadaveric cervical spine.

Careful control of the initial position of the base of the skull reveals that the injury mechanism is profoundly influenced by this variable in compressive loading. Defining the initial position of the spine as an erect (vertical) structure with the resting lordosis removed and using ram velocities of 64 cm/sec resulted in compression injuries. These included multipart atlas fractures, and lower cervical vertebral body compression and burst fractures. Figure 14.26 shows a typical compressive load to failure test.

Using the same test frame but moving the base of the skull 1 cm posteriorly resulted in an apex anterior buckle with posterior element fractures and anterior longitudinal ligament rupture. The injuries are consistent with the compression-extension injury classification. In contrast, moving the base of the skull 1 cm anteriorly produced a rearward buckle of the structure with lower cervical wedge compression fractures consistent with the compression-flexion injury classification.

Thus, by careful alignment of the initial

TABLE 14.12. Mean cervical bending stiffness (N-m/rad) for flexion (F), extension (E), and lateral bending (L) combined with compression (C) or tension (T), using two thoracic end conditions (fixed or pinned).

	Human											
	Fixed-pinned						Pinned-pinned					
	K_0			K_∞			K_0			K_∞		
Modes	Mean	σ	N	Mean	σ	N	Mean	σ	N	Mean	σ	N
CF	36.9	6.9	3	31.8	4.7	3						
TF							10.5		1	7.0		1
CE							2.4	0.4	3	1.8	0.3	3
TE	67.5		1	58.0		1	7.1		1	4.5		1
CL	6.0	1.7	3	3.3	0.4	3	2.0	0.5	3	1.0	0.2	2
TL							9.3		1	6.4		1

position over a range of 2 cm, it is possible to change the outcome from compression-extension to compression-flexion. Perhaps this is the reason there is such a wide range of responses to cervical spine compression in the relevant literature.

The flexion, extension, and lateral bending responses of whole cadaver cervical spines were investigated by McElhaney et al. (1988). Using a test frame, the bending stiffness was measured in six modes of loading from tension-extension through compression-flexion. Typical moment-angle curves are shown in Fig. 14.23, and Table 14.12 reports the mean bending stiffness for two thoracic end conditions, fixed and pinned.

Tension

A number of studies have been performed on isolated components and motion segments in the cervical spine. Isolated intervertebral disks were studied by Pintar (1986), who reported a mean tensile stiffness of 68 kN/m as the average stiffness of the cervical intervertebral disk. The results of Coffee et al. (1987), while insufficient to allow for statistical evaluation, show that tensile stiffness of one and two motion segment units are betweeen 10% and 20% of the measured compressive stiffness. Liu et al. (1980) report a tensile stiffness of single motion segments as 590 kN/m in data collected from young male cadavers. The effect of load magnitude on reported stiffness is apparent in the following studies. Panjabi et al. (1986) report single cervical motion segment

tensile stiffness of 53 kN/m when loaded with 25 N. Recent work by Shea et al. (1991) reports the tensile stiffness of midcervical (C2–C5) and lower cervical specimens (C5-T1) as 229 kN/m and 157 kN/m, respectively, when loaded with a 100-N load. The authors also note an increase in tensile stiffness with increasing applied load such that the midcervical stiffness increased to 433 kN/m with a tensile load of 300 N. While Panjabi et al. tested single motion segments and Shea et al. tested multiple motion segments, the stiffening effects with increasing load are apparent.

Few studies are available on the mechanical properties of the whole cervical spine in tension. Sances et al. (1982) report tensile load to failure of 10 cadaveric whole cervical spines (O-T3). Tensile axial load to failure varied from 1446 to 1940 N and load rates were varied from quasi-static to 142 cm/sec. Shea et al. (in press) in a soon-to-be-published study of combined extension-tension, report tensile load to failure in specimens with an initial 30° of extension tested at slow rates. Using peak load and peak deflection from this study, the tensile stiffness was 33.1 ± 18.6 kN/m.

Lateral Bending

Range of motion of the cadaver cervical spine were reported by Lysell (1969) and by White and Panjabi (1978a) as 8° for the occipito-atlantal joint, no lateral bending in the atlanto-axial joint, 10° in the middle cervical, and 4° and 8° in the lower cervical spine. Total range of motion and muscle strength measurements in lateral bending have been reported by Schneider et al. (1975) in volunteer studies. He reported a total of 71.0° of lateral bending; no significant differences were observed with sex, and a significant decrease was observed in range of motion with age from 86° at ages 18 to 24 to approximately 52° at ages 62 to 74.

Using volunteer deceleration data from the Naval Biodynamics Laboratory (NBDL), Bowman et al. (1984) reported the lateral bending stiffness of the cervical spine. Treating the cervical spine as pinned joints at the cranial-cervical and the cervical-thoracic junction connected by a rigid linkage, they determined the cranial-cervical stiffness as 3.74 N-m/degree, and the cervical-thoracic stiffness as 2.71 N-m/degree. Similar NBDL data presented by Wismans and Spenny (1983) show a lateral bending stiffness of approximately 1.6 N-m/degree for cranial-cervical junction. In a more recent study of volunteers, Wismans et al. (1986) reported a linear stiffness for the cervical-thoracic junction as 2.2 N-m/degree and the cranial-cervical junction as 0.4 N-m/degree. Goel et al. (1990) performed a study of isolated cadaver upper cervical spines and observed 4.2° and 3.4° of motion in the atlantoaxial and occipitoatlantal joints, respectively, when subjected to 0.3 N-m moment applied quasi-statically.

Torsion

Range of motion studies have been performed by various authors, using a variety of test systems. Total range of motion in rotation has been reported from 106° (Goldsmith, 1983) to 151° (Foust et al., 1971), with typical results near 130°. The occipitoatlantal joint is irrotational (Werne, 1957). In contrast, the atlantoaxial joint shows striking mobility at very low torques, accounting for more than 50% of cervical axial rotation, producing approximately 40° to 60° (White and Panjabi, 1978b). In the lower cervical spine, large variances in range of motion with spinal level, and from subject to subject, have been observed; however, a typical lower cervical segment rotates approximately 8° to 10° (White and Panjabi, 1978c).

While a considerable portion of the literature has been devoted to the characterization of the dynamic responses of the cervical spine to loading in the sagittal plane and in the coronal plane, only a few references are available that describe the axial rotation-torque responses of the head-neck system. Volunteer sled tests performed at the NBDL report a rotational stiffness of 0.339 N-m/degree (reported in Bowman et al., 1984). Wismans and Spenny (1983) report a piecewise linear representation of the torque-angle response produced from volunteer sled deceleration tests in the lateral direction. Mean stiffnesses were reported as 0 N-m/degree for 0° to 10° of axial rotation from the neutral position, 0.5 N-m/degree for 10° to 30°, and 0.25 N-m/degree for rotations greater than 30°. Subsequent reports from these authors list the stiffness as varying from 0.4 N-m/degree in lateral impacts to 0.75 N-m/degree in oblique impacts. Myers et al. (1989), using cadaveric specimens loaded dynamically to failure at 500°/sec, also represented the torque-angle response of the cervical spine with a piecewise linear model with an initial zero stiffness region, and a high stiffness region with a mean stiffness of 0.472 ± 0.147 N-m/degree beginning at 66.8° ± 6.2° of rotation. The influence of the musculature on the torsional response can be determined by comparing the results of Myers et al. (1989) with those of Wismans and Spenny (1983) (Fig. 14.27). Recognizing that the *in situ* response of a subject in a real accident will likely fall between the cadaver response and the prepared volunteer, this figure may be used as a window representing the range of potential responses.

The importance of viscous effects in cervical spine torsional responses has been shown to be significant. Specifically, torque relaxation has been shown to result in a decrease in measured torque on the order of 50% from hightest rates to quasi-static test rates. As this type of behavior has been observed in both bending and compression, the importance of reporting rate with spinal mechanical properties cannot be overstated. The nonlinear viscoelastic behavior observed in torsional loading has been successfully described with Fung's quasi-

FIGURE 14.27. Cervical spine torque-angle response for the isolated ligamentous spine (cadaver), and the volunteer response to lateral deceleration (Gy), showing the stiffening effects of the musculature.

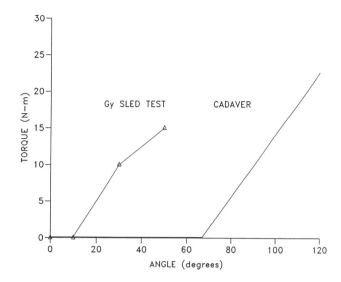

The Role of Head Constraint in Cervical Injury

The risk of injury from blows to the head has been studied extensively. Studies performed on the human cadaver have identified a large number of variables that influence neck injury. McElhaney et al. (1983b) noted that small changes in initial position of the head relative to the torso influenced injury mechanism from flexion injuries to extension injuries. Nusholtz et al. (1983) observed similar results in impacts of whole cadavers. Nusholtz et al. also stated that out-of-plane loading was necessary for the production of injury. Torg (1982) suggested that alignment of the cervical spine to remove the resting lordosis increased the ease with which the cervical spine was injured. Pintar et al. (1990) also noted the need for preflexion (i.e., removal of the resting lordosis) to create vertebral compression injuries. In contrast, Alem et al. (1984), impacting whole cadavers, noted that cervical injuries could be produced with the resting lordosis preserved. We believe these observations are due to the same phenomenon.

Mechanical analysis based upon the effective mass of the torso and the energy absorption of the neck reveals that the cervical spine is capable of managing impacts equivalent to vertical drop of 0.50 m when the neck is called upon to stop the torso (McElhaney et al., 1979). Unfortunately, most impact situations have considerably larger impact energies. In these situations, the head-neck complex must either move out of the path of, or be at risk for injury from, the energy of the impinging torso. The interaction of the head with the contact surface, the head constraint, or the end condition, plays a primary role in the ability of the head and neck to avoid the impinging torso, and plays a major role in the type of injury that results.

A group of studies have been performed to support this hypothesis. Roaf (1960) was unable to produce lower cervical ligamentous injury in unconstrained flexion. Hodgson and Thomas (1980) suggested that restriction of motion of the atlantoaxial joint greatly increased the risk of injury. Bauze and Ardran (1978) produced bilateral facet dislocation in the cadaver by constraining the rotation of the head and inserting a peg in the neural foramen. Yoganandan et al. (1986) noted that head constraint increased the measured axial load and the number of injuries in cadaver impacts. Liu and Dai (1989), based on a theoretical analysis of a beam column, suggested that the second-stiffest axis may play a role in injury, though the relationship between the second-

The linear viscoelastic model, and is reported by Myers et al. (1991a).

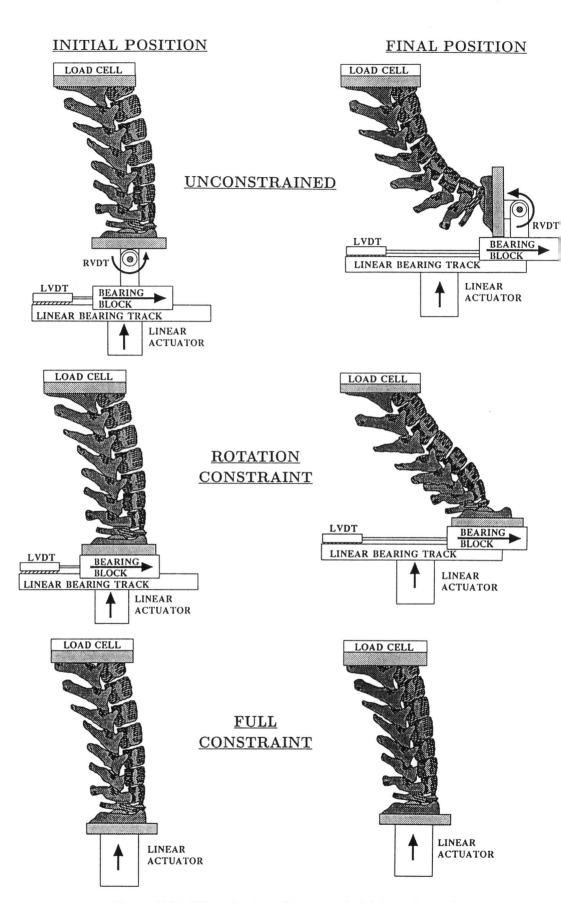

FIGURE 14.28. Effect of end conditions on spinal deformation mode.

TABLE 14.13. The effect of end condition on failure load and mechanism.

Specimen*	End condition	Peak axial load (N)	Axial deflection (cm)	Energy at failure (N-m)	Injury
A	Unconstrained	365	5.8	4.2*	None
B	Unconstrained	367	10.2	5.0*	None
C	Unconstrained	240	10.8	6.1*	None
D	Unconstrained	343	8.2	21.0*	None
E	Unconstrained	169	8.6	9.9*	None
F	Unconstrained	250	8.2	17.8*	None
Average	Unconstrained	289 ± 81.4	8.6 ± 1.8	11.5* ± 6.5	
G	Rotation constraint	3,590	3.6	14.6	BFD C5–C6
H	Rotation constraint	2,950	3.3	46.9	BFD C6–C7
I	Rotation constraint	1,130	2.9	20.7	BFD C7–T1
J	Rotation constraint	1,110	2.3	11.7	BFD C7–T1
K	Rotation constraint	600	1.5	4.8	BFD C7–T1
L	Rotation constraint	930	3.9	11.9	BFD C7–T1
Average	Rotation constraint	1,720 ± 1,234	2.9 ± 0.9	26.8 ± 23.7	
M	Full constraint	5,340	2.5	85.5	C2 comp. fx.
N	Full constraint	4,060	1.2	21.3	C3 comp. fx
O	Full constraint	6,840	1.2	42.0	C4 & C5 wedge comp. fx.
P	Full constraint	4,700	1.2	32.9	C4 & C5 comp. fx.
Q	Full constraint	3,000	1.7	26.1	C3 & C6 comp. fx.
R	Full constraint	4,940	1.1	21.5	C4 wedge comp. fx.
Average	Full constraint	4,810 ± 1,286	1.4 ± 0.4	32.9 ± 12.8	

BFD, bilateral facet dislocation.
* Values denote stored strain energy.

stiffest axis and the applied end condition has not been determined.

Following this line of reasoning, the authors performed cadaveric studies of isolated whole cervical spines to study the effect of an imposed end condition on the observed axial and flexural stiffness of the cervical spine. Figure 14.28 shows the end conditions and the resulting deformations the spine assumes subject to an axial deflection (a vertical motion of the head). Axial stiffness (defined by the secant method with a spatially fixed axis) was 3.6 kN/m in the unconstrained end condition, 28.4 kN/m in the rotation constraint end condition, and 41.0 kN/m in the full constraint end condition. Thus, stiffness increased 8.5-fold, and 12.2-fold with increasing constraint. Similar increases in the flexural rigidity have been observed by Doherty (1991).

Further, experimental work using 18 specimens distributed among the three end conditions demonstrates that increasing the degree of head constraint also increases the risk for, and type of, neck injury (Table 14.13). Full constraint, which might occur when the head pockets in the contact surface and the trajectory of the torso is colinear with the axis of the neck, resulted in compression and flexion-compression types of injury in six of six specimens. Mean axial load to failure was large (4,810 N); however, axial displacement was small and energy absorbed to failure was small compared to real-world impact energies. Rotation constraint, as might occur when the head pockets into the impact surface with the torso moving posteriorly, produces an S shape to the deforming spine, and bilateral facet dislocations in the lower cervical spine in six of six specimen studies. Mean axial load of bilateral facet dislocation was 1,720 N. As with full constraint, the energy absorbed to failure was small compared with the energy of impact, and the axial deflection to failure was also small.

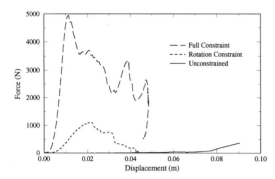

FIGURE 14.29. Force-deflection behavior to failure for three cervical spines, showing the influence of end condition on axial stiffness.

endhanced cervical injury potential. The reader should temper this concept realizing that the experiments discussed here were conducted at a low rate relative to real accidents. While the lower rate allowed for greater control over the end conditions, it neglected the potential contributions of inertial loading to the injury modes. Future work at the higher rate of real-world accidents is therefore recommended to validate this hypothesis.

Modeling and its Role in Understanding Injury

The complexity of the spine and the injury environment has created a need for repeatable, robust testing methods for the development of safety equipment. This need has been an impetus for the design and development of a group of mechanical models, the "car crash dummies," and a significant number of computational models of both cervical and total body dynamics.

These human surrogates have been refined over the last four decades to improve their simulation of human response, and, as a result of this effort, these tools now form the basis for much of the evaluation of injury potential. The absence of complete human tolerance data or a generalized cervical injury criterion poses a profound limitation on these models. Further, the rationale upon which these have devices have been developed is of primary importance in understanding the uses, limitations, and abuses of a particular tool. The following section gives a brief historical perspective on the development of these tools to define the settings in which they may be used. It also identifies the limitations in these areas and the need for further investigation into tolerance and injury mechanisms.

In the unconstrained group the applied axial displacement was sufficiently large (8.6 cm) of place the chin (if it were present) through the sternum and produce 96° of head flexion. Despite this large axial displacement, axial load remained small (289 N) and no injuries were detected by CT, magnetic resonance imaging, and physical dissection in six of six specimen studies. The unconstrained head-neck is thus able to move out of the way of the torso, allowing the torso to impact the contact surface and dissipate its energy without cervical injury. Figure 14.29 compares the axial load to failure for three specimens, illustrating the effect of end condition on injury. We believe this is the reason for the preponderance of compression-flexion injuries in shallow water diving, as the sand "pockets" the head on impact.

The experiments demonstrate that the greater the degree of constraint of the head imposed by the contact surface (i.e., the more restrictive the head end condition) the greater the risk for cervical injury for impacts where the neck is called upon to stop the torso. They also appear to be consistent with previous experimental results reported above, and relate well to the existing clinical classification schemes discussed in the section Injury Mechanisms and Classification, above. This suggests that safety equipment and injury environments that employ deformable contact surfaces that do not manage the energy to reduce the force of impact but rather impose a significant head constraint, may provide an

Physical Models

A group of mechanical devices has been developed to match the anthropometrics of a typical occupant, and the measured kinematics of volunteers to subinjurious, noncontact decelerations. These "crash dummies" have been used to predict the potential risk for injury from decelerations considered too large for volunteers. The risk of injury is assessed by comparing measured accelerations with the results of known human tolerance data and scaled animal studies. The additional design criteria for these devices include reproducibility, ease of fabrication, and durability; as such, these devices also provide a method for comparison of different injury-prevention strategies.

The initial devices were based on the 50th percentile male and had little biofidelity. Efforts to improve the biofidelity of these devices were sponsored largely by General Motors, the Motor Vehicle Manufacturers Association, and the National Highway Traffic Safety Administration, and have resulted in a number of designs and enhancements. In the 1970s, neckforms consisted of solid masses of butyl rubber. Culver et al. (1972) developed an articulated neckform with ball and socket joints in a butyl rubber housing for the lower cervical spine and a pin joint to mimic the action of the occipitoatlantal joint. Melvin et al. (1972) developed a similar neckform, with butyl rubber encased universal joints. Foster et al. (1977) introduced the Hybrid III Anthropometric Test Device, which incorporated a modification of Culver et al.'s device. The Hybrid III neckform included an occipitoatlantal joint force and moment transducer and a simplification of the articulations to reduce mechanical noise during testing. An increasing interest in side and oblique impact in motor vehicle accidents in the late 1970s and early 1980s has resulted in the design and experimental validation of a group of neckforms from a variety of institutions worldwire. While these devices provide improved biofidelity in side impact, development of a single "ultimate" dummy neck remains an area of continued research.

Understanding the origins for these devices defines to some extent their usefulness. These devices were designed and validated based on the kinematics of noninjurious, nonimpact decelerations of belted occupants. The devices have then been used to determine the kinematics of larger, potentially injurious, deceleration. Neglecting the effects of this extrapolation, it is apparent that these devices are *kinematic* simulators. Their utility is limited to determining velocity and accelerations of the head and neck in nonimpact decelerations. While this information provides the basis for determining the risk of noncontact head and neck injury (e.g., the "head injury criterion"), it does not provide insight into the risk of neck injury or head injury during impact except from the standpoint of a prediction of impact velocity. Indeed, a number of investigations have shown the Hybrid III neckform to be one to two orders of magnitude stiffer than the human volunteer and cadaver cervical spine in compression (Pintar et al., 1990). Realizing that load follows stiffness, data on neckform loading from impact of these devices cannot be directly related to human neck loads in real-world accidents.

To address this problem, Kabo and Goldsmith (1983) developed a head-neck model capable of three-dimensional motions that they instrumented and validated for sagittal plane impact loading. The device, in addition to being accurate from an anthropometric standpoint, was designed to provide data on intracranial fluid pressures, intervertebral disk pressures, and simulated muscle deformations. The impact testing, while above the threshold for injury as defined by the head injury criterion, represented relatively low impact accelerations (peak g's = 180). Accordingly, the performance of the device in high-energy impacts remains to be evaluated. Liang and Winters (1991) have recently produced a complete anthropometric head-neck replica from engineering materials, including individual vertebral bodies, disks, and passive and active muscle elements. The active muscle components are represented by a total of 10 pneumatic actuators. Preliminary data suggest that the device shows similar kinematic behavior to the cervical spine. The suitability of this device for impact studies has not been discussed, however. Clearly, continued effort to design a head-neck device with improved biofidelity for impact is necessary.

Computational and Finite Element Models

Computational models of the spine have evolved from three basic groups: continuum models, lumped or discrete parameter models, and finite element models. An extensive review on this subject is provided by Yoganandan et al. (1987).

The continuum or beam theory model of the spine was first developed in the aviation industry in the late 1950s to help understand the relationship between emergency pilot aircraft egress and the risk of spinal injury (Hess and Lombard, 1958). This model treated the spine as a straight, uniform, homogeneous, linearly elastic rod with free end conditions, subjected to an acceleration pulse at one end. This model evolved over subsequent years to include viscoelastic material properties (Terry and Roberts, 1968), an equivalent head mass (Liu and Murray, 1966), varying stiffness along the length of the column (Shirazi, 1971), an initial curvature of the beam (Li et al., 1971; Moffatt et al., 1971), the effects of transverse and rotary inertia (i.e., full 2-D analysis) (Cramer et al., 1976), and the contributions of the musculature (Soechting and Paslay, 1973). The goal of this approach is therefore the coupling of stress and acceleration determined from the models to the risk of spinal and head injury from estimates of human tolerance.

The most recent work using continuum models has been interested in determining the risk of cervical injury from eccentric loading. Using a curved homogeneous elastic beam, Liu and Dai (1989) suggested that the second-stiffest axis of loading of a column may represent the direction at which the spine is at its greatest risk for injury. The authors, acknowledging that the cervical spine is of considerably greater complexity than the proposed model, are currently seeking experimental validation of this hypothesis. Interestingly, this model allows for buckling, which may play a significant role in cervical injury (Myers et al., 1991c). It also remains useful in understanding and comparing the responses of the spine under different loading conditions by allowing the determination of the effective flexural stiffness (Doherty, 1991).

The obligatory simplification of the spine to a continuous beam is frequently cited as a limitation in this approach to modeling of injury mechanisms. The absence of load or acceleration-based criteria from cadaveric experimentation or actual injury data also limits the interpretation of these models. Thus, while these models are able to give insight into expected forces and accelerations from impact, as well as provide insight into experimental data, an accurate determination of the risk of cervical injury under the conditions modeled cannot be made.

The quasi-linear viscoelastic constitutive law hypothesized by Fung (1967) has also been used to predict the structural responses of the cervical spine. This model incorporates a continuous spectral reduced relaxation function, $G_r(t)$ together with a nonlinear stiffening elastic function, $F^e(\delta)$ in a hereditary integral formulation. Thus, the force time-history, $F(t)$, to an arbitarary deflection history, $\delta(t)$, is given by

$$F(t) = \int_{-\infty}^{t} G_r(t - \tau) \frac{dF^e(\delta(\tau))}{d\delta} \frac{d\delta(\tau)}{d\tau} d\tau \tag{14.1}$$

This model has been used to predict the structural responses of the cervical spine in compression, flexion, and torsion with a high degree of success (Doherty, 1991; McElhaney et al., 1983a; Myers et al., 1991a). Efforts to generalize this model to predict two- and three-dimensional coupled structural responses are currently under investigation, and will determine the future utility of this type of modeling.

The first lumped parameter model was developed in the late 1950s by Latham (1957), also with the goal of understanding pilot ejection injuries. It consisted of an undamped single degree of freedom, one-dimensional system that included the total body response to seat accelerations. This model was able to describe the linear motions of the end points (i.e., head and pelvis) with limited accuracy and was not able to describe local spinal loads or deformations. Subsequent work extended Latham's model to five and six degree of freedom systems and two dimensions (Kalips et al., 1971; McElhaney et al., 1983b; Orne and Liu, 1971; Sances et al., 1984; Vulcan and King, 1970; Zhu et al., 1990).

With the recognition that the posterior elements of the spinal column play an important role in load carrying in vertical loading of the spine, an increased interest in discrete parameter modeling developed (Prassad et al., 1974). These models, which include the individual structures of the spinal motion segment, have been developed to describe aircraft ejections, whiplash injuries, and the more general problem of the three-dimensional dynamics of the spine to an arbitrary loading history (Belytschko et al., 1978; Panjabi, 1973; Prassad and King, 1974; Reber and Goldsmith, 1979). They typically treat the components of the spine as pure elements (i.e., massless springs and ideal dampers connecting rigid bodies) or as combinations of elements (e.g., Kelvin solids). Historically, the large number of parameters used in these models has required the use of simplified material properties, given the limitations of existing computation facilities. Recent efforts, however, have become increasingly complex, and include elements that prescribe facet joint kinematics, and muscle tractions (Gudavalli and Triano, 1990; Liu and Murray, 1966; Seireg and Arvikar, 1975; Williams and Belytschenko, 1983). Efforts to measure the mechanical behavior of the individual components of the spine (Pintar, 1986) and incorporate this data into these models will no doubt improve the utility of this type of modeling.

Total body models based on numerical solutions to multibody equations of motion, either Lagrangian or Eulerian, have also been developed. These include the Crash Victim Simulator, the Articulated Total Body Model, PAM-Crash, Madymo3D, and others (Belytschko and Privitzer, 1978; Bowman, 1971; McHenry and Naab, 1967; Robbins et al., 1991; Wismans et al., 1982). Anthropometric data sets including joint characteristics are provided for these models using a body dimension set originally developed by Baughman (1983). These models incorporate cervical spines of varying complexity including rigid linkages, Kelvin elements, and multi-segmented components. Efforts have also been made to incorporate Hybrid III mechanical

properties into the models. As discussed above, these cervical models are kinematic in origin and thus their use should be restricted to nonimpact cervical simulations.

The recent availability of relatively affordable, higher speed computation has resulted in an increased popularity and complexity of computational spinal modeling. In particular, the use of finite element modeling is enjoying increased popularity throughout the field of biomechanics. Finite element models of the spine have been used by a number of authors to assess a variety of problems. These include the performance of spinal instrumentation, the influence of surgical intervention on spinal stability, the role of torsional loading on injury, and the influence of disk degeneration on spinal kinetics (Balasubramanian et al., 1979; Kim et al., 1991; Shirazi-Adl et al., 1986; Ueno and Liu, 1987). The bulk of this effort has been limited to the lumbar and thoracic spine, however (Yoganandan et al., 1987). Finite element models of the cervical spine are currently being developed by Kleinberger at NHTSA, following the work of Williams and Belytschko (1983).

Interestingly, the finite element method has been used by a number of authors to solve the inverse problem (Lin et al., 1978). Given a known geometry and global response of the structure, the authors determine the material properties. These techniques couple finite element techniques with optimization techniques based on minimizing error in the predicted responses of an arbitrarily selected set of points on the body. Given the statically indeterminate nature of the problem and the influence of the optimization technique on the solution, the uniqueness and validity of material properties determined in this method is questionable (Yoganandan et al., 1987).

Hybrid modeling techniques are also being developed that couple solutions from different modeling techniques. Of particular interest is the use of the finite element method for describing local stresses and deformations with numerical solutions of rigid multibody dynamic systems (Hoffmann et al., 1990). Such a system offers the advantages of both methods, namely a faster solution to large-scale dynamics problems coupled with a more accurate understanding of the local stresses and deformations in the components of interest.

It is important to recognize that finite element solutions are limited to the accuracy with which the constitutive equations of the materials, the geometry, the structural organization, and the injury criterion arc known. The behavior of the spine as a whole, and of its constituent components, has been shown to be nonlinear and viscoelastic. These responses do not conform to simple viscoelastic models, but instead require the computationally more complex spectral viscoelastic models like the quasi-linear exponential integral Maxwell-Weichert model (Doherty, 1991; McElhaney et al., 1983; Myers et al., 1991a). In addition, the spine's response to physiologic loads typically produces large strains. While several finite element software packages are able to handle large strains, nonlinear elasticity, anisotropy, and simple viscoelasticity, the absence of a rate-insensitive, quasi-linear viscoelastic element for use in finite element packages is a current limitation in this type of modeling. The development and use of poroelastic and hyperporoelastic elements may ultimately solve the problem of spinal viscoelasticity (Pflaster et al., 1990; Simon et al., 1990). The geometric complexity of the spine and the difficulty in defining the geometry experimentally is also a restriction in the use of finite element methods. Recent efforts to integrate the results of CT imaging with finite element mesh generation techniques may overcome this problem for the bony components of the spine (Kim et al., 1991; Levy and Palmer, 1987). However, a method for characterization of soft tissue geometry remains a significant challenge. The development of an injury criterion suitable for the spine or its constituents will also increase the accuracy of this method. Clearly, finite element modeling promises to play an increasing role in the study of the behavior of the spine. The limitations discussed create the need for continued research in this area. Finally, as with all modeling efforts, experimental validation provides the only way to assess their useful-

ness. Therefore, a continued effort to experimentally validate these models will be required if they are to be successful.

Summary

Physical and computational models of the cervical spine are becoming important elements in safety engineering. It is evident that much progress has been made with both physical and computational modeling; however, it is also evident that much remains to be done. By understanding the origins of each type of model, we are able to understand the uses and limitations of each. In order for these tools to have appropriate biofidelity for understanding impact and risk for neck injury from impact, a significant research and development effort is still required.

From the experimental community, better information of cervical injury mechanisms and human tolerance is required. From the modeling community, continued development and refinement of these models to better incorporate the complexity of the cervical spine and define the limitations of a given model is required. Most importantly, however, is the need for close collaboration between the two groups, to continue to develop and validate these tools.

Tolerance of the Cervical Spine

Characterization of the tolerance of the human cervical spine to injury remains a challenge to biomechanical engineering. The spine is a multisegmented column with nonlinear structural properties. Its geometry is complex, it produces large strains at physiologic loading, and its constituent elements have nonlinear material properties. Cervical injury mechanisms have been shown to be sensitive to the initial position of the neck, the direction of loading, the degree of constraint imposed by the contact surface, and possibly the rate of loading. In addition, a variety of host-related factors contribute to injury biomechanics. These include the bone mineral content of the vertebra, the presence of degeneration, the degree of muscular stimulation at the time of impact, and the variance associated with the geometric differences within the population. An additional limitation is posed by the lack of availability of cadaveric tissue for the study of injury, this being the primary limitation on the size of most studies and perhaps the greatest limitation to our understanding of injury biomechanics. Despite these limitations, a great deal has been learned about the tolerance of the neck to injury. The following is a summary of a number of studies reporting data relevant to the question of human tolerance.

One of the most frequently cited studies is the work of Mertz and Patrick (1971). Reporting data from both volunteer and cadaver decelerations, the authors determined a lower bound for the risk for neck injury based on the bending moment estimated at the occipital condyles for flexion and extension loading. For extension, the authors report noninjurious loading of 35 ft-lbs (47.3 N-m) with ligamentous injury expected above 42 ft-lbs (56.7 N-m). For flexion, the authors report initiation of pain at 44.0 ft-lbs (59.4 N-m), a maximum voluntary loading of 65 ft-lbs (87.8 N-m), and the risk for structural injury above 140 ft-lbs (189 N-m) in the cadaver following contact of the chin on the chest. The authors note, however, that muscular injury may occur below 140 ft-lbs. Clemens and Borow (1972), in deceleration studies of isolated cadaver torsos with a synthetic instrumented cranium coupled to the base of the skull, report that anteroposterior accelerations of 15g to the thorax (frontal collisions) can produce cervical injury. Interestingly, the injury was a recoil extension of the head that occurred after the head had flexed due to the deceleration, and thus, was fully preventable with a head rest. Instrumented studies of chiropractic cervical manipulations reported by Triano and Schultz (1990) show upper cervical moments of 22 to 24 N-m, and resultant forces of 120 to 130 N without injury. Notably, these manipulations are performed with great constraint of the resulting motions, and loads are frequently applied directly to the cervical spine. Thus, their role in determining tolerance is uncertain.

A large number of studies have reported compressive load to failure. While it is readily accepted that this parameter alone is a poor predictor of the risk for neck injury, it still remains a readily measurable and useful biomechanical parameter. Understanding and interpreting reported compressive load data can reduce the observed scatter and provide some insight into the problem of compression tolerance.

Differences in axial load to failure have been shown to depend on the injury produced, and therefore on the degree of constraint imposed by the contact surface. From a tolerance standpoint, these injuries should be evaluated separately. As an example, it has been observed by Maiman et al. (1983) and Myers et al. (1991c) that compression-flexion and compression-extension injuries produced in the cadaver require smaller axial loads than pure compressive injuries. Indeed, bilateral facet dislocations reported in Myers et al. occurred at 1,720 ± 1,230 N, and flexion injuries reported in Maiman et al. occurred at approximately 2,000 N. In contrast, compression injuries reported in these studies occurred at 4,810 ± 1,290 N and 5,970 ± 1,049 N, respectively. Given the importance of the musculature in resisting flexion and extension in the lower cervical spine, these values should be considered as a lower bound for human tolerance in compression-flexion and compression-extension injuries. In contrast, the compressive loads associated with pure compression injuries may represent a reasonable estimate of cervical compressive tolerance because the muscles are probably not involved in this type of injury.

Further reduction in the scatter of compression data may be gained by considering the effects of rate on axial load to failure. This concerns two primary effects. One, increasing rates of loading from quasi-static to dynamic (loading durations of 200 ms) will result in increases in measured axial load of as much as 50% due to viscous effects. Two, increasing loading rate to impact velocities (loading durations of approximately 20 ms or less) will include inertial effects of the head. Impactor load data must then be interpreted with the realization that neck loading will depend heavily on the inertial characteristics and accelerations of the head. This effect was observed by Yoganandan et al. (1986), who noted that in unrestrained and restrained cadaver impacts, impactor loads varied considerably from 3,000 to 7,000 N, and 9,800 to 14,600 N, respectively. In contrast, measured neck loading to failure remained between 1,100 and 2,600 N (mean = 1,730 ± 565 N). Thus, with considerations of the rate of loading, the degree of constraint imposed by the contact surface, and the injury mechanism, considerable insight into cervical compressive tolerance can be gained. Alem et al. (1984) suggested that impulse, the integral of the impactor force time-history, may correlate more closely with the risk of cervical injury than other impact parameters, but a larger number of tests would be necessary to validate this hypothesis.

Tensile loading of the cervical spine has been performed by a few authors producing both lower and upper cervical injuries in the cadaver. Mean load to produce occipitoatlantal ligmentous injuries of five complete cervical spines reported in Sances et al. (1982) was 1,537 ± 509 N. Shea et al. (1991) report a tensile load to failure of 500 ± 150 N in quasi-static cadaver tests of spines with an initial preextension of 30° and a mean extension moment of 3.9 ± 3.1 N-m. Both these results must be considered as a lower bound on the tolerance, however, given the absence of passive muscle tone. Mertz and Patrick (1971) suggest a tensile tolerance of 1,160 N in tension during extension loading (i.e., posteroanterior acceleration of the torso). Clemens and Burow (1972) suggest a value of 1,600 to 2,000 N, based on the experiments described above. Using the cadaver axial displacement data and the tensile stiffness reported by Bowman et al. (1984) from volunteer tests conducted at the NBDL, an estimate of the tensile tolerance of the injury victim may be determined. Specifically, using a tensile stiffness of 1,644 N/cm and a mean tensile displacement to failure reported in Shea et al. of 1.88 cm, we estimate that the human tolerance to tension may be as high as 3,100 N.

Estimates of the lower bound of torsional tolerance are available from Myers et al.

(1991b). Axial torque of 17.2 ± 5.1 N-m produced upper cervical injury in cadaver whole cervical spines (occiput to T1). Goel et al. (1990) report a slightly lower value of 13.6 ± 4.5 N-m in isolated upper cervical spine studies; however, the rates of loading in these experiments were considerably lower than in the previous study (4°/sec versus 500°/sec). Extrapolating piecewise linear torsional stiffness data from volunteer decelerations reported by Wismans and Spenny (1983) to the 114° ± 6.3° of rotation required to produce injury in the cadaver, we obtain an estimate of human torsional tolerance of approximately 28 N-m. We also suggest that the 114° of axial rotation from the neutral position required to produce upper cervical injury in whole cervical spines mitigates the role of small axial rotations as a mediator of lower cervical injuries.

Tolerance data for horizontal shear is limited and stems from data collected on occipito-atlantoaxial injuries. In particular, loading required to produce transverse ligament failure and odontoid fracture have been reported by a number of authors. Fielding et al. (1974) observed transverse ligament rupture at 824 N when the atlas is driven anterior relative to the axis in the isolated cadaver upper cervical spine. Doherty et al. (1992) produced odontoid fractures at 1,510 ± 420 N by applying posterior and lateral directed loads directly to the odontoid process. Understanding the relationship between these results, and the neck loads that develop dynamically in impact has not been determined. Based on the volunteer data in flexion, Mertz and Patrick (1971) suggest a lower bound of tolerance of 847 N. Cheng et al. (1982), in a cadaveric study of neck injury from decelerations produced by a distributed load to the chest, report cervical injuries in four specimens with estimated shear loads of 2,820 ± 1,760 N, in the presence of total resultant loads of 5,500 ± 2,500 N.

Discussion

The summary of the literature presented in this chapter shows that much has been written about the biomechanical aspects of cervical injury. Most of what we know comes from two sources: clinical studies, including accident reconstruction and analysis, and cadaver or cadaveric material studies. Mathematical models of structural behavior are currently quite primitive in terms of predicting failure modes and injury criteria. However, kinematic models are able to accurately predict head motion from torso motion.

Automotive accidents account for a high percentage of catastrophic neck injuries. The speeds can be high and forces or accelerations can occur in almost any direction. Thus, the injury mechanisms involve a wide range of modes with various combinations of tension, torsion, compression, extension, flexion, and lateral bending. Catastrophic neck injuries from sports, however, clearly cluster around the flexion-compression mechanism. This is probably because the impact speeds are usually below the levels that cause structural failures in shear, extension, or lateral bending. Diving and football accident reconstructions demonstrate that flexion-compression injuries can occur at head impacts as low as 10 feet per second when the head is suddenly arrested and the neck must stop the torso. These injuries seldom occur when the head is free to slide and the neck is not trapped between the head and torso. Because of the frequency of flexion-compression injuries, most of the cadaver work has been designed to study this injury mode. However, recent work has demonstrated that the flexion-compression injury mechanism is very sensitive to the initial conditions of head fixation, head linear and angular motions, and orientation of the head, neck, and torso. This makes it difficult to compare various laboratories' data and requires nonlinear modeling.

Much work needs to be done before we can understand the structural and material responses of the human cervical spine at a level that would allow evaluation of injury potential in extreme environments and the rational design of protective equipment.

Basic questions that need answers include:

1. What are the injury criteria and mechanisms for the human neck when the head is impacted in an arbitrary direction?

2. What is the effect of neck musculature?
3. What is the effect of age, size, shape, and density?
4. What structural and geometrical properties must be developed for finite element analysis?
5. Are the failure responses so nonlinear that mathematical modeling is not feasible?

These are but a few of the questions that research can answer and we encourage all who work in this area to carefully consider the theoretical and experimental problems discussed above.

Acknowledgment. This work was supported by the Department of Health and Human Services, Center for Disease Control grant R49/CCR402396-06 and the Virginia Flowers Baker Chair at Duke University.

References

Alem NM, Nusholtz GS, Melvin JW. Head and neck response to axial impacts. 28th Stapp Car Crash Conference. pp 275–287, 1984.

Allen BL, Ferguson RL, Lehmann TR, O'Brien RP (1982) A mechanistic classification of closed indirect fractures and dislocations of the lower cervical spine. Spine 7(1):1–27.

Anderson LD, D'Alonzo RT (1974) Fractures of the odontoid process of the axis. J Bone Joint Surg 56–A(8):1663–1674.

Babcock JL (1976) Cervical spine injuries. Arch Surg 111:646–651.

Balasubramanian K, Ranu HS, King AI (1979) Vertebral response to laminectomy. J Biomech 12:813.

Barnes R (1948) Paraplegia in cervical spine injuries. J Bone Joint Surg 30–B(2):234–244.

Baughman LD. Development of an interactive computer program to produce body descriptive data. Dayton Ohio University Research Institute, NTIS #AD-A133 720: Report #AFAMRL-TR-83-058, 1983.

Bauze RJ, Ardran GM (1978) Experimental production of forward dislocation of the human cervical spine. J Bone Joint Surg 60B:239–245.

Belytschko TB, Schwer L, Privitzer E (1978) Theory and application of a three-dimensional model of human spine. Aviat Space Environ Med 1:158.

Belytschko TB, Privitzer E. Refinement and validation of a 3-D head spine model. contract

AF33615-76-C506, AMRL, WPAFB, Dayton Ohio, 1983.

Blockey NJ, Purser DW (1956) Fractures of the odontoid process of the axis. J Bone Joint Surg 38B:794–817.

Bowman BM. An analytic model of a vehicle occupant for use in crash simulation. PhD Dissertation. Dept of Eng Mech, University of Michigan, 1971.

Bowman BM, Schneider LW, Lustak LS, Anderson WR, Thomas DJ. Simulation analysis of head and neck dynamic response. 28th Stapp Car Crash Conference. p 173, 1984.

Braakman R, Penning L. Injuries of the cervical spine, chapter III, causes of spinal lesions. In *Causes of spinal lesions*. Exerpta Medica, pp 53–63, 1971.

Braakman R, Vinken PJ (1967) Unilateral facet interlocking in the lower cervical spine. J Bone Joint Surg 49B(2):249–257.

Bucholz RW, Burkhead WZ (1979) The pathological anatomy of fatal atlantooccipital dislocations. J Bone Joint Surg 61A:248–250.

Chester JB (1991) Whiplash, postural control, and the inner ear. Spine 16(7):716–720.

Coffee MS, Edwards WT, Hayes CV, White AA III (1987) Biomechanical properties and strength of the human cervical spine. Trans ASME Bioeng Div 3:71.

Cramer HJ, Liu YK, Von Rosenberg DU (1976) A distributed parameter of the inertially loaded human spine. J Biomech 9:115.

Culver CC, Neathery RF, Mertz HJ. Mechanical necks with human-like responses. 16th Stapp Car Crash Conference. SAE 720959, pp 61–75, 1972.

Dai QG, Liu YK. Failure analysis of a beam-column under two-dimensional oblique eccentric loading with simulated muscle tractions as a model of spinal trauma. Injury prevention through biomechanics. Symposium Proceedings, Wayne State, pp 16–171, April 12, 1991.

Doherty BJ. The Responses of spinal segments to combined bending and axial loading. PhD Dissertation. Duke University, 1991.

Doherty BJ, Esses SI, Heggeness MH. A biomechanical study of odontoid fractures and fracture fixation. Cervical Spine Research Society in review, 1992.

Dolen KD (1977) Cervical spine injuries below the axis. Radiol Clin North Am 15(2):247–259.

Ewing CL, Thomas DJ, Beeler GW, et al. Dynamic response of the head and neck of the living human to $-G_x$ impact acceleration. 12th Stapp Car Crash Conference. Society of Automotive Engineers, New York, pp 424–439, 1968.

Ewing CL, Thomas DJ, Lustick L, et al. The effect of duration, rate of onset, and peak sled acceleration on the dynamic response of the human head and neck. 20th Stapp Car Crash Conference. Society of Automotive Engineers, Warrendale, Pennsylvania, pp 1–42, 1976.

Fielding JW, Cochran GVB, Lawsing JF III, Hohl M (1974) Tears of the transverse ligament of the Atlas. J Bone Joint Surg 56-A(8):1683–1691.

Foster JK, Kortge JO, Wolanin MJ. Hybrid III—a biomechanically-based crash test dummy. 21st Stapp Car Crash Conference. SAE 770938, pp 975–1014, 1977.

Foust DR, Chaffin DB, Snyder RG, Baum JK. Cervical range of motion and dynamic response and strength of cervical muscles. 17th Stapp Car Crash Conference. p 285, 1971.

Fung YC (1967) Elasticity of soft tissues in single elongation. Am J Physiol 213(6):1532–1544.

Gallie RL, Spaite DW, Simon RR. *Emergency orthopaedics of the spine*. Appleton and Lange, Norwalk, 1989.

Gehweiler JA, Osborne RL, Becker RF. *The radiology of vertebral trauma*. WB Saunders, Philadelphia, 1980.

Gershon-Cohen J, Budin E, Glauser F (1954) Whiplash fractures of cervicodorsal spinous processes; resemblance to shoveler's fracture. JAMA 155:560.

Goel VK, Winterbottom JM, Schulte KR, et al. (1990) Ligamentous laxity across the C0-C1-C2 complex: axial torque-rotation characteristics until failure. Spine 15:990–996.

Goldsmith W. Structure, mechanical properties, motion and models of the human neck. University of California, Berkeley, 1983.

Gosch HH, Gooding E, Schneider RC (1972) An experimental study of cervical spine and cord injuries. J Trauma 12:570–576.

Greeley PW (1930) Bilateral (ninety degrees) rotatory dislocation of the atlas upon the axis. J Bone Joint Surg 12:958–962.

Gudavalli MR, Triano JJ (1990) An analytical model for the estimation of loads and strains in the posterior ligaments of the lumbar spine. Adv Bioeng 231–234.

Harris JH Jr, Edeiken-Monroe B, Kopaniky DR (1986) A practical classification of acute cervical spine injuries. Orthop Clin North Am 17(1):15–30.

Hess JL, Lombard CV (1958) Theoretical investigations of dynamic response of man to high vertical accelerations. J Aviat Med 29:66.

Hodgson VR, Thomas LM. Mechanisms of cervical spine injury during impact to the protected head

Society of Automotive Engineers Transactions, #801300, pp 17–42, 1980.

Hoffmann R, Ulrich D, Protard J-B, Wester H, Jaehn N, Scharnhorst T. Finite element analysis of occupant restraint systems interaction with PAM-CRASH. 34th Stapp Car Crash Conference. pp 289–300, 1990.

Hohl M (1974) Soft-tissue injuries of the neck in automobile accidents. J Bone Joint Surg 56-A(8):1675–1682.

Huelke DF, Moffett EA, Mendelshon RA, Melvin JW. Cervical fractures and fracture dislocations—an overview SAE 790131, pp 462–468, 1980.

Kabo JM, Goldsmith W (1983) Response of a human head-neck model to transient sagittal plane loading. J Biomech 16(5):313–325.

Kalips I, Von Gierke HE, Weis EB. A five degree of freedom mathematical model of the body. Symposium on Biodynamic Models and their Applications. Aerospace Medical Research Laboratory (AMRL-TR-71-29), WPAFB, Ohio, p 211, 1971.

Kallieris D, Schmidt G. Neck response and injury assessment using cadavers and the US-SID for far-side lateral impacts of rear seat occupants with inboard-anchored shoulder belts. 34th Stapp Car Crash Conference. pp 93–99, 1990.

Kim YE, Goel VK, Weinstein JN, Lim TH (1991) Effect of disc degeneration at one level on the adjacent level in axial mode. Spine 16(3):331–335.

Kleinberger M, Personal communication. July, 1991.

Latham F (1957) A study of body ballistics: seat ejections. Proc R Soc London B147:121.

Levy MS, Palmer JF (1987) Three-dimensional computerized modeling of the occipital-atlanto-axial spine. Adv Bioeng pp 69–70.

Li TF, Advani SH, Lee YC. The effect of initial curvature on the dynamic response of spine to axial acceleration. Symp biodynamic models and their application. AMRL-TR71-29, WPAFB, Dayton Ohio, p 553, 1971.

Liang D, Winters JM. Mechanical response of an anthropomorphic head-neck system to external loading and muscle contraction. First World Congress of Biomechanics, II. San Diego, CA, August 30–September 4, p 316, 1990.

Lin HS, Liu YK, Ray G, Nikravesh P (1978) Systems identification for material properties of the intervertebral Joint. J Biomech 11:1–14.

Liu YK, Dai QG (1989) The second stiffest axis of a beam column: implications for cervical spine trauma. J Biomech Eng 111:122–127.

Liu YK, Murray A. Theoretical study of the effect of impulse on the human torso. In Fung YC (ed) Biomechanics. New York, ASME, pp 167–186, 1966.

Lysell E (1969) Motion in the cervical spine. Acta Orthop Scand S123:1.

Maiman DJ, et al. (1983) Compression injuries of the cervical spine; a biomechanical analysis. Neurosurgery 13:254–260.

Marar BC (1974) Hyperextension injuries of the cervical spine, the pathogenesis of damage to the spinal cord. J Bone Joint Surg 56-A(8):1655–1662.

McElhaney JH, Doherty BJ, Paver JG, Myers BS, Gray L. Combined bending and axial loading responses of the human cervical spine. 32nd Stapp Car Crash Conference, pp 21–28, 1988.

McElhaney JH, Paver JG, McCrackin HJ, Maxwell GM. Cervical spine compression responses. 27th Stapp Car Crash Conference. SAE 831615:163–177, 1983a.

McElhaney JH, Roberts VL, Paver JG, Maxwell GM. Etiology of trauma to the cervical spine. In Ewing CL, Thomas DL, Sances A Jr, Larson SJ (eds) Impact injury of the head and spine. CC Thomas, Springfield, Mass, 1983b.

McElhaney JH, Snyder RG, States JD, Gabrielson MA. Biomechanical analysis of swimming pool injuries. Society of Automotive Engineers, 790137, pp 47–53, 1979.

McHenry RR, Naab KN. Computer simulation of the crash victim a validation study. 10th Stapp Car Crash Conference. SAE 660792, 1967.

Melvin JW, McElhaney JH, Roberts VL. Improved neck simulation for anthropometric dummies. 16th Stapp Car Crash Conference. SAE 720958, pp 45–60, 1972.

Mertz HJ, Patrick LM. Strength and response of the human neck, 15th Stapp Car Crash Conference. SAE 710855, 1971.

Moffatt CA, Advani SH, Lin CJ. Analytical end experimental investigations of human spine flexure. Am Soc Mech Eng, 71-WA/BHF-7, 1971.

Montane I, Eismont FJ, Green BA (1991) Traumatic occipitoatlantal dislocation. Spine 16(2):112–116.

Myers BS, McElhaney JH, Doherty BJ (1991a) The viscoelastic responses of the human cervical spine in torsion: experimental limitation of quasi-linear theory and a method for reducing these effects. J Biomech 24(9):811–817.

Myers BS, McElhaney JH, Doherty BJ, Paver JG, Gray L (1991b) The role of torsion in cervical spinal injury. Spine 16(8):870–874.

Myers BS, McElhaney JH, Doherty BJ, Paver JG, Nightingale RW, Ladd TP, Gray L. Responses of the human cervical spine to torsion. 33rd Stapp Car Crash Conference. pp 215–222, 1989.

Myers BS, McElhaney JH, Richardson WJ, Nightingale R, Doherty BJ. The influence of end condition on human cervical spine injury mechanisms. The 35th Stapp Car Crash Conference. pp 391–400, 1991c.

Norton WL (1962) Fractures and dislocations of the cervical spine. J Bone Joint Surg 44A(1):115–139.

Nusholtz GS, Huelke DE, Lux P, Alem NM, Montalvo F. Cervical spine injury mechanisms. 27th Stapp Car Crash Conference. pp 179–197, 1983.

Ommaya AK, Hirsh AE (1971) Tolerances for cerebral concussion from head impact and whiplash in primates. J Biomech 4:13.

Orne D, Liu YK (1971) A mathematical model of spinal response to impact. J Biomech 4(1):49–71.

Panjabi MM (1973) Three-dimensional mathematical model for the study of the mechanics of the human vertebral column. J Biomech 6(6):671–680.

Panjabi MM, Summers DJ, Pelker RR, Vidoman T, Friedlander GE, Southwick WO (1986) Cervical spine biomechanics. J Orthop Res 4:152–161.

Pflaster D, Liable J, Krag MH, Johnson C, Pope MH, Simon BR. A three-dimensional poroelastic finite element model for lumbar spinal motion segments with experimental verification. First World Congress of Biomechanics, II. San Diego Ca, August 3–September 4, p 40, 1990.

Pintar F. The biomechanics of spinal elements. PhD Thesis. Market University, Milwaukee, December, 1986.

Pintar F, Sances A Jr, Yoganandan N, Reinartz J, Maiman DJ, Suh JK, Unger G, Cusick JF, Larson SJ. Biodynamics of the total human cervical spine. 32nd Stapp Car Crash Conference. pp 55–72, 1990.

Prassad P, King AI (1974) An experimentally validated dynamic model of the spine. J Appl Mech 41:546.

Prassad P, King AI, Ewing CL (1974) The role of artricular factors during $+G_z$ acceleration. J Appl Mech 41:321.

Reber JG, Goldsmith W (1979) Analysis of large head-neck motions. J Biomech 12:211–222.

Reid DC, Staboe LA (in press). Can J Sports Med.

Reid DC, Staboe LA (1987) Phys Sports Med.

Reid DC, Staboe LA, Allan DG (1989) Can J Sports Med.

Roaf R (1960) A study of the mechanics of spinal injury. J Bone Joint Surg 42B:810–823

Roaf R (1963) Lateral flexion injuries of the cervical spine. J Bone Joint Surg 45B:36–38.

Robbins DH, Bowman BM, Bennett RO. MVMA two-dimensional crash victim simulation. 18nd Stapp Car Crash Conference. pp 657–677, 1991.

Rogers WA (1957) Fractures and dislocations of the cervical spine. J Bone Joint Surg 39A:341–376.

Sances A Jr, et al. Head and spine injuries. AGARD Conference on Injury Mechanism, Prevention and Cost. Koln, Germany, pp 13–1 to 13–33, 1982.

Sances A Jr, Myklebust JB, Maiman DJ, Larson SJ, Cusick JF, Jodat RF (1984) The biomechanics of spinal injuries. CRC Crit Rev Bioeng 11(1):1.

Schneider LW, Foust DR, Bowman BM, Snyder RG, Chaffin DB, Abdelnovr TA, Baum, JK. Biomechanical properties of the human neck in lateral flexion. SAE, 751156:3212, 1975.

Schneider RC. Head and neck injuries in football. Williams and Wilkins, Baltimore, 1973.

Schneider RC, Cherry G, Pantek H (1959) The syndrome of acute central cervical spinal cord injury. J Neurosurg 27:546–577.

Schneider RC, Kahn EA (1956) Chronic neurologic sequel of acute trauma to the spine and spinal cord. Part I: The significance of the acute-flexion or "tear-drop" fracture-dislocation of the cervical spine. J Bone Joint Surg 38-A(5):985–997.

Seireg A, Arvikar RJ. A comprehensive musculo-skeletal model for the human vertebral column. ASME Biomechnaics Symposium. Houston TX, p 74, 1975.

Shea M, Edwards WT, White AA, Hayes WC (1991) Variations of stiffness and strength along the human cervical spine. J Biomech 24(2):95–107.

Shea M, Wittenberg RH, Edwards WT, White AA III, Hayes WC. In vitro hyperextension injuries in the human cadaveric cervical spine. Clin Orthop Rel Res In press.

Shirazi M. Response of the spine in biodynamic environments. symposium on biodynamic models and their applications. Aerospace Medical Research Laboratory AMRL-TR-71-29, WPAFB, Ohio, p 843, 1971.

Shirazi-Adl A, Ahmed AM, Shrivastave SC (1986) Mechanical response of a lumbar motion segment in axial torsion alone and combination with compression. Spine 11(9):914–927.

Simon BR, Gaballa MA, Yuan Y. Porohyperelastic finite element models including finite strains and swelling. First World Congress of Biomechanics, II. San Diego CA, August 30–September 4, p 201, 1990.

Soechting JF, Paslay PR (1973) A model for the human spine during impact including musculature influence. J Biomech 6:195.

Stapp JP. Human response to linear decelerations: part I and II. AF Technical Report No. 5915, 1949.

Stedman TL. Stedman's medical dictionary. 24th ed. Williams and Wilkins, Baltimore, 1982.

Taylor AR (1951) The mechanism of injury to the spinal cord in the neck without damage to the vertebral column. J Bone Joint Surg 33-B:543–547.

Taylor AR, Blackwood W (1948) Paraplegia in hyperextension cervical injuries with normal radiographic appearances. J Bone Joint Surg 30-B(2):245–248.

Terry CT, Roberts VL (1968) A viscoelastic model of the human spine subjected to G_z accelerations. J Biomech 1:161–168.

Torg JS. (ed) Atheletic injuries to the head neck and face. Lea & Febiger, Philadelphia, 1982.

Torg JS, Pavlov H. Axial load "teardrop" fracture, in atheletic injuries to the head, neck and face. 2nd ed. Lea & Febiger, Philadelphia, 1991.

Triano JJ, Schultz AB (1990) Cervical spine manipulations: applied loads, motions and myoelectric responses. Adv Bioeng 249–250.

Ueno, Liu YK (1987) A three-dimensional nonlinear finite element model of lumbar intervertebral joint in torsion. J Biomech Eng 109:200–209.

Vulcan AP, King AI. Forces and moments sustained by lower vertebral column of seated human during seat-to-head acceleration. In Dynamic response of biomechanical systems. ASME, New York, 1970.

Werne S (1957) Studies in spontaneous atlas dislocation. Acta Orthop Scand S23:1–150.

White AA III, Panjabi MM (1978a) The basic kinematics of the human cervical spine. A view of past and current knowledge. Spine 3:12.

White AA, Panjabi MM (1978b) The clinical biomechanics of the occipitoatlantoaxial complex. Orthop Clin North Am 9:867–878.

White AA, Panjabi MM. *Biomechanics of the Spine*. Lippincott, Philadelphia, 1978c.

Whitley JE, Forsyth HF (1960) The classification of cervical spine injuries. Am J Roentgenol 83:633.

Williams JL, Belytschko, TB (1983) A three-dimensional model of human cervical spine for input simulation. J Biomech Eng 105:321–32.

Wismans J, Philippens M, van Oorschot E, Kallieris D, Mattern R. Comparison of human volunteer and cadaver head-neck response in frontal flexion. 31st Stapp Car Crash Conference. SAE 872194, pp 1–11, 1987.

Wismans J, Maltha J, van Wijk JJ, Janssen EG. MADYMO—a crash victim simulation program for biomechanical research and optimization of designs for impact injury prevention. AGARD—Cologne, Germany, April, 1982.

Wismans JS, Spenny C. Performance requirements of mechanical necks in lateral flexion. 27th Stapp Car Crash Conference. p 137, 1983.

Wismans JS, Van Dorschot H, Walttring HJ. Omni directional human head-neck response. 30th Stapp Car Crash Conference. p 313, 1986.

Yoganandan N, Haffner MM, Maiman DJ, Nichols H, Pintar FA, Jentzen J, Weinshel SS, Larson SK, Sances A Jr. Epidemiology and injury biomechanics of motor vehicle related trauma to the human spine. 33nd Stapp Car Crash Conference. pp 22–242, 1989a.

Yoganandan N, Myklebust JB, Ray G, Sances A Jr (1987) Mathematical and finite element analysis of spine injuries. CRC Crit Rev Biomed Eng 15(1):29–93.

Yoganandan N, Sances A Jr, Maiman DJ, Myklebust JB, Pech P, Larson SJ (1986) Experimental spinal injuries with vertical impact. Spine 11(9):855–860.

Yoganandan, Sances A Jr, Pintar F (1989b) Biomechanical evaluation of the axial compressive responses of the human cadaveric and manikin necks. J Biomech Eng 111:250–255.

Zhu Y, Yang-He X, Zhu D-M, Sun C-Z. A lumped-parameter dynamic model of parachuter's head-neck system. First World Congress of Biomechanics, I. San Diego, CA, August 30–September 4, p 161, 1990.

15
The Biomechanics of Thoracic Trauma

John M. Cavanaugh

Introduction

During impact with an automobile, the thorax can interact with various components of the automobile interior and with several types of restraint. The types of interactions include unrestrained driver or passenger with steering wheel or instrument panel, and interactions with active or passive restaints, including three-point lap/shoulder belts, two-point shoulder belts, knee bolsters, and air bags. Injury to the thorax commonly occurs in frontal and side impacts and in impact directions intermediate to these two. In automotive accidents chest injury ranks only second to head injury in overall number of fatalities and serious injuries. It ranks second to head injury in overall economic cost using the Harm concept of Malliaris et al. (1982, 1985) as shown in Table 15.1.

Anatomy of the Thorax

The thorax consists of the rib cage and the underlying soft tissue organs. The thorax is bounded inferiorly by the diaphragm, a thin muscular sheet that separates the thoracic contents from the abdominal contents.

Rib Cage

The rib cage (Fig. 15.1) consists of 12 thoracic vertebrae (T1 through T12), 12 pairs of ribs, and the sternum. Posteriorly, each of the 12 ribs is joined to its corresponding thoracic vertebra at the costal facet joints. Anteriorly, each of the first seven ribs join the sternum at a condrosternal junction. Ribs 8 through 10 join the bottom of the sternum by cartilaginous attachments to the seventh rib. Ribs 11 and 12, called the floating ribs, have no anterior attachment to the sternum or other skeletal structures.

Lungs and Mediastinum

The left lung consists of two lobes—the upper (superior) and lower. The right lung consists of three lobes—the upper, middle, and lower (Fig. 15.2). The lungs are covered in a serous

TABLE 15.1. The ranking of the regions of the body according to Harm, an indicator of the economic cost of injury (from Malliaris et al., 1982).*

Body region	1980 and 1981	
	NASS	NCSS
Head	35.5	33.0
Face	2.8	3.6
Neck	4.6	13.8
Chest	26.7	20.0
Abdomen	18.2	14.7
Upper extremities	4.1	5.1
Lower extremities	5.1	7.9
Other	2.7	2.0
Unknown	0.4	0.0
Total	100	100

* Injuries to the thorax rank second in Harm. NASS, National Accident Sampling System; NCSS, National Crash Severity Study.

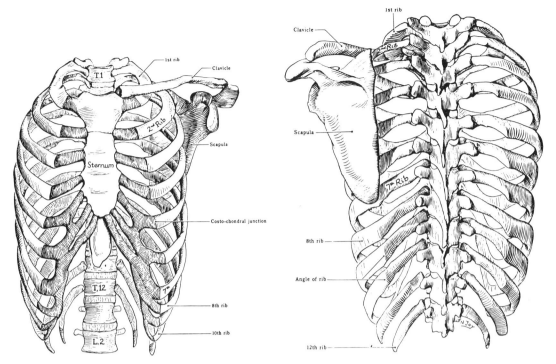

FIGURE 15.1. Illustration of the skeletal anatomy of the thorax. A. Anterior (front) view. B. Posterior (back) view. (From Anderson: Grant's Atlas of Anatomy, 8th Edition. Williams & Wilkins, Baltimore, 1983.)

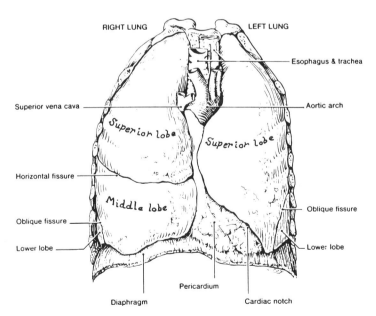

FIGURE 15.2. Diagram of the lungs. The right lung has upper, middle, and lower lobes. The left lung has upper and lower lobes. The mediastinum, in the central region of the thorax, contains the heart and great vessels and other structures as illustrated. (From Anderson: Grant's Atlas of Anatomy, 8th Edition. Williams & Wilkins, Baltimore, 1983.)

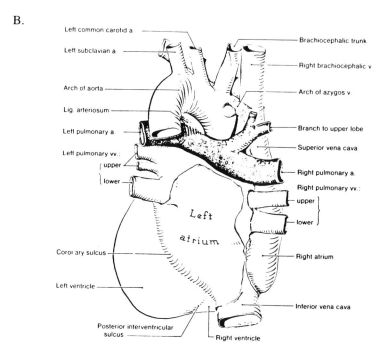

A.

Left common carotid a.
Brachiocephalic trunk
Left subclavian a.
Right brachiocephalic v.
Left brachiocephalic v.
Ligamentum arteriosum
Aortic arch
Superior vena cava
Left pulmonary a.
Asc. aorta
Pulm. artery
Left pulmonary vv.
Right pulmonary a.
Right pulmonary vv.
Auricle of left atrium
Coronary sulcus
auricle
Right atrium
Left ventricle
Right border of heart
Right ventricle
Left border of heart
Coronary sulcus
Ant. interventricular sulcus
Inferior vena cava
Inferior border of heart
Apex of heart

B.

Left common carotid a.
Brachiocephalic trunk
Left subclavian a.
Right brachiocephalic v.
Arch of aorta
Arch of azygos v.
Lig. arteriosum
Left pulmonary a.
Branch to upper lobe
Superior vena cava
Left pulmonary vv.:
upper
lower
Right pulmonary a.
Right pulmonary vv.:
upper
Left atrium
lower
Coronary sulcus
Right atrium
Left ventricle
Inferior vena cava
Posterior interventricular sulcus
Right ventricle

FIGURE 15.3. Diagram of the heart showing right and left atrium, right and left ventricles and great vessels. A. Anterior view. B. Posterior view. a, artery; v, vein; vv, veins. (From Anderson: Grant's Atlas of Anatomy, 8th Edition. Williams & Wilkins, Baltimore, 1983.)

membrane called the visceral pleura. The parietal pleura lines the inner surface of the chest wall, covers the diaphragm, and encloses the structures in the middle of the thorax. The central region of the thoracic cavity is called the mediastinum (Fig. 15.2, middle region), and contains the heart, the great vessels entering and leaving the heart, the thymus gland, the esophagus and lower portion of the trachea, the thoracic duct and thoracic lymph nodes, and nerves passing into and through the thorax, including the vagus and phrenic nerves. The mediastinum is bordered in front by the sternum and in back by the thoracic vertebrae.

Heart and Great Vessels

The heart (Fig. 15.3) is a hollow muscular organ that lies in the lower part of the thoracic cavity in the middle mediastinum. It is roughly the size of a man's fist, weighing 300 g in the adult male and 250 g in the female. The heart is divided into four chambers—left and right atria, and left and right ventricles. The right atrium receives the returning deoxygenated blood from all body tissues except the lungs. This returning blood comes in through the superior and inferior venae cavae. The right ventricle pumps the deoxygenated blood to the lungs through the pulmonary artery. In the lungs the blood is reoxygenated. The oxygenated blood from the lungs is returned to the left atrium through four pulmonary veins. From the left atrium, the oxygenated blood

goes to the thick-walled left ventricle, which pumps it out through the aorta to all parts of the body except the lungs.

Thoracic Injury

Cohen (1987) reported that for the thorax and abdomen, most of the contact for the driver is to the steering assembly, while for the passenger, it is to the instrument panel. The National Accident Sampling System (NASS) database from 1979 to 1984 was reviewed by Haffner for passenger cars in nonejection and nonrollover cases and published by Schneider et al. (1990). For both drivers and passengers, skeletal injury represented the highest percentage of the injury to the thorax (Table 15.2) as measured by the Abbreviated Injury Scale (AIS). This was followed by pulmonary/lung injuries for the driver, and then liver and heart injuries. The liver and spleen are located under the diaphragm, but are bounded by the lower lateral rib cage. The rim of the steering wheel or the instrument panel can produce soft tissue injuries to these areas. Although arterial injuries accounted for only 6% to 8% of AIS >2, they accounted for 27% to 30% of estimated Harm.

Flail Chest

Rib fracture and flail chest occur with blunt impact to the rib cage. It is probable that the ribs fail in bending, with the failure occurring

TABLE 15.2. The ranking of thoracic AIS and Harm by type of organ injury (compiled by Haffner in Schneider et al. 1990, p. 6).

Injury	Driver AIS 3 or greater	Passenger AIS 3 or greater	Driver HARM	Passenger HARM
Arterial	8	6	27	30
Heart	10	4	18	4
Joints	7	6	1	1
Liver	10	11	20	21
Pulmonary/lung	21	9	9	7
Spleen	6	8	3	9
Skeletal	25	30	10	10
Vertebral	3	6	1	4
Other and unknown	10	20	11	14
Total	100	100	100	100

on the tensile side of the ribs. Stalnaker and Mohan (1974) and Melvin et al. (1975) concluded that maximum compression of the chest is the determining factor for rib fracture. In their review of injury and response data from cadaveric studies, rib fractures were more frequent with chest deflections over 3 inches, while none occurred at deflections less than 2.3 inches. Thus, it appears that the number of rib fractures depends on the magnitude of rib deflection, rather than the rate of deflection. However, the amount of force depends on the rate at which the force is applied, due to the viscous nature of the thorax. Thus, for a given loading rate, force appears to be related to the number of rib fractures. Eppinger (1976) developed a relationship between the number of rib fractures and upper torso shoulder belt force, age, and weight of cadaveric subject.

Lung Contusions

Unlike rib fractures, lung contusion is rate dependent. Fung and Yen (1984) determined that it was a velocity-dependent phenomenon. At high velocities, a compression or pressure wave is transmitted through the chest wall to the lung tissue, causing damage to the capillary bed of the alveoli. Lacerations of lung tissue can also occur at sites of rib fractures.

Hemothorax and Pneumothorax

Hemothorax (bleeding into the lung tissue) is due to injury to the blood vessels of the lungs with consequent bleeding into the lung tissue. The blood vessels are often lacerated by broken ribs.

If a hole is created in the pleural sac between the lungs and the rib cage, a pneumothorax occurs. The puncture or laceration can be in the parietal pleura lining the inside of the rib cage or in the visceral pleura surrounding the lungs. The pneumothorax is often the result of rib fracture. Thus, rib fracture, hemothorax, and pneuomothorax appear to be deflection dependent, while lung contusion is velocity dependent.

Heart and Great Vessels

During high-speed thoracic impact the heart can be subject to contusion, laceration, or cardiac arrest. Lasky et al. (1968) in a review of 67 cases of frontal and side impact collisions by the Vehicle Trauma Research Group at UCLA found that in frontal collisions, energy-absorbing steering wheel hubs and columns resulted in reduced cardiovascular injury. Side impact collisions were shown to produce a large proportion of the cardiovascular injury in this study. Contusion appears to be due to compression and the velocity of compression, while cardiac laceration may be due to high magnitudes of compression over the sternum. At high rates of loading, the heart may undergo fibrillation or arrest. High-speed blunt impacts (>15 to 20 m/sec) appear to interrupt the electromechanical transduction of the heart wall. Cooper et al. (1982) reported on 38 midsternal impacts to the chest of pigs by a cylindrical mass of 0.14 to 0.38 kg and 3.7 and 10 cm in diameter at velocities of 20 to 74 m/sec. Acute ventricular fibrillation (AVF) appeared to be associated with midsternal blows during the T-wave of the electro-cardiogram (ECG). Kroell et al. (1986) reported 11 cases of ventricular fibrillation (VFB) in impacts to the midsternum of 23 anesthetized swine. Eight of the VFBs were immediate and five of these were in impacts that occurred during the T-wave of the ECG.

Aortic rupture is often seen in automotive accidents and is often fatal. Viano (1983) proposed several mechanisms for aortic injury, depending on the site of injury. Sites of laceration include the aortic isthmus, root, and aortic insertion into the diaphragm. The isthmus is a portion of the aorta between the ligamentum arteriosum and left subclavian artery (Fig. 15.3) that is narrowed during fetal development. During fetal development the ligamentum arteriosum is open and is called the ductus arteriosus. Aortic lacerations generally have a transverse orientation. The tearing strength of the aorta is higher in the longitudinal than the transverse direction according to work by Mohan and Melvin (1983), who showed that the descending midthoracic aorta failed in the transverse rather than longitudinal direction under uniform biaxial stretch. In their study, Lasky et al. (1968) postulated that large fluid pressures resulting in a water hammer effect may be important in causing vessel rupture. On the other hand, in another study Newman and Rastogi (1984) observed that in all 12 cases of aortic rupture, the impact was not directly frontal, suggesting that a transverse component of impact is required to produce aortic wall laceration between fixed and mobile sections of the aorta. In fact, in a series of 12

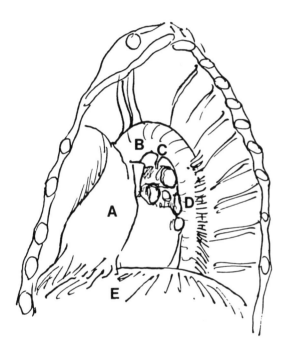

A. HEART IN PERICARDIAL SAC.

B. AORTIC ARCH.

C. LIGAMENTUM ARTERIOSUM.

D. DESCENDING THORACIC AORTA TIED DOWN
   TO POSTERIOR CHEST WALL WITH FASCIA

E. DIAPHRAGM.

FIGURE 15.4. Diagram showing the aortic arch and descending aorta which is attached to the posterior chest wall. The area between the junction of the aortic arch and descending aorta is where aortic ruptures were seen in the side impact study of Cavanaugh et al. (1990). (Reproduced with permission from Society of Automotive Engineers.)

cadaveric sled side impacts, Cavanaugh et al. (1990) reported five aortic lacerations, with the site of injury being distal to the ligamentum arteriosum, and at the top of the descending aorta, where it starts to become firmly attached to the posterior chest wall. They hypothesized that the more mobile heart and aortic arch translated laterally, producing tears at the top of the more firmly anchored descending aorta (Fig. 15.4). Thus, tears in the aorta and other great vessels branching from the heart may be due to a deformation that twists or tears the vessel wall in a transverse direction, due to high internal pressures, or to a combination of both. The tears have been observed to be in the transverse direction.

AIS and Other Scaling Methods

AIS

The standard method for classifying the level of injury to a body region or organ is the Abbreviated Injury Scale (AIS) of the Association for the Advancement of Automotive Medicine (AAAM) and periodically updated by the Committee on Injury Scaling. The last update was in 1990 with previous updates in 1985 and 1980. The numerical rating system ranges from 0 (no injury) to 6 (maximum, virtually unsurvivable). The higher the AIS level, the higher the mortality or threat to life. The scale does not quantify long-term disability or medical and societal costs of injury. Typical AIS (1990) injuries to the rib cage and to thoracic soft tissues are shown in Table 15.3.

A major difference in maximum AIS (MAIS) can occur because of modifications to AIS in 1980, 1985, and 1990. In 1980, severe flail chest was assigned AIS 4, while in the 1985 guide, severe flail chest requiring respiratory support was assigned AIS 5. In 1990, AIS 4 was again the maximum level for flail chest, except when it is bilateral, in which case AIS is 5. A flail chest is an unstable chest wall in which a portion of the rib cage does not rise on inspiration because of loss of structural rib cage integrity. In a cadaveric specimen this is dif-

TABLE 15.3. Typical skeletal and soft tissue injuries to the thorax ranked by AIS (1990 Revision).

AIS Skeletal injury	AIS Soft tissue injury
1 1 rib fracture.	1 Contusion of bronchus.
2 2–3 rib fractures. Sternum fracture.	2 Laceration of pericardium.
3 4 or more rib fractures. 2–3 rib fractures with hemothorax or pneumothorax.	3 Contusion of heart. Contusion of lung. Unilateral lung laceration.
4 Flail chest. 4 or more rib fractures with hemothorax or pneumothorax.	4 Bilateral lung laceration. Minor aortic laceration.
5 Bilateral flail chest.	5 Major aortic laceration. Lung laceration with tension pneumothorax.
6	6 Aortic laceration with hemorrhage not confined to mediastinum.

ficult to evaluate, but nine or more rib fractures to a hemithorax has been considered flail chest and assigned AIS 4, as per Viano (1989) and used by Cavanaugh et al. (1990).

ISS and PODS

The Injury Severity Scale (ISS) is a measure of the probability of survival. It is obtained by summing the square of the highest AIS in each of three body regions and was developed to account for the effect of injuries to multiple body regions. The ISS uses six body regions: (1) head and neck, (2) face, (3) chest, (4) abdomen and pelvis, (5) extremities and bony pelvis, and (6) external (Baker et al., 1974).

The Probability of Death Score (PODS) and PODSa (which accounts for subject age) were developed for the same purpose (Somers, 1983). The equation for PODS is as follows:

$$PODS = e^x/(1 + e^x) \qquad (15.1)$$

For PODS, $x = 2.2(AIS_1) + 0.9(AIS_2) - 11.25 + C$.

For PODSa, $x = 2.7(AIS_1) + 1.0(AIS_2) + 0.06 \times AGE - 15.4 + C$, where $C = -0.764$ for cars. AIS_1 = highest AIS code and AIS_2 = second highest AIS code.

The advantages of PODS over ISS are that PODS has a better goodness-of-fit to real data than ISS and has an inherent definition of health outcome (probability of death) (Somers, 1982).

Whereas AIS, ISS, and PODS quantify injury in terms of threat to life, other concepts have been developed to quantify injury in terms of additional factors, such as quality of life or societal cost of injury. These methodologies include Harm and the Injury Priority Rating (IPR). Harm establishes an economic value to each level of injury (Malliaris et al., 1982, 1985). Using Harm, chest injury ranks second only to head injury in overall number of fatalities and serious injuries (Table 15.1). Hirsch et al. (1983) used AIS to rank injuries by impairment. Impairment severity ranged from one to four, with four being most severe. Six different aspects of impairment (mobility, cognitive/psychological, cosmetic, sensory, pain, and daily living) for three different durations (0 to 1 year, 1 to 5 years, >5 years) were thus ranked. Carsten and O'Day (1984) developed the IPR to evaluate overall impairment. Carsten (1986) modified this and developed the Multi-Injury Priority Rating (MIPR) to express overall injury impairment. The IPR provides for postaccident survival and can distinguish the impairment due to injuries with the same AIS value. Marcus and Blodgett (1988) extended impairment studies to more recent data and reviewed IPR and impairment methodologies.

Biomechanics of Frontal Impact

Many biomechanical tests have been performed on human cadavers under controlled laboratory conditions to carefully measure biomechanical response (forces, accelerations, deformations, pressures) and to obtain details of resulting injury through necropsy of the body after impact. Pendulum and sled tests have been performed to ascertain these data for frontal and lateral impacts. These data have been used to develop frontal and side impact dummies and to develop injury criteria. A description of these tests follows.

Frontal Impact: Biomechanical Response of the Thorax

Pendulum Impacts to the Sternum

Some of the most extensive testing was published and analyzed in the 1970s and involved 6-inch diameter rigid pendulum impacts to the sternum of unembalmed cadavers (Fig. 15.5). The data were presented by Kroell et al. (1971, 1974), Nahum et al. (1970, 1971, 1975), and Stalnaker et al. (1973), and have also been analyzed by Lobdell et al. (1973) and Neathery (1974). In the Kroell tests the impactor contacted the sternum at the level of the interspace between the fourth and fifth ribs. Figure 15.6 shows force-deflection curves for 4.02 to 5.23 and 6.71 to 7.38 m/sec Kroell tests.

The total chest deflection including the flesh overlying the sternum was included by Kroell et al. (1971, 1974). Neathery (1974) developed corridors of skeletal chest deflection, based on

the Kroell data. Lobdell et al. (1973) showed that lower-impactor masses resulted in lower deflections. Patrick (1981) developed force-deflection curves under conditions similar to the Kroell unrestrained back conditions, but used himself as a volunteer and a padded (2.4-cm thick Rubatex R310V) 10 kg, 6-inch diameter striker at velocities of 2.4 to 4.6 m/sec. Forces in the tensed condition were slightly higher than in the relaxed condition for the same impact velocity. Apparent initial stiffnesses were as follows: 79 N/mm at 2.4 m/sec tensed, 57 N/mm at 2.4 m/sec relaxed, and 250 N/mm at 4.6 m/sec tensed. Peak skeletal deflections were 44 to 46 mm (16% to 17% deflection of the rib cage).

The idealized force-deflection curves derived from these responses can be divided into a loading and an unloading phase (Fig. 15.7), with the loading phase having three components (Melvin et al., 1988). An initial rapid rise or apparent initial stiffness (A) is due in large part to the viscous properties of the thorax. The force plateau (B) is also due to a viscous response. At maximum deflection (C), the impactor and subject are moving at a common velocity and the forces are due to inertial forces caused by whole-body acceleration, and the elastic forces are due to tissue compression. The unloading portion of the curve (D), is due to unloading of the compressed tissues, and follows the elastic nonlinear unloading of the thorax seen in quasi-static tests. Based on the Kroell data, Melvin et al. have developed the following equation to characterize these thoracic responses in pendulum impacts:

$$F(t) = KD^2(t) + CV(t) + mA(t)$$
$$(15.2)$$

where K = elastic spring constant, $47 N/m^2$ $(68.2 lb/in^2)$
  C = coefficient of viscous damping, 5.45 N-s/cm (3.11 lb-s/in)
  m = average effective mass, 0.286 kg (0.630 lb)
  D = chest deflection
  V = chest velocity of deformation
  A = chest acceleration
  F = impact force.

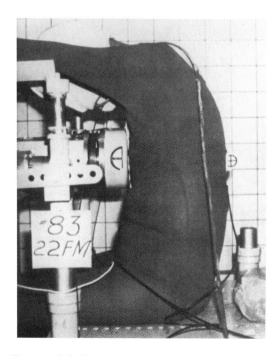

FIGURE 15.5. Photograph showing a frontal pendulum impact applied to the sternum. (From Kroell et al., 1971. Reproduced with permission from Society of Automotive Engineers.)

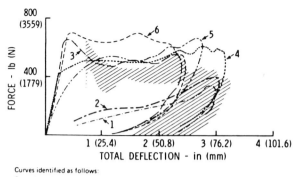

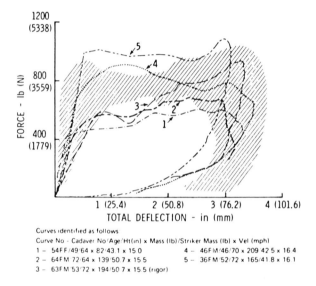

Force versus total deflection; nominal 43 and 51 lb (19.5 and 23.1 kg) strikers at 9.0–11.7 mph (4.02–5.23 m/s)

FIGURE 15.6. Force-deflection plots generated by Kroell et al. (1974) for frontal impacts to the sternum. (Reproduced with permission from Society of Automotive Engineers.) A. 4.02 to 5.23 m/sec impacts. Shaded area represents a corridor of three tests at 5.14 m/sec with 19.3 kg mass. B. 6.71 to 7.38 m/sec impacts. Shaded area represents a corridor of seven tests at 6.7 to 7.4 m/sec with 23.1 kg mass. The impactor had a 6-inch diameter flat, rigid surface, and a mass of 19.5 or 23.1 kg.

D, V, A, and F are for any moment in time (t). The values of K, C, and m (Melvin et al., 1988) are the average of idealized 4.2, 6.7, and 10.2 m/sec Kroell corridors using a 23.4-kg (51.5-lb) impactor mass. Using the Kroell data (1971, 1974) and the Patrick (1981) volunteer data, Melvin et al. (1988) developed equations for A (the initial rise or apparent stiffness

in Fig. 15.7) and B (the plateau force of Fig. 15.7).

$$A = 0.263 + 0.603 (V - 1.3) \quad (15.3)$$
$$B = 1 + 0.75 (V - 3.73)$$

where A is in kN/cm, B is in kN, and V is in m/sec.

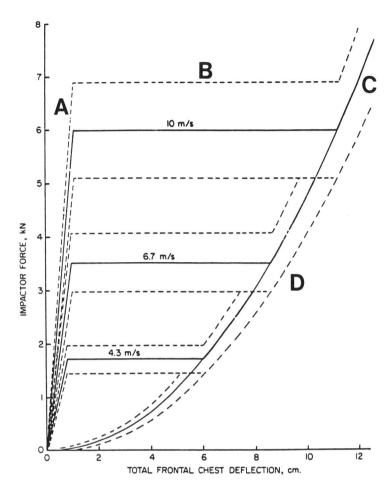

FIGURE 15.7. Plot of pendulum impact force-deflection curve illustrating the various components of the curve. A. Rise. B. Plateau. C. Maximum deflection. D. Unloading. Based on pendulum impacts using 15.2-cm diameter rigid flat disc and 23.4-kg impact mass. (Modified from Melvin et al., 1988).

Belt Loading

Three-Point Belt Loading

In a Canadian study of injury to 121 belted occupants, Dalmotas (1980) found that shoulder/chest injuries constituted 22% of AIS 2 and greater injuries. For those drivers who did not contact the steering assembly, injuries were skeletal fractures of clavicle, sternum, and ribs in the belt line in six drivers. No intrathoracic or abdominal injuries were attributed to belt loading. Patrick et al. (1974) reported similar results in crash investigations of drivers wearing three-point belts. Fourteen of 169 accident victims (8.3%) had rib or sternal fractures. Barrier equivalent velocity was 2 to 53 miles per hour (1 to 24 m/sec). At 0 to 9 miles per hour (0 to 4 m/sec) 29 of 32 occupants had no

injury. Three of three occupants had AIS 2 to 3 at velocities greater than 50 miles per hour. Two of these were AIS 3. All rib fractures occurred on the inboard side and followed the belt line. In a test series with 49 cadavers, Schmidt et al. (1974) reported similar fracture patterns.

Fayon et al. (1975) calculated the resultant normal force from the geometry and tension forces at belt anchorages and determined that sternal thoracic stiffness was 166.4 N/mm (951 lb/in). Walfisch et al. (1982) came up with slightly smaller values of 70 to 116 N/mm (mean 119.4 N/mm, 682 lb/in). L'Abbe et al. (1982) conducted static and dynamic tests of belt loading and consequent chest deflection in human volunteers (Fig. 15.8). The dynamic loads were up to 3,600 N and produced mid-

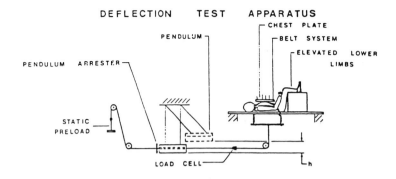

FIGURE 15.8. Diagram of the belt loading methodolgy of L'Abbe et al. (1982).

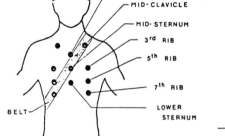

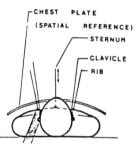

sternal stiffnesses of 137 N/mm, right seventh rib stiffnesses of 123 N/mm and 200 N/mm at the left clavicle. The Hybrid III frontal impact crash dummy tended to produce stiffer responses than in relaxed volunteers, with better agreement to tensed volunteers, particularly at midsternum. Backaitis and St. Laurent (1986), in similar tests, showed greatest deflections at the seventh rib in volunteers and least in the shoulder, while Hybrid III showed maximum deflections at the shoulder.

Two-Point Belt Loading Plus Knee Bolster

Cadaver data is available from work by Cheng et al. (1984), who performed 11 cadaver tests with a Volkswagen two-point belt and knee bolster in the right-front passenger position (Fig. 15.9). The belt crossed from the right shoulder to the left side. There were more rib fractures on the left in seven cadavers. The number of rib fractures ranged from 0 to 14, with seven subjects having seven or more rib

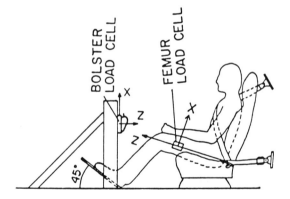

FIGURE 15.9. Diagram of the two-point belt loading plus knee bolster test setup of Cheng et al. (1984). (Reproduced with permission from Society of Automotive Engineers.)

fractures. Peak upper shoulder belt load was 5.1 to 7.6 kN for 48 km/h impacts with peak sled deceleration of 22 g's. The peak belt loads ranged from 3.6 to 9.7 kN for four runs with peak sled deceleration of $35\,g$'s. The ratio of lower to upper belt peak loads was approximately 0.9.

Air-Bag Tests

Human response to air-bag deployment and loading has been studied only relatively recently. There has been a concern for injury to the child and the out-of-position occupant (Aldman et al., 1974; Takeda and Kobayashi, 1980). Situations of concern include the shorter stature older subject who sits close to the steering wheel, the subject leaning over during an impact, or the subject brought closer to the steering wheel during a relatively minor first impact who is then hit by the air bag during a major second impact. Bag slap from high-velocity impacts (15 m/sec) can injure the lungs and heart. It is hypothesized that these injuries could be due to stress waves. At Wayne State University, Cheng et al. (1982) conducted a series of frontal impact sled tests with a pressurized air bag (Fig. 15.10). Peak bag pressure was 93 to 139 kPa (13.5 to 20.2 psi).

Chest AIS was 0 to 2 but overall MAIS was 2 to 6 due to cervical spine injury.

A detailed study of the effect of air-bag deployment on the Hybrid III was performed for the bag opposite head, neck, and thorax (Horsch et al., 1990). Highest response amplitudes occurred with the body part directly against the air-bag module. Additional tests were performed with the module opposite the sternum of anesthetized swine. Severe to critical injuries were seen in all tests where the swine's torso covered the module. Injuries included heart contusions and perforations. Injury was related to internal bag pressure. As long as bag volume was greater than gas volume generated, there would be minimal pressure and thus minimal force to the subject. There are two main times when available volume is less than generated volume: (1) "punch out" during initial pressurization of the module, and (2) "membrane-force" phases when the subject is in the path of the bag and the force is due to bag pressure on the subject. This includes tension forces from bag wraparound. Hybrid III test conditions in which the maximum value of velocity times

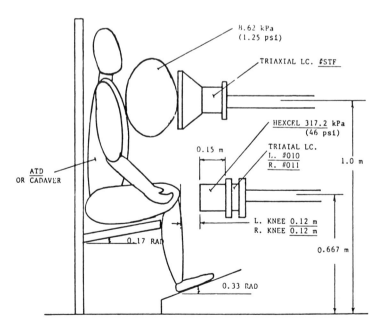

FIGURE 15.10. Diagram of the pressurized air-bag test set up of Cheng et al. (1982). (Reproduced with permission from Society of Automotive Engineers.)

compression (VC$_{max}$, otherwise known as the viscous criterion) was less than 1 m/sec resulted in no chest injury to the swine, and Hybrid III tests in which VC$_{max}$ was greater than 1 m/sec resulted in severe chest injury to swine. Chest compression velocities were as high as 14 m/sec.

Quasi-Static Tests

As three-point belts and air bags become more frequently used, lower rate loading will become more important in frontal impact. Also the distributed loading to the ribs due to the air bag, and rib and clavicle loading due to the shoulder belt, make the biomechanical response of the ribs and clavicle (in addition to the sternum) increasingly important. Thus, in addition to the dynamic pendulum data from sternal impacts, quasi-static chest loading data is also important. These data are described below.

Stalnaker et al. (1973) loaded the sternum of volunteers and cadavers with a 153-mm (6-inch) diameter rigid plate with the subject's back against a rigid wall. Stiffnesses averaged 12.2 N/mm for unembalmed cadavers, 40.2 N/mm for relaxed volunteers, and

114 N/mm in tensed volunteers (Fig. 15.11). Lobdell et al. (1973) showed much less stiffness under similar loading conditions: 7 N/mm for relaxed volunteers and 23.7 N/mm for the tensed subject (Fig. 15.12).

Tsitlik et al. (1983) measured force versus deflection due to loading the sternum of 11 patients with a 48 × 64 mm rubber thumper. The average stiffness was 9.1 N/mm (range: 5.25 to 15.9 N/mm) for deflections of 30 to 61 mm. At Wayne State University, Cavanaugh et al. (unpublished data) loaded the sternum and rib cage of three unembalmed cadavers with 1-inch strokes at quasi-static loading rates. The thorax stiffnesses were as follows: upper and midsternum, 8.6 to 12.3 N/mm; lower sternum, 5.7 to 11.4 N/mm; 2nd rib, 5.6 to 7.3 N/mm; 5th rib, 5.1 to 8.4 N/mm; and 7th rib, 3.4 to 5.2 N/mm. Weisfeldt (1979) loaded the chest of volunteers at 60 cycles/sec with a 22 × 64 mm pad. The mean stiffness was 6.3 N/mm. On one subject loading the chest with a 153-mm (6-inch) diameter pad resulted in a stiffness of 21 N/mm. Melvin et al. (1985), after reviewing the quasi-static load-deflection literature, concluded that at deflections up to 41mm the thorax has an approximate linear stiffness of 26.2 N/mm and for deflections greater than 76 mm, 120 N/mm. Melvin also

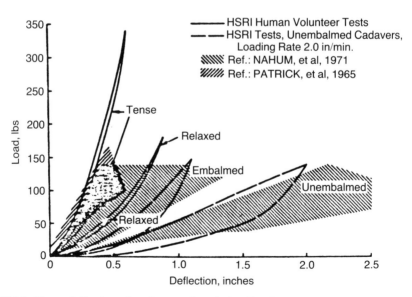

FIGURE 15.11. Force-deflection plots for quasi-static loading from Stalnaker et al. (1973, p. 195).

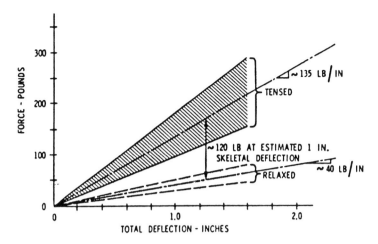

FIGURE 15.12. Force-deflection plots for quasi-static loading of Lobdell et al. (1973, p. 217).

modeled these force-deflection relationships with a quadratic equation:

$$F = Kd^2 \qquad (15.3)$$

where $K = 47.6 \, \text{N/mm}^2$.

Fayon et al. (1975) demonstrated stiffnesses of 17.5 to 26.3 N/mm due to sternal deflections up to 25 mm for static belt loading to supine volunteers. This compared to 8.8 to 17.5 N/mm for disk loading up to 38 mm. At the second rib, estimated stiffness was 17.5 to 35 N/mm and 8.8 to 17.5 N/mm at the ninth rib. Melvin and Weber (1985) estimated an apparent stiffness from the static belt tests of L'Abbe et al. (1982). These results were 67.5 N/mm at mid-sternum, 40 N/mm at right seventh rib, and 95 N/mm at left clavicle for deflections up to 10 mm and estimated normal forces up to 667 N. Melvin has suggested that these data may be significantly higher than those of Fayon et al. (1975) because spinal curvature may have reduced stiffness in the tests by Fayon et al.

Frontal Impact: Injury Tolerance of the Thorax

Much of the early work on frontal impact tolerance was reviewed by Mertz and Kroell (1970). Some of these data and later data are summarized below. These data have been used in the development of the Hybrid III frontal impact dummy (Foster et al., 1977).

Acceleration Criteria

Human tolerance for severe chest injury is often stated as the peak spinal acceleration (sustained for 3 ms or longer) not to exceed $60g$'s in a frontal crash. The Hybrid II and III dummies are used for assessment of frontal impact crashworthiness per the Code of Federal Regulations 571.208 (FMVSS 208). The Hybrid II dummy measures thoracic spinal acceleration but not chest compression, while the Hybrid III also measures chest compression.

Early acceleration tolerance data was obtained by Stapp (1951, 1970), who demonstrated the human tolerance to rocket sled acceleration when belt restraints were worn. Thoracic accelerations up to $40g$'s for 100 ms or less were tolerated. In one subject a maximum of $45g$'s was tolerated, which resulted in a calculated pressure of 252 kPa (36.5 psi) under the harness. Peaks of $30g$'s reached at a rate of $1,000g$'s/sec were not tolerated. Eiband (1959), in an analysis of the Stapp data, showed that the acceleration tolerance decreased as duration of exposure increased. Spinal acceleration is a general indicator of the overall severity of whole-body impact, but is sensitive to changing impact conditions (Lau and Viano, 1986).

Force Criteria

Patrick et al. (1965) performed a series of sled tests with embalmed cadavers to simulate the response of an unrestrained occupant. The head, chest, and knees impacted padded load cells. These studies were used as the basis for the design of the energy-absorbing steering column. Gadd and Patrick (1968) and Patrick et al. (1969) used a prototype energy-absorbing steering column in unrestrained cadaveric sled tests; 3.3 kN hub load to the sternum and 8.8 kN distributed load to the shoulders and chest resulted in only minor trauma in centered impacts. The reactive force is due to the inertial, elastic, and viscous components of the torso.

Bierman et al. (1946) tested young male volunteers with a drop-weight device that loaded a lap/double–shoulder belt harness 490 cm^2 (76 inches^2) in area. Painful reactions and minor injury occurred when loads exceeded 8.9 kN (2,000 pounds). When load area was increased to 1,006 cm^2 (156 inches^2), loads of 8.0 to 13.3 kN (1,800 to 3,000 pounds) were sustained without injury.

Energy Criterion

Eppinger and Marcus (1985) examined the results of 82 laboratory impact tests and concluded that severity of injury to the thorax was proportional to the amount of specific energy that the thorax must absorb. The severity of injury was found to be inversely proportional to the impacted area and the duration of time over which the energy was transferred.

Compression Criteria

Kroell et al. (1971, 1974) analyzed a large number of blunt thoracic impact experiments and determined that chest compression correlated well with AIS ($r = 0.730$), while maximum plateau force did not ($r = 0.524$). The linear equation relating AIS to compression was:

$$\text{AIS} = -3.78 + 19.56\,C \qquad (15.4)$$

where C is chest deformation divided by chest depth. C equals 0.3 (30%) for AIS 2 and 0.4

(40%) for AIS 4. Thus, for the 230-mm chest depth of the 50th percentile male, 30% compression or 69-mm (2.71-inch) deflection predicts AIS 2 and 40% compression or 92-mm (3.62-inch) deflection predicts AIS 4.

The integral of spinal acceleration, which is a measure of the velocity of deformation, and chest compression correlated well to injury severity (Nahum et al., 1975). In 5- to 7-m/sec sternal impacts to cadavers, compressions >20% regularly produced rib fractures. Compressions of 40% produced flail chest. Neathery et al. (1975) further analyzed the cadaver data base and recommended a sternal deflection of 75 mm for AIS 3 for the 50th percentile male. Viano (1978b) reported that severe injury to internal organs occurred at an average maximum compression (C_{max}) of 40% and recommended C_{max} of 32% to maintain enough rib cage stability to protect internal organs. The Code of Federal Regulations, Federal Motor Vehicle Standard 208 (Code of Federal Regulations, 571.208), allows a maximum 76-mm (3-inch) chest deflection in the 50th percentile Hybrid III dummy in frontal impact crashworthiness testing of automobiles.

Viscous Criterion

Soft tissue injury is compression dependent and rate dependent (Lau and Viano, 1986). Lau and Viano (1981a), in impacts over the liver of anesthetized rabbits, found that when C_{max} was held to 16%, liver injury increased as impact velocity increased from 5 to 20 m/sec. In frontal thoracic impacts to anesthetized rabbits at 5, 10, and 18 m/sec, severity of lung injury was found to increase with C_{max} at each level of velocity (Lau and Viano, 1981b). The alveolar region was more sensitive to the rate of loading than regions of vascular junctions. Data from 123 frontal impacts to anesthetized rabbits were used to define the viscous tolerance (Viano and Lau, 1983). This led to the development of the viscous criterion (Viano and Lau, 1985), which states that VC_{max}, the maximum product of velocity of deformation and compression, is an effective predictor of injury risk, and is a measure of the energy dissipated by the viscous elements of the thorax. Kroell et al. (1981, 1986) verified the validity of the viscous criterion in blunt thoracic frontal impacts to anesthetized swine. In Kroell et al. (1986), 23 swine (53.3 kg average mass) were impacted at 15 and 30 m/sec with a 4.9-kg striker mass with a 150-mm diameter striker plate. In a logistic regression analysis, VC_{max} and $V_{max}C_{max}$ were good predictors of the probability of heart rupture and thoracic MAIS >3, while C_{max} was not. Lau and Viano (1986) concluded that the viscous criterion is the best indicator for soft tissue injury to many body regions for velocities of deformation of 3 to 30 m/sec. The velocity of impact of automobile occupants to various parts of the automobile interior is in this 3 to 30 m/sec range, which is intermediate to the high-velocity pressure waves of a pure blast (in which injury occurs with little compression) and the pure crushing injuries of quasi-static loading (in which injury is due to compression alone). In an analysis of the 39 unembalmed cadaver sternal impacts (average age 62) performed by Kroell and others, VC_{max} of 1.3 m/sec was the value for 50% probability of thoracic AIS >3, and VC_{max} of 1.0 m/sec for a 25% probability of AIS >3,

based on probit analysis (Fig. 15.13) (Viano and Lau, 1985).

Biomechanics of Lateral Impact

Side impact is a most serious automotive injury problem, second only to frontal impact in terms of injury and fatality in the United States. Each year, about 8,000 automobile occupants are killed and thousands more injured due to side impact. In a recent review of fatality data by Viano et al. (1989), it was found that 31.8% of passenger car fatalities occur in crashes with the principal direction of force lateral to the vehicle. Of those, two-thirds of the fatalities are due to multivehicle crashes and the remainder involved the impact of a single vehicle with a fixed object. Multi-vehicle crashes frequently involve the older victim. Viano et al. reported that 76% of side impact victims were over age 50 and 28% over age 70. In single vehicle frontal crashes, 26% of fatalities were over age 50 and 8% over age 70.

Drop Tests

Stalnaker et al. (1979) analyzed force-deflection data of the struck-side half-thorax in a series of 15 lateral drop tests from a height of 1 to 3 m onto an unpadded or padded force plate using unembalmed cadavers. A corridor of normalized force versus relative deflection (%) of the half-thorax was formulated (Fig. 15.14). It was proposed that this be a corridor for the development of a side impact dummy; 35% compression was the value for AIS of 3 or less. Tarriere et al. (1979) analyzed this and additional data (16 1- to 2-m drop tests in which force and deflection were measured, and nine 3-m drop tests in which force was measured but not deflection). The test setup is shown in Fig. 15.15. Maximum normalized force for AIS 0 was 7.40 kN and for AIS 3, 10.20 kN. Compression of approximately 30% of the whole chest width was the tolerance for AIS 3 or less. Compresson of 35% for the struck-side half-thorax was the tolerance for AIS 3 or less. Maximum 3-ms lateral acceleration of the

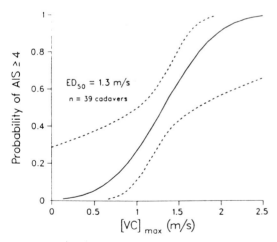

FIGURE 15.13. Curve showing the probability of thoracic AIS >3 as a function of VC_{max} (from Lau and Viano, 1986, p. 112). These data were derived from unembalmed cadaver impacts run at University of California, San Diego. (Reproduced with permission from Society of Automotive Engineers.)

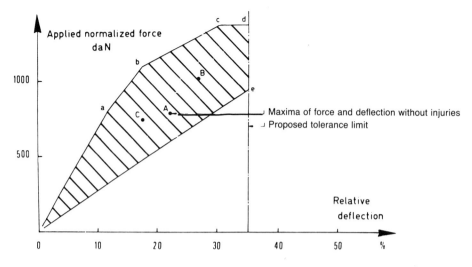

FIGURE 15.14. Normalized force versus deflection corridor of Stalnaker et al. (1979, p. 857) based on a series of lateral drop tests with unembalmed cadavers. (Reproduced with permission from Society of Automotive Engineers.)

fourth thoracic vertebra did not show a close relation to the number of rib fractures, but the maximum 3-ms acceleration averaged 49g in nine subjects with AIS 3 and 60g in 11 subjects with AIS 4 and 5 (Table 15.4).

Sacreste et al. (1982) analyzed bone condition factor (BCF) in 62 cadavers in an attempt to reduce the scatter in injury severity in cadaveric side impact tests. Using rib samples from these cadavers, eight parameters were measured: ash mass/total mass, ash mass per unit length, shear strength, bending strength, initial slope of force-deflection curve, shear energy, maximum bending stress, and Young's modulus. These data were examined in a factorial analysis and BCF, an indicator of bone resistance that integrates these factors,

was formulated using each of these parameters. The linear relationship of BCF to subject age had a 0.60 correlation coefficient.

Sled Tests

Starting in 1980, an extensive series of side impact sled tests were sponsored by the National Highway Traffic Safety Administration (NHTSA) and performed at the University of Heidelberg. The subjects (unembalmed cadavers) were placed on a seat of low coefficient of friction and 2 to 3 ft from the impacted wall. The sled was accelerated slowly and suddenly decelerated, so that the subject slid across the seat at the same speed as the sled and impacted the padded or unpadded

TABLE 15.4. Peak T4$_y$ accelerations in cadaveric lateral drop tests (from Tarrierre et al. 1979).*

AIS	No. of subjects	Average age	Resultant maximum acceleration			Resultant maximum acceleration (at 3 ms)		
			Minimum	Maximum	Average	Minimum	Maximum	Average
0	4	45	27	48	38	26	40	34
1,2	1	25	—	—	73	—	—	55
3	9	49	40	83	60	32	65	49
4,5	11	59	42	84	70	38	74	60

* Peak values of thoracic response versus injury.

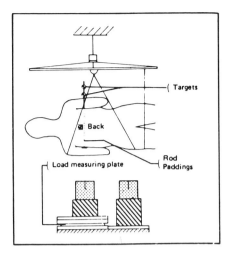

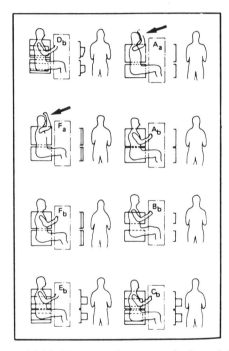

FIGURE 15.15. Diagram of test setup for lateral drop tests. (From Tarriere et al., 1979, p. 362).

sidewall. In the earliest tests the subjects were instrumented with the 12-accelerometer array developed by Robbins et al. (1976) and by Eppinger et al. (1978). This array measures accelerations at the ribs, sternum, and thoracic vertebrae (Fig. 15.16). Forces were not measured in the earlier tests. In the first series of these tests Kallieris et al. (1981) concluded

that acceleration responses were identical, but injury varied greatly, for the same response, leading to the conclusion that the injury function must have physical descriptors of the population as well as kinematic parameters. Eppinger et al. (1982) analyzed 30 side impact cadaver tests, 27 of them being the Heidelberg sled tests. The 12-accelerometer array was used and the analysis concentrated on the lateral responses of the fourth rib and the 12th thoracic vertebra. Injury could be successfully partitioned by using the variables of subject age versus struck-side fourth rib acceleration or rib relative velocity. Marcus et al. (1983) analyzed data from 11 Heidelberg sled tests, most of which included force measurements on the impacted wall (Fig. 15.17). A normalized thoracic AIS of AIS − 0.025 (age − 45) was proposed to normalize the injury to a 45-year-old subject. Eppinger et al. (1984) further analyzed the Heidelberg sled data and proposed the Thoracic Trauma Index (TTI). This index is the sum of an age factor (1.4 times subject age) and a thoracic acceleration term. In Eppinger et al. the acceleration term averaged the sum of the peak values of fourth struck-side rib (RIBy) and lateral twelfth thoracic vertebra (T12y) accelerations. The acceleration term is scaled by dividing the subject mass (MASS) by a standard 75 kg mass (MASS standard). The accelerations are first sampled and filtered per the authors.

$$TTI = 1.4 \times Age$$
$$+ \tfrac{1}{2}(Rib_y + T12_y)\,(Mass/Mass_{standard})$$
$$(15.5)$$

Morgan et al. (1986) analyzed the Heidelberg data and the Forschungsvereinigung Automobiltechnik (FAT) side impact test series in which a moving deformable barrier struck an Opel Kadett car body in which a cadaver was seated. They proposed a revised TTI that utilized the maximum of either a scaled fourth or unscaled eighth struck-side rib acceleration for Rib_y in the equation above. Figure 15.18 is a plot of maximum hard thorax AIS versus TTI for left-sided impact tests, and Fig. 15.19 is a curve of probability of AIS 4 versus TTI for left- and right-sided impacts. The "hard thorax" includes those structures in the upper

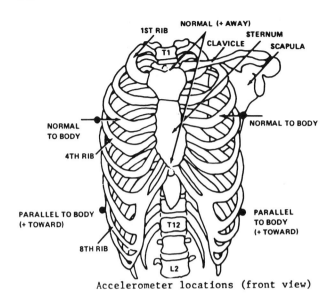

FIGURE 15.16. Diagram of 12-accelero-
meter thoracic array of Eppinger et al.
(1978).

Accelerometer locations (front view)

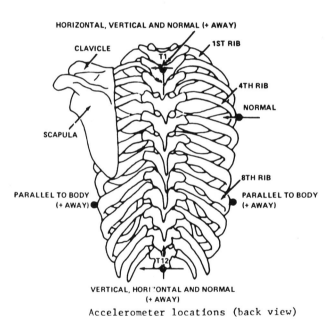

Accelerometer locations (back view)

abdomen bounded by the lower portion of the rib cage (Eppinger et al., 1982). Thus, the organs of the hard thorax include the liver and spleen. The side impact dummy (SID) was developed to measure upper and lower lateral rib accelerations and thoracic spine accelerations so that TTI can be measured to assess side impact crashworthiness (Morgan et al., 1986). The SID dummy will be used as the test measuring device in assessing side impact

crashworthiness of automobiles in FMVSS 214 (49 CFR, Part 571, 1990).

Cavanaugh et al. (1990) performed 12 sled tests with unembalmed cadavers in which the side wall was divided into shoulder, thoracic, abdominal, and pelvic beams (Fig. 15.20), and found that compression and velocity times compression (viscous criterion) were more predictive of thoracic injury than acceleration and force-based criteria. The efficacy of

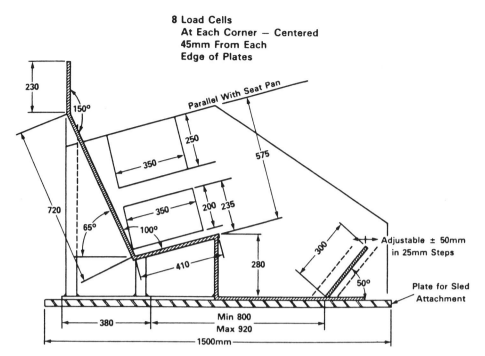

FIGURE 15.17. Diagram of instrumented side wall in Heidelberg side-impact sled test series. (From Marcus et al., 1983, p. 420. Reproduced with permission from Society of Automotive Engineers.)

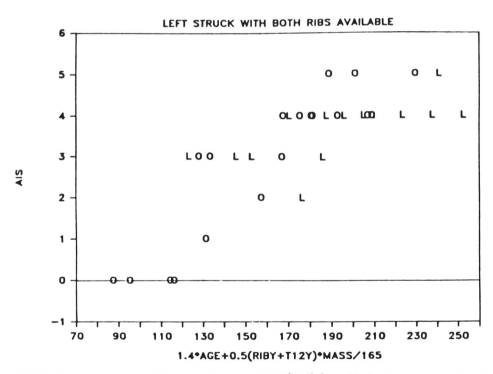

FIGURE 15.18. Plot of maximum AIS to the thorax versus the Thoracic Trauma Index (TTI) for left-sided impacts. O's are primarily from the Heidelberg sled test series and L's from the Forschungsvereinigung Automobiltechnik (FAT) test series in which a moving deformable barrier struck on Opel Kadett car body in which a subject was seated. (From Morgan et al., 1986, p. 36. Reproduced with permission from Society of Automotive Engineers.)

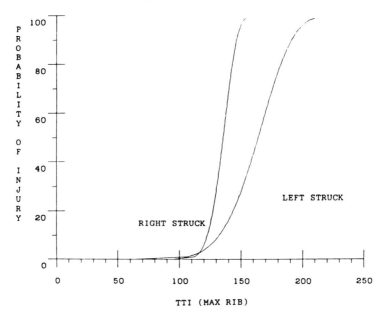

FIGURE 15.19. Probability curve of AIS 4 or greater to the thorax versus TTI. (From Morgan et al., 1986, p. 37. Reproduced with permission from Society of Automotive Engineers.)

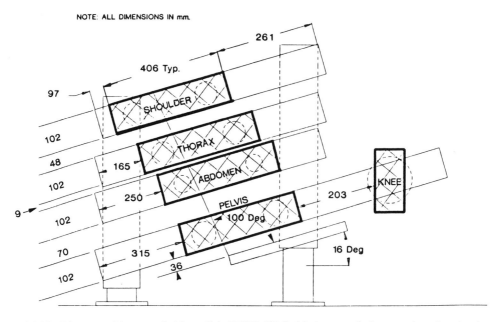

FIGURE 15.20. Diagram of impacted side wall in WSU-CDC side impact sled test series, showing beams at shoulder, thorax, abdomen, pelvis, and knee, instrumented with nine load cells. (From Cavanaugh et al., 1990, p. 24. Reproduced with permission from Society of Automotive Engineers.)

the viscous criterion was also borne out after analyzing an additional five padded wall tests. In general, the padded tests in which VC_{max} was kept below 1 m/sec resulted in AIS of 2 or less to the thorax, and tests in which VC_{max} was greater than 1 m/sec resulted in AIS of 4 or 5 to the thorax (unpublished data).

Impactor Tests

Viano (1989) performed a series of impactor tests with unembalmed cadavers at Wayne State University. The pendulum mass was 23.4 kg and direction of impact 30° anterior to lateral. Compression and VC_{max} were found to be good predictors of thoracic injury. Logist analysis indicated that peak compression (C_{max}) and the peak viscous response (VC_{max}) were better predictors of thoracic MAIS than peak $T8_y$ and $T12_y$ accelerations. For MAIS 4+, peak impactor force was also a good injury function. The Logist probability curves are shown in Fig. 15.21 for VC_{max}, C_{max}, and $T8_y$ acceleration. The force-deflection and force-time curves for 4.4, 6.5, and 9.5 m/sec impacts are shown in Fig. 15.22. The BIOSID side impact dummy was developed by a society of Automotive Engineers (SAE) task force in response to the perceived need for a dummy that could measure thoracic compression and rate of compression (Beebe, 1990) and also the perceived need for a dummy with more bifidelity than SID. At this time, BIOSID is

not allowed for assessing side impact crashworthiness in FMVSS 214 (49 CFR Part 571, 1990)

Mathematical Modeling of Thoracic Response

Lobdell et al. (1973) published a lumped-mass model of the thorax for use in frontal impact. The model (Fig. 15.23) utilized masses, springs, and dashpots, and the model's force-deflection response was matched to the frontal impact data of low- and high-velocity corridors of Kroell et al. (1971, 1974). Viano (1978a) modified this model to include kinetic energy, power, and momentum of the lumped masses, and energy stored in springs and dissipated in dashpots.

Mathematical modeling is playing an integral role in the development of side impact crashworthiness. Viano (1987a,b) modified his model for use in side impact. Using these models Viano (1987a) evaluated the benefit of constant crush force padding and constant stiffness padding (1987b). Based on reduction of the peak viscous response, a constant stiffness material was predicted to be more effective than a constant-force pad for a wide range of crash severity because the constant stiffness pad would be effective in low-severity as well as high-severity crashes, while a constant-force pad has a specific velocity range of effectiveness. For constant crush-force material, he

CHEST

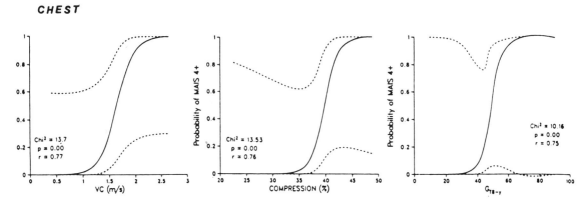

FIGURE 15.21. The Logist probability curves for VC_{max}, C_{max} and $T8_y$ acceleration from the pendulum impacts of Viano (1989, p. 136. Reproduced with permission from Society of Automotive Engineers.)

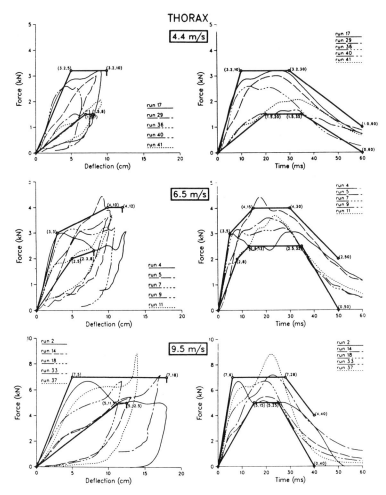

FIGURE 15.22. Force-deflection and force-time curves for 4.4, 6.5 and 9.5 m/sec impacts to the thorax with the center of impact at the xiphoid process and the impact 30° anterior to lateral. The pendulum was 23.4 kg, with a flat 15-cm diameter surface. (From Viano, 1989, p. 129. Reproduced with permission from Society of Automotive Engineers.)

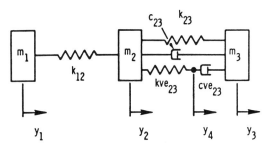

FIGURE 15.23. Lumped-mass model of the thorax for frontal impact (Lobdell, 1973, p. 233).

concluded that a rate-sensitive material that increased in crush strength with velocity of deformation would be most beneficial. For 50-mm thick padding the optimum crush force fit the following equation:

$$Fc = 0.50 \times (V - 2.0) \qquad (15.6)$$

and for 100 mm thickness:

$$Fc = 0.42 \times (V - 2.5) \qquad (15.7)$$

where Fc is in kN and V in m/sec.

At the time of the Viano study the Hybrid III chest was the closest simulation to human lateral response. With more recent cadaveric side impact data in which force and compression has been measured (Cavanaugh et al., 1990; Viano, 1989) development of new side impact models of the thorax would be quite useful, and an aid in understanding the potential benefit or harm of various types of padding being studied for side impact protection. Such a model has recently been published by King et al. (1991) based on the cadaveric sled data in Cavanaugh et al.

Deng (1988), using a CAL3D simulation program, showed that there are critical differences between free-flight impacts and velocity-pulse impacts. Typical laboratory lateral impact studies are free-flight impacts represented by a moving mass into a stationary subject (pendulum impacts) or a moving subject into a stationary mass (sled tests). Car-to-car side impacts are velocity-pulse impacts in which the impacting car imparts a velocity pulse to the struck door, which after traversing the space between struck door and occupant, strikes the occupant with little decrease in door velocity because of the large amount of energy behind the impact. Deng's velocity-pulse simulation showed that (1) a stiffer side door structure can reduce injury, (2) increasing the spacing between occupant and door is beneficial, and (3) the use of padding on the inner door panel reduces occupant acceleration but increases occupant deformation. Thus, TTI predicts that padding on the inner door panel is beneficial in side impact, and C_{max} and VC_{max} predict that padding is harmful in side impact. This conclusion has been borne out in full-scale side impacts analyzed by Campbell et al. (1990) in which 3 inches of ARCEL 512^{Tm} padding on the inner door panel of a midsized, four-door passenger car decreased TTI in the SID and increased VC_{max} in the BIOSID.

Future Research Needs

Future research needs in frontal impact include the deflection response of various portions of the rib cage to dynamic belt loading and air bag loading. These data are needed to develop a frontal impact dummy with biofidelity for these restraint conditions. The classic work done by Kroell and others in the 1970s addresses impact of the sternum with the steering wheel but not the distributed loading to other portions of the rib cage that occurs with air bag and three-point belt loading. The mechanism of injury to the heart and great vessels also needs further study, perhaps through controlled impacts using high-speed fluoroscopy and radiopaque dye in the heart and great vessels.

Future research needs in side impact include a lumped-mass model that responds with biofidelic force-deflection and force-time responses at the neck, shoulder, thorax, abdomen, and pelvis. Further development of side impact dummy biofidelity is required,

TABLE 15.5. Frontal impact injury tolerances.

Tolerance level	Injury level	Reference
Force		
3.3 kN to sternum	Minor injury	Patrick et al. (1969)
8.8 kN to chest and shoulders	Minor injury	Patrick et al. (1969)
Acceleration (g's)		
60	3 ms limit for Hybrid II & III	FMVSS 208
Deflection (mm)		
58	No rib fracture	Stalnaker and Mohan (1974)
76	Limit for Hybrid III	FMVSS 208
Compression (%)		
20	Onset of rib fracture	Kroell et al. (1971, 1974)
40	Flail chest	Kroell et al. (1971, 1974)
32	Tolerance for rib cage stability	Viano (1978)
VC_{max} (m/s)		
1.0	25% probability of AIS >3	Viano and Lau (1985)
1.3	50% probability of AIS >3	Viano and Lau (1985)

TABLE 15.6. Lateral impact injury tolerances.

Tolerance level	Injury level	Reference
Force (kN)		
7.4—drop test	AIS = 0	Tarrierre et al. (1979)
10.2—drop test	AIS = 3	Tarrierre et al. (1979)
5.5—pendulum impact	25% probability of AIS 4	Viano (1989)
Acceleration (g's)		
45.2 g T8$_Y$	25% probability of AIS 4	Viano (1989)
31.6 g T12$_Y$	25% probability of AIS 4	Viano (1989)
27.7 g Upper sternum-X	25% probability of AIS 4	Cavanaugh et al. (1990)
TTI(d) (g's)		
85	Max. in SID dummy for 4-door cars	FMVSS 214
90	Max. in SID dummy for 2-door cars	FMVSS 214
Compression (%) to half thorax		
35	AIS 3	Stalnaker et al. (1979)
35	AIS 3	Tarrierre et al. (1979)
31 (includes arm)	25% probability of AIS 4	Cavanaugh et al. (1990)
Compression (%) to whole thorax		
38.4	25% probability of AIS 4	Viano (1989)
VC$_{max}$ (m/s) to half thorax		
<1.0	AIS 0–2	
>1.0	AIS 4,5	Cavanaugh et al. (1990) and unpublished data
VC$_{max}$ (m/s) to whole thorax		
1.47	25% probability of AIS 4	Viano (1989)

perhaps through modifications of BIOSID. Particular areas that need to be addressed include head-neck response, shoulder-arm response, and the softer response of the thorax seen in older subjects. In side impact, controlled laboratory studies must also be performed in which the space between impactor and subject is varied using a velocity-pulse impactor of limited stroke. The influence of padding of various material properties in this interspace needs to be evaluated.

Summary and Conclusions

Forces, accelerations, and deflections of human cadavers have been measured in controlled laboratory tests to ascertain the biomechanical response of the thorax under a variety of test conditions. Test types include impactor tests, sled tests, drop tests, and quasi-static tests. Injury criteria have been developed to relate biomechanical response to probability of injury for these various test conditions. Table 15.5 summarizes the injury criteria obtained from these various tests for frontal impact and Table 15.6 for side impact.

References

49 CFR Part 571. Federal Motor Vehicle Safety Standards; Side Impact Protection. Federal Register, Docket No. 88-C6, Notice 8, RIN 2127-AB86, Vol 55(210), Oct. 30, 1990, pp 45721–45780, 1990.

Abbreviated Injury Scale (AIS)—1980 Revision Association for the Advancement of Automotive Medicine, Morton Grove, IL.

Abbreviated Injury Scale (AIS)—1985 Revision Association for the Advancement of Automotive Medicine, Morton Grove, IL.

Abbreviated Injury Scale (AIS)—1990 revision Association for the Advancement of Automotive Medicine, Morton Grove, IL.

Aldman B, Anderson A, Sexmark O. Possible effects of air bag inflation on a standing child. Proc 18th Conference of the American Association for Automotive Medicine, 1974.

Anderson JE. Grant's Atlas of Anatomy, 8th edition. Williams and Wilkins, Baltimore, 1983.

Backaitis SH, St. Laurent A. Chest deflection characteristics of volunteers and HYBRID III dummies. Proc 30th Stapp Car Crash Conference. SAE 861884, pp 157–166, 1986.

Baker SP, O'Neill B, Haddon W, Long WB. The injury severity score: a method for describing patients with multiple injuries and evaluating emergency care. J Trauma 14:187–196, 1974.

Beebe MS. What is BIOSID? SAE 900377, 1990.

Bierman HR, Wilder RM, Hellems HK. The physiological effects of compressive forces on the torso. Report No. 8, Naval Medical Research Institute Project X-630, Bethseda, MD, 1946.

Campbell KL, Wasko RJ, Henson SE. Analysis of side impact test data comparing SID and BIOSID. Proc 34th Stapp Car Crash Conference. SAE 902319, pp 185–205, 1990.

Carsten O. Relationship of accident type to occupant injuries. Report No. UMTRI-86-15, General Motors Research Laboratories, 1986.

Carsten O, O'Day J. Injury priority analysis. Report No. UMTRI-84-24, NHTSA, 1984.

Cavanaugh JM, Walilko TJ, Malhotra A, Zhu Y, King AI. Biomechanical response and injury tolerance of the thorax in twelve sled side impacts. Proc 34th Stapp Car Crash Conference. SAE 902307, pp 23–38, 1990.

Cheng R, Yang KH, Levine RS, King AI, Morgan R. Injuries to the cervical spine caused by a distributed frontal load to the chest. Proc 26th Stapp Car Crash Conference. SAE 821155, pp 1–40, 1982.

Cheng R, Yang KH, Levine RS, King AI. Dynamic impact loading of the femur under passive restrained condition. Proc 28th Stapp Car Crash Conference. SAE 841661, pp 101–118, 1984.

Code of Federal Regulations, 571.208, FMVSS 208, Occupant Crash Protection.

Cohen DS. The safety problem for passengers in frontal impacts: analysis of accidents, laboratory and model simulation data. Presented at the 11th International Technical Conference on Experimental Safety Vehicles, Washington, DC, 12–15 May, 1987.

Cooper GJ, Pearce BP, Stainer MC, Maynard RL. The biomechanical response of the thorax to non-penetrating trauma with particular reference to cardiac injuries. J Trauma 22(12):994–1008, 1982.

Dalmotas DJ. Mechanism of injury to vehicle occupants restrained by three-point seat belts. Proc 24th Stapp Car Crash Conference. SAE 801311, pp 439–476, 1980.

Deng YC. Design considerations for occupant protection in side impact—a modeling approach. Proc 32nd Stapp Car Crash Conference. SAE 881713, pp 71–79, 1988.

Eiband AM. Human tolerance to rapidly applied acceleration. A survey of the literature. National Aeronautics and Space Administration, Washington, DC. NASA Memo No. 5-19-59E, 1959.

Eppinger RH. Prediction of thoracic injury using measurable experimental parameters. Report 6th International Technical Conference on Experimental Safety Vehicles, pp 770–779. National Highway Traffic Safety Administration, Washington, DC, 1976.

Eppinger RH, Augustyn K, Robbins DH. Development of a promising universal thoracic trauma prediction methodology. Proc 22nd Stapp Conference. SAE 780891, pp 211–268, 1978.

Eppinger RH, Marcus JH. Prediction of injury in blunt frontal impact. Tenth International Conference on Experimental Safety Vehicles, Oxford, England, pp 90–104, 1985.

Eppinger RH, Marcus JH, Morgan RM. Development of dummy and injury index for NHTSA's thoracic side impact protection research program. Government/Industry Meeting and Exposition, Washington, DC. SAE 840885, 1984.

Eppinger RH, Morgan RM, Morgan RM. Side impact data analysis. Ninth International Conference on Experimental Safety Vehicles, 1982.

Fayon A, Tarriere C, Walfisch G, Got C, Patel A. Thorax of three-point-belt wearers during a crash (experiments with cadavers). Proc 19th Stapp Car Crash Conference. SAE 751148, pp 195–223, 1975.

Foster JK, Kortge JO, Wolanin MJ. Hybrid III—a biomechanically-based crash test dummy. Stapp Car Crash Conference Proceedings. Warrendale, PA, SAE 770938, pp 975–1014, 1977.

Fung YC, Yen MR. Experimental investigation of lung injury mechanisms. Topical Report, U.S. Army Medical Research and Development Command. Contract No. DAMD 17-82-C-2062, 1984.

Gadd CW, Patrick LM. Systems versus laboratory impact tests for estimating injury hazard. Society of Automotive Engineers, New York, SAE 680053, 1968.

Hirsch A, Eppinger R, Shams T, Nguten T, Levine R, Mackenzie J, Marks M, Ommaya A. Impairment scaling from the Abbreviated Injury Scale. Report No. DOT HS 806 648, NHTSA, 1983.

Horsch J, Lau I, Andrzejak D, Viano D, Melvin J, Pearson J, Cok D, Miller G. Assessment of air bag deployment loads. Proc 34th Stapp Car Crash Conference. SAE 902324, pp 267–288, 1990.

Kallieris D, Mattern R, Schmidt G, Eppinger R. Quantification of side impact responses and injuries. Proc 25th Stapp Car Crash Conference. SAE 811009, pp 329–366, 1981.

King AI, Huang Y, Cavanaugh JM. Protection of occupants against side impact. Thirteenth International Conference on Experimental Safety Vehicles, Paris, France, Nov. 4–7, 1991.

Kroell CK, Allen SD, Warner CY, Perl TR. Interrelationship of velocity and chest compression in blunt thoracic impact to swine II. Proc 30th Stapp Car Crash Conference. SAE 861881, pp 99–121, 1986.

Kroell CK, Pope ME, Viano DC, Warner CY, Allen SD. Interrelationship of velocity and chest compression in blunt thoracic impact. Proc 25th Stapp Car Crash Conference. SAE 811016, pp 549–579, 1981.

Kroell CK, Schneider DC, Nahum AM. Impact tolerance and response to the human thorax. Proc 15th Stapp Car Crash Conference. SAE 710851, pp 84–134, 1971.

Kroell CK, Schneider DC, Nahum AM. Impact tolerance and response to the human thorax II. Proc 18th Stapp Car Crash Conference. SAE 741187, pp 383–457, 1974.

L'Abbe RJ, Dainty DA, Newman JA. An experimental analysis of thoracic deflection response to belt loading. Seventh International IRCOBI Conference on the Biomechanics of Impacts, Bron, France, pp 184–194, 1982.

Lasky II, Siegel AW, Nahum AM. Automotive cardio-thoracic injuries: a medical-engineering analysis. Automotive Engineering Congress, Detroit, MI, SAE 680052, January 8–12, 1968.

Lau IV, Viano DC. Influence of impact velocity on the severity of nonpenetrating hepatic injury. J Trauma 21:115–123, 1981a.

Lau IV, Viano DC. Influence of impact velocity and chest compression on experimental pulmonary injury severity in an animal model. J Trauma 21:1022–1028, 1981b.

Lau IV, Viano DC. The viscous criterion—bases and applications of an injury severity index for soft tissues. Proc 30th Stapp Car Crash Conference. SAE 861882, pp 123–142, 1986.

Lobdell TE, Kroell CK, Schneider DC, Hering WE, Nahum AM. Impact response of the human thorax. In King WF, Mertz HJ (eds) *Human impact response measurement and simulation*. Plenum Press, New York, pp 201–245, 1973.

Malliaris AC, Hitchock R, Hedlund J. A search for priorities in crash protection. SAE 820242, 1982.

Malliaris AC, et al. Harm causation and ranking in car crashes. SAE 850090, 1985.

Marcus JH, Blodgett R. Priorities of automobile crash safety based on impairment. Proc 11th International Technical Conference on Experimental Safety Vehicles, Report No. DOT HS 807223, NHTSA, pp 257–269, 1988.

Marcus JH, Morgan RM, Eppinger RH, Kallieris D, Mattern R, Schmidt G. Human response to injury from lateral impact. Proc 27th Stapp Crash Conference. SAE 831634, pp 419–432, 1983.

Melvin JW, King AI, Alem NM. AATD system technical characteristics, design concepts, and trauma assessment criteria. AATD Task E-F Final Report in DOT-HS-807-224 U.S. Department of Transportation, National Highway Traffic Safety Administration, Washington, DC, 1988.

Melvin JW, Mohan D, Stalnaker RL. Occupant injury assessment criteria. SAE 750914, 1975.

Melvin JW, Weber K (eds). Review of biomechanical response and injury in the automotive environment. AATD Task B Final Report in DOT-HS-807-224 U.S. Department of Transportation, National Highway Traffic Safety Administration, Washington, DC, 1988.

Mertz HJ, Kroell CK. Tolerance of thorax and abdomen. In *Impact injury and crash protection*. Charles C. Thomas, Springfield, IL, pp 372–401, 1970.

Mohan D, Melvin JW. Failure properties of passive human aortic tissue II: biaxial tension tests. J Trauma 16:31–44.

Morgan RM, Marcus JH, Eppinger RH. Side impact—the biofidelity of NHTSA's proposed ATD and efficacy of TTI. 30th Stapp Car Crash Conference. SAE 861877, 1986.

Nahum AM, Gadd CW, Schneider DC, Kroell CK. Deflection of the human thorax under sternal impact. 1970 International Automobile Safety Conference Compendium, SAE, pp 797–807, 1970.

Nahum AM, Gadd CW, Schneider DC, Kroell CK. The biomechanical basis for chest impact protection: I. Force-deflection characteristics of the thorax. J Trauma 11(10):874–882, 1971.

Nahum AM, Schneider DC, Kroell CK. Cadaver skeletal response to blunt thoracic impact. Proc 19th Stapp Car Crash Conference. SAE 751150, pp 259–293, 1975.

Neathery RF. Analysis of chest impact response data and scaled performance specifications. Proc 18th Stapp Crash Conference. SAE 741188, pp 459–493, 1974.

Neathery RF, Kroell CK, Mertz HJ. Prediction of thoracic injury from dummy responses. 19th Stapp Car Crash Conference. SAE 751151, pp 295–316, 1975.

Newman RJ, Rastogi S. Rupture of the thoracic aorta and its relationship to road traffic accident characteristics. Injury 296:296–299.

Patrick LM. Impact force-deflection of the human thorax. Proc 25th Stapp Car Crash Conference. SAE 811014, pp 471–496, 1981.

Patrick LM, Bohlin NI, Anderson A. Three-point harness accident and laboratory data comparison. Proc 18th Stapp Car Crash Conference. SAE 741181, pp 201–282, 1974.

Patrick LM, Kroell CK, Mertz HJ. Forces on the human body in simulated crashes. Proc Ninth Stapp Car Crash Conference. University of Minnesota, pp 237–260, 1965.

Patrick LM, Mertz HJ, Kroell CK. Cadaver knee, chest and head impact loads. Proc Eleventh Stapp Car Crash Conference. Society of Automotive Engineers, New York, SAE 670913, pp 168–182, 1969.

Robbins DH, Melvin JW, Stalnaker RL. The prediction of thoracic impact injuries. Proc 20th Stapp Car Crash Conference. SAE 760822, pp 699–729, 1976.

Sacreste J, Brun-Cassan F, Fayon A, Tarriere C, Got C, Patel A. Proposal for a thorax tolerance level in side impacts based on 62 tests performed with cadavers having known bone condition. Proc 26th Stapp Car Crash Conference. SAE 821157, pp 155–171, 1982.

Schmidt G, Kallieris D, Barz J, Mattern R. Results of 49 cadaver tests simulating frontal collision of front seat passengers. Proc 18th Stapp Car Crash Conference. SAE 741182, pp 283–291, 1974.

Schneider LW, King AI, Beebe MS. Design requirements and specifications; thorax-abdomen development task. Interim report: trauma assessment device development program. Report No. DOT-HS-807-511, 1990.

Somers RL. New ways to use the 1980 Abbreviated Injury Scale. Accident Analysis Group, Laboratory for Public Health and Health Economics, Odense University Hospital, Odense, Denmark, 1982.

Somers RL. The probability of death score: an improvement of the injury severity score. Accid Anal Prev 15:247–257, 1983.

Stalnaker RL, McElhaney JH, Roberts VL, Trollope ML. Human torso response to blunt trauma. In King WF, Mertz HJ (eds) *Human impact response measurement and simulation*. Plenum Press, New York, pp 181–199, 1973.

Stalnaker RL, Mohan D. Human chest impact protection criteria. Proc 3rd International Conference on Occupant Protection. Society of Automotive Engineers, New York, pp 384–393, 1974.

Stalnaker RL, Tarriere C, Fayon A, Walfisch G, Balthazard M, Masset J, Got C, Patel A. Modification of part 572 dummy for lateral impact according to biomechanical data. Proc 23rd Stapp Car Crash Conference. SAE 791031, pp 843–872, 1979.

Stapp JP. Human exposure to linear decelerations. Part 2. The forward-facing position and the development of a crash harness. AFTR 5915, pt. 2. Wright-Patterson AFB, Dayton, Ohio, 1951.

Stapp JP. Voluntary human tolerance levels. In Gurdjian ES, Lange WA, Patrick LM, Thomas LM (eds) *Impact injury and crash protection*. Charles C. Thomas, Springfield, IL, pp 308–349, 1970.

Takeda H, Kobayashi S. Injuries to children from airbag deployment. Proc 8th International Technical Conference on Experimental Safety Vehicles. SAE 806030, 1980.

Tarriere C, Walfisch G, Fayon A, Rosey JP, Got C, Patel A, Delmus A. Synthesis of human tolerances obtained from lateral impact simulations. 7th International Conference on Experimental Safety Vehicles, Paris, France, pp 359–373, 1979.

Tsitlik JE, Weisfeldt ML, Chandra N, Effron MB, Halperin HR, Levin HR. Elastic properties of the human chest during cardiopulmonary resuscitation. Crit Care Med 11(9):685–692, 1983.

Viano DC. Evaluation of biomechanical response and potential injury from thoracic impact. Aviat Space Environ Med 49(1):125–135, 1978a.

Viano DC. Thoracic injury potential. Proc 3rd International Meeting on Simulation and Reconstruction of Impacts in Collisions, IRCOBI, Bron, France, pp 142–156, 1978b.

Viano DC. Biomechanics of non-penetrating aortic trauma: a review. Proc 27th Stapp Car Crash Conference. SAE 831608, pp 109–114, 1983.

Viano DC. Evaluation of the benefit of energy-absorbing material in side impact protection: part I. Proc 31st Stapp Car Crash Conference. SAE 872212, 1987a.

Viano DC. Evaluation of the benefit of energy-absorbing material in side impact protection: part II. Proc 31st Stapp Car Crash Conference. SAE 872213, 1987b.

Viano DC. Biomechanical responses and injuries in blunt lateral impact. Proc 33rd Stapp Car Crash Conference. SAE 892432, pp 113–142, 1989.

Viano DC, Culver CC, Evans L, Frick M, Scott R. Involvement of older drivers in multi-vehicle side impact crashes. Proc 33rd Annual Proc AAAM, 1989.

Viano DC, Lau IV. Role of impact velocity and chest compression in thoracic injury. Aviat Space Environ Med 54:16–21, 1983.

Viano DC, Lau IV. Thoracic impact: a viscous tolerance criterion. Tenth International Conference on Experimental Safety Vehicles, Oxford, England, pp 104–114, 1985.

Walfisch G, Chamouard F, Lesrelin, Fayon A, Tarriere C, Got C, Guillon F, Patel A, Hureau J. Tolerance limits and mechanical characteristics of the human thorax in frontal and side impact and transposition of these characteristics into protection criteria. Proc 7th International Conference on the Biomechanics of Impacts, IRCOBI, Bron, France, pp 122–139, 1982.

Weisfeldt ML. Compliance characteristics of the human chest during cardiopulmonary resuscitation. Final Report No. DOT-HS-805-800, 1979.

16
Biomechanics of Abdominal Trauma

Stephen W. Rouhana

Introduction

The abdominal organs, in general, lack the relatively well-protected environment afforded the thoracic organs by the rib cage. Trauma to the abdomen may be caused by penetrating objects or blunt impact, and can be life-threatening by any measure (American Association for Automotive Medicine, 1980; Borlase et al., 1990; Croce et al., 1991; Moore et al., 1989; Kumar et al., 1989). While trauma from penetrating objects is typically apparent, that from blunt impact initially may lack symptoms, leading to delayed diagnosis, with resultant high morbidity and mortality (Harris et al., 1991). This chapter will deal exclusively with blunt trauma such as that experienced by motor vehicle occupants in automotive collisions.

A description of the pertinent anatomy will serve as the starting point for this discussion on abdominal trauma, and as a reference for the rest of the chapter. Then a review of the clinical and field accident experience will be used to define the magnitude of the problem and to gain insights as to what contact points in the motor vehicle have been associated with abdominal trauma. Following an overview of work on the biomechanical response of the abdomen, which is essential for crash test dummy design, we will examine the published work on the mechanisms of injury and human tolerances to blunt abdominal trauma. The chapter will end with a short discussion regarding future avenues for research.

Anatomy

The abdomen is the largest "cavity" in the body, yet it can hardly be considered a cavity because the organs within normally fill the entire space (Gray, 1977). The abdominal viscera include two main types of organs, *viz.* the "solid" and the "hollow" organs, which behave quite differently under the various types of mechanical loading. The solid organs include the liver, spleen, pancreas, kidneys, adrenal glands, and ovaries; the hollow organs include the stomach, small and large intestines, urinary bladder, and the uterus.

The relative positions of the organs are shown in Fig. 16.1 (Zuidema, 1977). Note that the liver occupies most of the space enclosed by the lower rib cage on the right side of the body, while the spleen and stomach occupy the space within the lower rib cage on the left side. The pancreas is oriented transversely on the posterior wall of the abdomen.

Classical anatomy separates the abdomen into three rows and three columns as in Fig. 16.2 (Gray, 1977). The rows are derived by dividing the abdomen using two transverse planes: one at the level of the junction of the ninth rib and its costal cartilage (transpyloric), the other at the level of the superiormost point of the pelvis on the iliac crests (transtubercular). The top row includes the organs beneath the diaphragm and above the transpyloric plane (liver, stomach, spleen, pancreas, durdenum, part of the kidneys). The second row includes organs from the transpyloric plane to the

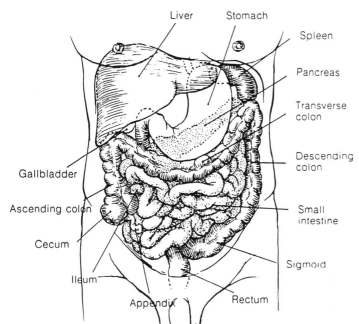

FIGURE 16.1. The abdominal organs. (From Zuidema, 1977. Reprinted with permission.)

transtubercular plane (ascending, descending, and transverse colon, part of the small intestine, the rest of the kidneys, and the gravid uterus). The bottom row includes all the abdominal organs below the iliac crests (cecum, sigmoid colon, bladder, and the rest of the small intestine, and the uterus).

The columns are derived by dividing the above rows into middle and lateral zones using two sagittal planes through the center of the right and left Poupart's ligament (also called the inguinal ligament), respectively. The names of the nine resulting regions of the abdomen are given in Fig. 16.2.

The abdomen is bounded above by the diaphragm, which forms a dome over the viscera, extending high into the thorax, up to the level of the junction of the fourth costal cartilage with the sternum (Gray, 1977). It is bounded below by the bony pelvis and the muscles attached to it. The top row of the abdomen is bounded anteriorly and laterally mainly by the lower rib cage, and posteriorly by the ribs and vertebral column (which is not usually considered as part of the abdomen). The middle row is bounded anteriorly and laterally by musculature, and posteriorly by musculature and the vertebral column.

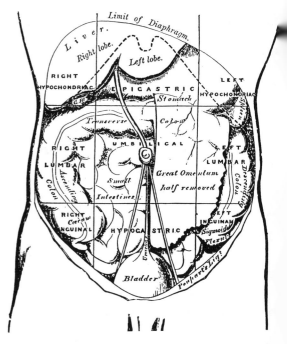

FIGURE 16.2. Classical separation of the abdomen (Gray, 1977).

The bottom row of the abdomen is bounded posteriorly by the sacrum and coccyx, laterally by the ilia, and anteriorly by musculature.

The major vessels of the abdomen are the abdominal aorta and inferior vena cava. They lie at the back of the abdominal cavity, and are located, respectively, in front of and slightly to the right of the vertebral column. There are major branches from each of these vessels at many points. They enter from the thoracic cavity through separate openings in the diaphragm, and bifurcate into left and right common iliac arteries and veins at the level of the fourth of fifth lumbar vertebra (just below the umbilicus).

Anatomic Features that Influence Mechanical Properties, Injury Mechanisms, and Tolerances

Gross density of the organ (i.e., not the tissue density), may be considered as the main characteristic that delineates a "solid" organ from a "hollow" organ. The liver and spleen, for example, are solid organs and are denser than hollow organs like the stomach and intestines. The main reason for the lesser density of the hollow organs is the presence of a large cavity within the organ itself (large relative to the size of the whole organ). While the solid organs have fluid-filled vessels within them, the hollow organs can have air, digestive matter, or even a fetus (in the case of the uterus) within them. The stomach and uterus have thicker walls than the intestines. Clearly, physical properties such as density, structure, material within, are major factors determining the mechanisms of injury for the organs.

A thin, serous membrane called the peritoneum covers the inner abdominal walls and surrounds each organ within the abdominal cavity (also called the peritoneal cavity). This membrane is smooth and lubricated by a small amount of serous fluid. One result of this membrane and its lubrication is low friction between the organs and the walls of the abdominal cavity, and between the organs themselves. This low friction between abdominal organs is one factor causing the relatively high mobility of many of the abdominal organs. Another

factor is that many of the organs are not rigidly fixed within the peritoneal cavity (Hollinshead, 1971). Some organs (such as the liver, spleen, and intestines) are tethered by folds of the peritoneum that form ligaments, omenta, and mesenteries, but are able to move within the limits of the tethers. Each kidney, for example, is encapsulated in fat on either side of the vertebral column, behind the peritoneum, and is tethered by its renal artery or vein.

The relatively high degree of mobility of the abdominal organs means that posture or body orientation can change the relative positions of some of the organs within the body (Pope et al., 1979). This can have a profound effect on the outcome of experiments examining injury mechanisms or mechanical response. For example, experiments performed with the subjects in a supine position may have entirely different results than experiments performed with the subjects seated or standing upright because the target organ may be in two entirely different orientations during the respective impacts.

Location of the organs also plays a role in the biomechanics of injury. For example, organs directly in front of the spine, may be at greater risk of being crushed in a frontal impact than organs lateral to the spine. Similarly, the right kidney is typically at a slightly lower level than the left kidney probably due to the presence of the liver (Gray, 1977). Then the right kidney may be more or less at risk compared to the left kidney.

In addition, the abdominal organs located within the confines of the lower rib cage, may be afforded some protection by the ribs. While not as stiff as the upper ribs (because of the indirect coupling to the sternum), the lower ribs still provide a load distributing surface for blunt impacts, and do offer some resistance to deformation, especially from the side or rear. These considerations have led some researchers to classify the region that contains the organs within the lower rib cage as the "hard thorax" (Eppinger et al., 1982, 1984). The impact response and tolerance of this region, in general, may indeed be different from the rest of the abdomen because of the presence of the ribs, but the mechanisms of injury to the organs themselves are probably the same.

Huelke et al. (1986) examined the anatomical differences between humans and human surrogates commonly used in injury biomechanics testing. They found a number of significant differences that may affect interpretation of the results of some experiments. For example, although the liver of a human moves with the diaphragm during respiration, it is not as well coupled in some surrogate species. In addition, the organs of human surrogates may have very different geometry when compared to the same organ in the human (e.g., the porcine spleen is long and "tongue-like" in appearance compared with the more globular human spleen). Therefore, anatomical considerations may be important when extrapolating the results of injury biomechanics experiments to the living human population.

Manifestation of Blunt Abdominal Trauma

Field Accident Data

Nahum et al. (1970) analyzed data from the accident files of the UCLA Trauma Research Group. The files contained data on collisions of 604 vehicles produced in the 1960–1969 model years. There were 972 occupants involved in the collisions, of whom 20% were lap belted and 1% were shoulder belted. The abdomen was injured in 3.5% of all occupants. The authors calculated injury rates for the abdomen-pelvis area in association with specific contact points. In the 1960–1966 vehicles 19.8% of the drivers received abdominal injuries that were associated with the steering system (55%), side interior (22%), "impact" (9%), seat belts (3.6%), and other contacts. In the 1967–1969 vehicles, after the introduction of energy-absorbing steering systems, the abdominal injury rate decreased to 16.5% of the drivers. The steering system association decreased dramatically to 21%, side interior increased (33%), "impact" (11%), seat belts (11%), and the rest from other contacts. The severity of the abdominal injuries was moderate to fatal for 73% of the 1960–1966 group, and for 52% of the 1967–1969 group.

Nearly one in ten (9.8%) passengers had abdominal injuries in the 1960–1966 group, as did 15.3% in the 1967–1969 group. For the 1960–1966 group, these injuries had contact associated with the lower instrument panel (38%), the side interior (23%), "impact" (15%), ejection (8%), the A-pillar (8%), the seat belt (8%), and other contacts. In the 1967–1969 group, the injuries were associated with contact to the lower instrument panel (30%), the seat belt (15%), the upper instrument panel (10%), side interior (10%), and other contacts.

Rear seat occupants saw a dramatic reduction in abdominal injury rate from 12.5% to 2.2% when comparing the 1960–1966 and 1967–1969 groups. The associated contacts were the seat back (57%), side interior (29%), and side glass (14%) in the 1960–1966 group, and the seat belt (100%) in the 1967–1969 group. Note, there was a dramatic change in abdominal injury severity from 71% moderate to fatal injury in the 1960–1967 group, to 100% minor injury in the 1967–1969 group.

Danner and Langwieder (1979) and Danner et al. (1979) analyzed data from 2,545 pedestrian collisions with passenger cars investigated by German motor vehicle insurers. They found that 19.8% of all pedestrian injuries, and 6.5% of all serious through fatal pedestrian injuries [Abbreviated Injury Scale (AIS) ≥3] were to the abdomen (only the head and tibia had greater frequency). Children and the elderly appeared to be overrepresented in terms of serious abdominal injury, with 22.7% of all the serious injuries to children in the abdominal region (only head and femur have more), and 24.8% of all serious injuries to the elderly in the abdominal region (only head and tibia have more).

Ricci (1980) analyzed data from the National Crash Severity Study (NCSS) that reported information for collisions in which the most severe injury occurred to an occupant of a towed passenger car. The study dates were

January 1977 through March 1979, and included a stratified sampling scheme in seven different areas of the United States. The NCSS includes data on approximately 25,000 actual vehicle occupants, and over 106,000 occupants if weighted data is used. Ricci found that 3.8% of all injuries in the NCSS database were to the abdominal region. However, when severity was taken into account, injury to the abdomen was overrepresented, accounting for 8.3% of all AIS ≥3, 29.9% of all AIS ≥4, and 30.7% of all AIS ≥ 5 injuries.

Hobbs (1980) reported on a two-year, in-depth investigation of collisions involving approximately 2,500 occupants in the United Kingdom. He found that while less than 1% of belted occupants were fatally injured, 8.4% of all unbelted occupants were fatally injured; 0.5% of the belted occupants, and 1.7% of the unbelted occupants received AIS ≥3 abdominal injuries in pure frontal and oblique frontal impacts. For injury of all severities, contact was associated with the seat belt, instrument panel, and door for belted occupants, and the steering system, instrument panel, and side door for the unbelted occupants. For rollovers, none (0%) of the belted occupants and 3% of the unbelted occupants sustained serious abdominal injuries.

Galer et al. (1985) studied 261 collisions in the United Kingdom that involved 297 vehicles and 506 occupants. They analyzed the data for belted occupants, and found that 14.6% of all injuries to drivers and 17.8% of all injuries to front seat passengers were to the abdomen/pelvis (they did not examine the abdomen alone). These represented 6.4% of the nonminor (AIS = 2 to 6) injuries to drivers and 18.1% of those to front seat passengers.

The main contacts associated with minor injury (AIS = 1) to the abdomen/pelvis of vehicle drivers were seat belt webbing (59%) and the side door (12%), and those associated with nonminor injury were the steering system (30%) and side door (70%). For front seat passengers seat belt webbing was the principal contact for minor injury (91%), while the side door (50%) and other vehicle contacts (50%) were associated with nonminor injury to the abdomen/pelvis.

Rouhana and Foster (1985) analyzed the NCSS data (the same data set set as Ricci above) specifically for side impact collisions. They found that 15.6% of all AIS ≥3 unjuries, and 24.2% of all AIS ≥4 injuries were abdominal. The main contact points associated with serious abdominal injury in left-side impacts were the side interior (39%), the armrest (30%), and the steering system (18%). The main contacts associated with serious abdominal injury in right-side impacts were the glove compartment (39%), side interior (28%), and the armrest (28%). The curious appearance of the glove compartment as an injury factor in side impacts reflects the large percentage of struck cars with forward velocity at the time of impact. The occupants on the side opposite the impact continue moving forward in those cases as described by Newton's first law.

Using the concept of "severity weighted frequency" of injury, the abdominal organs seriously injured for drivers in left-side impacts were ordered as kidneys (4.5%), liver (4.0%), spleen (3.7%), digestive (2.0%), and urogenital (0.8%). For passengers in right-side impacts, the injuries were ordered as liver (7.0%), spleen (3.2%), kidneys (2.5%), urogenital (2.5%), and digestive (1.2%). The near doubling of the proportion of liver injuries in right-side impacts when compared to left-side impacts makes sense from anatomical considerations.

Bondy (1980; cited in King, 1985) also analyzed the statistics in the NCSS database. His analysis showed that in frontal impact the order of serious abdominal injury was liver (39%), spleen (25%), digestive (16%), kidney (14%), and urogenital (2.6%). The contact points associated with serious abdominal injury were the steering system (51%), side interior/armrest (26%), instrument panel/glove compartment (17%), front seat back (5%), and belt webbing (1%). It is interesting to note that the restraint system was not associated with injury to any of the solid abdominal organs.

Summary

These field accident studies have shown that blunt abdominal trauma is a common result of motor vehicle–related collisions. In general, there is a preponderance of abdominal injuries to the solid organs compared to hollow organs. When age is accounted for, children and the elderly are overrepresented in terms of incidence of serious abdominal injuries. The order of organs injured was significantly different when comparing side and frontal impacts. There appears to be greater risk of renal injury for drivers in left-side impacts than for those in frontal impacts, or for passengers in right-side impacts.

The contact points associated with injury to unbelted occupants include many of the structures within the vehicle (steering system, side door, instrument panel, etc.). While safety-belt use is associated with an increase in minor abdominal injury compared to the unbelted occupant, there is a clear decline in serious injury to the abdomen when safety belts are used.

Clinical Data

Griswold and Collier (1961), in their very thorough collective review, found the frequency of blunt injury to the abdominal viscera to be, in descending order, spleen (26.2%), kidney (24.2%), intestines (16.2%), liver (15.6%), abdominal wall (3.6%), retroperitoneal areas (2.7%), mesentery (2.5%), pancreas (1.4%), and diaphragm (1.1%).

Baxter and Williams (1961) examined 158 patients with blunt abdominal trauma and found the following order: kidneys (34%), spleen (22%), liver (8%), and pancreas (8%). In a series of experiments with canine subjects they saw a different order, *viz.* spleen (48%), kidney (19%), liver (17%), and no pancreatic injuries. Half the large number of splenic injuries were subcapsular hematomas, which might not be noticed clinically unless a laparotomy was performed. When they accounted for those injuries, the experimental data were very similar to the clinical data.

Perry (1965) studied 152 cases of abdominal injury and reported that 70% to 76% were diagnosed clinically, but 22% to 24% were first recognized at autopsy. Of the blunt injuries, 79% were from motor vehicle–related in-

cidents. The frequency of organ injury was spleen (45%), liver (21%), intestines (13%), bladder (9%), mesentery (4%), kidney (3%), pancreas (2%), vena cava (2%), and stomach (1%). Most patients (84%) had injury to only one abdominal organ, but 11% had two organs injured, 4% had three organs injured, and 1% had four organs injured. The mortality rate was 45.7%, which was in stark contrast to a mortality rate of 6.7% for the patients with penetrating trauma in the same study. Of the deaths from blunt trauma, 26% were due to the abdominal injury itself; in 35% the abdominal injury contributed significantly to the mortality; and in 39% the mortality was a result of other injuries.

Tonge et al. (1972; cited in Nahum, 1973) analyzed data from 908 injured occupants of motor vehicles. They found that the liver was most commonly injured (32% of all drivers; 28% of all passengers), followed by the spleen (21% of all drivers; 26% of all passengers). Other organs injured, in descending order, were the kidneys, small bowel, colon, urinary bladder, urogenital organs, pancreas, adrenal glands, stomach, and duodenum.

Cox (1984) reported an analysis of 870 patients who required celiotomy for blunt abdominal trauma over a 5-year period. Ninety percent (90%) of the injuries were from motor vehicle–related collisions. The injury distribution was spleen (42%), liver (36%), retroperitoneal hematoma (15%), serosa and mesentery (13%), diaphragm (5%), bowel (5%), bladder (3%), vascular (3%), kidney (3%), and others. Mortality over the 5-year period was 25% of those patients with blunt abdominal trauma. Over 38% of the patients who died had two or more systems injured, and over 50% had associated injuries that required surgical intervention.

Bergqvist et al. (1985) compared abdominal injuries in children with those of adults in a study of 1,407 patients admitted over a 30-year period. Of these patients, 348 were children (≤14 years of age). The frequency of organ injury in the children was kidneys (18%), spleen (11%), liver (5%), small intestine (4%), and others. The frequency of organ injury to occupants of all ages was kidneys (29%), spleen (13%), liver (9%), retroperitoneal hematoma (5%), small intestine (4%), and others. Only 3% of the children, but 10% of the occupants of all ages, had two or more intra-abdominal injuries. Almost half of the injuries were sustained in motor vehicle collisions. Falls and sports injuries accounted for most of the rest.

Summary

While blunt trauma to the abdomen has a significantly higher mortality rate than penetrating trauma, mortality rates have declined from 46% in 1965 to 25% in 1984. This decrease is largely associated with improved diagnostic techniques and especially with diagnostic peritoneal lavage (Cox, 1984). The large number of patients with major associated injuries is a major factor in the mortality remaining. Although there is considerable variability in the frequency and order of organ injury among the reviews included here, the three most-frequently injured organs in blunt abdominal trauma appear to be the spleen, liver, and kidneys. The reader will note that these are all "solid" organs. As will be shown in the section Injury Mechanisms, Criteria, and Tolerances, the "solid" organs are injured much more readily than the "hollow" organs.

Mechanical Impact Response of the Abdomen

Relatively few studies have addressed the mechanical impact response of the human abdomen (Melvin et al., 1975). The studies that have been performed have examined different regions of the abdomen, using different loading surfaces, loading rates, and loading directions. As such it is difficult to define *one* response curve for the abdomen. In addition, as discussed previously, the abdomen is not a homogeneous region of the body (i.e., some organs are "solid" while others are "hollow," and some are located within the lower parts of the rib cage while others are surrounded only by soft tissue). Therefore, information pertaining to the appropriate region of the abdomen, the impacting surface, and the direction of loading need to be specified when an abdominal response corridor is given.

In the following discussion, the reader is referred back to the classical division of the anatomy (Fig. 16.2). From this figure, one could postulate that there may be 15 unique response curves made up of a frontal impact response curve for each of the nine regions, plus a lateral impact response curve for the three regions on the left and three on the right side of the abdomen (nine frontal + three right lateral + three left lateral = 15). In practice, not all of the classical anatomical regions of the abdomen have been examined individually. But, certain qualitative assumptions can be made to define the response of some regions of the abdomen in the absence of quantitative data. As shown in the following discussion, this will reduce the 15 possible abdominal response curves to eight possibly different response curves.

All of the published *frontal* impact response studies have used impact surfaces that were wider than the width (left of right) of the subjects tested. None have applied to a single classical region of the abdomen. Therefore, all of the response curves discussed here will be for one of the three rows of the abdomen. For example, in frontal impact, there may be a unique response corridor for each column of the top row of the abdomen (right and left hypochondriac, and epigastric regions), because of the presence of the liver on the right side, the spine in the central region, and the stomach/spleen on the left side. However, data exist only for the test condition in which all three columns of the top row were impacted at the same time. The response of the middle and bottom rows is expected to be different from that of the top row. The response of the region covered by the bottom row has not been published, but it is reasonable to assume that it is similar to that of the region covered by the middle row (except in pregnancy). Then, lacking quantitative data, the abdomen will be divided into two regions, *viz.* the upper abdomen (top row) and the lower abdomen (middle and bottom rows).

In *lateral* impact, there may be unique response corridors for the right and left regions of the top row of the abdomen, which consists mainly of the liver on the right side and the stomach and spleen on the left side, with over-laying ribs on both sides. It is well known that the tolerance of the right and left sides differ in lateral impact, so the responses may also differ. The lower abdomen again probably differs from the upper abdomen, but one may expect the right and left regions of the lower abdomen to have similar response characteristics.

Then, instead of 15 different response curves for frontal and lateral impacts to correspond to the classical anatomical division of the abdomen, the anatomic similarity of the various regions suggests that there could be eight unique response curves for pure frontal and lateral abdominal impacts. These would include one for each region shown in Table 16.1.

Frontal impact response work has examined the different rows of the abdomen, but has not made the distinction between the columns. In contrast, lateral impact response work has addressed the left-side versus right-side impact (left column versus right column), but has not addressed upper abdomen versus lower abdomen (top row versus middle and bottom rows). The following sections present the known abdominal response data for frontal and lateral impacts, to the upper and lower abdomen, and left and right side of the abdomen, using rigid impact surfaces and safety belts.

Frontal Impact Response

Lower Abdomen

Cavanaugh et al. (1986) performed studies of frontal impact to the lower abdomen of unembalmed human cadavers using a rigid cylindrical impactor. The impactor was an aluminum bar, 381 mm long and 25.4 mm in diameter, which was oriented with the long axis parallel to the width of the subject at the level of the third lumbar vertebra (L3). Each subject was seated upright, on a table, in the

TABLE 16.1. Unique nondegenerate response curves.

Frontal impact	Upper abdomen	Left region
		Central region
		Right region
	Lower abdomen	Left/right region
		Central region
Lateral impact	Upper abdomen	Left side
		Right side
	Lower abdomen	Left/right side

free-back condition, with legs straight out on the table (at 90° to the torso). The torso was held upright by straps under the arms that were released at the time of impact. A 32-kg or 64-kg impactor was accelerated using a pneumatic piston and translated 250 mm before striking the subject. Impact velocities varied from 4.9 m/sec to 13.0 m/sec. The maximum deflection of the subject was not limited by the impactor because it was essentially free-flying (but guided) during the impact. Abdominal deflection data (relative to the spine) was obtained by film analysis.

Figure 16.3 shows the high and low velocity, rigid impactor force-deflection response from Cavanaugh's tests ($|v| = 10.4 \pm 1.5$ m/sec, and $|v| = 6.1 \pm 1.1$ m/sec, respectively). Note that four of the seven high velocity impacts were done with the 64-kg pendulum, and all other tests were done with the 32-kg pendulum.

Nusholtz et al. (1988) also performed frontal impacts to the lower abdomen of unembalmed human cadavers using a "rigid lower rim of a steering wheel attached to a rigid column support" as the impact surface. The wheel was mounted to a 25-kg pendulum that was driven by a pneumatically accelerated piston, and was free-flying at the time of impact. The subject was seated on a table covered by polyethylene sheets (for low friction) with legs hanging down, and back free to move during the impact (free-back condition). An upright posture was established by suspending the subject from the ceiling using a parachute harness that was released at the time of impact. The impactor was positioned so that the bottom of the rim was "halfway between the most inferior point on rib 10 and the iliac crest" (approximately L3). Impact velocities varied from 3.9 to

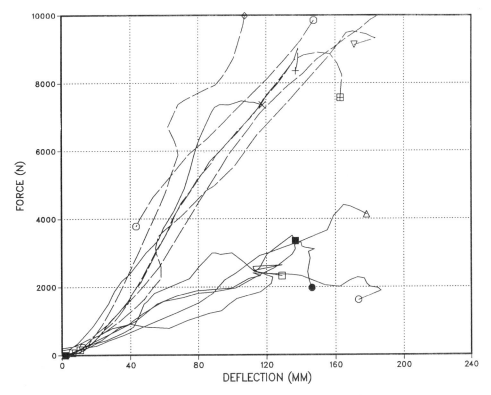

FIGURE 16.3. Rigid impactor, frontal response of the lower abdomen. (From Cavanaugh et al., 1986. Reprinted with permission © 1992, Society of Automotive Engineers, Inc.)

10.8 m/sec. Deflection was measured using string potentiometers and accelerometers affixed to the 12th thoracic vertebra and to the rigid impactor.

Figure 16.4 shows the rigid impactor force-deflection response from Nusholtz's tests ($|v| = 8.0 \pm 2.6$ m/sec). Note that although Nusholtz's velocity range spans both Cavanaugh's high- and low-velocity ranges, the two sets of experiments give different results in the low-velocity range. The reasons for these differences are not readily apparent.

Miller (1989) performed experiments with anesthetized porcine subjects lying supine in a V-shaped support. The tests were done on a closed-loop hydraulic test machine that controlled the stroke of a vertically moving piston. The top of a yoke that was shaped like an arch was connected to the piston, and 50-mm-wide belt webbing was connected to the bottom ends of the yoke (the bottom of the arch). The subject was positioned beneath

the belt webbing. The ends of the yoke were wider than the abdominal width of the test subject, and the V-support had notches cut out to prevent interference with the lap belt. The impact location was at the level of the fourth lumbar vertebra on the porcine subject, which is approximately the same relative location as the level of the third lumbar vertebra on the human, and is approximately the midpoint between the top of the pelvis and the bottom of the rib cage. Impact velocities were varied from 1.6 to 6.6 m/sec, and compressions were varied from 6% to 67% of the subject's anteroposterior dimension.

Miller reported the axial piston force and piston stroke data. The actual deflection of the abdomen in the midsagittal plane (directly beneath the piston) may have been different from the piston stroke because of belt stretch and changes in belt geometry. The raw force and deflection data was normalized by Rouhana et al. (1989, 1990) to determine

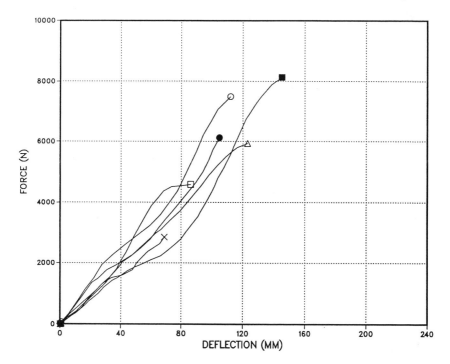

FIGURE 16.4. Rigid impactor, frontal response of the lower abdomen. (From Nusholtz et al., 1988.)

force-deflection curves. Normalization was performed using equal stress/equal velocity scaling to account for differences between subject masses and anteroposterior dimensions. Miller's experiments were performed at many different velocities, but the force-deflection curves appeared to be separable into a "low" (3.7 m/sec) and a "high" (6.3 m/sec) velocity group, based on stiffness.

Figure 16.5 shows the belt impact, normalized force-deflection response determined by Rouhana from Miller's tests ($|v|$) = 3.7 ± 0.84 m/sec).

Upper Abdomen

Stalnaker and Ulman (1985) reanalyzed data from previous experiments, which used various primate subjects, to establish abdominal response corridors. These impacts were performed with rigid impactors driven by a pneumatically operated piston. Six impact surfaces were used, including three different bars and three different wedges. Three different impact locations were used, including the central regions of the upper, middle, and

lower abdomen (mostly upper abdomen). All of the response data from the three different regions and six different impact surfaces was plotted on the same graph to define a single abdominal response corridor for $|v|$ = 12.1 m/sec. Scaling was used to define corridors for other velocities. Because the upper and lower abdominal response curves from different impact surfaces and different impact locations cannot be separated using the information in the publications, and since the data in general are close to the response for the lower abdomen, it is recommended that the lower abdominal response be used for the upper abdomen until more data become available.

Lateral Impact Response

Upper Abdomen

Walfisch et al. (1980) dropped unembalmed human cadaver subjects from 1- and 2-m drop heights to examine lateral impact response and injury. The surface impacted was a rigid or a

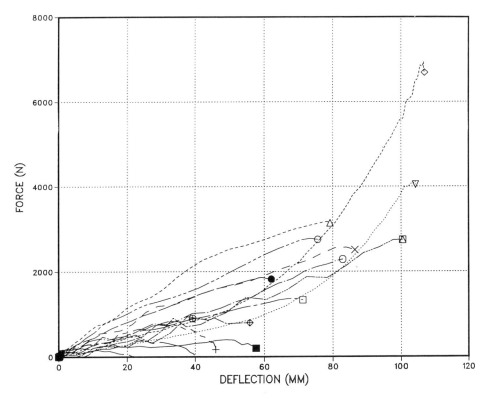

FIGURE 16.5. Lap belt impactor, frontal response of the lower abdomen. (From Rouhana et al., 1989, based on Miller, 1989.)

deformable simulated armrest that was struck by the right side of the subject at the level of the ninth rib. Contact velocities were 4.5 m/sec for the 1-m drop, and 6.3 m/sec for the 2-m drop. Deflection data was determined by film analysis, where deflection was defined as intrusion of the armrest relative to the spine (not the opposite side of the subject). Force data was obtained from load cells located beneath the simulated armrest.

Figure 16.6 shows the force-time curves for the rigid armrest data from Walfisch's tests after normalization using the method proposed by Mertz (1984). The corridors are those proposed for lateral impact by the International Standards Organization (ISO) (1989), with the upper and lower bounds given by the average of the curves plus and minus 25%, respectively.

Viano et al. (1989) reported the results of oblique lateral impacts to unembalmed human cadaver subjects using a pneumatic, power-assisted, pendulum impactor. In these tests, the pendulum was brought up to impact speed by the pneumatic device, after which it became a free mass supported only by two cables. The impactor surface was a 152-mm diameter rigid disk with rounded edges, and the impactor mass was 23.4 kg. The subjects were suspended upright, with hands and arms overhead. To minimize rotation of the torso, the subjects were positioned so that the line of action of the impactor was through the estimated center of gravity of the torso and was in a plane that was rotated 60° from the midsagittal plane (clockwise, as viewed from above, for right-side impacts or counterclockwise for left-side impacts). The impactor contacted the subject 75 mm below the xiphoid process and covered approximately ribs 6 through 10. Deflection data were obtained analysis of high-speed movies.

Figure 16.7 shows the force-deflection and force-time corridors for Viano et al.'s (1989) tests at 4.3, 6.7, and 9.5 m/sec. Since deflec-

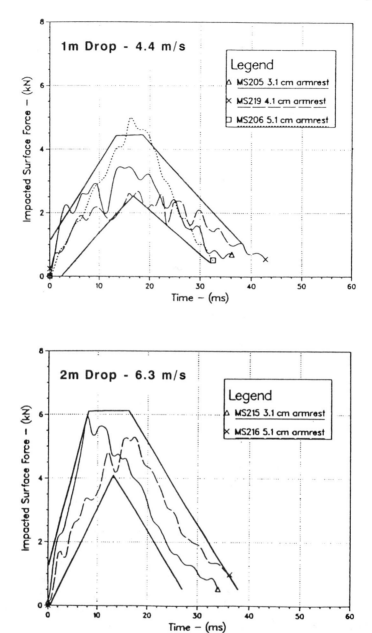

FIGURE 16.6. Rigid surface, lateral response of the upper abdomen from 1-m (top) and 2-m (bottom) drop tests. (Reproduced with permission from the International Organization for Standardization, Technical Report 9790-5, copyright 1989.)

tion data is very difficult to obtain using film analysis, the force-time curves are probably the most accurate. This data was also normalized to account for differences in subject mass, anthropometry, and test velocity. The reader will note that the units in scaling Equation 6 of Viano et al. (1989) do not work out correctly. It is not known whether that is due to a typographical error or if the scaling factors are in error.

RENORMALIZED ABDOMEN

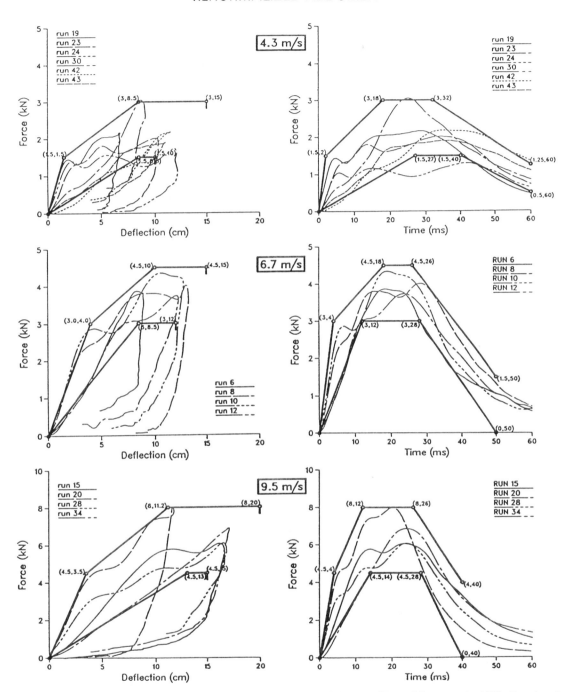

FIGURE 16.7. Rigid impactor, lateral response of the upper abdomen. (From Viano et al., 1989. Reprinted with permission © 1992, Society of Automotive Engineers, Inc.)

Injury Mechanisms, Criteria, and Tolerances

A mechanism of injury from blunt trauma can be defined as a description of the cause of organ injury. That is, it is a description of how the state of stress or strain that produced injury was set up in the organ. For example, one injury mechanism for intestinal rupture may be increased intraluminal pressure. This intraluminal pressure may occur because of compression of the abdomen. But, regardless of its etiology, the pressure may cause stretching of the intestinal walls, and injury can occur if that stretching exceeds the material strength of the walls.

An injury criterion is a mathematical relationship, based on empirical observation, which formally describes a relationship between some measurable physical parameter interacting with a test subject and the occurrence of injury that directly results from that interaction. This description is typically in the form of an equation representing a dose-response relationship. For example, the force or compression applied to the abdomen may be correlated with liver injury. In general, there are typically many physical parameters that have some correlation with the injury outcome.

Statistical analyses are typically used to define injury criteria. One such approach, logistic regression (Kroell et al., 1986), produces a continuous function relating the amount of the input physical parameters (the dose) to the probability of a certain type and severity injury (the response). A graph of the resulting function typically has a sigmoidal shape, starting as a horizontal line with zero probability of injury at zero input, curving to a steep slope at a transition region, and curving again to a plateau at 100% probability of injury for points above some level of input parameter.

The tolerance to injury can be defined as the value of some known injury criterion that delineates a noninjurious event from an injurious event. Or, phrased another way, the tolerance is the minimum dose associated with a specified probability of producing injury of a specified severity.

In automotive safety studies, the injury criteria and tolerances are determined using human surrogates (human cadavers, anesthetized animals, etc.). The criteria become the basis for instrumentation in another human surrogate, the crash test dummy. Automotive safety engineers utilize crash test dummies in an attempt to measure the important physical parameters during a crash test of a vehicle under development. These measurements are then compared to the human tolerance values to interpret how well a design performs.

There have been many studies performed that address the mechanisms of injury, injury criteria, and human tolerance for the abdominal region of the body. The results indicate that there are a number of different criteria and mechanisms of injury, and that different organs respond to different physical inputs. Some of the studies have examined the organs after removal from the body, but the majority have examined the organs in situ, that is, in their normal state in the body (surrounded by other organs, complete with attachments, and in an intact peritoneal cavity). Each type of experiment adds to a general understanding of the underlying physical processes that are associated with abdominal injury.

In actual vehicle crashes, there are many different ways in which energy is input to the body. Unbelted occupants clearly have many more possible sources of abdominal injury than belted occupants (these include the steering system, armrest, side door, shift levers, instrument panels, other occupants, external sources from ejection, and others). Belted occupants, on the other hand, have relatively few sources of abdominal injury (the side door, armrest, improperly worn safety belts).

The following discussion centers on the various criteria and mechanisms of abdominal injury from blunt trauma, first in general, and then as they apply to particular abdominal organs.

General Limitations on Injury Mechanism Data

Early studies of blunt abdominal trauma resulted in the hypothesis that the liver and spleen are less able to absorb energy from impact than the hollow organs because of their anatomic vulnerability to direct impact, "limited mobility," pedicle attachments, and proximity to the margins of the lower ribs (Stapp, 1971; Widman, 1969; Nusholtz et al., 1980).

Walker (1969) suggested that injury to the elderly or intoxicated can occur from a relatively minor blow because of weakened or relaxed muscles. This has been supported by clinical observations of severe internal injury from apparently innocuous contact in the presence of a relaxed abdominal wall (Walt and Wilson, 1973). Others have shown that elevated blood alcohol levels do increase injury probability to the heart and spine when comparing similar exposures with and without ethanol in the blood (Desiderio, 1987, 1988; Ridella and Anderson, 1986).

The pathological or normal physiological state of organs can also have a marked effect on the injury outcome in blunt trauma. For example, biomechanical experiments have shown that cirrhotic livers are stiffer and less extensible before failure in tension than non-cirrhotic livers (Yamanaka et al., 1985). Other considerations include liver fibrosis (see below), splenomegally associated with mononucleosis, a full bladder, or presence of gas or chyme in the intestines (chyme is a mixture of partially digested food and digestive secretions). (Clemedson et al., 1969; Schmidt, 1979; Walt and Wilson, 1973).

The location of impact on the body can have a dramatic effect on the injury outcome (Baxter and Williams, 1961; Nusholtz, 1985). Baxter and Williams (1961) found a fivefold increase in hepatic injury, and a twofold increase in renal injury when the impact location was the side as opposed to the front of their subjects.

Age as a Factor in Abdominal Injury

Yamada (1970) has shown that the tensile strength of the stomach, large and small intestines, kidneys (renal fibrous capsule, renal parenchyma, renal calyx), ureters, and urinary bladder all decrease with age. He noted that

the tensile strength for these organs decreased by 28%, 42%, 42%, 17% (6%, 24%, 22%), 15%, and 30%, respectively, when comparing strength at age 20 versus age 70.

Barancik et al. (1986) studied hospital admissions for emergency room patients who had been in motor vehicle collisions, and found a higher probability of admission for the elderly (age >65) and the very young (<20) (Barancik et al., 1986; Lau and Viano, 1986).

Sturtz (1980) found that the "loadability" of the liver and spleen is higher at the age of 10 than at ages over 15. He also observed that the abdominal region is proportionally larger and that the liver is more exposed in children than in adults.

Schmidt (1979) analyzed the work of Fazekas et al. (1971a,b, 1972) on isolated fresh human cadaver livers, kidneys, and spleens. Fazekas et al. found a decrease in the amount of pressure before failure in elderly fibrotic livers, but an increase in pressure before failure of the kidneys. Schmidt, in contrast, found increased pressure necessary to injure a fibrotic liver.

Laboratory Studies

Acceleration

Acceleration of the body has long been regarded as an important parameter in the etiology of human organ injury (Eppinger et al., 1982, 1984; Stapp, 1971). Eppinger et al. (1982), in the development of the Thoracic Trauma Index (TTI) for side impact, included the upper abdominal organs (liver, kidneys, and spleen) in what they termed the "hard thorax." Using statistical techniques they developed a mathematical relation between thoracic AIS and a weighted sum of the input acceleration and the age of the cadaver subject tested. The accelerations used are those of the left upper or lower rib (whichever is larger), and the 12th thoracic vertebra. TTI has shown limited predictive ability for upper abdominal organs, but it does not apply to the middle or lower abdominal organs.

In contrast, Horsch et al. (1985) and Lau et al. (1987) found "no correlation between abdominal injury and maximum lower spinal acceleration measured directly opposite to the impact site." The lack of correlation between spinal acceleration and abdominal injury in this study is not surprising, however, since the accelerometer was located on the spine of the subject, while the impact was to the front of the subject's abdomen. Accelerations for the TTI calculation are from accelerometers located on the spine and on a rib on the same side of the subject that is impacted. One might expect different biomechanics in the thorax and abdomen due to the presence and absence of the rib cage, respectively. The accelerometer on the back of the subject will only pick up the whole body acceleration from a frontal abdominal impact, while the accelerometer on the impacted side of the rib cage will pick up both the whole body and local acceleration in a thoracic impact. It is reasonable to expect the local acceleration to be related to injury production.

Brun-Cassan et al. (1987) showed that "protection criteria based solely on thoracic acceleration measurements cannot account for the occurrence and severity of . . . abdominal injuries." They also question the classification of the upper abdominal organs as thoracic, stating that since the "lower part of the rib cage is considered . . . softer than the . . . upper part . . . It is difficult to consider that some abdominal organs could be protected by the . . . hard-thorax."

More recently, Viano et al. (1989) found that spinal acceleration was not well correlated to abdominal injury in lateral pendulum impacts to human cadavers.

Compression

Crushing of organs can occur in blunt impact situations when the body surface deforms, and the organs interior to the impact site are compressed against an opposing surface. Crushing injury can occur at very low speeds. For example, crushing injury of the liver might occur in a low-speed collision when an unbelted occupant strikes the instrument panel. During the event, the anterior surface (front) of the occupant is stopped by the instrument panel

which causes local deformation. But, the posterior surface (back) of the occupant continues moving forward until enough force is built up to stop the entire body. Alternatively, an occupant in a collision with a lap belt improperly worn can sustain an abdominal injury when the lap belt stops the anterior abdominal wall, and the inertia of the rest of the body compresses the intestines between the belt/abdominal wall and the spinal column.

In a series of 45 lower abdominal impact experiments using anesthetized canine subjects, Williams and Sargent (1963) concluded that the mechanism of injury to the intestines in blunt impact is compression of the intestines against the spinal column. These were "fixed-back" tests with the subjects supine.

Melvin et al. (1973), in tests with surgically mobilized organs from anesthetized primates, showed that a related parameter, *viz.* compressive strain (change in length per unit length), was related to the severity of kidney injury. These could also be considered fixed-back tests.

In experiments with primates and human cadavers, Stalnaker et al. (1973a) found that abdominal compression was related to abdominal injury severity. In lateral impacts, they showed that different tolerance values apply for right- versus left-side impacts.

Rouhana et al. (1986) saw no correlation between compression and probability of either hepatic or renal injury in 117 experiments with rigid lateral impacts to anesthetized rabbits in a "free-back" condition (i.e., subjects suspended prone in a sling with no surface behind them). However, in similar experiments with a crushable impactor there was a positive correlation for hepatic injury and compression ($r = 0.97$; $p < 0.03$), but not for renal injury.

Miller (1989) found that maximum compression was well correlated with the severity of abdominal injury in 25 experiments using a safety belt to load the lower abdomen of anesthetized porcine subjects ($r = 0.69$; $p = 0.0002$; $x^2 = 12.1$). These experiments were performed at relatively low velocities (mean = 3.6 m/sec; range = 1.6 to 6.6 m/sec).

Viano et al. (1989) showed poor correlation between compression and abdominal injury severity in lateral abdominal pendulum impacts.

Rate Effects and Viscous Injury

Rate of impact loading has long been recognized as a factor in injury outcome (Kroell et al., 1981). Many of the solid abdominal organs are fluid-filled. It is well known that fluid systems (e.g., shock absorbers) exhibit different mechanical characteristics under different rates of loading.

Impact studies by McElhaney et al. (1971), using live anesthetized primates, showed that small changes in impact velocity had a profound effect on the injury level. Melvin et al. (1973, see the section Compression) also noted that the liver and the kidneys were both sensitive to rates of loading.

Lau and Viano (1981a) held abdominal compression constant and varied the preimpact velocity in experiments with anesthetized rabbits. They noted a significant increase in hepatic injury with increasing impact velocity.

Rouhana et al. (1984, 1985) found that the product of maximum impact velocity (V) and maximum abdominal compression (C) was well correlated with the severity of abdominal injury from analysis of 117 abdominal impacts to anesthetized rabbits. They called this product, $V * C$, the Abdominal Injury Criterion (AIC). Viano and Lau (1983) had previously found the same quantity was related to thoracic injury severity.

Citing the work by Rouhana et al. (1984), Stalnaker and Ulman (1985) reexamined the data from 1973 studies on primates and human cadavers. They concluded that the "$V * C$ is a relevant parameter for predicting injury in subhuman primates," and that the "values obtained from primates appear to be useful in predicting abdominal injury in man." When frontal and side impacts were considered separately, and each abdominal region was considered separately, the correlation of $V * C$ with AIS $\geqslant 3$ injury was very high ($r = 0.92$ to 0.99).

Up to this point the interrelationship between velocity and compression used preimpact velocity, and maximum compression ($V_{max} * C_{max}$). In 1985, Viano and Lau extended the previous work by measuring the compression as a function of time (t). This allowed the product of the velocity-time history and compression-time history to be compared with injury outcome. A strong correlation was found between the maximum of the product, $VC(t)$, and the injury produced. This time-varying product was called the Viscous Response and was used to define a Viscous Tolerance Criterion for thoracic impact (Viano and Lau, 1985).

In a study of injury to 17 porcine subjects from steering system impacts, Horsch et al. (1985) showed good correlation of the abdominal injury outcome with the maximum of $VC(t)$. They did not examine the relationship between $V_{max} * C_{max}$ and injury.

Kroell et al. (1986) examined the interrelationship between velocity and chest compression in blunt impact to 23 porcine subjects. Their results showed better correlation of $V_{max} * C_{max}$ than $VC(t)_{max}$ for probability of heart rupture and for probability of AIS $\geqslant 4$ injury.

The Viscous Criterion was further refined in 1986 by Lau and Viano (1986) and compared to other criteria. When compared to $V_{max} * C_{max}$ the authors noted that a time-varying function gives one the ability to discriminate the timing of injury production, which may help in the development of countermeasures. They also proposed that a time-varying function could account for changes in velocity caused by collapse of the surface being impacted. While this is true, the velocity environment of the subject (in this case a test dummy) will never be greater than the preimpact velocity, and the probability that a structure will fail is also likely related to the impact velocity (since force, energy available, and impact velocity are very well correlated). Therefore, the main advantage of the viscous response is the time history it gives.

Much research has taken place since the AIC and the Viscous Criterion were proposed. While some research has shown that there is little difference in the end result (Kroell et al., 1986), other research has shown the utility of knowledge of the time of injury occurrence (Lau and Viano, 1988). Therefore, the viscous response is probably the more desirable function to measure, but in cases where it cannot be measured, the AIC is a good substitute.

More recent data by many researchers has provided supporting evidence of the correlation of abdominal injury with the AIC and the Viscous Tolerance Criterion (Lau and Viano, 1988; Miller, 1989; Rouhana, 1987; Viano et al., 1989).

Wave Motion

Cooper and Taylor (1989) and Cooper et al. (1991) present evidence that stress waves and shear waves play a role in the production of injury in blast and impact loading of the body. They propose wave phenomena as the manner in which injury occurs at locations that are remote from the impact site. The velocity of deformation is the predominant factor in determining the magnitude of the wave created.

In higher velocity phenomena such as non-penetrating projectiles (50 m/sec), the authors suggest that stress waves emanate from the impact site, traveling at the speed of sound in the tissues. Injury occurs at interfaces between unlike tissues or tissue/air boundaries (e.g., intestinal wall/intraluminal gas). Mechanisms proposed include (a) stress wave–induced compression and reexpansion of the stressed wall, (b) production of a pressure differential across the boundary, or (c) "spalling," where energy is released as the wave attempts to propagate from a dense to a much less-dense medium (the reflected wave is tensile, which may injure the tissue because many materials have lower strength in tension than compression).

In lower-velocity phenomena such as those encountered in automotive collisions (<15 m/sec), displacements of external body surfaces may be propagated as a transverse wave of low velocity and long duration, i.e., a shear ware. Injury may result from (a) dif-

ferential motion of connected adjacent structures, (b) strain at the sites of attachments, or (c) collision of viscera with stiffer structures.

These stress wave/shear wave postulates are similar to those proposed by von Gierke et al. (1952, 1964), who based his postulates on a mechanical model of the human body exposed to impact.

Impact Force

Force is such a normal a part of everyday life that its effects are taken for granted. Gravitational force keeps us firmly attached to terra firma, weak and strong nuclear forces bind the matter of the world, and electromagnetic forces are used by man for all sorts of conveniences (electric motors, etc). Force is defined as "that which changes the state of rest or motion in matter, measured by the rate of change of momentum" (Weast et al., 1984). Newton's first law states that an object will remain at rest unless acted upon by an external force, and an object in motion will remain in motion at a constant velocity unless acted upon by an external force.

When a vehicle is in a collision, the state of motion of the occupants within the vehicle may be changed drastically depending on the severity of the collision. To do this, according to Newton's laws, forces are exerted on the occupant. The actual etiology of these forces may be from inertia/acceleration, compression of elastic bodies, compression of viscous bodies, or other means. As such one might expect that the impact force an occupant experiences, whatever its origin, should be well correlated with injury outcome.

In 85 impacts to primate and porcine subjects, Trollope et al. (1973) found the manner in which the force is applied to be important. For intact animals, over 1.6 kN was needed to produce an "Estimated Severity of Injury" (ESI) = 2 liver injury (similar to AIS = 3 or 4), whereas only 0.67 kN was necessary to produce injury of the same severity in a surgically exposed liver.

Stalnaker et al. (1973a,b) found that the severity of abdominal injury was proportional to the logarithm of the impact force and time duration squared.

Gogler et al. (1977) studied impacts with mini-pigs at velocities of 9.8 to 16.9 m/sec and saw a transition from AIS = 3 abdominal injury to AIS = 4 at 1.5 kN. They also noted a transition from subacute shock to acute shock over a force range of 0.6 to 1.0 kN.

Peak force of 0.35 kN was associated with AIS ≥4 abdominal injury in impacts to the abdomen of anesthetized rabbits (Lau and Viano, 1981a). The peak force was very well correlated to velocity of impact.

Rouhana et al. (1986) performed 214 experiments of lateral abdominal impacts to anesthetized rabbits using rigid and crushable impacting surfaces. Their analysis showed that peak force was very well correlated with probability of AIS ≥3 renal injury, but not with probability of hepatic injury. They were able to reduce the number of renal lacerations by a factor of 3 by use of a force-limiting material, but the material used had no effect on hepatic lacerations. They postulated that the renal lacerations occurred at the time of peak impact force. It is possible that the force limiting did not reduce hepatic injury because the force limit was too high.

Peak force was the best correlate with AIS ≥4 abdominal injury of all the biomechanical measures compared in a study by Viano et al. (1989). The values given in Table 11 of that publication show that the correlation coefficient, significance, and goodness of fit were better for peak force ($r = 0.75$; $p = 0.004$; $\chi^2 = 8.5$), than for the viscous response ($r = 0.60$; $p = 0.013$; $\chi^2 = 6.1$), maximum compression, and acceleration measurements. Although the authors concluded that the viscous response was the best correlate with AIS ≥3 thoracic injury, the correlations were not statistically significant. The statistics presented for AIS ≥4 thoracic injury were significant, and showed much better correlation, goodness of fit, and significance for the peak force than for the viscous response.

Miller (1989) showed that peak force was well correlated with the probability of AIS ≥3 and AIS ≥4 lower abdominal injury in belt loading ($r = 0.67$; $p = 0.0003$; $\chi^2 = 12.8$).

Pressure

Many researchers have examined the pressure applied during impact as a way to account for impact surfaces of different shape and size. Williams and Sargent (1963, see the section Compression) found that the average peritoneal pressure was greater than the intraluminal pressure in the intestine during impact. In addition, the presence of air or water in the intestine did not affect the injury outcome. They concluded that intestinal rupture was not caused by intraluminal pressure exceeding the intraperitoneal pressure.

Analysis by McElhaney et al. (1971, see the section Rate Effects) led to an estimate of 131 kPa for the tolerable pressure applied by "an armrest-like striker" to the midabdominal region. This value was independent of the side of the body struck, and was associated with ESI = 3 injury (similar to AIS = 4 or 5). For a "flat rigid striker of larger cross-section than the animal struck," the tolerable value was 386 kPa.

Fazekas et al. (1971a,b, 1972) studied isolated cadaver organs and found that a pressure of 168.5 kPa was necessary to cause superficial laceration of the liver, while 319.8 kPa caused multiple ruptures. They also found that 44.0 kPa caused superficial laceration of the spleen.

In their work on surgically exposed livers and kidneys, Melvin et al. (1973, see the section Compression) found that "moderate trauma [ESI ≥3, similar to AIS = 4 or 5] under dynamic loading occurs at a threshold stress level of approximately 310 kPa in the liver." They noted that kidney injury severity was not ordered by stress level.

Analysis by Stalnaker et al. (1973a,b) and Trollope et al. (1973) gave conflicting tolerance numbers from the same data, but all showed a relationship between impact pressure and injury outcome.

Walfisch et al. (1980) performed tests with eight cadavers dropped on their sides from various heights onto simulated armrests. They found that the average pressure on the armrest was a reliable indicator of injury severity ($r = 0.93$). They found that a pressure of

260 kPa was associated with AIS $\geq$ 3 injury severity.

In a study of belt loading to anesthetized canine subjects, Lau and Viano (1981b) saw the initiation of "hepatic surface injury" when the pressure was 350 kPa.

Rouhana et al. (1986) found that by using force-limiting honeycomb material beneath the impact surface, renal lacerations were prevented when the crush strength was 231 kPa. Liver injury was not affected by honeycomb of the same crush strength.

Miller (1989, see the section Compression) found that the peak pressure was well correlated with the probability of AIS $\geq$3 injury ($r = 0.67$; $p = 0.0003$; $\chi^2 = 12.6$), and also correlated (although not as well) with probability of AIS $\geq$4 injury ($r = 0.60$; $p = 0.0004$; $\chi^2 = 13.2$).

Energy Input and Force Times Compression ($F_{max} * C_{max}$)

Baxter and Williams (1961) performed a series of blunt abdominal impact experiments with anesthetized canine subjects. They found that the number of abdominal injuries increased from 1.5 to 2.65 per subject as the impact energy increased from 271 to 407 J.

Mays (1966) dropped cadaver livers onto a concrete surface from varying heights in an attempt to reproduce clinically relevant bursting injuries. He found that great heights were needed (this author estimates a maximum drop height of 35.7 m). Flaccid organs did not produce bursting injuries unless they were repressurized before the test by filling them with barium and saline. Mays found that 36 to 46 J was associated with tears and superficial lacerations of the Glisson's membrane (AIS = 4 injury), 144 to 182 J was associated with deep lacerations without vascular involvement (AIS = 5 injury), and 386 to 488 J was associated with extensive pulpefaction of the parenchymal tissue "as seen clinically in bursting injury," and "severe disruption of the tertiary divisions of the portal vein, hepatic artery, and bile ducts" (AIS = 5 injury).

Williams and Sargent's experiments (1963, see the section Compression), dropping

weights onto the abdomen of anesthetized canine subjects, showed that 542 J produced clinically relevant intra-abdominal injuries.

The drop tests by Walfisch et al. (1980, see the section Pressure) showed that serious injury (AIS = 3) was produced when both a force of 4.5 kN, and a compression of 28% of the half abdomen (or 14% of the whole abdomen) were simultaneously attained.

Rouhana (1987) reanalyzed the Walfisch data, and showed that the product of the maximum force (F) and maximum abdominal compression ($F_{max} * C_{max}$) was well correlated with the probability of AIS $\geq$4 abdominal injury ($r = 0.89$; $p = 0.002$; $\chi^2 = 9.6$). He proposed this measure as another injury criterion for abdominal injury.

That $F_{max} * C_{max}$ was well correlated with probability of abdominal injury makes sense from intuition. It is related to the amount of work done on the subject during impact, and hence is also related to the amount of energy lost in the impact. Tissue and organ disruption is certainly an energy dissipative process. Therefore, the larger the $F_{max} * C_{max}$ product, the more energy loss and tissue destruction one might expect. A logical next step would be to measure force and compression as a function of time during impact. One could then investigate the correlation of the maximum of $F(t) * C(t)$ with probability of injury in a manner analogous to the viscous criterion.

Miller (1989, see the section Compression) confirmed the predictive ability of $F_{max} * C_{max}$ in seat belt impacts to the lower abdomen of anesthetized porcine subjects. In fact, $F_{max} * C_{max}$ was better correlated than the viscous response with the probability of AIS $\geq$4 injury to the lower abdomen. (Note the error in Miller's Table V. The correct values for $F_{max} * C_{max}$ are given on her Figure 6 as $r = 0.71$, $p = 0.0002$, and $\chi^2 = 14.0$; while for VC_{max} they are $r = 0.67$, $p = 0.0005$, and $\chi^2 = 15.1$.)

Clinical Studies

Clinical studies have tended to look more at injury to specific organs, but some have examined abdominal injury in general. The following review is not meant to be exhaustive, but rather to give an overview of what has been done.

Liver

The liver is the largest of the solid organs in the abdomen, which when subjected to blunt trauma is associated with the highest morbidity and mortality rates (Frey, 1970; Frey et al., 1973; Lim, 1982; Singleton, 1963; Walt and Wilson, 1973). The right lobe of the liver is the most frequently injured part of the organ (Moar, 1985; Rivkind, 1989). Many of the deaths attributed to liver injury are due to hemorrhage. However, the vast majority of patients with hepatic injury have one or more associated injuries (Frey et al., 1973). Rivkind et al. found that 69% of the patients with blunt hepatic injury who died had significant brain injury (Glasgow Coma Score of 6).

Arnold et al. (1977) have shown that the liver capsule (Glisson's membrane), under tensile loading, exhibits significant initial compliance followed by high resistance after approximately 1 mm of extension. The same experiments demonstrated stress relaxation, a phenomenon that occurs in viscoelastic materials, and is indicative of a dependence of mechanical properties on the rate of loading.

The liver may be injured by direct trauma or indirect trauma. With direct trauma several injury patterns have been described. Minor injuries include subcapsular hematoma (in which Glisson's membrane remains intact but there is an area of hemorrhage underneath) or superficial lacerations (tears that do not extend into the parenchyma of the organ). Moderate injuries include "bear-claw" markings caused by multiple linear lacerations. More significant injuries include crushing or bursting injuries manifested as stellate lacerations, both of which may be associated with massive tissue destruction and pulpefaction or shattering of the parenchyma (Frey et al., 1973; Hardy, 1972; Lau and Viano, 1981a,b; Lim, 1982; Mays, 1966; Melvin et al., 1973).

The mechanisms of blunt liver injury range from simple compression against the spine or posterior wall of the abdomen in low-velocity impacts, to viscous injury caused by build up of internal fluid pressure at high rates of loading leading to excessive tensile or shear strains (similar to a water balloon bursting) (Mays, 1966; Melvin et al., 1973). In addition, the liver may be injured by motion relative to the rest of the body during rapid deceleration. In this case, injury is typically at points of attachment and is caused by stretching the ligaments or blood vessels beyond their tensile strength. Finally, the liver may be lacerated by penetration of ribs that are fractured due to blunt trauma.

It is interesting to note that liver injury can also occur from impacts at remote body regions. Stein et al. (1983) delivered blunt cardiac impacts to anesthetized canine subjects, and found hepatic congestion in 100%, and laceration in 18% of the subjects. Subcapsular splenic hematoma was observed in 44% of the subjects. The mechanism of this remote site injury production was believed to be "extraordinarily high venous pressure that develops at the instant of impact."

Spleen

The spleen is an extremely well-vascularized organ situated in the upper left part of the abdomen, directly underneath the diaphragm and posterior and to the left of the stomach. The highly vascular nature of the spleen carries with it a significant risk of mortality (10% to 25%) from traumatic disruption of the organ (Frey, 1970; Mustard et al., 1984; Singleton, 1963; Teniere et al., 1985; Walt and Wilson, 1973). The manifestations of injury are several. One result of trauma to the spleen is subcapsular hematoma with or without parenchymal hemorrhage. This can lead to delayed rupture of the spleen days or even weeks after the traumatic event. There may be superficial lacerations, which could lead to progressive hemorrhage, or deep lacerations and transection of the parenchyma, which can result in extensive blood loss and shock.

The two classical mechanisms of injury to the spleen include a blow to the left upper abdomen that strikes the spleen directly, and indirect trauma caused by rapid deceleration of the body and large displacement of the spleen relative to its point of attachment. The former mechanism would be associated with deep lacerations and parenchymal disruption probably by a crushing mechanism in low-velocity impacts, and a viscous mechanism in higher-velocity impacts. The latter would be associated with tears at the pedicle or hilar regions of the spleen as the attachments stretch beyond their limits during deceleration (Teniere et al., 1985).

Although treatment is beyond the scope of this chapter, it is noteworthy that treatment of traumatic injury to the spleen has undergone a revolution in thought in the past decade. While in the 1960s and 1970s the treatment of choice for splenic trauma was universally splenectomy (Frey et al., 1973; Singleton, 1963; Wooldridge, 1969), current wisdom suggests that the spleen can be salvaged in at least one-third of all trauma cases. This change in thought has been brought about by increasing evidence and awareness of the spleen's place in the immunologic armament of the body (Messinger and Schreiber, 1985; Mucha, 1986; Mustard et al., 1984, Teniere et al., 1985; Trunkey, 1982).

Kidneys

The kidneys are located between the 12th thoracic and second lumbar vertebrae, and are actually behind the peritoneum. The renal parenchyma is surrounded by a strong, adherent, fibrous capsule that itself lies within a layer of fat. This perirenal fat is encapsulated by Gerota's fascia, which is important in trauma because of its ability to contain hematomas (McAninch, 1982). The kidneys are bounded by muscles on the sides and back of the abdomen, the vertebral column medially, and by the other abdominal organs anteriorly. While judging from this anatomical location one would assume that the kidneys are fairly well protected from blunt trauma, injury to the kidneys appears to be overrepresented in side impacts to the abdomen. However, generally as much as 85% to 90% of all non-penetrating renal trauma is of minor severity.

Injuries such as renal contusion and shallow cortical lacerations are deemed minor as long as the capsule remains intact (Pranikoff

et al., 1990). Other renal injuries include renal pedicle injuries, deep parenchymal lacerations, and macerated kidneys. While most minor injuries are managed conservatively and heal spontaneously, major lesions require surgical intervention (McElhaney et al., 1976; Pranikoff et al., 1990). Renal pedicle injuries may result from relative motion during deceleration because of renal mobility and the tethering effect of the hilum. Parenchymal lesions are more likely the result of direct impact to the kidneys (McAninch, 1982).

Pancreas and Duodenum

Injury to the pancreas and duodenum accounts for less than 5% of the injuries seen at most trauma centers. Of these injuries, less than 25% are from blunt trauma (Booth and Flint, 1990; Freeman, 1985). Nevertheless, the mechanism of injury in the blunt trauma cases is most likely due to crushing of the organs between some struck object and the vertebral column (Crohn, 1964). Injury to the pancreas may range from superficial contusion to complete transection or maceration. Mortality from isolated pancreatic injury is as low as 3%, but because of associated injuries, overall mortality approaches 30% (Booth and Flint, 1990).

Injury to the duodenum may involve duodenal hematoma or perforation, with or without associated pancreatic injury. Duodenal injury may include contusion or laceration caused by crushing against the spine, tears caused by shear of the duodenum relative to its fixed attachment points, or blowout rupture caused by increased intraluminal pressure if two ends of the duodenum become pinched and occluded during impact (McElhaney et al., 1976).

Intestines

Automobile-related accidents account for a large percentage of intestinal injuries (Dauterive et al., 1985; Farthmann and Kirchner, 1990; Strate and Grieco, 1983). Most injuries to the colon (as many as 96%) are from penetrating trauma (Perry, 1965; Schrock,

1982). Blunt intestinal injuries consist of contusion to the wall, perforations or transections, and mesenteric lesions, including avulsion of the root. Proposed mechanisms of injury differ and there are numerous papers that allude to a single mechanism (Braun et al., 1985; Mays and Noer, 1966; Shapiro and Wolverson, 1989; Singleton, 1963; Stalnaker, 1973b; Williams and Sargent, 1963).

In reality, there are probably many different mechanisms of intestinal injury that vary with the type of trauma experienced by the organ. For example, punctures in the wall opposite the mesenteric border without significant surrounding hemorrhage may be from a blowout due to increased intraluminal pressure, while those with surrounding hemorrhage may be from shearing or crushing against the spine, and mesenteric root avulsion may be from motion relative to fixed attachments during severe deceleration (Christensen, 1982; Dauterive et al., 1985; McElhaney et al., 1976). Perforation has also been caused by fracture of the pelvis and by fracture of the sacroiliac joint (Farthmann and Kirchner, 1990; Shapiro and Wolverson, 1989).

Mortality in blunt intestinal trauma is well correlated with the number and severity of associated injuries (Strate and Grieco, 1983). The study by Strate and Grieco showed that patients who died with isolated colon injury had nearly twice as many associated injuries as those who lived.

Williams and Sargent (1963) definitively showed that crushing of the intestine against the vertebral column is one mechanism of intestinal injury. In their experiments, the presence of air or fluid within the intestines, when impacted, had no effect on the injury outcome.

Mays and Noer (1966) showed that a small amount of energy (1.2 J) is enough to cause injury to the isolated small intestine. By dropping small masses onto the isolated intestines, they were able to elicit graded traumatic responses, from tears of the outer layers to complete ruptures. They also showed that the effects of blunt impact to the intestine can be delayed and very serious (acute intestinal obstruction by hematoma, or chronic obstruction by scarring due to tissue necrosis). Unfortunately they do not give enough information to adequately describe the biomechanics of the impact and injury response.

Urinary Bladder

While major bladder trauma is not a frequent injury (Carroll and McAninch, 1984), it is associated with significant mortality in the range of 9% to 22% (Carroll and McAninch, 1984; Cass, 1984; McAninch, 1982; Pranikoff et al., 1990). This mortality is attributed to the large number of associated injuries (94% to 97%). In addition, the urinary bladder is well protected within the pelvis and rarely succumbs to blunt trauma without associated pelvic fracture (84% to 97%) (Carroll and McAninch, 1984; Cass, 1984). Carroll and McAninch found that the most frequently injured areas of the bladder are the dome (34%) and the lateral wall (29%), with the remainder to the neck, anterior, and posterior areas in roughly equal proportions.

Rupture may be intra- or extraperitoneal, depending on the mechanism of injury. Extraperitoneal injuries are usually the result of a bone fragment piercing the bladder wall. Intraperitoneal ruptures typically result from a blow to the lower abdomen of a person with a distended bladder. Such an impact may result in high internal pressures that exceed the breaking strength of the walls or dome (Pranikoff et al., 1990).

Diaphragm

Injury to the diaphragm occurs in 0.8% to 1.6% of all patients admitted to the hospital after blunt trauma. Motor vehicle collisions are associated with over 90% of these injuries (Kearney et al., 1989; Voeller et al., 1990). Of these, lateral impact motor vehicle collisions are more highly associated with diaphragmatic rupture than frontal collisions. The mechanisms of injury postulated for diaphragmatic rupture include shearing of the stretched membrane, avulsion of the diaphragm from its points of attachment, and transmission of pressure through the viscera acting as a fluid.

However, there is no experimental evidence to validate any of these proposed mechanisms (Kearney et al., 1989).

Uterus

The nongravid uterus is rarely injured by blunt trauma because of its location surrounded by the pelvis (Frey, 1970). However, the gravid uterus because of its increased size and fluid-filled state has greater potential for injury (Oni et al., 1984). Reported injuries to the gravid uterus include uterine rupture, placental separation, placental laceration (Lane, 1977; Matthews, 1975; Stuart et al., 1980; Cheteuti and Levene, 1987; Civil et al., 1988; Svendsen and Morild, 1988).

Several mechanisms of injury to the gravid uterus have been postulated. Crosby et al. (1968, 1972) reported on a series of experiments with anesthetized primate subjects, which revealed up to a tenfold increase in intrauterine pressure during impact with subjects restrained by a lap belt only and those restrained by a lap-shoulder belt. This pressure increase was not opposed by equal pressure increase in the abdominal cavity and it is believed that in some cases the pressure differential may lead to uterine rupture. Alternatively, rapid compression (probably accompanied by shear at the placenta/uterine junction) may be the mechanism of placental abruption or separation.

Another mechanism of the uterine rupture and placental abruption relates to occupant kinematics during a collision while restrained by a lap belt only. Kinematic data reported by Crosby et al. (1968) showed that the chest of occupants restrained only by a lap belt moved first, and that motion of the head and abdomen lagged behind. This led to hyperextension of the cervical spine and a simultaneous peak in intrauterine pressure. The torso then pivoted forward and jackknifed around the lap belt such that the abdomen was compressed against the seat and intrauterine pressure again peaked. Of note is that the intrauterine pressure reached the same peak level with a shoulder belt restraint as it did when only a lap belt restraint was used (Crosby et al., 1968).

There is incomplete information in the publications regarding the condition of the uterus, although 5 of 10 fetuses died as a direct result of the impact when the mother was restrained only by a lap belt, compared with 1 of 12 when the mother was restrained by a lap-shoulder belt.

It has been well established that the best way to prevent fetal death in a motor vehicle collision is to prevent maternal injury and death, and the seat belt is recognized as a major positive factor in reducing maternal injury and fatality (Attico et al., 1986; Bowdler et al., 1987; Crosby, 1974; Crosby and Costiloe, 1971; Crosby et al., 1968; Drost et al., 1990; Herbert and Henderson, 1977). Crosby et al. (1972) concluded that lap-shoulder belt restraint offers better protection than a lap-belt alone, but that both forms of restraint are better than no restraint at all for the pregnant occupant. This conclusion is well supported by the literature (Esposito et al., 1991; King et al., 1971; Lane, 1977; Matthews, 1975; Stafford et al., 1988; van Kirk and King, 1969; Wiechel et al., 1989).

Of paramount importance is that whatever restraint system is used, it be used correctly. This means keeping the belt taut, and wearing the lap belt beneath the anterior-superior iliac spines of the pelvis ("low as possible, below the bulge") (Matthews, 1975).

Major Vessels

Blunt trauma causing injury to major abdominal vessels is extremely rare (Clyne and Ashbrooke, 1985), probably because of their relatively protected location adjacent to the vertebral column in the retroperitoneum. The results of trauma to these vessels can be contusion, laceration, transection, or avulsion, which can lead to hemorrhage, thrombosis, false aneurysm, or arteriovenous fistula.

Trauma to the abdominal aorta is potentially fatal, with a reported mortality of 28% (Holcroft, 1982; Reisman and Morgan, 1990). The mechanisms of injury to the aorta and other major vessels include direct impact and indirect effects of impact. In particular, direct application of force, for example, by the lower rim of the steering wheel can cause rupture or laceration by either shearing of the vessel against the spine, or by laceration from a vertebral fracture.

Indirect mechanisms may be associated with increased intraluminal pressure beyond the ability of the vessel to resist (1,000 to 2,500 mm Hg), or deceleration injury where an organ such as the kidney moves relative to its arterial attachment point, causing avulsion of the renal artery. This mechanism plays more of a role in the branch vessels than in the abdominal aorta itself.

Blunt traumatic injury to the abdominal veins is even more rare than that to the arteries. However, the mortality in one study was 38% (Robbs and Costa, 1984). The mechanisms of blunt traumatic injury to the abdominal veins parallel those of the arteries, but the outcome may be significantly different. This difference comes about because of difficulty controlling hemorrhage due to the rich collateral network of veins, and difficulty in repair due to the thin-walled, fragile nature of veins (Campbell et al., 1981; Conti, 1982; Van De Wal et al., 1990).

Safety Belt – Associated Injury

No discussion of abdominal injury would be complete without a discussion of injury associated with safety belts. Ever since the "seat belt syndrome" was first published, a well-established clinical literature has developed describing blunt abdominal injuries associated with the interaction of the safety belt and abdomen (Anderson et al., 1991; Appleby and Nagy, 1989; Asbun et al., 1990; Clyne and Ashbrooke, 1985; Garrett and Braunstein, 1962; Harms et al., 1987; Huelke and Lawson, 1976; Huelke and Sherman, 1987; Legay et al., 1990; King, 1985; Langwieder et al., 1990; Leung et al., 1982; Marsh et al., 1975; McElhaney et al., 1972; Newman et al., 1990; Reid et al., 1990; Rutledge et al., 1991; Sivit et al., 1991; Stylianos and Harris, 1990; Williams, 1970; Williams et al., 1966; Woelfel et al., 1984). This could easily be the subject of a chapter by itself, and so only a few important points will be addressed here.

Two of the phenomena proposed to explain belt-associated injury are misplacement of the belt and submarining. Wells et al. (1986) examined the placement of lap belts in 198 adult passengers in a normal, seated posture. They found that 42% had placed the center lines of the belt above the anterior-superior iliac spine (ASIS) of the pelvis and 89% had part of the belt above the ASIS. They also found that slouching significantly increased the proportion of occupants with malpositioned belts. Other researchers have also identified belt misplacement as a major factor in injury to belted occupants in motor vehicle collisions (Cocke and Meyer, 1963; States et al., 1987; Agran et al., 1987).

Lap belt submarining occurs when the occupant's pelvis uncouples from the lap belt causing the occupant's abdomen, not the pelvis, to load the lap belt (Leung et al., 1982; Rouhana et al., 1989, 1991).

The evidence supporting the overall effectiveness of safety belts is overwhelming, typically showing that unbelted occupants have twice the risk of fatal injury when compared to their belted counterparts (Anderson et al., 1991; Asbun et al., 1990; Garrett and Braunstein, 1962; Harms et al., 1987; Huelke and Lawson, 1976; Huelke and Sherman, 1987; King, 1985; Langwieder et al., 1990; Leung et al., 1982; Marsh et al., 1975; McElhaney et al., 1972; Rutledge et al., 1991; Williams, 1970; Williams et al., 1966). However, the pattern of injuries to vehicle occupants may also change with the use of seat belts such that the more severe head, neck, or chest injuries of the unbelted occupant are traded off for more frequent but less serious abdominal injuries (Arajarvi et al., 1987; Harms et al., 1987). Studies have shown that up to 90% of the restraint-associated injuries are minor (AIS = 1) in nature (Marsh et al., 1975; Langwieder et al., 1990).

Bohlin (1967, cited in Asbun et al., 1990) reported on a series of 37,500 passengers in more than 28,500 collisions with no mortality for a restrained occupant at any collision speed under 60 mph. The same study showed fatal injuries to unrestrained occupants at speeds as low as 12 mph. Leung et al. (1982) showed that most submarining occurs at high Δv (≥ 30 mph), and that 60% of all AIS ≥ 3 abdominal injuries to restrained occupants were at Δv greater than 30 mph.

Huelke and Lawson (1976) studied 6,154 occupants in frontal collisions, of whom 202 were belted occupants who sustained lower torso injuries. Most of the lower torso injuries were minor (72% were AIS = 1). While restrained occupants had greater risk of abdominal injury of *any* severity (10% risk for restrained, 6% for unrestrained), restrained occupants had half the risk of *serious* abdominal injury (13% risk for restrained, 27% for unrestrained).

In a study of 3,901 patients in the North Carolina Trauma Registry by Rutledge et al. (1991) the risk of sustaining any abdominal injury, or hepatic or splenic injury was the same for belted versus unbelted occupants. However, the risk of gastrointestinal injury doubled, and the risk of "other" abdominal injury decreased by a factor of two for belted occupants. At the same time, the risk of head injury for belted occupants decreased by 40%.

The main types and mechanisms of injuries that have been associated with abdominal interaction with the lap belt were described by Williams et al. (1966) and Williams (1970). Injuries to the abdominal wall include hematoma, transection of the rectus abdominis muscle, full-thickness skin necrosis (seen in obese individuals only), and delayed hernia. The mechanisms proposed were direct force of impact and shear by the belt.

Intestinal injuries were discussed earlier, but one postulated belt-associated mechanism not mentioned is the pinching of the walls of the bowel, trapping gas within a small segment. Then, as the loading of the occupant continues, the pressure built up in the segment may cause bursting of the wall.

The most appropriate end to this discussion of belt-associated injury comes from the original authors who brought these injuries to light. "It is concluded from the data examined in this report that under conditions of low severity, where the vast majority of all accidents occur, the seat belt presents no hazard to occupants. . . . Only in the most severe crash conditions are serious injuries likely to be associated with seat belt application . . . [and] even under these conditions . . . [the] automobile occupants are better off *with* a seat belt than without one" (Garrett and Braunstein, 1962).

Proposed Human Tolerance Values

One of the most important results of the experimental studies on the mechanisms of injury and injury criteria are values for human tolerance to the physical parameters shown to correlate with injury. The studies presented above are replete with such values, which are presented in Tables 16.2 to 16.9. Most of these values need to be qualified, because none of them are the results of experiments on living human beings. They represent data from anesthetized animal studies or human cadaver studies. In addition, human tolerance is known to vary because of differences in size, strength, physical conditioning, etc. Therefore, the values given must be interpreted carefully in light of these qualifiers.

Suggested Future Research

The coverage by the published reports that detail the response of the abdomen is coarse at best when compared to the classical division of the abdomen. Of course, there may be no reason that abdominal trauma studies need follow the classical separation of the abdomen, but even by making assumptions about the relative similarity of the various divisions, the known response of the abdomen is incomplete.

In addition, the effects of muscle tension have not been included in any of the abdominal response corridors proposed, but have been included in previously proposed thoracic response curves. In thoracic impact with the muscles relaxed, the rib cage response will undoubtedly govern the response of the region. In abdominal impact, there is no overlaying shell structure like the rib cage. Therefore, one might expect consideration of

TABLE 16.2. Correlations of peak force with injury.

Author	(Year)	Peak force	Injury severity	Organ injured	Comments
Trollope et al.	(1973)	1.56 kN	ESI >2	Liver	Intact animal
		0.67 kN	ESI >2	Liver	Exposed liver
					$N = 85$ primates; $N = 15$ *Sus scrofa*
Stalnaker et al.	(1973a)	3.11 kN (R & L)	ESI >3	Upper abdomen	
					$N = 96$ primates & human cadavers; free side; scaled armrest; belt
Gogler et al.	(1977)	0.59–0.98 kN	N/A	Abdomen	Subacute shock—acute shock
		1.47 kN	AIS 3–4	Abdomen	AIS 3–4 transition
					$N = 12$; *Sus scrofa*; projectile tests; frontal abdominal impacts; free back; 11.4–15.5 kg
Lau and Viano	(1981)	0.24 kN	AIS >3	Liver	Contusion
					$N = 26$; oryctolagus cuniculus; fixed back; compression = 16% for all experiments
Rouhana et al.	(1986)	0.82 kN	AIS >3	Liver	ED_{50}
		1.14 kN	AIS >3	Kidney	ED_{50}
					$N = 214$; oryctolagus cuniculus; side impacts; 107 with force-limiting Hexcel; free side; area = 7.0 in. sq.
Miller	(1989)	2.93 kN	AIS >3	Lower abdomen	ED_{25}
		3.96 kN	AIS >3	Lower abdomen	ED_{50}
		3.76 kN	AIS >4	Lower abdomen	ED_{25}
		4.72 kN	AIS >4	Lower abdomen	ED_{50}
					$N = 25$; *Sus scrofa*; lap belt impacts; fixed back; all energy into subject
Viano et al.	(1989)	6.73 kN	AIS >4	Upper/ midabdomen	ED_{25}
					$N = 14$; unembalmed cadavers; rigid pendulum; side impact; free back; some energy into whole body motion

TABLE 16.3. Correlations of maximum compression with injury.

Author	(Year)	C_{max}*	Injury severity	Organ injured	Comments
Stalnaker et al.	(1973a)	60% (L)	ESI >3	Upper abdomen	
		54% (R)	ESI >3	Upper abdomen	
					$N = 96$ primates & human cadavers; free side; scaled armrest; belt
Lau and Viano	(1981)	16% at 12 m/sec	AIS >3	Liver	Contusion
					$N = 26$; oryctolagus cuniculus; fixed back; compression = 16% for all experiments
Rouhana et al.	(1986)	29%	AIS >3	Liver	ED_{50}
					$N = 214$; oryctolagus cuniculus; side impacts; 107 with force-limiting Hexcel; free side; area = 7.0 in. sq.
Miller	(1989)	37.8%	AIS >3	Lower abdomen	ED_{25}
		48.4%	AIS >3	Lower abdomen	ED_{50}
		48.3%	AIS >4	Lower abdomen	ED_{25}
		54.2%	AIS >4	Lower abdomen	ED_{50}
					$N = 25$; *Sus scrofa*; lap belt impacts; fixed back; all energy into subject
Viano et al.	(1989)	43.7%	AIS >4	Upper/midabdomen	ED_{25}
					$N = 14$; unembalmed cadavers; rigid pendulum; side impact; free back; some energy into whole body motion

* % of entire A-P or lateral dimension of subject.

TABLE 16.4. Correlations of $V_{max} * C_{max}$ with injury.

Author	(Year)	$V_{max}C_{max}$	Injury severity	Organ injured	Comments
Rouhana et al.	(1984, 1985)	1.75 m/sec (R)	AIS >3	Upper/midabdomen	ED_{25}
		2.71 m/sec (R)	AIS >3	Upper/midabdomen	ED_{50}
		2.10 m/sec (L)	AIS >3	Upper/midabdomen	ED_{25}
		3.31 m/sec (L)	AIS >3	Upper/midabdomen	ED_{50}
					$N = 117$; oryctolagus cuniculus; free side; lateral abdominal impacts
Stalnaker et al.	(1985)	Frontal 3.0 m/sec	AIS = 3	Upper abdomen	
		Frontal 3.8 m/sec	AIS = 3	Midabdomen	
		Frontal 3.0 m/sec	AIS = 3	Lower abdomen	
		Right side 3.5 m/sec	AIS = 3	Abdomen	
		Left side 4.7 m/sec	AIS = 3	Abdomen	
					$N = 42$; primates from previous studies; 6 diff. impactors; 4 diff. locations; from linear regression of VC with AIS
Rouhana et al.	(1986)	3.15 m/sec (R & L)	AIS >3	Liver	ED_{50}
		5.5 m/sec (R & L)	AIS >3	Kidney	ED_{50}
					$N = 214$; oryctolagus cuniculus; side impacts; 107 with force-limiting Hexcel; free side; area = 7.0 in. sq.
Rouhana et al.	(1987)	0.75 m/sec	AIS >3	Liver	
					$N = 8$; human cadavers; right-side impacts; analysis of Walfisch data; probability of injury not stated

TABLE 16.5. Correlations of $[V*C]_{max}$ with injury.

Author	(Year)	$[VC]_{max}$	Injury severity	Organ injured	Comments
Lau and Viano	(1986)	1.2 m/sec	AIS >5	Liver	ED_{25}
		1.4 m/sec	AIS >5	Liver	ED_{50}
					$N = 20$; *Sus scrofa*; chest/abdomen contact; steering wheel
Lau and Viano	(1988)	1.20 m/sec	AIS >4	Liver	Laceration ED_{25}
		1.24 m/sec	AIS >4	Liver	Laceration ED_{50}
					Same as Lau (1986) + 9 more subjects with "punch pulled"
Miller	(1989)	1.40 m/sec	AIS >4	Lower abdomen	ED_{25}
					$N = 25$; *Sus scrofa*; lap belt impacts; fixed back; all energy into subject
Viano et al.	(1989)	1.98 m/sec	AIS >4	Upper/midabdomen	ED_{25}
					$N = 14$; unembalmed cadavers; rigid pendulum; side impact; free back; some energy into whole body motion

TABLE 16.6. Correlations of pressure with injury.

Author	(Year)	Pressure	Injury severity	Organ injured	Comments
Williams	(1963)	50 kPa	AIS >3	Lower abdomen	$N = 45$; canidae; 50 lb wt. dropped 8 ft onto a board over lower abdomen; 28 of 49 subjects had intestinal injury
McElhaney et al.	(1971)	131 kPa (WS)	ESI >3	Midabdomen	
		386 kPa (LF)	ESI >3	Midabdomen	$N = 13$; primates; pneumatic impactor; free back/side; bar, belt, large flat block (LF), wedge shape (WS)
Fazekas et al.	(1971, 1972)	44 kPa	AIS = 4	Spleen	Rupture
		169 kPa	AIS = 4	Liver	Superficial lacerations
		320 kPa	AIS = 5	Liver	Multiple ruptures $N = $ unknown; human cadaver; isolated livers
Melvin et al.	(1973)	310 kPa	ESI >3	Liver	Exposed, perfused liver $N = 17$ liver; $N = 6$ kidney; *Macaca mulatta*; MTS type; fixed back; V = 2.5 m/sec
Trollope et al.	(1973)	600 kPa (CB)	ESI >3	Upper abdomen	
		152 kPa (LF)	ESI >3	Upper abdomen	$N = 85$ primates; $N = 15$ *Sus scrofa*; cylindrical bar (CB); large flat block (LF)
Stalnaker et al.	(1973a)	214 kPa	ESI >3	Upper abdomen	$N = 96$; primates & human cadavers; free side; scaled armrest; belt
Stalnaker et al.	(1973b)	669 kPa (CB)	ESI >3	Upper abdomen	
		193 kPa (LF)	ESI >3	Upper abdomen	$N = 96$; primates & *Sus scrofa*; cylindrical bar (CB); large flat block (LF); free side; scaled armrest
Walfisch et al.	(1980)	260 kPa	AIS >3	Liver	$N = 8$; human cadavers; drop tests; right side impacts only
Lau and Viano	(1981)	67 kPa	AIS >3	Liver	Contusion $N = 26$; oryctolagus cuniculus; fixed back; compression = 16% for all experiments
Rouhana et al.	(1984, 1985)	276 kPa	AIS >4	Kidney	Laceration ED_{50} $N = 117$; oryctolagus cuniculus; free side; lateral abdominal impacts
Rouhana et al.	(1986)	180 kPa	AIS >3	Liver	ED_{50}
		251 kPa	AIS >3	Kidney	ED_{50} $N = 214$; oryctolagus cuniculus; side impacts; 107 with force-limiting Hexcel; free side; area = 7.0 in. sq.
Miller	(1989)	166 kPa	AIS >3	Lower abdomen	ED_{25}
		226 kPa	AIS >3	Lower abdomen	ED_{50}
		216 kPa	AIS >4	Lower abdomen	ED_{25}
		270 kPa	AIS >4	Lower abdomen	ED_{50} $N = 25$; *Sus scrofa*; lap belt impacts; fixed back; all energy into subject

TABLE 16.7. Correlations of $F_{max} * C_{max}$ with injury.

Author	(Year)	$F_{max}C_{max}$	Injury severity	Organ injured	Comments
Walfisch et al.	(1980)	4.5 kN 14% deflection (See Rouhana, 1987)	AIS = 3	Liver	$N = 8$; human cadavers; drop tests; right side impacts only
Rouhana et al.	(1987)	0.63 kN	AIS >3	Liver	4.5 kN; 14% deflection whole abdomen
		0.88 kN	AIS >3	Liver	4.5 kN; 19.5% deflection whole abdomen
					$N = 8$; human cadavers; right-side impacts; analysis of Walfisch data; probability of injury not stated
Miller	(1989)	1.33 kN	AIS >3	Lower abdomen	ED_{25}
		1.96 kN	AIS >3	Lower abdomen	ED_{50}
		2.00 kN	AIS >4	Lower abdomen	ED_{25}
		2.67 kN	AIS >4	Lower abdomen	ED_{50}
					$N = 25$; *Sus scrofa*; lap belt impacts; fixed back; all energy into subject

TABLE 16.8. Correlations of velocity with injury.

Author	(Year)	Velocity	Injury severity	Organ injured	Comments
McElhaney et al.	(1971)	(MM) 11.3 m/sec (L)	ESI >3	Midabdomen	
		(PC) 14.5 m/sec (L)	ESI >3	Midabdomen	
		(MM) 9.8 m/sec (R)	ESI >3	Midabdomen	
		(PC) 12.5 m/sec (R)	ESI >3	Midabdomen	
					$N = 13$; primates [Papio cynocephalus (PC), *Macaca mulatta* (MM)]; pneumatic impactor; free back/side; bar, belt; large flat block, wedge shape
Stalnaker et al.	(1973a)	(Pr) 7.3 m/sec (L)	ESI >3	Upper abdomen	
		(Pr) 6.1 m/sec (R)	ESI >3	Upper abdomen	
					$N = 96$ primates (Pr) & human cadavers; free side; scaled armrest; belt
Lau and Viano	(1981)	8–10 m/sec	AIS >3	Liver	Contusion
		12–14 m/sec	AIS >4	Liver	Bursting injury
					$N = 26$; oryctolagus cuniculus; fixed back; compression = 16% for all experiments

TABLE 16.9. Correlations of energy with injury.

Author	(Year)	Energy	Injury severity	Organ injured	Comments
Williams	(1963)	542 J	AIS >3	Lower abdomen	
					$N = 45$; canidae; 50 lb wt dropped 8 ft onto a board over lower abdomen; 28 of 49 subjects had intestinal injury
Mays	(1966)	37–46 J	AIS = 4	Liver	Superficial lacerations
		144–182 J	AIS = 5	Liver	Deep lacerations, no vascular injury
		386–488 J	AIS >5	Liver	Macerated
					$N = 15$; human cadaver livers; drop tests; livers injected with saline & barium; h = 2.1 m to 35.7 m; M = 1.4 kg to 1.8 kg

muscle tension to be even more important for abdominal response than for thoracic response.

Similarly, the correlations of the injury mechanisms proposed, to date, with probability of injury from blunt impact are not perfect. Many of the proposed mechanisms have no empirical evidence of being correct. A multivariate analysis similar to Stalnaker's (1973a,b) may be required to be able to equate cause and effect or dose and response in the complex interactions that occur in blunt loading. Statistical techniques have improved in the years since the first automotive-related research took place, thanks in large part to the improvement and proliferation of computers. Whatever research is done in the future, more rigorous analyses would improve the state of knowledge.

Knowledge of the biomechanics of the injury process is also not comprehensive. There is a mixture of data including some from human cadavers for rigid loading surfaces, and some from belt loading to living anesthetized animal subjects. Impactor shapes, sizes, and methods of impact have varied, leaving many gaps in basic knowledge.

While there have been advances in the development of surrogates to measure abdominal loading which occurs during submarining (Beebe, 1990; Czernakowski and Klanner, 1987; Daniel, 1974; Daniel et al., 1982; Janssen and Vermissen, 1988; Leung et al., 1979; Maltha and Stalnaker, 1981; Melvin and Weber, 1986; Mooney and Collins, 1986; Rouhana et al., 1989, 1990), a surrogate abdomen that provides biofidelity and risk of occupant injury for any degree of loading, impact direction, speed, and type of loading surface does not exist (Rouhana et al., 1989, 1990; Schneider et al., 1989). The development of such a device would greatly enhance the design of automobiles in regard to abdominal injury protection.

Finally, a broad research program with basic biomechanical studies addressing the missing or vague areas mentioned above, coupled with a laboratory recreation of accidents from the field, may help to fill in the gaps in our knowledge. This could lead to a better understanding of the biomechanics of blunt traumatic injury to the abdomen, enhance the ability to determine when abdominal injury would occur in vehicle testing by allowing development of improved test devices, and ultimately lead to safer automobiles for those who will inevitably be involved in collisions.

References

Agran PF, Dunkle DE, Winn DG (1987) Injuries to a sample of seatbelted children evaluated and treated in a hospital emergency room. J Trauma 27(1):58–63.

American Association for Automotive Medicine. *The Abbreviated Injury Scale—1980 Revision.* Morton Grove, Illinois, AAAM:1980.

Anderson PA, Rivara FP, Maier RV, Drake C (1991) The epidemiology of seatbelt-associated injuries. J Trauma 31(1):60–67.

Appleby JP, Nagy AG (1989) Abdominal injuries associated with the use of seatbelts. Am J Surg 157:457–458.

Arajarvi E, Santavirta S, Tolonen J (1987) Abdominal injuries sustained in severe traffic accidents by seatbelt wearers. J Trauma 27(4): 393–397.

Arnold G, Gressner AM, Clahsen H, Kronchen A (1977) On the biomechanical function of the liver capsule. Experientia—Specialia 33:1089–1091.

Asbun HJ, Irani H, Roe EJ, Bloch JH (1990) Intra-abdominal seatbelt injury. J Trauma 30(2): 189–193.

Attico NB, Smith III RJ, FitzPatrick MB, Keneally M (1986) Automobile safety restraints for pregnant women and children. J Reprod Med 31(3): 187–192.

Barancik JI, Chatterjee BF, Greene-Cradden YC, Michenzi EM, Kramer CF, Thode HC, Fife D (1986) Motor vehicle trauma in northeastern Ohio. I: incidence and outcome by age, sex, and road-use category. Am J Epidemiol 123(5): 846–861.

Baxter CF, Williams RD (1961) Blunt abdominal trauma. J Trauma 1:241–247.

Beebe MS. What is BioSID? SAE 900377, 1990.

Bergqvist D, Hedelin H, Lindblad B, Matzsch T (1985) Abdominal injuries in children: an analysis of 348 cases. Br J Accident Surg 16(4):217–220.

Blaisdell FW, Trunkey DD (eds). *Trauma Management: volume I—abdominal trauma.* Thieme-Stratton, New York, 1982.

Bohlin NI. A statistical analysis of 28,000 accident cases with emphasis on occupant restraint value. 11th Stapp Car Crash Conference Proceedings, SAE 670925, pp 455–478, 1967.

Bondy N. Abdominal injuries in the National Crash Severity Study. *National Center for Statistics and Analysis Collected Technical Studies, Vol. II: Accident data analysis of occupant injuries and crash characteristics*, National Highway Traffic Safety Administration, Washington DC, pp 59–80, 1980.

Booth, FV, Flint LM. Pancreatico-duodenal trauma. In Border JR, Allgower M, Hansen ST, Ruedi TP (eds) *Blunt multiple trauma—comprehensive pathophysiology and care*. Marcell Dekker, New York, pp 497–509, 1990.

Border JR, Allgower M, Hansen Jr ST, Ruedi TP (eds) *Blunt multiple trauma: comprehensive pathophysiology and care*. Marcel Dekker, New York, 1990.

Borlase BC, Moore EE, Moore FA (1990) The abdominal trauma index—a critical reassessment and validation. J Trauma 30(11):1340–1344.

Bowdler N, Faix RG, Elkins T (1987) Fetal skull fracture and brain injury after a maternal automobile accident. J Reprod Med 32(5):375–378.

Braun BH, Breen PC, Brotman SR (1985, March) Small bowel injury following blunt trauma. Pennsylvania Med.

Brun-Cassan F, Pincemaille Y, Mack P, Tarriere C. Contribution and evaluation of criteria proposed for thorax-abdomen protection in lateral impact. Eleventh International ESV Conference Proceedings. SAE 876040, pp 289–301, 1987.

Campbell DN, Liechty RD, Rutherford RB (1981) Traumatic thrombosis of the inferior vena cava. J Trauma 21(5):413–415.

Carroll PR, McAninch JW (1984) Major bladder trauma: mechanisms of injury and a unified method of diagnosis and repair. J Urol 132:254–257.

Cass AS (1984) The multiple injured patient with bladder trauma. J Trauma 24(8):731–734.

Cavanaugh JM, Nyquist GW, Goldberg SJ, King AI. Lower abdominal tolerance and response. 30th Stapp Car Crash Conference Proceedings. SAE 861878, pp 41–63, 1986.

Chetcuti P, Levene MI (1987) Seat belts: a potential hazard to the fetus. J Perinat Med 15:207–209.

Christensen N. Small bowel and mesentery. In Blaisdell FW, Trunkey DD (eds) *Trauma management: volume I—abdominal trauma*. Thieme-Stratton, New York, pp 149–163, 1982.

Civil ID, Talucci RC, Schwab CW (1988) Placental laceration and fetal death as a result of blunt abdominal trauma. J Trauma 28(5):708–710.

Clemedson C-J, Frankenberg L, Jonsson A, Pettersson H, Sundqvist A-B (1969) Dynamic response of thorax and abdomen of rabbits in partial and whole-body blast exposure. Am J Physiol 216(3):615–620.

Clyne CAC, Ashbrooke EA (1985) Seat-belt aorta: isolated abdominal aortic injury following blunt trauma. Br J Surg 72:239.

Cocke WM, Meyer KK (1963) Splenic rupture due to improper placement of automotive safety belt. JAMA 183(8):693.

Conti S. Abdominal venous trauma. In Blaisdell FW, Trunkey DD (eds) *Trauma management: volume I—abdominal trauma*. Thieme-Stratton, New York, pp 253–278, 1982.

Cooper GJ, Taylor DEM (1989) Biophysics of impact injury to the chest and abdomen. J R Army Med Corps 135:58–67.

Cooper GJ, Townend DJ, Cater SR, Pearce BP (1991) The role of stress waves in thoracic visceral injury from blast loading: modifications of stress transmission by foams and high-density materials. J Biomech 24(5):273–285.

Cox E (1984) Blunt abdominal trauma—a 5-year analysis of 870 patients requiring celiotomy. Ann Surg 199(4):467–474.

Croce MA, Fabian TC, Kudsk KA, Baum SL, Payne LW, Mangiante EC, Britt LG (1991) AAST Organ Injury Scale: correlation of CT-graded liver injuries and operative findings. J Trauma 31(6):806–812.

Crohn BB (1964) Trauma and the lower gastrointestinal tract. Trauma 5(5):63–125.

Crosby WM (1974) Trauma during pregnancy: maternal and fetal injury. Obstet Gynecol Surv 29(10):683–699.

Crosby WM, Costiloe JP (1971) Safety of lap-belt restraint for pregnant victims of automobile collisions. N Engl J Med 284(12):632–636.

Crosby WM, King AI, Stout LC (1972) Fetal survival following impact: improvement with shoulder harness restraint. Am J Obstet Gynecol 112(8):1101–1106.

Crosby WM, Snyder RG, Snow CC, Hanson PG (1968) Impact injuries in pregnancy. Am J Obstet Gynecol 101(1):100–110.

Czernakowski W, Klanner W. Development of a two-dimensional sensor determining abdominal loading on TNO-dummies. Eleventh International ESV Conference Proceedings. SAE 876044, pp 323–332, 1987.

Daniel RP. Test dummy submarining indicator system. United States Patent 3,841,163, October 15, 1974.

Daniel RP, Koga MS, Prasad P, Yost CD. A force measuring mechanical test device for estimating and comparing the energy absorbing characteristics of vehicle interior side panels. Ninth International ESV Conference Proceedings. SAE 826058, pp 465–469, 1982.

Danner M, Langwieder K. Collision characteristics and injuries to pedestrians in real accidents. Seventh International ESV Conference Proceedings. pp 587–610, 1979.

Danner M, Langwieder K, Wachter W. Injuries to pedestrians in real accidents and their relation to collision and car characteristics. 23rd Stapp Car Crash Conference Proceedings. pp 161–198, 1979.

Dauterive AH, Flancbaum L, Cox EF (1985) Blunt intestinal trauma—a modern-day review. Ann Surg 201(2):198–203.

Desiderio MA (1987) The effects of acute, oral ethanol on cardiovascular performance before and after blunt cardiac trauma. J Trauma 27(3): 267–277.

Desiderio MA (1988) The effect of the rate of rise of blood alcohol on the outcome of cardiac injury. J Trauma 28(6):765–771.

Drost TF, Rosemurgy AS, Sherman HF, Scott LM, Williams JK (1990) Major trauma in pregnant women: maternal/fetal outcome. J Trauma 30(5): 574–578.

Eppinger RH, Morgan RM, Marcus JH. Side impact data analysis. Ninth International ESV Conference Proceedings. pp 244–250, 1982.

Eppinger RH, Marcus JH, Morgan RM. Development of dummy and injury index for NHTSA's thoracic side impact protection research program. SAE 840885, 1984.

Esposito TJ, Gens DR, Smith LG, Scorpio R, Buchman T (1991) Trauma during pregnancy—a review of 79 cases. Arch Surg 126:1073–1078.

Farthmann EH, Kirchner RJ. Small and large bowel injuries. In Border JR, Allgower M, Hansen ST, Ruedi TP (eds) Blunt multiple trauma—comprehensive pathophysiology and care. Marcel Dekker, New York, pp 511–526, 1990.

Fazekas IG, Kosa F, Jobba G, Meszaros E (1971a) Die Druckfestigkeit der menschlichen Leber mit besonderer Hinsicht auf die Verkehrsunfalle. Z Rechtsmed 68:207.

Fazekas IG, Kosa F, Jobba G, Meszaros E (1971b) Experimentelle Untersuchungen uber die Druckfestigkeit der menschlichen Niere. Zacchia 46:294.

Fazekas IG, Kosa F, Jobba G, Meszaros E (1972) Beitrage zur Druckfestigkeit der menschlichen Milz bei stumpfen Krafteinwirkungen. Arch Kriminol 149:158.

Freeman CP (1985) Isolated pancreatic damage following seat belt injury. Br J Accident Surg 16(7):478–480.

Frey CF. Injuries to the thorax and abdomen. In Huelke DF (ed) Human anatomy, impact injuries, and human tolerances, P-29, Society of Automotive Engineers, New York, pp 69–76, 1970.

Frey CF, Trollope M, Harpster W, Synder R (1973) A fifteen-year experience with automotive hepatic trauma. J Trauma 13:1039–1049.

Galer M, Clark S, Mackay GM, Ashton SJ. The causes of injury in car accidents—an overview of a major study currently underway in britain. Tenth International ESV Conference Proceedings. pp 513–525, 1985.

Garrett JW, Braunstein PW (1962) The seat belt syndrome. J Trauma 2:220–238.

Gogler E, Best A, Braess HH, Burst HE, Laschet G. Biomechanical experiments with animals on abdominal tolerance levels. 21st Stapp Car Crash Conference Proceedings. SAE 770931, pp 712–751, 1977.

Gray H. Anatomy, descriptive and surgical. Bounty Books, New York, 1977.

Griswold RA, Collier HS (1961) Blunt abdominal trauma: collective review. Surg Gynecol Obstet 112:309.

Hardy KJ (1972) Patterns of liver injury after fatal blunt trauma. Surg Gynecol Obstet 134: 39–43.

Harms PL, Renouf M, Thomas PD, Bradford M. Injuries to restrained car occupants; what are the outstanding problems? Eleventh International ESV Conference Proceedings. SAE 876029, pp 183–201, 1987.

Harris LM, Booth FV, Hassett JM (1991) Liver lacerations—a marker of severe but sometimes subtle intra-abdominal injuries in adults. J Trauma 31(7):894–901.

Herbert DC, Henderson JM (1977) Motor-car accidents during pregnancy: 2. Med J Aust 1: 670–671.

Hobbs CA. Car occupant injury patterns and mechanisms. Eighth International ESV Conference Proceedings. pp 755–768, 1980.

Holcroft JW. Abdominal arterial trauma. In Blaisdell FW, Trunkey DD (eds) Trauma management: volume I—abdominal trauma. Thieme-Stratton, New York, pp 229–251, 1982.

Hollinshead, WH. *Anatomy for surgeons: volume 2—the thorax, abdomen, and pelvis.* 2nd ed. Harper and Row, New York, 1971.

Horsch JD, Lau IV, Viano DC, Andrzejak DV. Mechanism of abdominal injury by steering wheel loading. 29th Stapp Car Crash Conference Proceedings. SAE 851724, pp 69–78, 1985.

Huelke DF, Lawson TE. Lower torso injuries and automobile seat belts. SAE 760370, 1976.

Huelke DF, Nusholtz GS, Kaiker PS (1986) Use of quadruped models in thoraco-abdominal biomechanics research. J Biomech 19(12):969–977.

Huelke DF, Sherman HW (1987) Seat belt effectiveness: case examples from real-world crash investigations. J Trauma 27(7):750–753.

International Standards Organization. Road vehicles—anthropomorphic side impact dummy—part 5: Lateral abdominal impact response requirements to assess biofidelity of dummy. Technical Report, ISO TR 9790-5, 1989.

Janssen EG, Vermissen ACM. Biofidelity of the European side impact dummy—EUROSID. 32nd Stapp Car Crash Conference Proceedings. SAE 881716, pp 101–124, 1988.

Kearney PA, Rouhana SW, Burney RE (1989) Blunt rupture of the diaphragm: mechanism, diagnosis, and treatment. Ann Emerg Med 18(12):1326–1330.

King AI. Abdomen. In Melvin JW, Weber K (eds) Review of biomechanical impact response and injury in the automotive environment. UMTRI Report 85–3: Task B Final Report. National Highway Traffic Safety Administration, Washington, DC, 1985.

King AI, Crosby WM, Stout LC, Eppinger RH. Effects of lap belt and three-point restraints on pregnant baboons subjected to deceleration. 15th Stapp Car Crash Conference Proceedings. SAE 710850, pp 68–83, 1971.

Kroell CK, Allen SD, Warner CY, Perl TR. Inter-relationship of velocity and chest compression in blunt thoracic impact to swine II. 30th Stapp Car Crash Conference Proceedings. SAE 861881, pp 99–121, 1986.

Kroell CK, Pope ME, Viano DC, Warner CY, Allen SD. Interrelationship of velocity and chest compression in blunt thoracic impact. 25th Stapp Car Crash Conference Proceedings. SAE 811016, pp 547–580, 1981.

Kumar B, Paul G, Kumar Sharma A (1989) Injury Severity Score (ISS) as a yardstick in assessing the severity and mortality of various abdomino-pelvic trauma hospitalized victims—a clinical vis-a-vis autopsy study. Med Sci Law 29(4):333–336.

Lane JC (1977, April) Motor-car accidents during pregnancy: 1. Med J Aust (1):669–670.

Langwieder K, Hummel T, Felsch B, Klanner W. Injury Risks of children in cars—epidemiology and effect of child restraint systems. 23rd FISITA Conference Proceedings. SAE 905119, pp 905–919, 1990.

Lau IV, Horsch JD, Viano DC, Andrzejak DV (1987) Biomechanics of liver injury by steering wheel loading. J Trauma 27(3):225–235.

Lau VK, Viano DC (1981a) Influence of impact velocity on the severity of nonpenetrating hepatic injury. J Trauma 21(2):115–123.

Lau VK, Viano DC (1981b) An experimental study on hepatic injury from belt-restraint loading. Aviat Space Environ Med 52(10):611–617.

Lau IV, Viano DC. The viscous criterion—bases and applications of an injury severity index for soft tissues. 30th Stapp Car Crash Conference Proceedings. SAE 861882, pp 123–142, 1986.

Lau VK, Viano DC. How and when blunt injury occurs—implications to frontal and side impact protection. 32nd Stapp Car Crash Conference Proceedings. SAE 881714, pp 81–100, 1988.

LeGay DA, Petrie DP, Alexander DI (1990) Flexion-distraction injuries of the lumbar spine and associated abdominal trauma. J Trauma 30(4):436–444.

Leung YC, Tarriere C, Fayon A, Mairesse P, Delmas A, Banzet P. A comparison between part 572 dummy and human subject in the problem of submarining. 23rd Stapp Car Crash Conference Proceedings. SAE 791026, pp 675–720, 1979.

Leung YC, Tarriere C, Lestrelin D. Submarining injuries of 3 pt. belted occupants in frontal collisions—description, mechanisms and protection. 26th Stapp Car Crash Conference Proceedings. SAE 821158, pp 173–205, 1982.

Lim Jr. RC. Injuries to the liver and extra hepatic ducts. In Blaisdell FW, Trunkey DD (eds) Trauma management: volume I—abdominal trauma. Thieme-Stratton, New York, pp 123–147, 1982.

Maltha J, Stalnaker RL. Development of a dummy abdomen capable of injury detection in side impacts. 25th Stapp Car Crash Conference Proceedings. SAE 811019, pp 651–682, 1981.

Marsh JC, Scott RE, Melvin JW. Injury patterns by restraint usage in 1973 and 1974 passenger cars. 19th Stapp Car Crash Conference Proceedings. pp 45–78, 1975.

Martin Jr JD, Haynes CD, Hatcher CR, Smith III RB, Stone HH (eds) Trauma to the thorax and abdomen. Charles C. Thomas, Springfield, IL, 1969.

Matthews CD (1975) Incorrectly used seat belt associated with uterine rupture following vehicular collision. Am J Obstet Gynecol 121:1115–1116.

Mays ET (1966) Bursting injuries of the liver. Arch Surg 93:92–106.

Mays ET, Noer RJ (1966) Colonic stenosis after trauma. J Trauma 6(3):316–331.

McAninch JW. Injuries to the urinary system. In Blaisdell FW, Trunkey DD (eds) Trauma management: volume I—abdominal trauma. Thieme-Stratton, New York, pp 199–227, 1982.

McElhaney JH, Roberts VL, Hilyard JF. Handbook of human tolerance. Japan Automobile Research Institute, Tokyo, 1976.

McElhaney JH, Roberts VL, Melvin, JW. Biomechanics of seat belt design. 16th Stapp Car Crash Conference Proceedings. SAE 720972, pp 321–344, 1972.

McElhaney JH, Stalnaker RL, Roberts VL, Snyder, RG. Door crashworthiness criteria. 15th Stapp Car Crash Conference Proceedings. SAE 710864, pp 489–517, 1971.

Melvin JW, Mohan D, Stalnaker RL. Occupant injury assessment criteria. 1975 SAE Transactions. SAE 750914, pp 2483–2494, 1975.

Melvin JW, Stalnaker RL, Roberts VL, Trollope ML. Impact injury mechanisms in abdominal organs. 17th Stapp Car Crash Conference Proceedings. SAE 730968, pp 115–126, 1973.

Melvin JW, Weber K. Review of biomechanical impact response and injury in the automotive environment. UMTRI Report 85–3: Task B Final Report. National Highway Traffic Safety Administration, Washington, DC, 1985.

Melvin JW, Weber K. Abdominal intrusion sensor for evaluating child restraint systems. Passenger comfort, convenience and safety: test tools and procedures. P-174. SAE 860370, pp 249–256, 1986.

Mertz HJ. A procedure for normalizing impact response data. SAE 840884, 1984.

Messinger A, Schreiber P (1985, July–August) Associated injuries and alternatives in management of splenic trauma. Curr Surg.

Miller MA (1989) The biomechanical response of the lower abdomen to belt restraint loading. J Trauma 29(11):1571–1584.

Moar JJ (1985) Autopsy assessment of liver lacerations. S Afr Med J 68:180–182.

Mooney MT, Collins JA. Abdominal penetration measurement insert for the hybrid III dummy. Passenger Comfort, Convenience and Safety: Test Tools and Procedures, P-174. SAE 860653, pp 285–289, 1986.

Moore EE, Shackford SR, Pachter HL, McAninch JW, Browner BD, Champion HR, Flint LM, Gennarelli TA, Malangoni MA, Ramenofsky ML, Trafton PG (1989) Organ injury scaling: spleen, liver, and kidney. J Trauma 29(12): 1664–1666.

Mucha Jr P (1986) Changing attitudes toward the management of blunt splenic trauma in adults. Mayo Clin Proc 61:472–477.

Mustard Jr RA, Hanna SS, Blair G, Harrison AW, Taylor GA, Miller HAB, Maggisano R (1984) Blunt splenic trauma: diagnosis and management. Can J Surg 27(4):330–333.

Nahum AM, Schneider DC. Soft tissue injuries and injury tolerance levels. First International IRCOBI Conference Proceedings. pp 411–422, 1973.

Nahum AM, Siegel AW, Brooks S. The reduction of collision injuries: past, present and future. 14th Stapp Car Crash Conference Proceedings. SAE 700895, 1970.

Newman KD, Bowman LM, Eichelberger MR, Gotschall CS, Taylor GA, Johnson DL, Thomas M (1990) The lap belt complex: intestinal and lumbar spine injury in children. J Trauma 30(9): 1133–1140.

Nusholtz GS, Kaiker PS, Huelke DF, Suggitt BR. Thoraco-abdominal response to steering wheel impacts. 29th Stapp Car Crash Conference Proceedings. SAE 851737, pp 221–245, 1985.

Nusholtz GS, Kaiker PS, Lehman RJ. Steering system abdominal impact trauma. UMTRI Report No. 88–19, MVMA, 1988.

Nusholtz GS, Melvin JW, Mueller G, MacKenzie JR, Burney R. Thoraco-abdominal response and injury. 24th Stapp Car Crash Conference Proceedings. SAE 801305, pp 187–228, 1980.

Oni OOA, Okpere EE, Tabowei O, Omu EA (1984) Severe road traffic injuries in the third trimester of pregnancy. Br J Accident Surg 15(6):376–378.

Perry JF (1965) A five-year survey of 152 acute abdominal injuries. J Trauma 5:53–61.

Pope ME, Kroell CK, Viano DC, Warner CY, Allen SD. Postural influences on thoracic impact. 23rd Stapp Car Crash Conference Proceedings. SAE 791028, pp 765–795, 1979.

Pranikoff K, Golio A, Sufrin G. The management of urologic trauma. In Border JR, Allgower M,

Hansen ST, Ruedi TP (eds) Blunt multiple trauma—comprehensive pathophysiology and care. Marcel Dekker, New York, pp 527–533, 1990.

Reid AB, Letts RM, Black GB (1990) Pediatric chance fractures: association with intra-abdominal injuries and seatbelt use. J Trauma 30(4):384–391.

Reisman JD, Morgan AS (1990) Analysis of 46 intra-abdominal aortic injuries from blunt trauma: case reports and literature review. J Trauma 30(10):1294–1297.

Ricci L. NCSS Statistics: Passenger Cars. UM-HSRI Report 80–36, 1980.

Ridella SA, Anderson TE (1986) Compression of rat spinal cord in vitro: effects of ethanol on recovery of axonal conduction. CNS Trauma 3(3):193–205.

Rivkind AI, Siegel JH, Dunham CM (1989) Patterns of organ injury in blunt hepatic trauma and their significance for management and outcome. J Trauma 29(10):1398–1415.

Robbs JV, Costa M (1984) Injuries to the great veins of the abdomen. S Afr J Surg 22(4):223–228.

Rouhana SW. Abdominal injury prediction in lateral impact—an analysis of the biofidelity of the Euro-SID abdomen. 31st Stapp Car Crash Conference Proceedings. SAE 872203, pp 95–104, 1987.

Rouhana SW, Foster ME. Lateral impact—an analysis of the statistics in the NCSS. 29th Stapp Car Crash Conference Proceedings. SAE 851727, pp 79–98, 1985.

Rouhana SW, Jedrzejczak EA, McCleary JD. Assessing submarining and abdominal injury risk in the Hybrid III family of dummies: part II—Development of the small female frangible abdomen. 34th Stapp Car Crash Conference Proceedings. SAE 902317, pp 145–173, 1990.

Rouhana SW, Kroell CK. The effect of door topography on abdominal injury in lateral impact. 33rd Stapp Car Crash Conference Proceedings. SAE 892433, pp 143–151, 1989.

Rouhana SW, Lau IV, Ridella SA. Influence of velocity and forced compression on the severity of abdominal injury in blunt, nonpenetrating lateral impact. GMR Research Publication No. 4763, 1984.

Rouhana SW, Lau IV, Ridella SA (1985) Influence of velocity and forced compression on the severity of abdominal injury in blunt, nonpenetrating lateral impact. J Trauma 25(6):490–500.

Rouhana SW, Ridella SA, Viano DC. The effect of limiting impact force on abdominal injury:

a preliminary study. 30th Stapp Car Crash Conference Proceedings. SAE 861879, pp 65–79, 1986.

Rouhana SW, Viano DC, Jedrzejczak EA, McCleary JD. Assessing submarining and abdominal injury risk in the Hybrid III family of dummies. 33rd Stapp Car Crash Conference Proceedings. SAE 892440, pp 257–279, 1989.

Rutledge R, Thomason M, Oller D, Meredith W, Moylan J, Clancy T, Cunningham P, Baker C (1991) The spectrum of abdominal injuries associated with the use of seat belts. J Trauma 31(6):820–826.

Schmidt G. The age as a factor influencing soft tissue injuries. Fourth International IRCOBI Conference Proceedings. pp 143–150, 1979.

Schneider LW, King AI, Beebe MS. Design requirements and specifications: thorax-abdomen development task. Interim report. Trauma Assessment Device Development Program. UMTRI Report 89–20, Washington, DC, National Highway Traffic Safety Administration, 1989.

Schrock TR. Trauma to the colon and rectum. In Blaisdell FW, Trunkey DD (eds) Trauma management: volume I—abdominal trauma. Thieme-Stratton, New York, pp 165–184, 1982.

Shapiro MJ, Wolverson MK (1989) Perforation of the retroperitoneal sigmoid colon secondary to fracture-dislocation of the left sacroiliac joint: case report. J Trauma 29(5):694–696.

Singleton Jr AO (1963) Blunt trauma to the abdomen. Trauma 5(2):39–72.

Sivit CJ, Taylor GA, Newman KD, Bulas DI, Gotschall CS, Wright CJ, Eichelberger MR (1990) Safety-belt injuries in children with lap-belt ecchymosis: CT findings in 61 patients. AJR 157:111–114.

Stafford PA, Biddinger PW, Zumwalt RE (1988) Lethal intrauterine fetal trauma. Am J Obstet Gynecol 159(2):485–489.

Stalnaker RL, McElhaney JH, Roberts VL, Trollope ML. Human torso response to blunt trauma. In King WF, Mertz HJ (eds) Human impact response: measurement and simulation. Plenum Press, New York, 1973b.

Stalnaker RL, Roberts VL, McElhaney JH. Side impact tolerance to blunt trauma. 17th Stapp Car Crash Conference Proceedings. SAE 730979, pp 377–408, 1973.

Stalnaker RL, Ulman MS. Abdominal trauma—review, response, and criteria. 29th Stapp Car Crash Conference Proceedings. SAE 851720, pp 1–16, 1985.

Stapp JP. Biodynamics of deceleration, impact, and

blast. In Randel HW (ed) Aerospace medicine. 2nd ed. Williams & Wilkins, Baltimore, pp 118–166, 1971.

States JD, Huelke DF, Dance M, Green RN (1987) Fatal injuries caused by underarm use of shoulder belts. J Trauma 27(7):740–745.

Stein PD, Sabbah HN, Hawkins ET, White HJ, Viano DC, Vostal JJ (1983) Hepatic and splenic injury in dogs caused by direct impact to the heart. J Trauma 23(5):395–404.

Strate RG, Grieco JG. Blunt injury to the colon and rectum. J Trauma 23(5):384–388.

Stuart GCE, Harding PGR, Davies EM (1980) Blunt abdominal trauma in pregnancy. CMA Journal 122:901–905.

Sturtz G. Biomechanical data of children. 24th Stapp Car Crash Conference Proceedings. SAE 801313, pp 513–559, 1980.

Stylianos S, Harris BH (1990) Seatbelt use and patterns of central nervous system injury in children. Pediatr Emerg Care 6(1):4–5.

Svendsen E, Morild I (1988) Fetal strangulation following uterine rupture. Am J Forensic Med Pathol 9(1):54–57.

Teniere P, Janer R, Michot F (1985) Les contusions de la rate. Rev Practicien 35:19–26.

Tonge JI, O'Reilly MJ, Davison A, Johnston NG (1972) Traffic crash fatalities: injury patterns and other factors. Med J Aust 2(1):5–17.

Trollope ML, Stalnaker RL, McElhaney JH, Frey CF (1973) The mechanism of injury in blunt abdominal trauma. J Trauma 13(11):962–970.

Trunkey DD. Spleen. In Blaisdell FW, Trunkey DD (eds) Trauma management: volume I—abdominal trauma. Thieme-Stratton, New York, pp 185–197, 1982.

Van De Wal HJCM, Draaisma JM, Vincent JG, Goris RJA (1990) Rupture of the supra-diaphragmatic inferior vena cava by blunt decelerating trauma: case report. J Trauma 30(1):111–113.

Van Kirk DJ, King AI. A preliminary study of an effective restraint system for pregnant women and children. 13th Stapp Car Crash Conference Proceedings. SAE 690814, pp 353–364, 1969.

Viano DC, Lau VK (1983) Role of Impact Velocity and Chest Compression in Thoracic Injury. Aviat Space Environ Med 54(1):16–21.

Viano DC, Lau IV. Thoracic impact: a viscous tolerance criteria. Tenth International ESV Conference Proceedings. 1985.

Viano DC, Lau IV, Asbury C, King AI, Begeman P. Biomechanics of the human chest, abdomen, and pelvis in lateral impact. Proceedings of the 33rd Association for the Advancement of Automotive Medicine. 1989.

Voeller GR, Reisser JR, Fabian TC, Kudsk K, Mangiante EC (1990) Blunt diaphragm injuries. Am Surg 56(1):28–31.

von Gierke HE (1964) Biodynamic response of the human body. Appl Mech Rev 17(12):951–958.

von Gierke HE, Oestreicher HL, Franke EK, Parrack HO, von Wittern WW (1952) Physics of vibrations in living tissues. J Appl Physiol 4:886–900.

Walfisch G, Fayon A, Tarriere C, Rosey JP, Guillon F, Got C, Patel A, Stalnaker RL. Designing of a dummy's abdomen for detecting injuries in side impact collisions. Fifth International IRCOBI Conference Proceedings. pp 149–164, 1980.

Walker LG. Mechanisms of injury. In Martin Jr JD, Haynes CD, Hatcher CR, Smith III RB, Stone HH (eds) Trauma to the thorax and abdomen. Charles C. Thomas, Springfield, IL, pp 47–58, 1969.

Walt AJ, Wilson RF. Blunt abdominal injuries: An overview. Biomechanics and its application to automotive design, P-49. Society of Automotive Engineers, New York, 1973.

Weast RC, Astle MJ, Beyer WH (eds) CRC handbook of chemistry and physics. 65th ed. CRC Press, Inc.; Boca Raton Florida, 1984.

Wells RP, Norman RW, Bishop P, Ranney DA (1986) Assessment of the static fit of automobile lap-belt systems on front-seat passengers. Ergonomics 29(8):955–976.

Widman WD (1969) Blunt trauma and the normal spleen; peacetime experience at a military hospital in Europe. Milit Med 134:25–35.

Wiechel JF, Sens MJ, Guenther DA. Critical review of the use of seat belts by pregnant women. Automotive frontal impacts, SP-782. SAE 890752, pp 61–69, 1989.

Williams JS. The nature of seat belt injuries. 14th Stapp Car Crash Conference Proceedings. SAE 700896, pp 44–65, 1970.

Williams JS, Lies BA, Hale HW (1966) The automotive safety belt: in saving a life may produce intra-abdominal injuries. J Trauma 6(1):303–315.

Williams RD, Sargent FT (1963) The mechanism of intestinal injury in trauma. J Trauma 3:288–294.

Woelfel GF, Moore EE, Cogbill TH, Van Way CW (1984) Severe thoracic and abdominal injuries associated with lap-harness seatbelts. J Trauma 24(2):166–167.

Wooldridge BF (1969) Traumatic rupture of the spleen. Missouri Med 66:804–806.

Yamada H. Strength of biological materials. Williams and Wilkins, Baltimore, 1970

Yamanaka N, Okamoto E, Toyosaka A, Ohashi S, Tanaka N (1985) Consistency of human liver. J Surg Res 39(3):192–198.

Zuidema GD (ed). The Johns Hopkins atlas of human functional anatomy. The Johns Hopkins University Press, Baltimore, 1977.

17
Injury to the Thoraco-Lumbar Spine and Pelvis

Albert I. King

Injury to the bony portion of the thoracolumbar spine is rare in automotive collisions. Soft tissue injuries appear to be more common. Major modes of injury to the spine are described, followed by a discussion of the biomechanical response of the spine to vertical $(+g_x)$ and horizontal $(-g_x)$ acceleration. A form of spinal injury due to the wearing of shoulder belts is discussed. The biomechanics and neurophysiology of low back pain form the foundation for an understanding of soft tissue injury. The relationship between disc rupture and impact loading is considered to be remote as disc rupture is a degenerative process that occurs over a long period of time. Mathematical models of the spine are also reviewed.

The pelvis is a bony structure that transmits the weight of the torso to the lower extremities during normal locomotion and supports the torso in the seated position. In an automotive impact environment, it can sustain injury from both frontal and side impact, and, during aircraft ejection or vertical falls, it is called upon to take the entire inertial load from seat-to-head acceleration. Injuries to the pelvis, however, contribute only about 1% to the total Injury Priority Rating (IPR). This structure is important in this discussion, therefore, primarily for its response during load transmission.

The Spine

Functions of the Spine

The human vertebral column is the principal load-bearing structure of the head and torso.

There are also secondary functions performed by each portion of the spinal column. The cervical spine provides the head with a limited degree of mobility and a protected pathway for the proximal segment of the spinal cord. The thoracic spine offers the same protection to the cord, while it offers mobility to the upper torso and rib cage. The lumbar segment provides the lower torso mobility and encloses the distal end of the spinal cord. The protective role of the vertebral column is analogous to the function served by the skull to protect the brain. However, anatomic requirements dictate that the spine be flexible and yet strong so that it can serve a multitude of functions. Like the skull, it is strong but not strong enough to withstand mechanical insults of modern day transportation systems. Injuries that affect the function of the spinal cord can result in death, quadriplegia, or paraplegia. Those who survive suffer permanent disabilities that cannot be restored as yet by modern medicine. Other biomechanical motivations to study the mechanical response of the spine include neckache and backache, osteoporosis, and scoliosis.

This chapter deals in part with the biomechanics of the spine, with particular emphasis on injury mechanisms and mechanical response to impact acceleration. Although spinal injuries are relatively uncommon in automotive accidents, they can often be rather severe and disabling. They are more common in aircraft accidents and constitute a special problem in aircraft ejection, which is the cause of anterior wedge fractures of the thoracolumbar spine.

In a review of 1988 National Accident Sampling System (NASS) data on thoracolumbar spinal injuries, it was found that the frequency of injury was about 2% if vertebral fracture and back muscle strain were included and 0.3% if only vertebral fractures were included. It is interesting to note that for an Abbreviated Injury Scale (AIS) range of 3 to 6, the frequency of spinal injury was 2.1% for lap-shoulder–belted occupants, while it was 1.5% for all cases and 1.3% for unrestrained occupants.

Anatomy of the Thoracolumbar Spine

Familiarity with the anatomy of the vertebral column is a necessary condition for the understanding of the biomechanics of the spine and its response to load. The ability to model this response also calls for an appreciation of the function of the various components of the column. From a macroscopic point of view, the vertebral column is made up of 24 individual bones, called vertebrae, that are joined together by several different types of soft tissue. The primary types of soft tissue are the intervertebral discs, ligaments, and skeletal muscle. As shown in Fig. 17.1, the 7 vertebrae supporting the head constitute the cervical spine, while the 12 vertebrae below it form the thoracic spine. The lumbar spine is the most inferior segment and is made up of 5 vertebrae. The entire column is supported by the sacrum, which is anatomically a part of the pelvic girdle. The thoracolumbar spine is located along the midline of the posterior aspect of the torso, and the cervical spine is along the posterior aspect of the neck. In general, each vertebra consists of a body, neural arch or pedicles, laminae, facet joints, spinous process, and transverse processes. The body is a cylindrically shaped bone consisting of a core of spongy bone surrounded by a thin layer of cortical or compact bone. The end-plates above and below the centrum are cartilaginous. The sides of the body are usually slightly concave and form a narrow waist at midlevel. Figure 17.2 shows a typical lumbar vertebra,

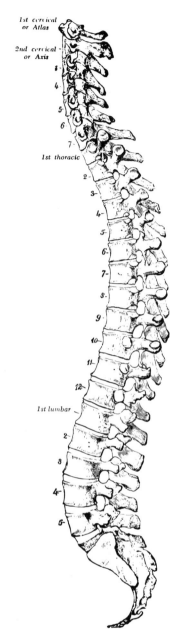

FIGURE 17.1. Lateral view of the spine. (From Gray, 1973).

viewed laterally and posteriorly. The pedicles arise from the posterolateral aspects of the body and are directed rearward. They form the lateral aspects of the spinal canal that surrounds the spinal cord and affords it mechanical

SUPERIOR ENDPLATE
VERTEBRAL BODY
INFERIOR ENDPLATE

SUPERIOR ARTICULAR FACET
POSTERIOR FACE OF
VERTEBRAL BODY
LAMINA
SPINOUS PROCESS

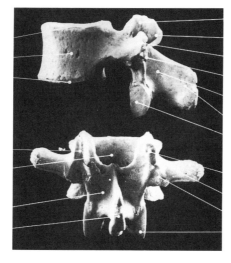

SUPERIOR ARTICULAR FACET
MAMMILLARY PROCESS
TRANSVERSE PROCESS
ACCESSORY PROCESS
SPINOUS PROCESS LAMINA
SPINOUS PROCESS
INFERIOR ARTICULAR FACET

MAMMILLARY PROCESS
TRANSVERSE PROCESS
ACCESSORY PROCESS
INFERIOR ARTICULAR FACET

FIGURE 17.2. Lateral and posterior view of a lumbar vertebra.

protection. The laminae are quadrilaterally shaped pieces of compact bone that form the posterior aspect of the spinal canal. At the junction between the pedicles and the laminae are the articular facets. Each vertebra has four facets, two superior and two inferior. The facets of a lumbar vertebra show that these bony projections articulate with mating projections (facets) of the vertebrae above and below. The joints formed by the facets are true synovial joints, encapsulated by capsular ligaments. The orientation of the facet joint surfaces varies from vertebra to vertebra and is of biomechanical interest because the facets form a load-bearing function of the spine with the vertebral bodies. The geometry of the facets will be described below.

Continuing with the general description of a typical vertebra, the transverse and spinous processes complete the posterior structure. They act as attachment points for muscles and ligaments and can be considered as short, cantilever beams with free ends. The vertebrae gradually increase in size caudally, roughly in proportion to the weight they are expected to support. The precise description of each vertebra can be found in a text on human anatomy. The lateral view of the entire column in Fig. 17.1 shows three principal spinal curves: the lordotic cervical and lumbar curves and the

kyphotic thoracic curve. The normal spine is straight when viewed frontally. Abnormal lateral curves found in scoliotic spines tend to develop in adolescence and are more common in females than males. Mechanical explanations for this form of instability are not completely satisfactory. It should also be noted that the thoracic spine supports the posterior section of the rib cage. A pair of ribs arise from each thoracic vertebra. These ribs articulate with the vertebrae near the junction of the pedicles with the vertebral bodies and at the tips of transverse processes.

A few of the special features of the spine will now be discussed. In particular, the orientation of the facets is of biomechanical significance. In order to describe the orientation of the facet joint surfaces, it is convenient to use a unit vector to establish the aproximate orientation of these surfaces. Some of the surfaces are slightly curved, and the description of their orientation assumes the unit normal to be located at the center of the surface. The unit normal for thoracic superior facets is directed generally posteriorly with a variable lateral component of about 30 deg and an upward tilt of about 20 deg. The lumbar surfaces are slightly curved, but the unit normal at the center is directed medially. Its orientation tends to shift to a posteromedial direction for the lower lumbar vertebrae. However, the vector tends to lie in a horizontal plane. A pictorial description of the orientation of facet surfaces can be found in Gray (1973). Another special feature of note is the inclination of the fifth lumbar vertebra (L5). The end-plates are inclined at the L4–5 and L5–S1 level due to the lordotic curvature of the lumbar spine. The forward inclination of L5 can be more than 30 deg in some individuals, resulting in high shear loads at these lower lumbar joints.

The vertebrae are joined together by soft tissue, anteriorly by ligaments and intervertebral discs, and posteriorly by ligaments and facet joint capsules. Intervertebral discs are cartilaginous in origin and consist principally of collagen, proteoglycans, and water. The disc can be divided into two main regions, the nucleus pulposus and the annulus fibrosus. The latter is a ring of primarily type I collagen (the type found in skin, tendon, and bone), made up of dense layers of collagen fibers that have an intricacy of pattern that almost defies description. In general, the direction of the fibers in adjacent layers cross each other at an oblique angle, but the direction of the fibers in any given layer can also change or the fibers can bifurcate and assume more than one direction. In the lumbar region, 12 to 16 layers can be found anteriorly. Type II collagen (the type found in hyaline cartilage) can be found in the nucleus, which has a higher concentration of proteoglycans, giving it a gel-like character. Proteoglycans have an affinity for water and are responsible for the maintenance of tension in the annular collagen fibers. The anatomy and function of the disc are affected by age. Disc degeneration begins at a very young age, and normal, healthy discs are the exception rather than the rule in spines over the age of 25. The number and size of collagen fibrils increase with age, and the distinguishing features of the nucleus disappear as age transforms the entire disc into fibrocartilage. A detailed description of the anatomy of the disc can be found in Peacock (1952) and in a more recent version by Buckwalter (1982).

A new finding regarding the microstructure of annular layers has been reported by Marchand and Ahmed (1990). They confirmed the fact that the fiber orientation within a single layer can indeed vary and that the change in orientation occurred at cleavage lines that are possibly sites of mechanical weakness where a disc herniation can occur.

The articular facets are enclosed by a joint capsule and appear to allow the spine to flex freely while acting as motion limiters in spinal extension or rearward bending. Schultz et al. (1988) reported that these capsules can undergo a large amount of stretch, particularly when the lumbar spine is placed in extension. There is also neurophysiological evidence provided by Yamashita et al. (1990) of pain fibers in the capsule that can be stimulated sufficiently to be set off, resulting in low back pain. The joint surfaces are lined with articular cartilage and are lubricated by synovial fluid.

There are three spinal ligaments that run along the entire length of the spine. They are the anterior and posterior spinal ligaments which line the anterior and posterior aspects of the vertebral bodies, and the supraspinous ligament, which joints the tips of the spinous processes. The ligamentum flavum, or yellow ligament, is a strong band that connects adjacent laminae behind the spinal cord. The interspinous ligament is a thin membrane located between adjacent spinous processes.

The spine is maintained in an erect posture with the help of the skeletal musculature. The extensor muscles of the thoracolumbar spine can be divided into two main groups: the superficial transversocostal and splenius group and the deeper transversospinal group. The former group contains muscles that arise from the pelvic region and insert at various levels from the 6th to the 12th rib. Others arise from the lower ribs and insert at the upper ribs or along the cervical spine. The deeper group contains muscles that join one vertebra to another or span one or more vertebrae. The principal flexors of the thoracolumbar spine are the internal oblique muscles and the rectus abdominis.

Injury Mechanisms

Injuries to the vertebral column can be roughly classified into seven different categories:

1. Anterior wedge fractures of vertebral bodies
2. Burst fractures of vertebral bodies
3. Dislocations and fracture-dislocations
4. Rotational injuries
5. Chance fractures
6. Hyperextension injuries
7. Soft tissue injuries

Anterior Wedge Fractures

These injuries occur at all levels of the spine and are common in both aircraft and automotive accidents. The mechanism of injury is combined flexion and axial compression. It is a mild form of spinal injury commonly identified with the pilot ejection problem. The region most susceptible to anterior wedge fractures during ejection is between T10 and L2, although they can occur in the upper thoracic region as well (T4–T6). Kazarian (1982) postulated that the mechanism of injury to the T4–T6 segment is forcible exaggeration of the normal upper spinal curvature. The fact that very little vertical ($+g_z$) acceleration is experienced in an automotive crash does not mean that wedge fractures cannot occur. Begeman et al. (1973) have shown that subjects restrained by a lap belt and an upper torso belt, in a $-g_x$ environment, develop high spinal loads that can cause wedge fractures similar to ejection seat injuries.

Burst Fractures

These injuries are due to higher levels of input acceleration or applied load, applied more directly over the vertebral body, causing it to break up into two or more segments. The integrity of the cord is threatened by the movement of the segments posteriorly into the spinal canal. The cord can also be injured by the retropulsion of the disc into the canal, particularly in the cervical spine. It should be noted that in many cases of paralysis, post-impact x-rays show a burst fracture with fragments that do not intrude into the spinal canal. This does not mean that the spinal cord was not injured or contused by these fragments because such x-rays do not reveal the full extent of their dynamic retropulsion and

because there is some retraction of the fragments after the impact.

Dislocations and Fracture-Dislocations

These are generally flexion injuries accompanied by rotation and posteroanterior shear. Unilateral dislocations require an axial rotational component, while bilateral dislocations can be due solely to flexion. The essential difference between a simple wedge fracture and a fracture-dislocation is, according to Nicoll (1949), the rupture of the interspinous ligament. This observation is biomechanically significant and will be discussed later. There are varying degrees of dislocation. The inferior facets can be simply moved upward relative to the superior facets of the vertebra below or the facets can be perched on top of each other. There can also be a forward dislocation with fracture of the facets or the neural arch, and forward dislocation with locking of the facets. That is, the inferior facets have moved up and over the superior facets of the vertebra below and come back down so that they are now anterior to the superior facets. There is a high probability of neurologic damage in this type of injury because the cord is subjected to high shearing and stretching forces. If there is dislocation without wedging, the mechanism of injury is a high shear load in the posteroanterior direction (Kazarian, 1982).

Rotational Injuries

If the spine is twisted about its longitudinal axis and is subjected to axial and/or shearing loads, lateral wedge fractures can occur (Nicoll, 1949). Other forms of injury include uniform compression of the vertebral body and fracture of the articular facets and lamina. Kazarian (1982) indicated that lateral wedge fractures seem to gravitate to two spinal regions: T2 to T6 and T7 to T10. The damage to the posterior intervertebral joint is on the concave side, and this injury is often accompanied by fracture of the transverse process on the convex side. Unlike the anterior wedge fracture, this injury may result in neurologic deficit, including paraplegia.

Chance Fractures

This injury was first described by Chance (1948) as being a lap belt–related syndrome in which a lumbar vertebra is split in the transverse plane, beginning with the spinous process. Subsequent studies, for example, by Smith and Kaufer (1967), attribute the injury to the improper wearing of the lap belt while involved in a frontal $(-g_x)$ collision. The belt rides over the iliac wings and acts as a fulcrum for the lumbar spine to flex over it, causing a marked separation of the posterior elements without any evidence of wedging (Steckler et al., 1969). When the lap belt is used in conjunction with an upper torso restraint, this injury does not occur.

Hyperextension Injuries

Hyperextension injuries of the cervical spine result in avulsion of the anterior aspect of the vertebral bodies, sometimes termed "teardrop fractures." Kazarian et al. (1979) reported the occurrence of hyperextension injuries of the thoracic spine resulting from ejection from F/FB-118 aircraft. The superior lip of one or more vertebrae is avulsed along with the rupture of the anterior longitudinal ligament. This injury is sometimes accompanied by loss of posterior vertebral body height. When this occurs, there may be injury to the articular facets, pedicles, and/or the laminae. The incidence was 23% over a 10-year period. The powered inertial reel and the seat back were considered responsible for this rare injury because of the large forces exerted on the front of the torso when the belts pulled the shoulders back.

Soft Tissue Injuries

The soft tissues involved are the intervertebral disc, the various ligaments around the intervertebral joint, the facet joints and their capsules, and the muscles and tendons attached to the vertebral column. The usual complaint of this type of injury is low back pain which is often associated with radiating pain down the buttocks and the lower extremities. The incident provoking this complaint can vary from a mild bump in the rear by another vehicle while the victim is stopped at the light to a bus going over a pothole to a relatively severe collision of two cars at an intersection. If the x-rays taken in the emergency room are negative, a diagnosis of lumbar sprain or strain is made and the patient is sent home with some pain killers. In some cases, the pain persists and eventually a diagnosis of disc rupture, disc bulge, or other specific syndromes is made and the incident in question is generally blamed to be the cause of the injury. This cause-and-effect relationship is invariably based on the history provided by the patient and not on the severity of the impact or the biomechanics of the loading on the spine.

Biomechanical Response of the Thoracolumbar Spine

Because of its flexibility, the vertebral column is frequently subjected to bending loads that are superimposed upon the axial load it bears to support the head and torso. There is no question that impact accelerations in the horizontal plane exert bending loads on the spine. However, vertical $(+g_z)$ acceleration is also capable of subjecting the spine to a high level of bending due to the fact that the vertebral column is located along the posterior aspect of the torso.

It is perhaps interesting to trace the progress made in experimental research on spinal injury, beginning with this bending hypothesis made by King et al. (1968). The development of countermeasures to prevent anterior wedge fractures from occurring in pilots who eject from disabled aircraft was somewhat hampered by simple spinal models of Latham (1957) and Hess and Lombard (1958). While they are admirable modeling efforts for their time and are sound from an engineering viewpoint, they unfortunately led subsequent researchers away from looking at the anatomy of the spine. The models were capable of simulating axial loading only. Experimental studies on the spine during whole-body acceleration of cadavers in the $+g_z$ impact acceleration mode revealed that the spine was subjected to high bending loads even though it was restrained by a shoulder harness, and the input acceleration was in the seat-to-head (vertical) direction. This led to a more detailed study of the load-carrying capacity of the spine during $+g_z$ acceleration. Ewing et al. (1972) tested a series of embalmed cadavers on the Wayne State University vertical accelerator, using three different restraint configurations: the hyperextended, erect, and flexed modes. In the hyperextended mode the spine was pulled back at the shoulders by a pair of military-type harnesses, while the thoracolumbar spine was placed in extension by inserting a block of wood 50 mm thick behind the spine at the L1 level. In the erect mode, the spine was in its natural configuration while seated in a rigid seat, with the shoulder belts tightened manually to a tension of approximately 300 N. The shoulder harness was loosened in the flexed mode, permitting the torso to flex forward freely. The objective of the study was to determine the fracture level of the spine as a function of its spinal configuration. The results are shown in Table 17.1. By hyperextending the spine, the fracture g-level increased some 80%, and the observed difference was significant at the 95% level. In a subsequent search for this

dramatic increase in spinal strength, it was determined that the spine did not received external support from the hyperextension block and that the reason was an internal redistribution of the load borne by the spine.

Prasad et al. (1974) embarked on a study to prove the hypothesis that the spine had two load paths and that the articular facets were indeed capable of transmitting load from one vertebra to the next. This facet load was difficult to measure directly but could be computed indirectly if the load borne by the disc was determined. An intervertebral load cell (IVLC) was designed to replace the inferior portion of a lumbar vertebra that was cut out by means of a double-bladed rotary saw. The IVLC shown in Fig. 17.3 is 10 mm thick and has a diameter of about 40 mm. It is capable

TABLE 17.1. Increase in g-level to fracture due to hyperextension of the lumbar spine.

Spinal configuration	No. of specimens	Average fracture g-level (g)
Hyperextended	4	17.6
Erect	5	10.4
Flexed	3	9.0

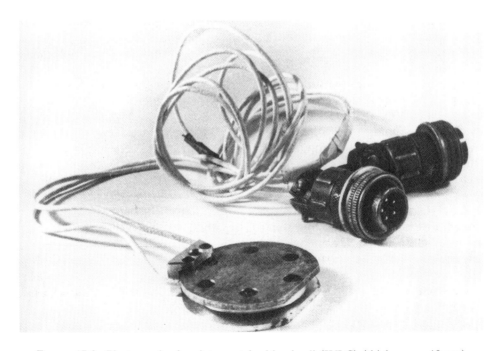

FIGURE 17.3. Photograph of an intervertebral load cell (IVLC) (thickness = 10 mm).

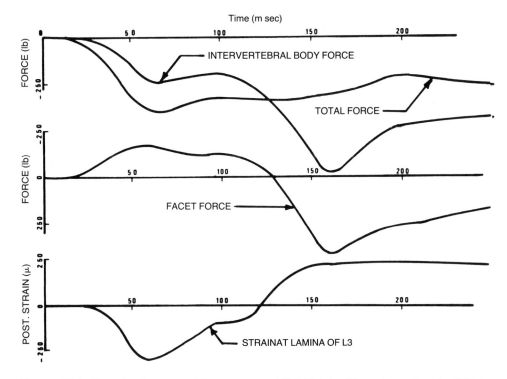

FIGURE 17.4. Facet load computed from measured IVLC data. (From Prasad et al., 1974.)

of measuring axial compression and the eccentricity of that load in the midsagittal plane. Figure 17.4 shows the facet load computed by subtracting the intervertebral load from the total load borne by the spine. The latter was assumed to be proportional to the measured seat pan load, with the proportionality constant equal to the ratio of the weight of the torso above the IVLC to the total weight of the body. At the beginning of the acceleration pulse, the facets were in compression, sharing the inertial load with the vertebral body and disc. As the head and torso flexed forward, the facets went into tension. These results were confirmed by Hakim and King (1976), who reproduced the IVLC loads on excised spinal segments in an MTS materials testing machine. By hyperextending the spine, the facets were prevented from going into tension, thus increasing the fracture level of the most vulnerable vertebral bodies in the thoracolumbar spine. Furthermore, the facet load hypothesis provided an explanation for the frequently observed anterior wedge fractures. The addi-

tional compression borne by the bodies was needed to balance the flexion moment caused by forward rotation of the head and torso. Since the moment arm is of the order of 25 mm and the flexion moment can be as high as 40 N.m, this additional compression is over 1,000 N. Such excessive compressive loads are the cause for anterior wedging of the vertebral bodies. Injury data from subhuman primates, obtained by Kazarian et al. (1971) indicate that derangement of facets was due to locking of the facet joints to act as load paths during $+g_z$ acceleration. Although injuries to the posterior elements are rare in pilot ejection, these observations corroborate the load-bearing hypothesis of the facets.

Patwardhan et al. (1982) measured contact pressure between the articular surfaces of lumbar facets and computed a facet force, reporting it to be the vertical facet force that was measured indirectly by Prasad et al. (1974). This was felt to be erroneous since the articular surfaces are quite incapable of transmitting large shear loads. Yang and King (1984)

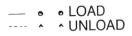

FIGURE 17.5. Response of an isolated facet joint to a compressive load. (From Yang and King, 1984.)

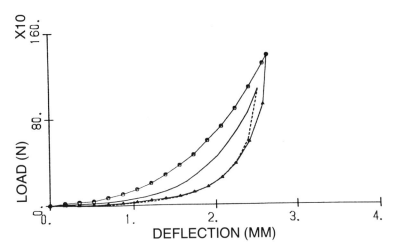

FIGURE 17.6. Response of an isolated facet joint to a tensile load. (From Yang and King, 1984.)

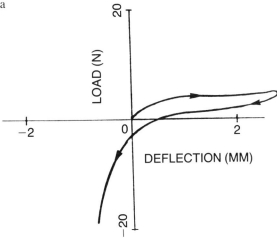

performed loading experiments on isolated facet joints and obtained results that can explain the mechanism of load transmission through the facet joint. The posterior elements were separated from the body by cutting through the pedicles. The two facets were then loaded axially in their normal configuration in an Instron testing machine. In compression, they acted as a stiffening spring, as shown in Fig. 17.5. In tension, however, they afforded very little resistance. Most of the tensile resistance was provided by the ligamentum flavum and the interspinous and supraspinous ligaments. Figure 17.6 shows the tensile load deflection curve of the isolated facets, with all ligaments severed. The mechanism of load transmission in compression is thus different from that in tension, and it is postulated that high compressive loads can be generated in the facet joint when the inferior tip of the inferior facet bottoms out on the pars interarticularis of the vertebra below it. In tension, the resistance is provided by soft tissues, such as the ligaments and the extensor muscles of the

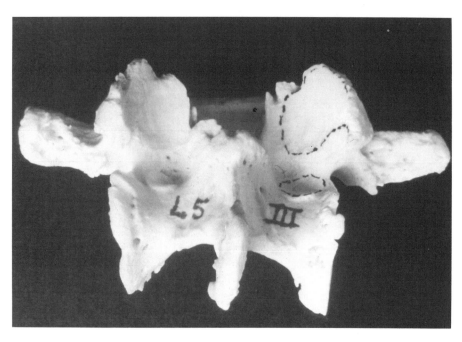

Figure 17.7. Heavy impression of facet tip contact with the lamina of a possible weight lifter. (Courtesy of Dr. Jacob, Balgrist Hospital, Zurich.)

back. Figure 17.7 is a photograph of a lamina, showing graphic evidence of facet loading due to a lifetime of heavy weight bearing. It should be noted that the axial loading experiment on isolated facet joints was carried out because very little rotation of the facet joint could be detected when complete spinal segments were subjected to combined axial compression and forward flexion. Thus, for the isolated facets, axial compression is equivalent to spinal extension and axial tension to spinal flexion. These results have a significant impact on the understanding of injury mechanisms of the spine. The observation made by Nicoll (1949) that dislocations occur if the interspinous ligaments are ruptured is equivalent to saying that the capsules cannot provide much resistance in flexion and that facets can be easily subluxed if the posterior ligaments are torn. In fact, the geometry of the facet surfaces can be an important consideration as far as dislocation is concerned. Those with surfaces that are almost horizontal would be easier to dislocate than those with vertical faces, particularly in the presence of torsional loads and horizontal

shear forces. The high frequency of dislocations at the C5–C7 level can be attributable to the facet geometry of those vertebrae.

As further evidence of facet loading, contact pressure between the tip of the inferior facet and the lamina was measured by El-Bohy et al. (1989). A miniature pressure transducer was inserted into the inferior facet through a predrilled hole so that its diaphragm was located at the very tip of the facet just above the lamina. The experimental setup is shown in Fig. 17.8. The spinal segment was subjected to three types of loading: a simulated body weight that acted some 14 mm anterior to the center of the top disc, a simulated extensor muscle load that acted 50 mm posterior to the center of the top vertebral body, and an anterior eccentric load of 45 N simulating a weight borne by an individual. The pressure transducer was set to read zero pressure with the spine completely unloaded. A body weight equal to 50% of the body weight of the cadaver was then applied, causing the segment to flex. A simulated extensor muscle load was applied until the spine was returned to its erect configuration

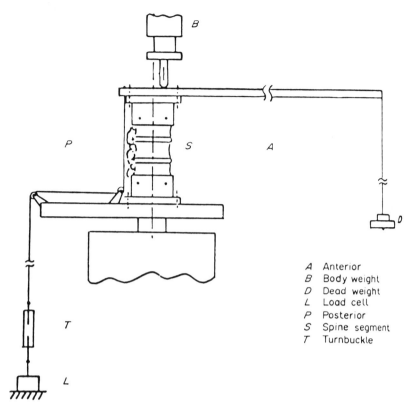

A   Anterior
B   Body weight
D   Dead weight
L   Load cell
P   Posterior
S   Spine segment
T   Turnbuckle

FIGURE 17.8. Schematic of the test setup for measuring facet contact pressure. (From El-Bohy et al., 1989.)

and the facet tip pressure was measured. In all six segments tested there was a measurable facet contact pressure. When the 45-N weight was applied at an anterior eccentricity of 340 mm, the segment again assumed a flexed configuration with no measurable facet pressure. However, when the extensor muscle force was used to bring the spine back to its erect position, a further increase in facet pressure was observed in five of the six segments tested. Statistically, this increase was significant at the 95% level.

The biomechanics of a compressive force being generated in the vertebral column during a frontal impact ($+g_x$) acceleration need to be discussed. This phenomenon was initially discovered when a two-dimensional model of the spine developed by Prasad and King (1974) was exercised to simulate a frontal impact. Cadaver tests were carried out by Begemen et al. (1973) to verify the existence of this force, since vertical forces are not expected to be generated in a horizontal crash. Large seat pan loads were measured if the subject was restrained by an upper torso restraint, such as a cross-chest belt. This was the net force after accounting for all lap belt forces. Dummies did not generate this seat pan load. Subsequent tests by Begeman et al. (1980) involving volunteer subjects confirmed these results. It was postulated that the seat pan load was a manifestation of spinal compression due to the tendency of the spine to straighten out during $-g_x$ acceleration. The reverse situation exists during a rear-end collision. The spine goes into tension and the body tends to ramp up the seat back. It may be necessary to increase the height of some of the head rests to prevent hyperextension of the neck.

There is now anecdotal evidence of an increase in the frequency of thoracolumbar injuries among automotive crash victims, after the enactment of seat belt use laws in the United States. States et al. (1989) reported a

TABLE 17.2. Change in lumbar injuries in Monroe Country, New York between 1983–84 and 1985–86.

	Subjects*			Controls**		
	83–84	85–86	% Change	83–84	85–86	% Change
AIS 1–2	15	27	+80	16	19	+18.8
3–5	9	7	−22	2	4	+100.0

* Subjects are injured automotive occupants treated at county hospitals.
** Controls are nonautomotive traffic accident victims treated at the same hospitals (motorcyclists and pedestrians).

significant increase in spinal injuries as a result of the belt law in New York State. Hospital data from all hospitals in the Rochester area were reviewed for injuries sustained 1 year before and 1 year after the effective date of the belt law. Assuming that the number of automotive-related victims remained the same, then there was a large increase in spinal injuries, as shown in Table 17.2. In addition, there is a case report by Miniaci and McLaren (1989) of four anterolateral wedge compression fractures that were attributed to the wearing of lap shoulder belts.

Soft Tissue Injuries to the Thoracolumbar Spine

Although the frequency of bony injuries to the thoracolumbar spine is relatively low as a result of vehicular crashes, that of soft tissue injuries to the intervertebral joints appear to be much higher. As mentioned earlier, the common complaint is low back pain (LBP), occasionally associated with pain radiating down the extremities. Since LBP is a very common complaint, inasmuch as eight out of ten persons will have at least one such attack in their lifetime, it becomes extremely difficult to pinpoint the cause of any particular attack or to relate it to any given incident.

A difficulty in the diagnosis and treatment of LBP is its etiology. It is often called idiopathic, meaning it has no known cause. Recent research is homing in on at least a few of the causes of LBP but by and large, it is still difficult to determine the exact etiology. The pain can come from many sources and depends on the duration of the symptoms. The major

culprits are believed to be the disc, the ligaments around the posterior structures of the spine, the facet joint capsules, and the tendons and muscles around the intervertebral joint. Current work by Yamashita et al. (1990) focuses on the source of pain, namely the presence and activation of pain-sensing nerve endings or nociceptors. The premise is that in order for someone to sense pain there are three basic requirements:

1. Presence of nociceptors in the soft tissue in question
2. Adequate deformation of the soft tissue containing the nociceptors
3. Firing of the nociceptors in response to the deformation.

The first requirement is self-evident and needs no elaboration. However, the morphological study of the distribution of nerve endings in the intervertebral joint is still very much a topic of current research. Notably, one can point to the work of Giles and Taylor (1987) and Bogduk and Twomey (1987) as well as to an ongoing study by King et al. (1990). There is some evidence that pain fibers are present in the outer layers of the intervertebral disc annulus. They are found in and around the capsules of the facet joints, extending to the borders of nearby ligaments and tendons.

The biomechanics of soft tissue deformation has also been studied. Stokes (1987) found that the strain of the anterior disc due to an applied compressive load was about 10% along the directions of the annular fibers. In Schultz et al. (1988), it was reported that the human facet joint capsule can undergo large deformations, particularly during spinal extension.

TABLE 17.3. Maximum tensile facet capsule stretch (%/N-m).

Cadaver no.	Extension tests			Flexion tests		
	X-axis	Y-axis	Z-axis	X-axis	Y-axis	Z-axis
400	7.1	8.7	5.3	0.6	0.2	0.1
464	4.8	5.5	8.2	0.1	0.4	0.3
807	3.3	2.5	6.4	0.4	0.6	0.3
329	7.4	6.3	0.2	0.8	2.6	1.9
455	1.3	3.9	1.3	0.3	1.3	0.3
490	0.8	2.5	4.7	2.2	4.5	1.2
002	0.8	7.4	7.0	1.3	3.5	6.4
117	0.8	6.6	6.6	0.9	7.1	1.3
034	12.4	21.0	21.1	2.0	0.3	2.0
SD	4.0	5.6	6.0	0.7	2.4	2.0
CV	93.8	78.4	88.7	77.5	104.5	122.8

The X-axis is directed anteriorly in the transverse plane.
The Y-axis is directed laterally to the left in the transverse plane.
The Z-axis is directed superiorly, normal to the transverse plane.
SD, standard deviation; CV, coefficient of variation.

In fact, during cadaveric experiments on spinal motion segments under static loading, the stretching of the superior lateral corner of certain facet capsules can be easily seen without optical magnification. The stretch can vary over a large range of strain, depending on the geometry of the facets. Table 17.3 shows some unpublished data, given in the form of stretch per unit moment (in N.m). The peak values of the flexion and extension moments applied were 24 and 18 N.m, respectively.

With respect to the third requirement, it is a well-known fact that nociceptors have high thresholds and do not go off unless stimulated vigorously. The large deformations noted in the facet capsules may be large enough but it is necessary to demonstrate this neurophysiologically. Yamashita et al. (1990) and Avramov et al. (1991) have mapped the distribution of nociceptors and other types of mechanoreceptors in and around the facet joint. They have also shown that spinal load and stretching of the facet capsule can cause the high threshold nociceptors to fire. This work confirms the previously reported facet syndrome by Mooney and Robertson (1976) and others. In fact, facet pain may be responsible for a large proportion of the LBP being reported. This combined neurophysiological and biomechanical technique is being extended to the disc,

which appears to be sensitive to a change in the pH of its contents (Nachemson, 1969).

With regard to the relationship between disc rupture and impact loading on the spine, it can be safely said that disc ruptures do not occur as the result of a single loading event, unless there are associated massive bony injuries to the spine. This statement is based on a review of the literature on spinal response by Henzel et al. (1968), who indicated that early researchers such as Ruff (1950), Brown et al. (1957), and Roaf (1960) observed that the vertebral body always broke before the adjacent disc incurred visible damage. Moreover, Brinckmann (1986) has shown that a severely weakened lumbar disc, with the posterior elements removed, could not be ruptured and hardly even bulged when loaded in compression to 1 kN. Additional loads causing fracture of the vertebral body did not result in herniation or excessive bulging. There are two reports of disc rupture due to a single loading event in the literature. Farfan et al. (1970) applied torsional loads to intact lumbar motion segments without any compressive preload and was able to cause posterior and anterior disc ruptures after a rotation averaging 22.9 deg for normal discs and a rotation averaging 15.2 deg for abnormal discs. They also tested facet joints and facet capsules to failure and found that the average angle at which they failed was 14 and 12 deg, respectively. This meant that if the facets were allowed to slide over each other or fracture, resulting in a large rotation, then the rupture can occur. Normally, in the presence of a preload of the facets, a single torsional load that does not disrupt the facets or tear the capsules does not cause rupture. The second report is by Adams and Hutton (1982) in which they caused spontaneous rupture of several discs by compressing the spine while it was hyperflexed both laterally and sagittally. If the disc did not rupture on the first try, it was flexed 1 or 2 deg more and loaded again with the same load. The average angle of flexion was 12.9 deg, implying that the lumbar spine alone was flexed a total of 64 deg. The average applied load was 5,449 N (1,225 lb). This situation is again not representative of a realistic loading condition as it is extremely rare that a large compressive force would be applied to a spine that is virtually

doubled over. Moreover, the herniation occurred between the disk and the end-plate due to extreme tension on the posterior aspect of the disc. There was no rupture of the annulus. In fact, both of these reports tend to reinforce the point of view that a single loading event is unable to cause disc rupture.

Under repeated loading, Yang et al. (1988) were able to produce disc herniation (extrusion of nuclear material to the outside of the disc) by the application of repetitive torsional loads combined with compression and flexion and with the facets removed. Figure 17.9 shows extrusion of nuclear material (white arrow) after approximately 20,000 cycles of torsional loading. In a subsequent study by Gordon et al. (1991) nuclear extrusion occurred in 4 of 14 specimens that were tested under combined axial load, flexion, and torsion, with the posterior elements intact. The average number of cycles of loading was 36,750. Previous attempts by Hardy et al. (1959) resulted in the

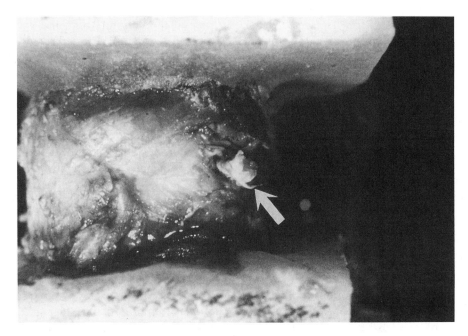

FIGURE 17.9. Photograph of extrusion of nucleus pulposus following several thousand cycles of torsional loading. (Courtesy of Dr. K.H. Yang, Wayne State University, Detroit.)

extrusion of the nucleus into the end-plates and compression fracture of the end-plates and the vertebral bodies. Only one unembalmed specimen was tested and failure occurred at 1.29 million cycles. Liu et al. (1983, 1985) performed fatigue tests on lumbar motion segments under axial and torsional loads. Under axial loading, failure occurred in the form of fracture of the vertebral body or of the end-plates. Under torsional loading there were some annular tears observed but no extrusion of disc material. Disc rupture appears to be the result of a slow degenerative process that can take a long time to develop.

Mathematical Models of the Thoracolumbar Spine

Mathematical models can often be used as an experimental tool to study the response of a system to a variety of input conditions. The premise is that the model must provide reliable predictions before this type of study can be of value. In other words, models that have been validated against experimental data are required. King and Chou (1976) reviewed mathematical models of impact developed before 1975 and discussed in detail models of the spine that were available at that time.

Two-dimensional models developed after 1975 include discrete parameter models by Tennyson and King (1976) and by Pontius and Liu (1976). Both were extensions of previous models without muscles, and both had a capability of simulating a delayed response of the musculature following a stretch stimulus. Validation against human volunteer impact data was provided by Tennyson and King (1976, 1977).

Since 1975, many three-dimensional (3-D) models have been developed to simulate the response of the spine to impact acceleration. Belytschko and Privitzer (1978) demonstrated the capability of a 3-D model of the entire spine. It is basically a discrete parameter model in which the vertebrae are represented by rigid bodies interconnected by deformable elements. It was capable of simulating ejection seat dynamics as well as spinal response to a horizontal crash ($-g_x$ impact acceleration). There was, however, no validation against experimental data.

A finite element model of a motion segment was developed by King and Yang (1985) to simulate the response to the articular facets, using the data detailed by Yang and King (1984). This model is based on that of Hakim and King (1979) for a single vertebra and computes stress distribution in the body, disc, and posterior structures. The disc has a fluid nucleus surrounded by a low modulus annular material. It is still a static model, which can be made to respond to dynamic inputs at a later date. The computed intradiscal pressure compared favorably with experimental data. In a parametric study, it was found that the sensitive variables were the modulus of elasticity of the annulus fibrosus and spongy bone.

More recent models include the work of Shirazi-Adl (1984), who developed a comprehensive 3-D finite element model of a lumbar motion segment and has been simulating a variety of static loading conditions, such as the prediction of facet load in the lumbar spine (Shirazi-Adl and Drouin, 1987).

Discussion

Because of the fact that spinal injuries are relatively infrequent in automotive accidents, research on the biomechanics of spinal injury and response is not as advanced as that for body regions that are frequently injured, such as the head or the thorax. For the thoracolumbar spine, the tolerance information is over 30 years old for $+g_z$ acceleration, and there has been no new information since the publication of the curves by Eiband (1959). The fact that tolerance is dependent upon the restraint system used and the age of the occupant renders the problem of defining it as a single parameter virtually impossible. Furthermore, the configuration of the spine plays an important role in the injury pattern it sustains as a result of an impact in a given direction. In the absence of a restraint system, more spinal injuries are likely to occur, especially for motorcycle riders and occupants involved in rollovers. Thus, it is also extremely difficult to arrive at a limited set of injury criteria for the spine, particularly since the failure of the spinal components is not restricted to the bony portions of the spine. Much of the spinal resistance to bending and torsional loads is provided by soft tissues—ligaments, muscles, and cartilage (disc). For each set of loading conditions, injury criteria need to be formulated. Such a task is indeed formidable.

The mechanisms of injury to the spine are relatively well understood. Failure of the various spinal components can be attributed to a combination of axial and bending loads. The central role played by the articular facets cannot be overemphasized. Together with the vertebrae, they provide a dual load path for the transmission of axial load. In forward bending, the compressive load may be borne entirely by the body. However, new data being acquired from spinal segments appear to indicate that the facets are load bearing until there is excessive flexion. In the living spine, the role of the musculature of the back acts to increase facet loading. Torsional loads and shear loads are also resisted to a great extent by the facets. In the lumbar region, Patwardhan et al. (1982) may have measured this torsional resistance, using pressure-sensitive Fuji film.

Conclusions

1. Spinal anatomy is extremely complex. A thorough knowledge of its construction and function is essential to understanding its biomechanical role in load bearing and protection of the spinal cord.
2. The articular facets play a central role in the mechanism of spinal support and in the mechanisms of injury to the spine. The orientation of the facet surfaces may explain the tendency of subluxation and dislocation of certain vertebrae. It should be noted that subluxation is an unstable condition that endangers the integrity of the cord.
3. The manner in which facets resist compressive and tensile loads has been studied by means of tests on isolated facet joints. It can be hypothesized that compressive resistance is generated by the bottoming out of the tip of the inferior facets onto the pars interarticularis of the vertebra below. Proof

of this hypothesis will require additional research. The facets offer virtually no resistance to tensile loads. The smooth surfaces of the facets and the relatively weak capsular ligaments are unable to provide the tensile resistance necessary for countering such loads. It is postulated that the ligaments and muscles along the posterior spine assume this role.
4. Impact loads are not likely to produce ruptures of the lumbar intervertebral disc. Injuries to the soft tissues of the intervertebral joint are, however, difficult to diagnose. At present, there is adequate evidence to state that the facet capsule is a source of low back pain.
5. Tolerance data are woefully lacking. A carefully worked-out research plan is needed to address this complex problem of injury tolerance and injury criteria. In particular, there is a need to study the tolerance of the facets to dislocation, which is a high-risk injury. The types of dislocation and the injury mechanisms involved need to be identified at each spinal level and for each combination of applied loads.
6. The use of mathematical models to study the response of the spine is a viable approach because of the flexibility of the models and the low cost involved in comparison with that incurred in experimental research. Whenever possible, the combined approach of using models and obtaining experimental data based on model predictions will enhance the understanding of spinal response.

The Pelvis

Anatomy of the Pelvis

The pelvis (Latin for "basin") is a ring of bone interposed between the flexible spinal column, which it supports, and the movable lower limbs, upon which it rests. Mechanically, it is the only load path for the transmission of the weight of the head, arms, and torso to the ground. Thus, the pelvic structure is more massive than that of the cranial or thoracic cavities. The pelvic ring or girdle is composed of four bones. Two hip bones form the side and front walls of the ring, while the sacrum and coccyx make up the rear wall. Figure 17.10 shows a frontal view of the male and female pelvis. There are many differences between the male and female pelvis, but the principal functional difference is the shape of the inner cavity that is completely surrounded by bone. This aperture is almost circular in the female, while it is wider in the side-to-side direction in the male. In the female, this aperture is the birth canal through which the fetus must pass. The orientation of the pelvis is less variable in the standing posture than that of the seated posture. A method for defining pelvic orientation will be discussed below.

The Hip Bone

The hip bone is a large, relatively flat, and irregularly shaped bone that forms the greater part of the pelvic girdle. It is formed by three fused bones called the ilium, ischium, and pubis. The fusion occurs around a cup-shaped articular cavity called the acetabulum (hip socket), which is situated near the middle of the outer surface of the bone. The ilium makes up the flank of the hip bone and is the upper broad and expanded portion that extends upward from the acetabulum. The ilium is divided into two parts, the large wing-like ala and the body of the ilium that forms a part of the acetabulum. Most of the landmarks and surface features are of little biomechanical sig-

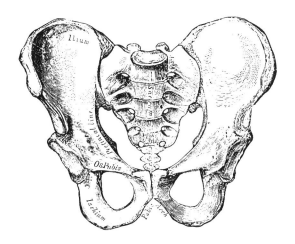

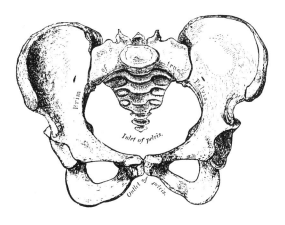

FIGURE 17.10. Frontal view of the male and female pelvis (From Gray, 1973.)

nificance and will not be discussed. However, it is necessary to point out the anterior-superior iliac spine (ASIS), which acts as an anatomical anchor point to prevent the lap belt from slipping over the top of the pelvis, a phenomenon called "submarining." The ilium is attached to the sacrum along its medial (inside) surface called the auricular surface. This surface is covered with cartilage, but the joint is not synovial. It is therefore postulated that only a limited amount of relative motion can occur here.

The ischium forms the lower and rearward part of the hip bone and is divided into two parts, a body and a ramus. The former constitutes the rearward third of the acetabular cup. The lowest portion of the body is the ischial tuberosity, which supports the upper torso in a seated posture. The ramus is a thin flattened part of the ischium that joins with the inferior pubic ramus. The pubic bone is an irregularly shaped bone composed of a body and two rami, the superior and inferior pubic rami. The body forms the front third of the acetabulum. The upper ramus extends from the body to the midsagittal plane, where it articulates with the corresponding ramus on the opposite side. The joint formed by the two superior pubic rami is called the pubic symphysis, which is a slightly movable joint containing a cartilaginous disc between the two bones. The lower pubic ramus joins with the ramus of the ischium to form the bottom arch of the obturator foramen. The inferior pubic rami likewise join each other through the pubic symphysis.

The Sacrum and Coccyx

The rear wall of the pelvic girdle is composed of the sacrum and the coccyx. The former is a fusion of five sacral vertebrae and is triangular in shape. Its auricular surfaces form a solid joint with the pelvis through which the weight of the upper torso is transmitted to the legs or the ischial tuberosities. The bone is concave toward the front and supports the lumbar spine at the top.

The coccyx is a vestigial tail made up of three to five fused vertebra. The vertebrae do not have all of the features of normal vertebrae, inasmuch as they are devoid of all the posterior structures, and the last vertebra is a mere nodule of bone. The sacral-coccygeal joint is a slightly movable joint, interposed by a thin disc of cartilage that is stiffer than a normal intervertebral disc.

Orientation of the Pelvis

This orientation varies from person to person and is different for the standing and seated posture. Quantification of orientation requires a plane of reference that appears as a straight line when the pelvis is viewed laterally. Nyquist and Murton (1975) proposed that the plane formed by the two ASIS's and the pubic symphysis can be used as a reference. The three landmarks are palpable, and x-ray is not needed to identify them. Although a method exists to define pelvic orientation, it is not known whether a large body of data exists for either the standing or seated posture. According to Gray (1973), the variation in pelvic orientation in the standing posture is about 10 deg.

The Proximal Femur

Since the femur articulates with the pelvis and injuries are often located in the vicinity of the hip joint, it is necessary to discuss briefly the anatomy of the proximal femur. The femur is the longest and strongest bone in the body and is roughly cylindrical in shape along its shaft. However, the shape of the two ends is different from that of the shaft. In particular, the proximal or upper portion of the femur is made up of a head, neck, and trochanteric region. A view of the proximal femur from the rear is shown in Fig. 17.11.

The head of the femur has a spherical shape, forming a synovial joint with the acetabulum. This joint is commonly known as the hip joint. The surface of the head is lined with a layer of hyaline cartilage, typical of a synovial joint. Its blood supply comes through the neck of the femur, which is the structure below the head.

The neck of the femur is shaped like a truncated cone and connects the head with the rest of the femur. It is almost cylindrical at the

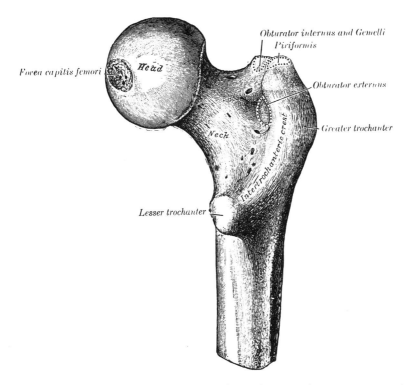

Obturator internus and Gemelli
Piriformis

Fovea capitis femori

Head

Obturator externus

Neck

Intertrochanteric crest

Greater trochanter

Lesser trochanter

FIGURE 17.11. Rear view of the proximal (upper) femur. (From Gray, 1973.)

base of the head, and its axis is at an angle of about 125 deg with the femoral shaft. In the female, this angle can be as low as 90 deg. The lower boundary of the neck is defined by the intertrochanteric crest in the rear and by the intertrochanteric line in the front. Both boundaries are well-defined ridges that act to demarcate the neck from the trochanteric region.

The trochanteric region is an enlarged portion of the proximal femoral shaft distinguished by two landmarks, the greater and lesser trochanter. The former is a prominence that extends laterally from the base of the neck and is easily palpable in most people. The level of its upper boundary corresponds to the center of the femoral head or the center of the hip joint. The lesser trochanter is a smaller prominence on the inside of the femur. It is visible on x-ray but not palpable.

The proximal femur is covered by a layer of cortical or compact bone and contains spongy or cancellous bone within. The strength and density of the spongy bone varies with age and sex. Impact trauma can cause fractures to the head, neck, or trochanter. As the fracture line moves downward from the head, the fracture type changes from subcapital to transcervical to intertrochanteric and peritrochanteric.

Pelvic Injuries from Clinical Experience

A survey of pelvic injury patterns as reported in the clinical literature was made in an effort to understand the various types of injuries to this body structure. Although the more recent clinical literature tends to report injuries to the pelvis due to auto-related accidents, the reports generally cover pelvic injuries from all causes, such as crushing injuries to miners, falls, and excessive muscular activity. Many of the papers describe injuries to the hip joint and the proximal femur along with those of the bony pelvis. The extension into the hip joint has a sound clinical basis, since the treatment of the hip and upper femur involves the pelvis, and the hip and pelvis are frequently injured simultaneously. This discussion will therefore include injuries to the hip joint and the upper femur.

This review is divided into pelvic injury types, hip injury types, and clinical incidence. A comprehensive summary of injuries sustained by the entire anatomical region was found in Watson-Jones (1976), and that classification is presented here.

Pelvic Injuries

Injuries to the pelvis, not involving the hip joint, can be classified under four distinct headings: avulsions of muscle insertions, isolated fractures of the pelvic ring, double or multiple fracture of the pelvic ring, and fractures of the sacrum and coccyx.

Avulsions of Muscle Insertions

Due to excessive muscular activity, a portion of the pelvis can be avulsed or separated from the main bone at the point of muscle insertion. For example, the ASIS can be avulsed by the sartorius muscle, or the hamstrings can avulse the ischial tuberosity. These injuries occur in young adults who are engaged in athletic activities, and they are not the result of impact-type accidents.

Isolated Fractures of the Pelvic Ring

If there is a single fracture around the pelvic ring, significant displacement of the fractured segments does not arise. Unilateral fractures of the superior or inferior pubic rami, or of both rami, are examples of isolated fractures that do not require surgical intervention. Other isolated fractures include single fractures of the ilium with minor separation of the pubic symphysis, separation of the pubic symphysis, and sacroiliac subluxation (slippage). These injuries appear to be the result of minor impacts. For example, in a side impact aimed at the greater trochanter, pubic rami fractures frequently occur.

Multiple Fractures or Fracture-Dislocations

With multiple fractures, the pelvic ring becomes unstable. Large displacements of the fragments are possible. The two main types of injury are fractures of the pubic segments only and fractures of the pubic bone associated with fractures of the ilium.

Multiple injuries of the pubis consist of two or more fractures of the rami with dislocation of the pubic symphysis. They occur in pedestrians struck on the side of the pelvis by an automobile. In general, fractures of the rami occur on the nonimpacted side. If there are bilateral multiple fractures of the rami, the impacted side cannot be firmly established. Although surgical intervention is not required, the patient can suffer urinary tract injuries, such as rupture of the urethra, a duct that conducts urine out of the body from the bladder (Wiggishoff and Kiefer, 1968).

The most common type of combined injuries of the iliac and pubic segments is the dislocation of the pubic symphysis with dislocation of the sacroiliac joint. Other types of injury include the fracture of the ilium accompanied by a dislocation of the pubic symphysis or fracture of both rami on one side with sacroiliac dislocation on the same side. Bladder and urethral injuries are common is these cases. The mechanism of injury is a force applied from the front to the back as opposed to a sideward force in the previous case.

Injuries to the Sacrum and Coccyx

Extensive injuries to the pelvis can result in fractures of the sacrum. These usually occur in regions of stress concentration; that is, across the foramina or holes through which the sacral nerves pass. There may be associated nerve injury. Vertical acceleration can cause compression of the sacrum with a loss in height. Coccygeal injuries are sustained in falls in a sitting position. The injury can be a contusion, fracture, or dislocation of the coccyx. Although it is not a serious injury, it can be extremely painful.

Associated Soft-Tissue Injuries

The most serious soft-tissue injury associated with pelvic fractures is hemorrhage. It comes from large blood vessels in the pelvic wall as well as from the fractured surfaces themselves. The amount of blood loss can be large, and one of the methods to stop the hemorrhage is to ligate the internal iliac arteries. Injuries to the bladder and urethra and to the abdominal viscera are also common. These injuries will be discussed in detail below.

Hip Injuries

These injuries occur in and around the hip joint. They involve one or more of the following structures: acetabulum, femoral head, and proximal femur. In the adolescent, damage to the epiphysis in the proximal femur can occur, and in the aged injuries to the hip are the result of bone loss and decreased resilience. Hip injuries can be grouped under three main headings: avulsions of the proximal femoral epiphysis, traumatic hip dislocations, and fractures of the neck of the femur.

Avulsions of the Epiphysis

These injuries occur in adolescents due to powerful muscular exertions. The greater and lesser trochanter can be avulsed by muscular violence during athletic competition.

Traumatic Hip Dislocations and Fracture-Dislocations

These injuries are described below according to whether the dislocations are accompanied by injuries to the pelvis (acetabulum), femoral head, femoral neck, and femoral shaft.

The easiest way to dislocate a hip is to flex and adduct the hip and to apply a force along the femur rearward. In this position the hip joint is not supported by any bony structure. Automobile occupants who undergo a frontal impact with their legs crossed are liable to sustain this dislocation injury. If the hip is not fully adducted, fracture of the lip of the acetabulum along the back of the hip joint can occur together with a backward dislocation of the hip joint. Central dislocation with fracture of the acetabulum occurs when the hip is struck from the side, such as in a side-impact collision. The near-side occupant is struck by the door at the level of the greater trochanter,

causing the femoral head to punch through the thin wall of the acetabulum. The mechanism of a central acetabular fracture due to a side impact to the greater trochanter has been reproduced in a series of cadaveric experiments by Pearson and Hargadon (1962), who used 56-lb (25.5-kg) and 150-lb (68.2-kg) pendulums to cause these fractures. Grattan and Hobbs (1969) reported that six out of seven cases of central acetabular fracture were due to side impact, while Eichenholtz and Stark (1964) asserted that the mechanism was a blow to the greater trochanter. This injury can also occur in the standing posture with the hip joint in a neutral position. A heavy blow to the shoulders or back can cause the hip to abduct, forcing the head of the femur into the acetabulum. If the hip is abducted, a rearward impact to the femur can cause an anterior (forward) dislocation. A rear seat passenger in a frontal crash can be forced into the seat back with the thighs abducted and suffer such a dislocation (Beaupre, 1973). If the knee is wedged between the front seat back and the wall of the vehicle, separation of the sacroiliac joint can result (Markham, 1972).

In rearward dislocations of the hip joint involving fracture of the rim of the acetabulum, the femoral head can also be fractured. There is the prospect of developing a long-term disability in the form of traumatic arthritis. According to Armstrong (1948), the incidence is as high as 60%.

Hip dislocations accompanied by injuries to the femoral neck are rarely seen and occur in the elderly group. Necrosis of the head of the femur due to loss of blood supply (avascular necrosis) tends to result from these injuries. The mechanism of injury is a high tensile bending stress applied to the femoral neck causing it to fracture as the joint is dislocated.

Dislocations with fracture of the femoral shaft are also rare and are easy to miss on x-rays (Schoenecker et al., 1978). The mechanism of injury is unknown, but bending of the shaft is involved because the fractures tend to be transverse.

Fractures of the Neck of the Femur

There are two major classes of femoral neck fractures, intracapsular and extracapsular. The hip joint capsule, or the fibrous tissues enclosing the joint, extends from the pelvis to the inter-trochanteric line of the femur. If a fracture occurs within the capsule, it can be a subcapital fracture of the head or a transcervical fracture of the neck. Extracapsular fractures can be either intertrochanteric or peritrochanteric.

Clinical Incidence of Pelvic Injuries

Six large series of clinical studies involving pelvic injuries are summarized. Three of the six were concerned with skeletal injuries, one with massive hemorrhage, and two with abdominal injuries.

Ryan (1971) surveyed 713 patients between 1956 and 1967 with fractures and fracture-dislocations of the pelvis. X-ray films of 387 patients admitted between 1958 and 1963 were studied in detail. A large majority (321 of the 387 patients) were traffic accident victims, including 154 pedestrians and a large group of 140 of unknown status. Only twenty were known to be occupants. The most common fracture was that of the pubic ramus (305), followed by the acetabulum (89), and the ilium (79). There were a total of 116 dislocations divided approximately equally among those of the hip, pubic symphysis, and sacroiliac joint.

Conolly and Hedberg (1969) reported on 200 patients with pelvic injuries. They classified them as being major or minor. Injuries that involve the line of weight transmission and bilateral fracture of the pubic rami were con-sidered major. A total of 109 patients sustained major injuries. The four major injuries were acetabular fracture (49), bilateral pubic rami fracture (34), multiple fracture of the hemi-pelvis (21), and separation of the pubic symphysis (5). Among the minor injuries, there were 82 cases of unilateral fracture of rami and an occasional case of isolated fracture of the ilium. In the third study by Kulowski (1962), he reported on 145 cases of hip, femur, and knee injuries sustained by automotive occupants. There were a total of 184 lesions, with 23 patients having multiple injuries. Twelve cases of hip injury were associated with femoral shaft fractures or knee injuries, and

there were only three cases of pelvic fractures.

Hauser and Perry (1966) looked at 196 patients with pelvic fractures and analyzed the role played by hemorrhage. About two-thirds of the patients were traffic accident victims. The total mortality rate was 19.4%. However, those with significant blood loss suffered a mortality rate of 30% (19 out of 63 patients). There was more blood loss in the more severely injured patients who required more trans-fusions. It was suggested that ligation of the hypogastric arteries saved three of four patients so treated.

As far as associated abdominal injuries are concerned, there were two surveys. Levine and Crampton (1963) reported on a series of 425 patients with pelvic girdle fractures. Only 35 patients had severe or major abdominal injuries (8.2%). This is much lower than the 22% to 29% rate reported previously. Thirty-three of the 35 patients had traffic-related injuries. A total of fifteen types of complicating injuries were listed. They can be grouped under the following categories:

Injuries to the bladder, urethra, and vagina with or without vascular injuries
Injuries to the hard abdominal organs (liver, spleen, and kidney)
Injuries to the small intestine, mesentery, and diaphragm
Hemothorax
Retroperitoneal hemorrhage
Nerve injuries (frequently to the sciatic nerve).

This survey shows a low percentage of urinary tract injuries (3.5%) compared to 9% to 21% in other surveys. This may be due to the heavy concentration of cases related to automotive trauma. In the other survey of 1,309 cases by Moore (1966), there were only twenty-six cases of intra-abdominal injuries not involving the urogenital organs. The paper was concerned with perforation of the large and small intes-tines and laceration of the mesentery. There were 11 patients with perforation of the in-testines and not other injuries. Ten of the 26 patients had multiple intra-abdominal injuries, including perforations and lacerations. No mechanisms of injury were proposed.

Pelvic Impact Response and Tolerance to Injury

Research on pelvic response to static and dynamic loads and associated injury thresholds can be categorized in terms of direction of loading: vertical, frontal, and lateral. Early work on pelvic response to vertical loading constituted a significant contribution to the literature, but, when viewed from current perspectives, it appears to be largely qualitative due to the lack of instrumentation at that time. Pelvic response to frontal loads applied via the femur was studied by several investigators. Although the data are rather sparse, it is possible to determine a response relationship between knee load and pelvic acceleration. In side impact, there are recent data that can be used to establish injury tolerance of the pelvis as a function of pelvic deformation, age, and body weight.

Vertical Loading

Data on pelvic response to vertical loads were provided by Evans and Lissner (1955) and Fasola et al. (1955), who performed vertical loading tests on human pelves. In the former study, stress-coat lacquer was used to determine the areas of high tensile strain during the application of static and dynamic loads to the pelvis. Input energies from 3.7 to 12.8 N.m (33 to 113 in-lb) were applied to the ischial tuberosities of 22 isolated pelves, 16 of which were embalmed. Tensile strain patterns were found on both surfaces of the iliac wing, around the acetabulum, and on the pubic rami. In a second series of test, the entire body was dropped vertically onto the ischial tuberosities resulting in input energy levels of 22.6 to 50.9 N.m (200 to 450 in-lb). Fracture of the ischiopubic ramus occurred in a 79-year-old male pelvis at 27.1 N.m (240 in-lb). The strain pattern was similar to that observed in the first series.

The study by Fasola et al. (1955) involved the dropping of a weight onto the lumbar spine of cadaveric specimens. The lower portion of the pelvis, including the proximal femur, was embedded in cement to hold the pelvis upright. A force of 3.7 kN (830 lb) was necessary to

cause a bilateral dislocation of the sacroiliac joint. The disjunction was due to avulsion of the bone at sites of ligamentous attachment near the joint. Static loading resulted in a fracture dislocation of the joint at a load of 3.5 kN (775 lb).

Frontal Loading

Evans and Lissner (1955) also carried out stress-coat studies on the pelvis, which was loaded frontally at the pubic symphysis, and identified regions of tensile strain. Fasola et al. (1955) produced bilateral fracture of the superior and inferior pubic rami with a load of 2.7 kN (595 lb).

Sled tests to elicit the response of the knee-thigh-pelvis complex to frontally applied impact loads were carried out by Patrick et al. (1966), using embalmed cadavers. Most of the study was concerned with the tolerance of the knee and femur, but there were data on the fracture loads of the proximal femur and the pelvis. The hip sustained fractures at loads ranging from 4.2 to 17.1 kN (950 to 3,850 lb) among the 10 cadavers tested. The load range for pelvic fractures was 6.2 to 11.8 kN (1,400 to 2,650 lb). The authors considered these load limits to be conservative because of the age of the cadavers. However, the wide range over a limited number of tests renders statistical analysis difficult. A normalization procedure for cadaver data needs to be formalized before these data can be used.

In a more recent study, Melvin and Nusholtz (1980) performed six sled tests on unembalmed cadavers during which knee loads and pelvic accelerations were measured. Two knee load cells were used, but they were tied together by a rigid plate to minimize errors due to excessive bending. Impact load peaks varying from 8.9 to 25.6 kN (2,000 to 5,760 lb) resulted in hip and/or pelvic fractures. There were also femoral shaft fractures and injuries to the patella and condyles. There was only one case in which the hip or pelvis was not involved, and in a lightweight individual the loads generated were insufficient to cause any fracture (6.2 to 8.1 kN, 1,400 to 1,820 lb). Pelvic accelerations were indicative of load transfer to the pelvis, and abrupt changes in the acceleration signal were representative of pelvic fractures occurring. Acceleration traces were provided in the report by Melvin and Nusholtz, but their peaks were not listed or correlated with injury. It is also interesting to note that the knee force curves showed a double peak if there was fracture of the femoral neck followed by that of the shaft. There was only a single peak if the shaft fractured first.

In another study by Nusholtz et al. (1982), 37 knee impacts were carried out on 16 cadavers, using a pendulum impactor. The test subject was suspended in a restraint harness and impacted frontally at the knee or laterally at the level of the greater trochanter. Only the frontal impacts are discussed here. The impactor surface was either rigid or padded by three different types of foam: 25 mm (0.5 in) of Styrofoam or 25 to 100 mm (0.5 to 4 in) of Ensolite. Impactor velocity varied from 3.4 to 21.3 m/s (11.2 to 69.9 ft/s). Pelvic and trochanteric acceleration were monitored along with impactor force. No pelvic or hip fractures occurred at force levels as high as 37 kN (8,300 lb). Response data in the form of pelvic linear and angular acceleration were provided. However, acceleration data were difficult to analyze. For example, the magnitudes of the three components of angular acceleration of the pelvis were inconsistent in that the component about the spinal axis (z-axis) was not always predominant. Initial rotation of the pelvis appeared to be about the contralateral trochanter, but subsequent motion of the pelvis and femur were rather complex. Peak pelvic accelerations were less than those of the greater trochanter and were found to lag the trochanteric acceleration. Mechanical impedance was used as an analytical tool, and resonance was estimated to occur between 180 and 280 Hz. Impedance corridors were plotted for both the pelvis and the trochanter. However, because of the large scatter in the data, it was difficult to obtain average values of mass and spring rate for the pelvis.

Brun-Cassan et al. (1982) conducted 10 whole-body impacts on unrestrained and unembalmed cadavers at collision speeds of 49.5 to 67.1 km/h (30.7 to 41.7 mph). Peak knee loads ranged from 3.7 to 11.4 kN (830 to 2,560 lb). There was only one fracture injury noted, that of the right patella and iliac crest at a knee load of 8.8 kN (1,980 lb). Finally, Doorly (1978) impacted isolated pelves with a drop weight causing acetabular and hip injuries. The impact force was not measured but was computed from energy considerations. The computed average force could not be correlated to the observed injuries.

Lateral Loading

Cadaveric research on lateral impact response of the pelvis was performed at Organisme National de Securite Routiere (ONSER), Association Peugeot-Renault (APR), University of Michigan Transportation Research Institute (UMTRI), the University of Heidelberg, and Wayne State University. Results from each laboratory will be discussed separately without regard to chronology. Repeated impacts were carried out on ONSER test subjects, while the APR studies were single drop tests on a variety of surfaces. The UMTRI lateral tests were single impacts. At the University of Heidelberg, whole-body sled tests were conducted in the side-impact mode. There were two series of tests at Wayne State University—pendulum impacts sponsored by General Motors (GM) and whole-body impacts sponsored by the Centers for Disease Control (CDC).

ONSER

Pendulum impacts on cadaveric subjects were reported by Ramet and Cesari (1979), Cesari et al. (1980), and Cesari and Ramet (1982). The latest report was given by Cesari et al. (1983), which contains all of the results reported since 1979. A total of 22 cadavers were used in this effort by ONSER. There were a total of 60 tests, using a 17.3-kg (38-lb) pendulum impactor with a 175-mm (6.9-in) diameter impact face having a spherical radius of curvature of 600 mm (23.6 in). The impact speeds ranged from 21 to 44.6 km/h (13.0 to 27.7 mph). Each cadaver sustained multiple (two to five) impacts that were administered at increasing velocities until fracture occurred. In

55 of these tests, a rigid impactor was used. The remaining tests were padded impacts. All impacts were aimed at the greater trochanter. Impact force and pelvic acceleration were measured. Peak force data as well as force and acceleration data, except for cumulative durations less than 3 ms (the so-called 3-ms clip), were provided.

Most of the injuries were multiple fractures of the pubic rami. In order of frequency of occurrence, these were followed by fractures of the proximal femur, dislocation of the sacroiliac joint, fractures of the iliac wing, and fractures of the acetabulum. The authors stated that this pattern of injury compared favorably with data from fourteen accidents, the source of which was not given. In general, the experimental injuries were less severe because the tests were suspended fractures of the rami while standing subjects (pedestrians) are more prone to acetabular fractures. No reason was given for the observed difference in injury pattern. There were three femoral neck fractures out of the 22 cadavers tested. This is more frequent than that in the accident data in which there was only one case of femoral neck fracture out of a total of 14 cases.

In terms of quantitative data, the results were separated into two groups by sex. For males, the force for fracture with the 3-ms clip, ranged from 4.9 to 11.9 kN (1,100 to 2,900 lb). The corresponding range for females was 4.4 to 8.2 kN (1,000 to 1,840 lb). The average force for an AIS-2 or -3 pelvic injury was 8.6 kN (1,930 lb) for males and 5.6 kN (1,260 lb) for females. The age range for males was 54 to 85 years, and that for females was 54 to 84. An index was introduced to correct for the body weight and height of the test subjects. It was termed the Livi Index, which is the ratio of the cube root of the body weight in kg and 10 times the standing height in meters. The Livi Index is used to obtain a corrected body weight. The Livi Index for a 50th percentile male is 23.5. Thus, the correction factor is the ratio of 23.5 to the computed Livi Index of the test subject. The corrected weight of the subject is the product of the correction factor and its actual weight. By plotting the fracture-producing force at 3 ms against actual body weight, the correlation coefficient was found to be 0.75. It increased to 0.89 if the corrected weight was used. The least squares line for impact force as a function of corrected body weight is given by:

$$\text{Impact Force} = 193.85\,Wc - 4{,}710.6$$

where Wc is the corrected body weight. For a 50th percentile male weighing 75 kg (165 lb), the impact force for fracture is 9.8 kN (2,210 lb), which is higher than that of the average of the male cadaver data. The measured acceleration values with the 3-ms clip were less than 100 G. The authors defended their multiple impact procedure vigorously, stating that the force-time histories were consistent in pattern for multiple impacts and that the impact force increased consistently with increasing impactor speed.

The effect of using a padded impactor was studied in five tests on three cadavers. Two of them sustained AIS-3 injuries while one had AIS-2 injuries. The force required to cause fracture was about the same as that for a rigid impactor, but the speed of the impactor could be increased by 40%.

Following dynamic testing, the nonimpacted hemipelvis was instrumented with nine strain gates and subjected to a static lateral load. High strains were measured in the pubic rami followed by strains in the ischiopubic rami. Strains were low in the acetabulum and ilium. Section moduli of the iliopubic rami were measured and plotted against the impact force at fracture. The resulting least squares line had a correlation coefficient of 0.96.

The proposed tolerance force with the 3-ms clip is 10 kN (2,250 lb) for a 75-kg (165-lb) person. This reduces to 4.6 kN (1,030 lb) for a 5th percentile female. The authors recommended that side-impact dummies should be fitted with a lateral force transducer. This transducer should be located in the anterior region of the pelvis, such as near the pubic rami where many injuries occur.

In a later paper presenting the development of an improved anthropomorphic test device (ATD) pelvis for lateral impact, Cesari et al. (1984) discussed the use of the ATD pelvic acceleration with the 3-ms clip as an injury criterion. They concluded that injury does not correlate with impactor maximum force as well as it does with maximum pelvic acceleration ($r = 0.891$ versus $r = 0.986$). However, their pelvis design was also shown to produce higher accelerations than those obtained with cadavers. A linear regression analysis of cadaver maximum pelvic lateral acceleration versus impactor force produced a correlation coefficient of 0.77.

APR

The bulk of the APR data are contained in reports by Fayon et al. (1977) and Tarriere et al. (1979). The latter contains all of the side impact data acquired at APR via a series of 26 cadaveric drop tests. The subjects ranged in age from 25 to 71 years and in weight from 41 to 75 kg (90 to 165 lb). Each subject was dropped only once, but there was a variety of test configurations and impact surfaces for the thorax as well as the pelvis. The subject was suspended with cables and dropped on its side onto a load-measuring plate. The arm was either at a 45 deg angle or was pulled out of the way during thoracic impact. The impact surfaces were rigid planes or padded surfaces. Some supported the shoulder at impact while others did not. When energy-absorbing pads were used, the thorax and pelvis impacted separate blocks. The thoracic impact load was measured by a load cell. Pelvic response was given in terms of pelvic acceleration, measured at the sacrum in the midsagittal plane, 90 mm (3.5 in) distal to the iliac crests. The condition of the bone was characterized by its ash content given as a percentage of wet weight (C/M) and ash content in 10 mm (0.4 in) of rib given in g/cm (C/L). Undamaged ribs were also subjected to standard bending and shear tests.

The drop height ranged from 0.5 to 3 m (20 to 118 in). Fractures of the pubic rami were observed in four subjects. There were multiple injuries in one subject who sustained fractures of the iliac wing and acetabulum in addition to the fractures of the rami. In the other 22 subjects, there were no pelvic or hip injuries. There were no femoral neck fractures. If data from a 68-year-old female subject are ignored, the lowest fracture level is 50 G with the 3-ms

clip and the highest is 90 G with the 3-ms clip. The proposed tolerance level is 80 to 90 G with the 3-ms clip. Note that this is pelvic acceleration and not that of the impactor.

UMTRI

Published UMTRI data consist of 12 tests reported by Nusholtz et al. (1982) using a flat pendulum impactor. Most of the impacts were aimed at the greater trochanter of a cadaver suspended in a restraint harness. Impact force and pelvic acceleration were measured. The peak force ranged from 3.2 to 14 kN (720 to 3,150 lb), and the peak linear acceleration varied from 38 to 135 G for impact speeds of 18.4 to 31.0 km/h (11.4 to 19.2 mph). Six of the 12 cadavers sustained pelvic fractures. Four of them had fractures of the pubic rami, and one sustained fractures to the ilium. These injuries did not occur at high force or acceleration levels. The absence of femoral neck fractures was again noted. The lack of correspondence between observed injuries and measured data was attributed to variation among subjects. It was also concluded that these data were not comparable to those of ONSER, since the test setup and impactor configurations were all different.

University of Heidelberg

Marcus et al. (1983) presented data from 11 cadaver tests carried out at the University of Heidelberg. They were whole-body side-impact tests in which the thoracic and pelvic impact surfaces were instrumented with load cells to measure contact force. Eight of the 11 tests were rigid wall impacts at 24, 32, and 40 km/h (15, 20, and 25 mph). The other three were padded impacts at 32 km/h (20 mph), using foam developed by APR. Subjects ranged in age from 17 to 61 years and in weight from 50 to 99 kg (110 to 218 lb). The body weight was corrected in the same manner as that proposed by Cesari and Ramet (1982), using the Livi Index. The pelvic impact force was then plotted against corrected body weight. Among the 11 data points, there were three pelvic injuries with an AIS rating of 2 or 3, but the type of injury was not disclosed. The range of pelvic forces at 3 ms was 3.6 to 28.9 kN (800 to 6,500 lb). It was concluded from this study that the tolerance limits proposed by Cesari and Ramet may be too conservative. It was also determined that 28% of the inertial force of impact was transmitted via the pelvis.

Wayne State University (GM Tests)

Viano et al. (1989) performed a series of 14 pendulum impact tests on unembalmed cadavers at Wayne State University. The mass of the 150-mm diameter pendulum was 23.4 kg and its speed varied from 16.2 to 33.8 km/h (10.0 to 21.0 mph). The impact location was the greater trochanter. Lateral pelvic response was reported in the form of force-deflection curves, as shown in Fig. 17.12. A variety of parameters was used to determine that suitability as a measure of tolerance. It was found that peak pelvic acceleration and pelvic deformation were not reliable measures. However, the ratio of pelvic deformation to pelvic width (percent compression) was found to correlate well with pubic rami fracture, which was the only type of injury observed. The tolerance level for 25% probability of serious injury to the pelvis was found to be 27% of pelvic compression, based on the entire width of the pelvis.

Wayne State University (CDC Tests)

A total of 16 whole-body side-impact tests have been run to date, using a modified University of Heidelberg setup in which the lateral impact force at the shoulder, thorax, abdomen, and pelvis were measured separately. It should also be noted that impact to the transmission of impact force to the pelvis was through the greater trochanter, as the pelvic load cell plate was only 100 mm high and was designed to miss the wing of the ilium. Cavanaugh et al. (1990) have already reported on data from the first 12 tests. The percent compression of the pelvis was again found to be the best measure of tolerance, based on a Logist analysis of the data. For a 25% probability of fracture, the tolerance is 32.6% of the struck side half width. Peak impact force and pelvic acceleration did not perform well as injury indicators. Pubic rami injuries were observed but again, there were no femoral neck fractures.

Pelvic Response to Frontal and Lateral Impacts

If pelvic response is defined as an acceleration output at the pelvis for a force input to either the knee, for frontal response, or the greater trochanter, for lateral response, the only published data that can provide this informa-

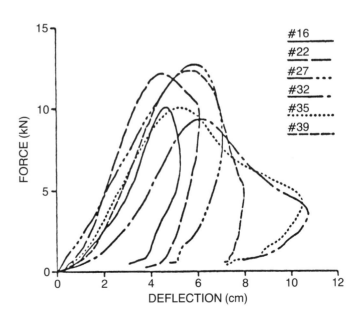

FIGURE 17.12. Force-deflection response of the pelvis during lateral impact. (From Viano et al., 1989.)

tion are found in Nusholtz et al. (1982). For frontal response, the peak force and acceleration data in Table 7 of Nusholtz et al. were analyzed by linear regression techniques. (Run 80L098 was considered to be an "outlier", and the data from this run were not used in the regression analysis.) For all 15 data points, including both rigid and padded knee impacts, the correlation coefficient is 0.78. If only rigid impacts are used, the result is a correlation coefficient of 0.80, a value similar to that obtained by Cesari et al. (1984) for lateral impacts. There is thus not a strong relationship between pelvic acceleration and knee loads.

A similar analysis was performed for all available lateral impact data provided by Nusholtz et al. (1982). A meaningful linear regression line could not be drawn for the lateral impact data. Its slope was almost zero, and the correlation coefficient was less than 0.1. The low correlation of maximum pelvic acceleration and peak input load was attributed to the highly variable response of the system to the point of load application and pelvis-leg orientation at the time of impact. However, in tests in which pelvic deformation was measured, there was excellent correlation of this variable with pelvic AIS, as was shown by Viano et al. (1989) and by Cavanaugh et al. (1990).

Summary and Conclusions

As a major load-bearing structure between the upper torso and the lower extremities, the pelvis plays an important role in controlling body kinematics. Injuries to the pelvis contribute only about 1% to the total Injury Priority Rating (IPR). Lateral response of the pelvis has been studied for both impactor and flat-wall impacts and has been described in terms of force-time histories and pelvic acceleration-time histories. Lateral loading tolerances for the pelvis are available in terms of peak deformation, force, and acceleration limits, with the deformation limit showing the best correlation to injury severity, as quantified by the pelvic AIS.

The infrequency of femoral neck fractures due to side impacts to the greater trochanter is a surprising finding. It has been hypothesized that the elderly sustain such injuries when they fall laterally and impact the greater trochanter. More research is necessary to determine if femoral neck fractures are spontaneous and if the fall is the result of the fracture and not the cause.

References

Adams MA, Huttan WC (1982) Prolapsed intervertebral disc. A hyperfletion injury. Spine 7: 184–191.

Armstrong JR (1948) Traumatic dislocation of the hip joint. J Bone Joint Surg 30B:430–445.

Avramov AI, Cavanaugh JM, Ozaktay AC, King AI. Effects of controlled mechanical loading on Group III and IV afferents from the lumbar facet joint: An in vitro study. In *Proceedings Eighteenth Annual Meeting of the Society for the Study of the Lumbar Spine*. University of Heidelberg, Heidelberg, pp 23–24, 1991.

Beaupre A. Trochanteric fractures. Proceedings Tenth Traffic Injury Research Foundation of Canada Annual Meeting. TIRF, Ottawa, pp 15–18, 1973.

Begeman PC, King AI, Levine RS, Viano DC. Biodynamic response of the musculoskeletal system to impact accelerations. In *Proceedings of the Twenty-fourth Stapp Car Crash Conference*. SAE 801312. Society of Automotive Engineers, Warrendale, PA, 1980.

Begeman PC, King AI, Prasad P. Spinal loads resulting from $-g_x$ acceleration. In *Proceedings of the Seventeenth Stapp Car Crash Conference*. SAE 730977. Society of Automotive Engineers, Warrendale, PA, 1973.

Belytschko T, Privitzer E. A three-dimensional discrete element dynamic model of the spine head and torso. In von Gierke HE (ed) *Models and analogues for the evaluation of human biodynamic response, performance and protection*. AGARD Conf Proc No. 253, pp A9-1 to A9-15, 1978.

Bogduk N, Twomey LT. *Clinical anatomy of the lumbar spine*. Churchill Livingstone, Melbourne, 1987.

Brinckmann P (1986) Injury of the annulus fibrosus and disc protrusions. An in vitro investigation on human lumbar discs. Spine 11:149–153.

Brown T, Hansen RJ, Yorra, AJ (1957) Some mechanical tests on the lumbosacral spine with particular references to the intervertebral discs. J Bone Joint Surg 39A:1135–1164.

Brun-Cassan F, Leung YC, Tarriere C, Fayon A, Patel A, Got C, Hureau J. Determination of knee-femur-pelvis tolerance from the simulation of car frontal impacts. Proceedings Seventh International Conference on the Biomechanics of Impacts. IRCOBI, pp 101–115, 1982.

Buckwalter JA. The fine structure of human intervertebral disc. In White AA, Gordon SL (eds) *Idiopathic low back pain*. Mosby, St. Louis, pp 108–143, 1982.

Cavanaugh JM, Walilko TJ, Malhotra A, Zhu Y, King AI. Biomechanical response and injury tolerance of the pelvis in twelve sled side impact tests. In *Proceedings Thirty-fourth Stapp Car Crash Conference*. SAE 902307. Society of Automotive Engineers, Warrendale, PA, 1990.

Cesari D, Bouquet R, Zac R. A new pelvis design for the European side impact dummy. In *Proceedings Twenty-eighth Stapp Car Crash Conference*. SAE 841650. Society of Automotive Engineers, Warrendale, PA, 1984.

Cesari D, Ramet M. Pelvic tolerance and protection criteria in side impact. In *Proceedings Twenty-sixth Stapp Car Crash Conference*. SAE 821159. Society of Automotive Engineers, Warrendale, PA, 1982.

Cesari D, Ramet M, Clair PY. Evaluation of pelvic fracture tolerance in side impact. In *Proceedings Twenty-sixth Stapp Car Crash Conference*. SAE 801306. Society of Automotive Engineers, Warrendale, PA, 1980.

Cesari D, Ramet M, Bouquet R. Tolerance of human pelvis to fracture and proposed pelvic protection criterion to be measured on side impact dummies. In *Proceedings Ninth International Technical Conference on Experimental Safety Vehicles*. Washington, DC, U.S. Department of Transportation, National Highway Traffic Safety Administration, pp 261–269, 1983.

Chance GO (1948) Note on a type of flexion fracture of the spine. Br J Radiol 21:452–453.

Conolly WB, Hedberg EA (1969) Observations on fractures of the pelvis. J Trauma 9:104–111.

Doorly TPG (1978) Forces imposed on the hip-joint in car collisions. J Traffic Med 6:44–46.

Eiband AM. Human tolerance to rapidly applied accelerations: A summary of the literature. NASA Memorandum No. 5-19-59E, 1959.

Eichenholtz SN, Stark RM (1964) Central acetabular fractures a review of thirty-five cases. J Bone Joint Surg 46:695–714.

El-Bohy AA, Yang KH, King AI (1989) Experimental verification of facet load transmission by direct measurement of facet/lamina contact pressure. J Biomechanics 22:931–941.

Evans FG, Lissner HR (1955) Studies on pelvic deformations and fractures. Anat Rec 121:141–165.

Ewing CL, King AI, Prasad P (1972) Structural considerations of the human vertebral column under $+g_z$ impact acceleration. J Aircraft 9:84–90.

Farfan HF, Cossette JW, Robertson GH, Wells RV, Kraus H (1970) The effects of torsion on the lumbar intervertebral joints: the role of torsion in the production of disc degeneration. J Bone Joint Surg 52A:468–497.

Fasola AF, Baker RC, Hitchcock FA. Anatomical and physiological effects of rapid decelerations. WADC-TR 54-218. Wright-Patterson AFB, Ohio, 1955.

Fayon A, Tarriere C, Walfisch G, Got C, Patel A. Contributions to defining the human tolerance to perpendicular side impact. Proc. Third International Conference on Impact Trauma, IRCOBI, pp 297–309, 1977.

Giles LGF, Taylor JR (1987) Innervation of lumbar zygapophysial joint synovial folds. Acta Orthop Scand 58:43–46.

Gordon SJ, Yang KH, Mayer PJ, Mace AH, Kish VL, Radin, EL (1991) Mechanism of disc rupture —a preliminary report. Spine 16:450–456.

Grattan E, Hobbs JA (1969) Injuries to hip joint in car occupants. Br Med J 11:71–73.

Gray H. *Anatomy of the human body*. Lea & Febiger, Philadelphia, 1973.

Hakim NS, King AI (1976) Programmed replication of in situ (whole-body) loading conditions during in vitro (substructure) testing of a vertebral column segment. J Biomech 9:629–632.

Hakim NS, King AI (1979) A three-dimensional finite element dynamic response analysis of a vertebra with experimental verification. J Biomech 12:277–292.

Hardy WG, Lissner HR, Webster JE, Gurdjian ES (1959) Repeated loading tests of the lumbar spine—a preliminary report. Surg Forum 9:690–695.

Hauser CW, Perry JF, Jr (1966) Massive hemorrhage from pelvic fractures. Minn Med 49:285–290.

Henzel JH, Mohr GC, von Gierke HE (1968) Reappraisal of biodynamic implications of human ejections. Aerospace Med 39:231–240.

Hess JL, Lombard CF (1958) Theoretical investigations of dynamic response of man to high vertical accelerations. Aviat Med 29:66–75.

Kazarian LE (1982) Injuries to the human spinal column: biomechanics and injury classification. Exerc Sport Sci Rev 9:297–352.

Kazarian LE, Beers K, Hernandez J (1979) Spinal injuries in the F/FB-111 crew escape system. Aviat Space Environ Med 50:948–957.

Kazarian LE, Boyd D, von Gierke H. The dynamic biomechanical nature of spinal fractures and articular facet derangement. AGARD Publication CP-88-71, Paper No. 19, 1971.

King AI, Chou CC (1976) Mathematical modelling, simulation and experimental testing of biomechanical system crash response. J Biomech 9:301–317.

King AI, Vulcan AP, Cheng LK. Effects of bending on the vertebral column of the seated human during caudocephalad acceleration. Proceedings of the Twenty-first Annual Conf Engg Med Biol, p 32, 1968.

King AI, Yamashita T, Ozaktay AC, Cavanaugh JM. A morphological study of the lumbar facet joint capsule and its innervation. Proceeding Sixth International Conference on Biomedical Engineering. National University of Singapore, Singapore, pp 32–35, 1990.

King AI, Yang KH. Biomechanics of the lumbar spine. In Schmid-Schonbein G (ed) *Frontiers in applied mechanics and biomechanics*. Springer-Verlag, New York, pp 210–224, 1985.

Kulowski J. Interconnected motorist injuries of the hip, femoral shaft and knee. In *Proceedings Fifth Stapp Automotive Crash and Field Demonstration Conference*. University of Minnesota, Minneapolis, pp 105–124, 1962.

Latham FA (1957) A study in body ballistics: seat ejection. Proc R Soc [B] 147:121–139.

Levine JI, Crampton RS (1963) Major abdominal injuries associated with pelvic fractures. Surg Gynecol Obstet 11:223–226.

Liu YK, Goel VK, Dejong A, Njus G, Nishiyama K, Buckwalter J (1985) Torsional fatigue of the lumbar intervertebral joints. Spine 10:894–900.

Liu YK, Njus G, Buckwalter J, Wakano K (1983) Fatigue response of lumbar intervertebral joints under axial cyclic loading. Spine 8:857–865.

Marchand F, Ahmed AM (1990) Investigation of the laminate structure of lumbar disc annulus fibrosus. Spine 15:402–410.

Marcus JH, Morgan RM, Eppinger RH, Kallieris D, Mattern R, Schmidt G. Human response to and injury from lateral impact. In *Proceedings Twenty-seventh Stapp Car Crash Crash Conference*. SAE 831634. Society of Automotive Engineers, Warrendale, PA, 1983.

Markham DE (1972) Anterior-dislocation of the hip and diastatis of the contralateral sacroiliac joint: the rear-seat passenger's injury? Br J Surg 59: 296–298.

Melvin J, Nusholtz G. Tolerance and response of the knee-femur-pelvis complex to axial impacts. UM-HSRI-80-27. University of Michigan, Highway Safety Research Institute, Ann Arbor, 1980.

Miniaci A, McLaren AC (1989) Anterolateral compression fracture of the thoracolumbar spine. A seat belt injury. Clin Orthop 240:153–156.

Mooney V, Robertson J (1976) The facet syndrome. Clin Orthop 115:149–156.

Moore JR (1966) Pelvic fractures: associated intestinal and mesenteric lesions. J Surg 9:253–261.

Nachemson A (1969) Intradiscal measurements of pH in patients with lumbar rhizopathies. Acta Orthop Scand 40:23–42.

Nicoll EA (1949) Fractures of the dorso-lumbar spine. J Bone Joint Surg 31B:376–393.

Nusholtz G, Alem NM, Melvin JW. Impact response and injury to the pelvis. In *Proceedings Twenty-sixth Stapp Car Crash Conference*. SAE 821160. Society of Automotive Engineers, Warrendale, PA, 1982.

Nyquist GW, Murton CJ. Static bending response of the human lower torso. In *Proceedings Nineteenth Stapp Car Crash Conference*. SAE 751158. Society of Automotive Engineers, Warrendale, PA, 1975.

Patrick LM, Korell CK, Mertz HJ, Jr. Forces on the human body in simulated crashes. Proceedings Ninth Stapp Car Crash Conference. University of Minnesota, Minneapolis, pp 237–259, 1966.

Patwardhan A, Vanderby R Jr, Lorenz M. Load bearing characteristics of lumbar facets in axial compressions. In Thibault L (ed) *1982 Advances in bioengineering*. ASME, 155–160, 1982.

Peacock A (1952) Observations on the postnatal structure of the intervertebral disc in man. J Anat 86:162–179.

Pearson JR, Hargadon EJ (1962) Fractures of the pelvis involving the floor of the acetabulum. J Bone Joint Surg 44B:550–561.

Pontius UR, Liu YK. Neuromuscular cervical spine model for whiplash. In SAE Publication No. SP-412, *Mathematical modeling biodynamic response to impact*. SAE 760770. Society of Automotive Engineers, Warrendale, PA, 1976.

Prasad P, King AI (1974) An experimentally validated dynamic model of the spine. J Appl Mech 41:545–550.

Prasad P, King AI, Ewing CL (1974) The role of articular facets during $+g_z$ accelerations. J Appl Mech 41:321–326.

Remet M, Cesari D. Experimental study of pelvis tolerance in lateral impact. Proceedings Fourth International Conference on the Biomechanics of Trauma. IRCOBI, pp 243–249, 1979.

Roaf R (1960) A study of the mechanics of spinal injuries. J Bone Joint Surg 42B:810–823.

Ruff S. Brief acceleration: less than one second. In German aviation medicine, World War II. U.S. Government Printing Office, Washington, DC, 1:584–597, 1950.

Ryan P (1971) Traffic injuries of the pelvis at St. Vincent's Hospital, Melbourne. Med J Aust 1: 475–479.

Schoenecker PL, Manske PR, Sertl GO (1978) Traumatic hip dislocation with ipsilateral femoral shaft fractures. Clin Orthop Rel Res 130:233–238.

Schultz A, Carter D, Grood E, King A, Panjabi M. Posterior support structures: basic science perspectives. In Frymoyer JW, Gordon SL (eds) *New perspectives on low back pain*. American Academy of Orthopedic Surgeons, Park Ridge, IL, 1988.

Shirazi-Adl A. Three-dimensional nonlinear finite element stress analysis of a lumbar intervertebral joint. PhD Thesis. McGill University, Montreal, 1984.

Shirazi-Adl A, Drouin G (1987) Load bearing role of facets in a lumbar segment under sagittal plane loadings. J Biomech 20:601–613.

Smith WS, Kaufer H. Lumbar seat belt fracture. In Selzer ML, Gikas PW, Huelke DF (eds) *The prevention of highway injury*. University of Michigan, Ann Arbor, MI, 1967.

States JD, Annechiarico RP, Good RG, Lieou J, Andrews M, Cushman L, Ingersoll G. A time comparison study of the New York State safety belt use law utilizing hospital admission and police accident report information. In *Proceedings Thirty-third Annual Conf of Assoc for the Advancement of Automotive Medicine*. AAAM, Des Plaines, IL, pp 265–281, 1989.

Steckler RM, Epstein JA, Epstein BS (1969) Seat belt trauma to the lumbar spine: an unusual manifestation of the seat belt syndrome. J Trauma 9:508–513.

Stokes IAF (1987) Surface strain on human intervertebral discs. J Orthop Res 5:348–355.

Tarriere C, Walfisch G, Fayon A, Rosey JP, Got C, Patel A, Delmas A. Synthesis of human tolerance obtained from lateral impact simulations. In *Proceedings Seventh International Technical Conference on Experimental Safety Vehicles*. U.S. Department of Transportation, National Highway Traffic Safety Administration, Washington, DC, pp 359–373, 1979.

Tennyson SA, King AI. A biodynamic model of the human spinal column. Trans SAE 760771, 1976.

Tennyson SA, King AI. Mathematical models of the spine. In Avala XJR (ed) *Proceedings of the First International Conference on Mathematical Modeling*. Vol 2, pp 977–985, 1977.

Viano DC, Lau IV, Asbury C, King AI, Begeman P. Biomechanics of the human chest, abdomen, and pelvis in lateral impact. In *Proceedings Thirty-third Annual Conference of Assoc. for the Advancement of Automotive Medicine*. AAAM, Des Plaines, IL, pp 367–382, 1989.

Watson-Jones R. *Fractures and joint injuries*. Churchill Livingstone, London, 1976.

Wiggishoff CC, Kiefer JH (1968) Urethral injury associated with pelvic fracture. J Trauma 8:1042–1048.

Yamashita T, Cavanaugh JM, El-Bohy AA, Getchell TV, King AI (1990) Mechanosensitive afferent units in the lumbar facet joint. J Bone Joint Surg 72A:865–870.

Yang KH, Byrd III AJ, Kish VL, Radin EL (1988) Annulus fibrosus tears—an experimental model. Orthop Trans 12:86–87.

Yang KH, King AI (1984) Mechanism of facet load transmission as a hypothesis for low back pain. Spine 9:557–565.

18
Injury to the Extremities

Robert Levine

An understanding of how bones respond to loads that cause failure (fractures) can help one understand the forces that cause the damage. Figure 18.1 is an injury not uncommonly seen in emergency rooms and orthopedic offices. It is not uncommon for a patient with this injury to state that it happened during a fall. However, if one asks this patient, "Who did you hit?" the patient usually looks at you sheepishly and says that he was in a fight or got angry and hit a wall. The x-ray shows what is known as a boxer's fracture, which usually results from hitting someone or something with a closed fist. The normal reaction when falling is to open one's hand and fall on the open hand, sustaining a wrist or elbow fracture. An understanding of the biomechanics of extremity injuries not infrequetly allows one to determine the trauma that caused an injury.

There are many classifications of injuries. Unfortunately the same group of injuries may have more than one classification associated with it. Sometimes a classification is of only historical interest, for a newer understanding of the injuries has led to a better classification system. The old one, however, should not be forgotten, for older literature and medical charts may use the old classification system. The classification system may vary from locale to locale. One center may believe that factor x is important in the understanding of a given problem and its treatment and therefore base its system on factor x, while another center may believe that the most relevant information is factor y and have a classification based on that factor. The same injuries may be classified differently in different countries. In the United States and Canada, growth plate injuries are usually classified with the Salter-Harris system, while in Switzerland and Germany, one commonly finds the same injuries classified by the Müeller method. A given system may change. The Abbreviated Injury Scale (AIS) was originally developed in 1959. In the past 20 years it has undergone several modifications; an injury that was AIS 3 in 1960 may be only AIS 2 today. The AIS levels of 7, 8, and 9[a] are no longer used. Classifications can be useful when used properly but can also cause confusion when used incorrectly.

Injury Scaling

There are several general classifications of injuries in common use and these attempt to categorize all injuries an extremity may sustain. One of the earliest is the AIS, which was originally published in the *Journal of the American Medical Association* in 1971.[1] In its original form it was a 10-point scale (0 to 9) and it was designed primarily to be used in motor vehicle accidents (impact or blunt trauma). In the past 20 years it has evolved to where it is

---

[a] Originally 9 indicted more than three fatal lesions within that patient. Revisions of AIS would code each AIS 6 lesion separately. AIS 9 currently means that the injury level is unknown; in the original AIS this would have been AIS 99.

FIGURE 18.1. Boxer's fracture, which usually results from hitting someone or something with a closed fist.

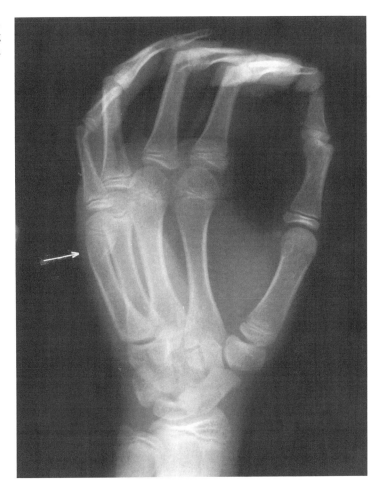

applied to all traumatic injuries including blunt & pennited. In its current form it is a 6-point scale that ranges from AIS 1 (minor) to AIS 6 (currently untreatable).[2] Table 18.1 summarizes the AIS 90 injury levels. The current format is a six-digit number followed by a decimal point and a digit after the decimal point. The six digits to the left of the decimal point identify the body region (first digit), type of anatomic structure (second digit), specific anatomic structure (third and fourth digits), and level of injury within the specific body region (fifth and sixth digits). The single digit to the right of the decimal point is the AIS level for the specific injury.

AIS has been proven to be an excellent measure of injury severity but it has not been as useful as a predictor of impairment and outcome. In AIS 90 there essentially is no

TABLE 18.1. Abbreviated Injury Scale (AIS) injury levels.

AIS code	Description
1	Minor
2	Moderate
3	Serious
4	Severe
5	Critical
6	Maximum
9	Unknown

skeletal injury with a severity level greater than AIS 3. The healing time of a significant skeletal injury is measured in months. A joint injury, even with optimum treatment, can cause a permanent impairment. Many injuries whose severity is greater than skeletal injuries have a far shorter recovery time. For example, splenic laceration is graded between AIS 2 and AIS 5.

Once one has recovered from the surgery, which takes only a few weeks, no significant long-term impairment is expected. The AIS 4 or 5 spleen injury means an impairment of a few weeks, while the AIS 2 or 3 skeletal injury could mean an impairment that could last a lifetime.

Many injury victims have more than one injury. Yet, AIS looks at each injury separately. It considers each injury as if the others did not occur. An open, grossly contaminated fracture of the tibia has a far different prognosis than a similar tibia fracture that is closed. The treatment and results of a given injury in patients with multiple system injuries are often different than those in patients who have only one system injured. To better evaluate the mortality rate for multiply injured patients, Baker et al.,[3] after noting the shortcomings of AIS, developed the Injury Severity Score (ISS). The ISS is the sum of the squares of the AIS for the three most-severely injured body regions. No region may be represented more than once in the calculation of ISS. ISS is considered to be 75 if an individual has an AIS 6 injury. ISS cannot be calculated if there is an AIS 9 (unknown) injury.[2] ISS correlates with mortality.

AIS is an anatomic injury scale; it does not consider preexisting disease, the patient's age, or the physiologic condition of the patient in the emergency room. The trauma score (TS) was developed in 1981 by Champion et al.[4] The 1981 TS was based on respiratory rate, respiratory effort, systolic blood pressure, periphery profusion (capillary refill), and the Glasgow Coma Scale (GCS). Values can range from 1 to 16. The higher the score, the greater the probability of survival. The probability of survival goes from 0.00 at a TS of 1 to 0.99 with a TS of 16. A combined anatomic and physiological score, TRISS, was found to correlate better with survival than either used alone. In 1989, due to the difficulty of evaluating respiratory effort, TS was simplified to a 13-point scale (0 to 12), the Triage Revised Trauma Scale (T-RTS), which was based on the GCS, systolic blood pressure (SBP), and respiratory rate (RR).[5] The probability of survival goes from 0.037 with a T-RTS of

0 to 0.995 with a T-RTS of 12. The RTS is defined as:

$$RTS = 0.9368\,GCS_c + 0.7326\,SBP_c + 0.2908\,RR_c.$$

The probability of surviving the injuries goes from 0.027 with an RTS of 0 to 0.988 with an RTS of 8.

Survival after injury depends not only on the severity of the injuries but upon the condition of the injured individual at the time of injury. An elderly, infirm individual is more likely to succumb to injuries than a young vigorous athlete. To improve the evaluation of outcome, Boyd et al.[6] used ISS, RTS, and the patient's age to develop the TRISS method of evaluating outcome. The TRISS method gives a probability of survival (P_s) based on TS or RTS, ISS, and the patient's age (A). The formula is:

$$P_s = \frac{1}{1 + e^{-b}}$$

where

$$b = b_0 + b_1(TS) + b_2(ISS) + b_3(A)$$
$$b = b_0 + b_1(RTS) + b_2(ISS) + b_3(A)$$

and where $b_{0...3}$ are constants that are derived from regression analysis and vary whether the trauma is blunt or penetrating and whether one is calculating P_s for TS or RTS. TRISS is more effective at predicting outcome than either ISS or TS/RTS.

An attempt to salvage an unsalvageable limb can be dangerous to the patient and can significantly increase medical expenses.[7,8] It is also very costly in terms of medical resources. The Mangled Extremity Syndrome Index (MESI) was developed by Gregory et al.[9] to predict limb salvageability. The score was based on patient and injury factors. These included ISS, skin injury, nerve injury, vascular injury, bony injury, time from injury, patient's age, preexisting disease, and presence of shock. It is complex in that each anatomic structure, for example, each nerve, is evaluated individually and can add to the MESI. Limbs with a MESI below 20 were salvageable and those with a MESI above 20 were not salvageable. Johansen et al.[8] described a

TABLE 18.2. Mangled Extremity Severity Score (MESS).

Energy Skeletal/soft tissue		Limb ischemia		Shock		Age	
		Normal pulse and profusion	0	Systolic BP always >90 mg Hg	0	<30	0
Low energy Stab wound Simple fracture Low velocity GSW (gunshot wound)	1	Decreased or absent pulse with normal perfusion	1*	Transient hypotensive episode	1	30–50	1
Medium energy Open fractures Multiple fractures Dislocations	2	Pulseless; parathesias, diminished capillary refill	2*	Persistent hypotension	2	>50	2
High energy Close-range shot-gun wound High velocity GSW Crush injury	3	Cool, paralyzed, insensate, numb	3*				
Very high energy High energy + gross contamination and/or skin avulsion	4						

Modified from Johansen et al.[8]
* Double score for ischemia >6 hours.

Mangled Extremity Severity Score (MESS), which is a simplification of MESI. It is a 14-point scale that is summarized in Table 18.2. The MESS differences between salvageable and unsalvageable lower extremities were significant. Limbs with a score of 6 or less were salvageable, and those with a score of 7 or greater could not be saved.

The anatomically based scales, such as the AIS, can be used to evaluate the effectiveness of safety measures. If a change is effective in mitigating injury, the average AIS for those protected by the new measure should be less than the average AIS before the commencement of the new measure. Physiologically based scales, such as TS, T-RTS, or RTS, and the combined scales, such as TRISS, are valuable because they allow us to evaluate how an injury is being treated. As treatment improves, the survival probability for a given RTS should improve or more patients should survive than the prediction of TRISS.

Classification of Injuries

Fractures

The most common type of skeletal component in the extremities are long bones. Figure 18.2 is a typical long bone. There are significant differences in the biomechanical properties of the diaphysis and metaphysis. Anatomically

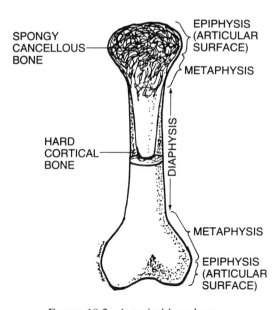

FIGURE 18.2. A typical long bone.

the metaphyseal region has a relatively thin cortex with a fairly significant intramedullary supporting structure of cancellous bone. The diaphysis has a thick cortex and almost no intramedullary cancellous structure. The failure (fracture) patterns of the diaphysis are similar to those of a hollow cylindrical tube. The failure patterns of the metaphysis are a bit more difficult to predict because of the variable composite of cancellous and cortical bone in this region. Most of the specialized classifications are for fractures that involve the metaphyseal and epiphyseal regions of long bones.

All fractures are either open or closed. A closed fracture is one in which the skin and soft tissues over the fracture are intact; hence, there has been no exposure of the bone to outside contamination. The old term for this type of injury, and one that will be found in older literature, is a "simple" fracture. This term was changed, as there can be some rather complicated "simple" fractures and "simple" does not always describe the injury accurately. An open fracture is one in which the skin and overlying soft tissues are damaged and there has been exposure of the bone to direct outside contamination. The old term for this type of injury is "compound" fracture. A fracture caused by an object penetrating the skin and contacting the bone, for example, a gunshot wound (GSW), is an open fracture.

The lack of a wound does not necessarily indicate that there is no damage to the skin and underlying soft tissues. It is possible to have significant injury between the skin and bone without having an open wound. The AO-ASIF has recognized the importance of the occult injury to the soft tissues beneath the intact skin and has categorized the potential occult soft tissue injuries. Müeller et al.[10] reported the AO-ASIF classification of skin and soft tissue injuries based on the fracture classification method of Maurice E. Müeller. It is a five-point anatomically based scale. For closed skin lesions, IC1 is normal, IC2 to IC4 indicate increasingly severe damage to the skin and subcutaneous tissues, and IC5 is a special injury in which there is traumatic necrosis of skin and subcutaneous tissue. IC is an

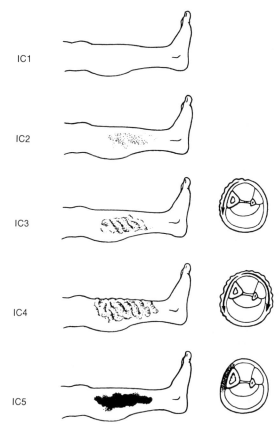

FIGURE 18.3. A summary of the AO classification of closed skin injuries.

abbreviation for integument closed. Figure 18.3 summarizes the AO-ASIF classification of closed skin injuries.

Open fractures are classified by the wound size. Originally open fractures were divided into three major types (Table 18.3). Gustilo et al.[11] noted that type I and type II open fractures rarely become infected and that infection occurs in approximately 20% of type III open fractures. They also noted that not all type III open fractures behaved alike; in fact, based on the behavior of the injuries, they were able to divide type III open fractures into three subgroups, types IIIA, IIIB, and IIIC.

The AO-ASIF open fracture classification is a four-grade system, IO1 to IO4. IO stands for integument open. This is very similar to the three-level classification of Gustilo et al.[11] The AO-ASIF open fracture classification is summarized in Fig. 18.4.

TABLE 18.3. Classification of open fractures.

Type	Wound
I	Less than 1 cm
II	Up to 1 cm with significant muscle, soft tissue contusion, or up to 10 cm without significant underlying soft tissue damage
IIIA	Extensive soft tissue laceratio, adequate bone coverage possible
IIIB	Extensive soft tissue laceration, inadequate bone coverage
IIIC	Open fracture with associated arterial injury

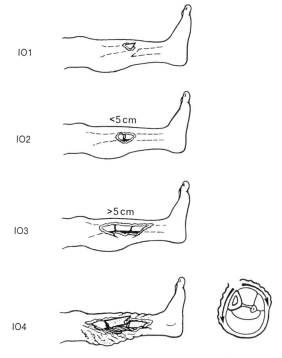

FIGURE 18.4. A summary of the AO-ASIF open fracture classification.

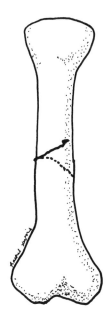

FIGURE 18.5. An undisplaced fracture, in which the bony fragments are still in their normal anatomic positions.

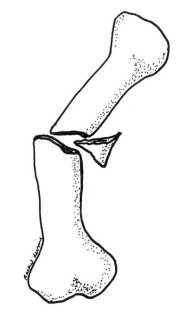

FIGURE 18.6. A displaced fracture, in which one or more pieces of bone has moved from its normal anatomic position.

A fracture is a break in the continuity of a bone. There are several descriptive terms used in the classification of a given fracture. All fractures are either displaced or undisplaced. An undisplaced fracture. (Fig. 18.5) is a fracture in which the bony fragments are still in their normal anatomic positions; there is simply a crack or cracks in the bone, but all pieces are exactly where they belong. A displaced fracture (Fig. 18.6) is one in which one or more of the pieces of bone has moved from its normal anatomic position. A frac-

ture may also be described as impacted or angulated. In an impacted fracture (Fig. 18.7) the bone is compressed, with essentially the only displacement being a slight shortening

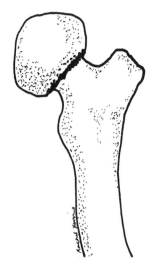

FIGURE 18.7. An impacted fracture, in which the bone is compressed.

of the bone. In an angulated fracture (Fig. 18.8), which is commonly seen in children who have fairly "plastic" bone, the only deformity is an angulation at the fracture site. Displacement can give a hint about the forces involved. Undisplaced fractures usually result from relatively low energy input, while displaced fractures need higher forces. An undisplaced fracture can be treated without reduction, while a displaced fracture not infrequently needs to be reduced (put into normal alignment).

Fractures can be described by their location along the bone. An intra-articular fracture involves the articular surface of a bone. An intracapsular fracture is one within a joint capsule but which does not necessarily involve the articular surface. A metaphyseal fracture

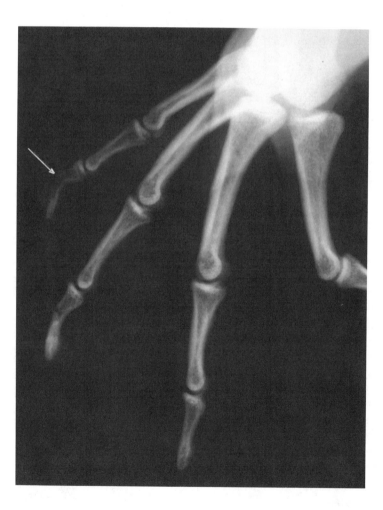

FIGURE 18.8. An angulated fracture, in which the only deformity is an angulation at the fracture site.

would be in the metaphysis of a long bone, while a diaphyseal fracture would be in the diaphyseal region. This terminology is not pure, for often a more specific anatomic location will be given. For instance, a supracondylar fracture of a femur is a metaphyseal fracture but it is more descriptively called supracondylar because it is above the condyles of the femur. A bimalleolar fracture would involve the medial and lateral malleoli of the ankle. A fracture is not infrequently described by its location in the diaphysis. For instance, a fracture may be described as being in the region of the junction of the proximal one-third and distal two-thirds of a long bone.

All fractures are either comminuted or noncomminuted. If the bone is broken into only two pieces, then the fracture is noncomminuted (Fig. 18.9). When the bone is broken into more than two pieces, the fracture is usually said to be comminuted. Comminution may be classified according to the method of Winquest and Hansen[12] using four grades. This classification was based on the stability of femur fractures after fixation with an intramedullary (IM) rod. The rods used were rods that could not be locked; hence, comminution could lead to loss of fracture alignment and/or femoral shorten-

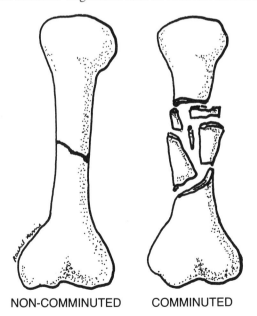

NON-COMMINUTED   COMMINUTED

FIGURE 18.9. A noncomminuted fracture, in which the bone is broken into only two pieces.

ing. In grade I injuries, there was only a very small fragment of comminution; the fracture could be essentially considered as transverse or short oblique. Long oblique and spiral fractures were not considered as a grade I injury because of the potential for shortening and/or rotation with IM rod fixation. In a grade II fracture, there was at least 50% of cortical abutment possible after reduction and IM rod fixation. In grade III injuries, some cortical contact was still possible, but it was less than 50%. The difference between grade II and grade III at the time was determined by the location of the comminution. A grade IV injury was one in which the comminution is such that for a section of bone, there was no possible contact of the cortices of the fragments. Grade IV would be subject to shortening when fixed with IM rods, for there was no cortex that could be approximated to maintain the normal length of the femur. Comminution is an indication of the bone strength and energy input. Comminution correlates fairly well with energy input: the higher the energy, the greater the comminution. However, energy is not the only factor in comminution. Bone strength is another factor; weaker bone tends to become comminuted with less energy.

How the fracture crosses the affected bone may also be used as a descriptor. A transverse fracture (Fig. 18.10) is essentially perpendicular to the long axis of the bone. A transverse fracture results from a direct load perpendicular to the long axis of the bone. A spiral fracture (Fig. 18.11) is one in which the fracture line spirals up the bone. A spiral fracture results from a torsional stress being placed on a long bone. An oblique fracture (Fig. 18.12) is one in which the fracture traverses the shaft at an angle. An oblique fracture will occur when there is axial loading of a long bone combined with torsional loading. A fracture may also be described as having a butterfly fragment (Fig. 18.13). The butterfly is a triangular-shaped fragment of bone involving one cortex of the injured bone. A fracture with a butterfly fragment results from a bending movement being placed on a long bone. The butterfly occurs on the side in which the bone is in compression. A fracture may also be described as being a

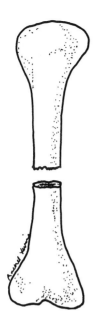

FIGURE 18.10. A transverse fracture, which is perpendicular to the long axis of the bone.

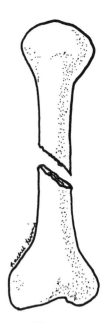

FIGURE 18.12. An oblique fracture, in which the fracture traverses the shaft at an angle.

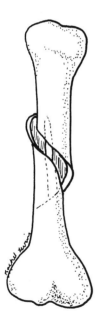

FIGURE 18.11. A spiral fracture, in which the fracture line spirals up the bone.

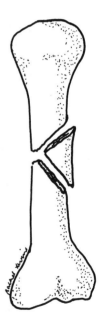

FIGURE 18.13. A butterfly fragment of bone.

segmental fracture (Fig. 18.14), which is a fracture in which there are two fractures in the shaft of the bone, creating a segment of bone that has fractures at each end. An avulsion fracture is a fracture in which a piece of bone is pulled (avulsed) out of position. The small avulsed fragment remains attached to a ligament or tendon. A transverse fracture may

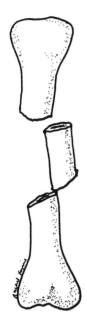

FIGURE 18.14. A segmental fracture, in which there are two fractures in the bone shaft.

occur in a sesamoid. The patella is the largest sesamoid in the human body. A strong contraction of the quadriceps, especially when the knee is rapidly flexing due to loading when one is starting to fall, will lead to a transverse patellar fracture. A stress fracture is an injury that results from repeated microtrauma. A stress fracture is a fatigue failure of a bone. It is the "march fracture" of a metatarsal not uncommonly seen in soldiers who have suddenly started training with long marches. A final type of fracture is a pathologic fracture. A pathologic fracture occurs through an area of abnormal bone, such as what would be found in a patient with a bone tumor or with metastatic tumors to bone.

Anatomically, the epiphysis is a specific location of a long bone. It is the region just under the articular surface at the ends of long bones. Epiphyseal fractures are found in the description of fractures in individuals who are skeletally immature. The fractures involve the

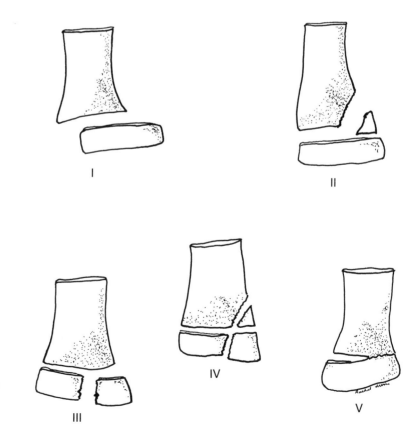

FIGURE 18.15. The Salter-Harris classification of epiphyseal fractures.

physis, and frequently, by convention, they are called epiphyseal fractures (physis).

Salter and Harris[13] classified epiphyseal injuries (Fig. 18.15). A Salter type I fracture is a shear fracture through the epiphyseal plate. There is no cancellous bone injury; the separation is through the germinal layer of the cartilaginous epiphyseal plate. A Salter type II fracture is similar to the Salter type I fracture except that in a Salter type II fracture, a piece of metaphysis remains attached to the epiphysis. A Salter type III fracture is an intra-articular fracture that extends from the articular surface to the epiphyseal plate and then courses along the plate to its periphery. A Salter type IV fracture is a fracture that crosses the epiphyseal plate, usually going from the metaphysis to the articular surface. A Salter type V fracture may be the most difficult to identify and usually has a poor prognosis. It is a compressive injury of the growth plate and will frequently destroy the germinal layer, leading to growth abnormalities. The Salter classification, although the most common in the United States and Canada, is not universal. Rang,[14] in a text on the growth plate, proposed a sixth type of injury (Fig. 18.16) in which there is a bit of separation of the periosteum over the physis, with hematoma between the physis and periosteum that eventually causes premature epiphyseal closure and growth abnormalities.

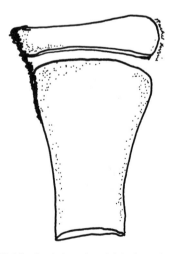

FIGURE 18.16. An injury in which there is a separation of the periosteum over the physis.

Müeller et al.[10] has developed a classification that is based not only on appearance but also on treatment and prognosis. Figure 18.17 summarizes Müeller's classifications. Type A fractures pass between the junction of the zone of hypertrophy and zone of provisional calcification within the epiphyseal plate. Type A1, which is equivalent to a Salter I fracture, is a shear fracture through the physeal plate. Type A2, which is the same as a Salter II, is partly a shear fracture through the plate but to which is attached a portion of the metaphysis.

Müeller type B injuries usually need to have an open reduction and internal fixation. Type B1, equivalent to a Salter III, is a fracture in which there is damage to the articular surface. It is a partial separation of the epiphysis from the metaphysis. The fracture line does not cross the physis. In type B2 fractures, Salter IV, the fracture line starts in the articular surface and involves the epiphysis, physis, and metaphysis. A type B3 injury is an avulsion fracture involving the perichondrial ring. The B4 injury is an abrasive injury to the periphery of the epiphysis with damage to the zone of Ranvier.

Müeller type C injuries are the same as Salter V fractures. These carry the worst prognosis as they are compressive injuries (crush) of the physis. Due to damage to the growth plate, growth abnormalities are expected. Müeller divided these into C1 and C2, where the amount of damage in a C2 injury is greater than that present in a C1 injury.

The Müeller classification indirectly suggests treatment and prognosis. Type A injuries have the best prognosis. The germinal layer of the physis is intact. These fractures usually heal and if there is any residual deformity, it will usually be corrected by remodeling as the child matures. Type A fractures rarely need open reduction and internal fixation. Type B fractures carry a poorer prognosis. Types B1 and B2 have an intra-articular component. Accurate reduction with internal fixation is usually needed to prevent a posttraumatic arthritis, especially in type B2 injuries, to prevent premature closure of a portion of the growth plate. Type B3 also needs an accurate reduction, but because there is damage to the

FIGURE 18.17. Müeller's classification of fractures.

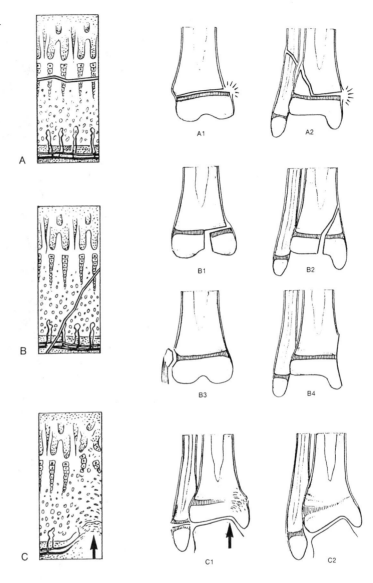

perichondral ring and zone of Ranvier, growth disturbances may follow. In type B4, an open abrasion of the physis, the damage is not repairable and premature epiphyseal closure is fairly common. Type C injuries have the worst prognosis. They are a crush of the germinal layer with a disorganization of the physis. In type C injuries, growth abnormality will almost always result. Unfortunately, there is no open procedure that can repair a type C injury.

Immature bone differs from adult bone in that the bone is more plastic and the periosteum, the soft tissue layer that is just superficial to the cortex, is thicker. The thick periosteum and greater plasticity allow for special types of fracture patterns that are present only in immature bone. Immature bones are somewhat flexible, like a greenstick freshly cut from a tree, and it is possible to angulate the bone and fracture only one cortex; this is a greenstick fracture. In immature bones one may also see a torus fracture, which is a wrinkle noted in the cortex.

Fractures may be identified by an eponym. Eponyms are not without problems. They are not universal and the same fracture may have different eponyms in different areas. Eponyms are often misapplied. A Colles' fracture is a specific fracture of the distal radius (wrist), described before there was roentgenogram diagnosis of fractures; yet one might find an emergency room record with "Colles' fracture"[b] as the final diagnosis of a displaced distal radial epiphyseal fracture when the fracture should be classified as a displaced Salter type I or type II fracture of the distal radial epiphysis. Yet, if eponyms are universal and used only for one specific injury, they may have some value. A Jones' fracture, a fracture about 1.5 cm distal to the proximal end of the fifth metatarsal, is a specific injury and is quite different than the much more common avulsion fracture of the base of the fifth metatarsal. Although these two fractures are positioned anatomically quite close, the end results, especially the probability of nonunion, differ considerably, with the true Jones' fracture having a far worse prognosis than the avulsion fracture of the base of the fifth metatarsal.

Fractures are predictable; specific loading causes specific injuries. The pattern of a long fracture can be explained by its response to the force that caused the failure. The behavior of bones to loading is fairly consistent and allows classification of fractures by mechanism of injury. This classification overlaps with pattern classification because a specific load causes a specific pattern of injury. An understanding of the behavior of bones to loading serves as a classification of fractures according to the mechanism of the injury. There are four possible types of injury mechanisms: (1) direct blows, (2) penetration, (3) indirect loading, and (4) repetitive loading.[15]

A fracture may be caused by a direct blow to the soft tissue overlaying the bone. Low-energy direct blows cause transverse fractures. Figure 18.18 is a nightstick fracture of the ulna, a typical low-energy direct-blow injury. The fracture is essentially transverse. Mechanically,

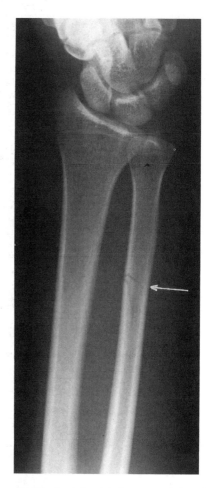

FIGURE 18.18. A nightstick fracture of the ulna.

the ulna is a beam being loaded in the middle with resistance to the load at the end of the beam (three-point bend). A high-energy direct blow will cause a markedly comminuted fracture. Figure 18.19 is a typical bumper injury of the proximal tibia, an injury that was first described by Cotton and Berg[16] in 1929 and has been called the Cotton fracture.

Fractures can also be caused by penetration, such as gunshot wounds (GSWs). Low-velocity GSWs, that is bullets with velocity less than 1,800 ft/sec, are considered low-energy injuries. Most of the injury is to the bone. There is usually little soft tissue injury unless the bullet happens to traverse a nerve or vessel in its path to the bone. Since these are low-energy injuries, they, like most low-energy

_____

[b] A fracture that by original description cannot occur through an open distal radial epiphysis, as it was a fracture of adults.

FIGURE 18.19. A typical bumper injury of the proximal tibia.

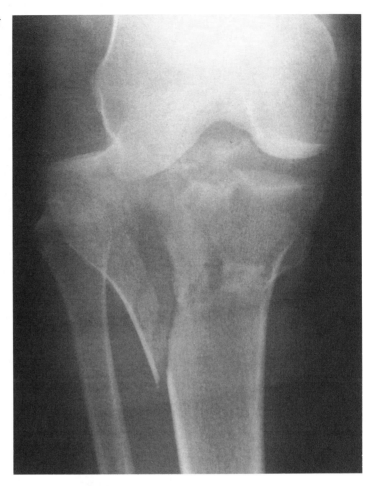

injuries, tend to have a fairly good prognosis. High-velocity GSWs, where the bullet velocity is greater than 1,800 ft/sec, are very different from low-velocity GSWs. In high-velocity GSWs, there is not only the bony injury, there is also significant injury to the soft tissues due to the energy transferred from the missile to the soft tissues.

Many fractures are caused by indirect loading. If the binding of a ski does not release when a skier falls, a torque is placed on the tibia causing a torsional fracture. Or if during a motor vehicle accident, the knee of a unrestrained passenger hits the dashboard, the forces may cause a fractured acetabulum. Injuries caused by indirect loading are injuries that occur away from the actual site of loading.

Traction on a bone will cause a transverse fracture perpendicular to the force. Avulsion

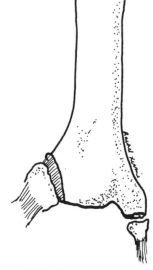

FIGURE 18.20. An avulsion fracture, in which a piece of bone is pulled off with a ligament or tendon.

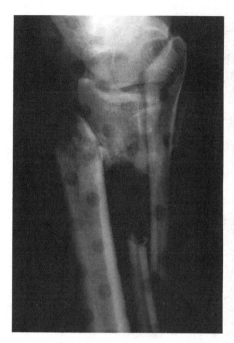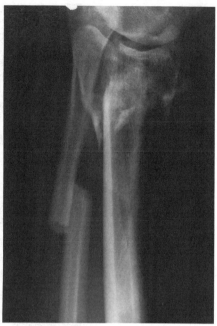

FIGURE 18.21. A pillion fracture, which is a longitudinal compression.

fractures (Fig. 18.20), in which a piece of bone is pulled off with a ligament or tendon, are also usually perpendicular to the line of load application. Angulation or bending of a long bone will cause a transverse fracture with a butterfly fragment (Fig. 18.13). Torque on a long bone will cause a spiral fracture. Compression along the long axis of the bone will cause a longitudinal split and an intra-articular compression fracture. Pylon fractures (Fig. 18.21) are typical longitudinal compression fractures. Oblique fractures result from combined loading, either axial loading with angulation or angulation with torsion and axial loading. Figure 18.22 summarizes the types of fractures according to loading.

Müeller et al.[17] have developed a comprehensive classification based on the morphology of the fracture. All fractures are divided in types (A, B, or C), groups (1, 2, and 3) and subgroups (0.1, 0.2, and 0.3) (Fig. 18.23). All bones are given a number. Each long bone is divided into three or four parts. Table 18.4 summarizes the identification number and number of segments of the various bones. All long bones, except the tibia/fibula, have three

segments, proximal (1),[c] middle (2), and distal (3). The tibia-fibula has four segments: proximal (1), middle (2), distal (3), and malleolar (4). The spine is divided into three segments: cervical (1), thoracic (2), and lumbar (3). The pelvis is considered to have two segments: extra-articular (1), and acetabulum (2).

All injuries are coded $BS\text{-}TG.S_g$ where B = bone, S = segment, T = type of fracture, G = group, and S_g = subgroup. If an injury involves two segments of a bone, the injury will be coded twice, with each segment coded as a separate injury. The total coding system is well illustrated in a comprehensive classification book, Classification of Fractures of Long Bones.[17] The system is excellent for long bone fractures. It is a useful system because it can easily be adapted to database storage, retrieval, and analysis. However, it needs further development because it fails to adequately classify fractures that do not involve long bones, that is, any bone with a code number

[c] Number in parentheses refers to the segment number in the classification system.

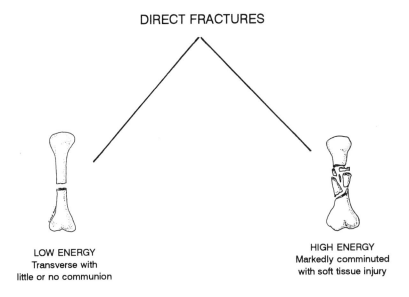

DIRECT FRACTURES

LOW ENERGY
Transverse with
little or no communion

HIGH ENERGY
Markedly comminuted
with soft tissue injury

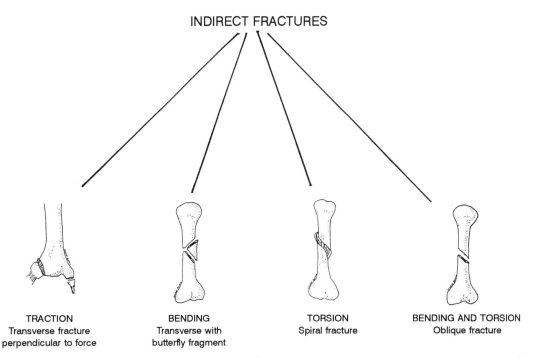

INDIRECT FRACTURES

TRACTION
Transverse fracture
perpendicular to force

BENDING
Transverse with
butterfly fragment

TORSION
Spiral fracture

BENDING AND TORSION
Oblique fracture

FIGURE 18.22. A summary of the types of fractures according to loading. (Modified from Harkess et al.[15])

greater than 4. It is less than perfect in that coding, for some of the bones need up to four bits. It would have been better for database storage if bones needed only two bits for their identification.

Dislocations

A dislocation (luxation) is a complete displacement of the articulating ends of bones. In a dislocation there is no remaining contact of the

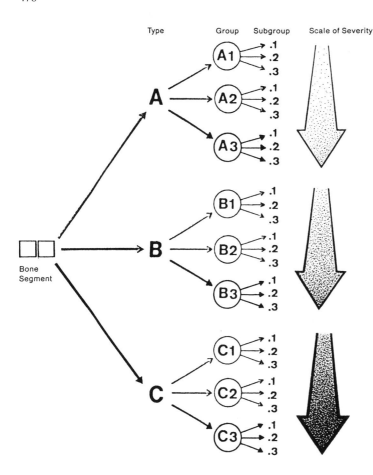

FIGURE 18.23. Müeller's general classification of long bone fractures.

TABLE 18.4. Müeller's numbering system for identification of bones.

ID number	Bone(s)	Number of segments
1	Humerus	3
2	Radius/ulna[a]	3
3	Femur	3
4	Tibia/fibula[b]	4
5	Spine	3
6	Pelvis	2
7	Hand	—
8	Foot	—
91.1	Patella	—
91.2	Clavicle	—
91.3	Scapula	—
92	Mandible	—
93	Facial bones and skull	—

[a] Radius and ulna considered as "one" bone.
[b] Tibia and fibula considered as "one" bone.

normally articulating surfaces. If some contact remains between the articulating surfaces, then the joint is said to be subluxed (less than a luxation). If there is a fracture close to and/or involving one of the articular surfaces and an associated dislocation, the injury is described as a fracture-dislocation. Like fractures, dislocations can be open or closed. If the skin is broken and the joint exposed, the dislocation is open. If the skin about the joint is intact, then the dislocation is closed.

Ligament Injuries

Ligaments consist of a dense, fibrous tissue and serve to hold joints together and prevent abnormal motion at a joint. They are usually closely associated with the joint capsule. Ligament injuries may be divided into three types. A sprain is an injury to a ligament.

Sprains are classified into three grades. A grade III ligament sprain is a complete tearing of the ligament. A grade II is a stretch of the ligament beyond its normal elastic range. The ligament is still intact but it has been elongated and probably has suffered significant internal damage. A grade I sprain is a stretch of the ligament within its elastic limit causing some local bleeding and inflammation. Grade II and grade III ligament injuries may lead to joint instability and eventual degenerative arthritis because of abnormal motions of the joint during loading. Instability may also predispose the individual to further sprains as is sometimes noted following lateral ankle sprains.

Nerve Injuries

A nerve, unlike many other tissues, is not for transmitting a mechanical force; rather, it is like an electrical wire, for its role is to transmit neural (chemical-electrical) impulses to and from the central nervous system. Nerves are long cells, up to about 1 m in length. The cell body is close to or within the vertebral column. The axon, which is a long extension from the cell, is bundled with other axons to form nerves. These axons are covered with various amounts of myelination. Seddon[18] classified nerve injuries into three types and Sir Henry Cohen proposed the naming of the three types: (1) neurapraxia, (2) axonotmesis, and (3) neurotmesis. Neurapraxis is the first level of nerve injury. The large motor fibers are predominately affected and anatomic continuity of the nerve is preserved. The prognosis for recovery is excellent and usually complete within a few days to weeks. The next level of injury is axonotmesis. The nerve is anatomically intact, but there is a complete interruption of all types of nerve fibers with essentially complete motor and sensory loss. The nerve has to recover by axonal regeneration and this starts at the cell body, near or in the spinal column, and progresses outward at approximately 1 mm per day. The most severe form of injury is neurotmesis, in which there is complete disruption within the nerve and/or an actual severing of the nerve. This injury needs surgical repair. There is wallerian degeneration of the nerve distal to the site of the injury and the prognosis for recovery is far poorer than in the other two classes of nerve injuries. A nerve may not always have only one type of injury. It is possible to have combined types of injuries within a given nerve.

Upper Extremity

The bones of the upper extremity include the clavicle, scapula, humerus, radius and ulna, eight carpal bones, five metacarpals, and the phalanges within the digits. The only bone attachment of the upper extremity to the trunk is at the sternoclavicular (SC) joint. The bony attachment of the upper extremity to the trunk is not of paramount importance, for it is possible to remove the distal end of the clavicle, thereby eliminating the bony attachment of the upper extremity to the trunk without significantly affecting function. However, excising the total clavicle may lead to a significant impairment of the extremity.[19]

The SC joint, clavicle, and acromioclavicular (AC) joint are injured by a loading on the extremity at the lateral aspect of the shoulder, which causes the shoulder to bend inward (medially) into the chest wall. The clavicle, like all bones, can be injured by a direct blow. In motor vehicle trauma, a typical mode of injury would be a side impact in which the victim moves laterally, striking the shoulder on the door and or its supporting structures. Injuries to the AC and SC joints are the result of a lateral compressive force on the shoulder applied through loading the lateral aspect of the acromion as would happen in a fall onto the point of the shoulder.[20]

Injuries of the AC joint are most generally classified into three levels of severity. In a grade I sprain, there is only a mild stretch or a disruption of a few of the fibers of the joint capsule and coracoclavicular ligament. There is no significant abnormality noted on x-ray. The diagnosis is made on history, complaints, and the finding of tenderness over the AC joint. In grade II injury, there is a disruption of the joint capsule, but the coracoclavicular ligament remains intact. There will be a slight elevation of the lateral end of the clavicle on x-ray. In a grade III injury, there is rupture of both the AC joint capsule and the coracoclavicular ligaments and there will be complete dislocation of the end of the clavicle noted on x-ray.

SC joint injuries are classified into three grades. In a grade I injury, there is no laxity of the supporting ligaments and only mild pain in the SC joint. In a grade II injury, there is a rupture of the sternoclavicular ligaments with intact costoclavicular ligaments. There is no more than minimal displacement of the medial end of the clavicle. There will be localized tenderness and swelling over the SC joint. In a grade III injury both ligaments, sternoclavicular and costoclavicular, are ruptured and the SC joint is dislocated. The clavicle will displace either anteriorly or posteriorly. The posterior dislocation, which is also referred to as a retrosternal dislocation, is rare and can result in sudden death because of damage to the great vessels or respiratory distress.

Clavicle fractures are classified according to their location along the bone. Group I fractures, the most common type, involve the middle third of this S-shaped bone. Group II fractures are distal to the attachment of the coracoclavicular ligament. Group II fractures are the result of a force on the point of the shoulder that drives the humerus and scapula downward.[20] Neer[21] has further classified group II fractures into two subgroups. In type I, the ligaments are intact and there is little displacement. In type II there is a coracoclavicular ligament with displacement of the proximal fragment. In a review of 215 clavicle fractures Sankarankutty and Turner[22] found that 91% resulted from a fall or direct blow on the point of the shoulder, 8% by direct trauma, and 1% from a fall on the outstretched arm.

The forces needed to fracture the clavicle have been reported by Messerer.[23] These are summarized in Table 18.5.

Klenermann[24] subjected proximal humeri to loading modes. Compression of the head in the vertical axis of the humerus showed a mean breaking failure load of 1,100 lbf (range 600 to 1,850 lbf). When the head was loaded to

TABLE 18.5. Clavicle strength.

	Male	Female
Torque (N = m)	15	10
Range	12–17	8–11
Bending (kN)	0.98	0.60
Range	0.78–1.18	0.49–0.69
Average maximum moment (N = m)	30	17
Long axis compression (kN)	1.89	1.24
Range	1.22–2.64	0.88–2.06

From Messerer, as reported in Naham and Melvin.[23]

simulate falling on the point of the shoulder, the failure force averaged 742 lbf (range 224 to 1,344 lbf).

Fractures of the diaphysis of the humerus can result from direct trauma, such as a direct blow, or from indirect trauma. The classification of fractures can be with any of the descriptive methods described in the beginning of this chapter. Figure 18.24 shows the AO-ASIF classification of humeral diaphyseal fracture.

Humeral fracture can occur without any contact. The muscle forces involved in overhand throwing have caused spiral fractures of the humerus. Clemons and Hammond[25] were first to report on humeral fractures resulting from muscular forces. Herzmark and Klune[26] reported four cases in 1952. They felt the fracture resulted from a powerful torque caused by the stabilization of the humerus by the deltoid in external rotation and the flexors of the arm, in combination with the leverage of the forearm which is at right angles to the humerus, internally rotating the bone. Several others have reported a few cases caused by the overhand throwing of baseballs, hand grenades, or javelins.[27–30] Chao et al.[29] calculated and then experimentally showed that a force of 7 ft-lb torque would fracture a humerus. This value was lower than the 488 lbf-inch (range 195 to 815 lbf-inch) found by Klenermann[24] as the torque needed to fracture humeral shafts.

Using a three-point bending model, Klenermann found that the mean bending moment at failure for 14 specimens was 1,066 lbf-inch. The fracture pattern was transverse until it was more than halfway through the bone and then it veered distally forming an

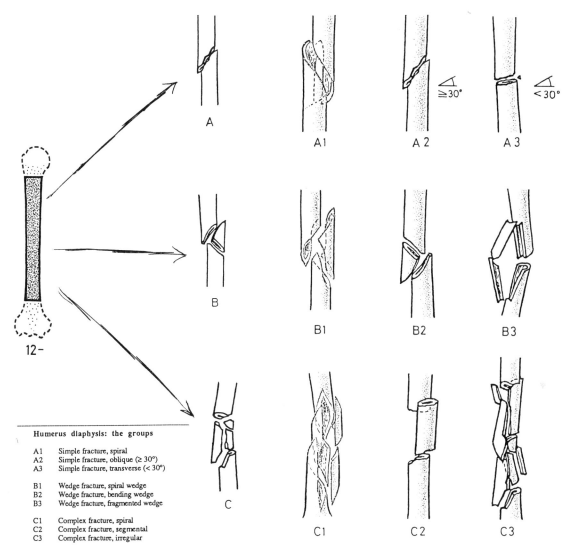

12−

Humerus diaphysis: the groups

A1 Simple fracture, spiral
A2 Simple fracture, oblique (≥ 30°)
A3 Simple fracture, transverse (< 30°)

B1 Wedge fracture, spiral wedge
B2 Wedge fracture, bending wedge
B3 Wedge fracture, fragmented wedge

C1 Complex fracture, spiral
C2 Complex fracture, segmental
C3 Complex fracture, irregular

FIGURE 18.24. AO-ASIF classification of humerus fractures.

L-shaped pattern. This pattern was constant whether the bone was loaded in the anterior-posterior or medial-lateral plane. In 20% of the specimens, there was an undisplaced butterfly fragment in the proximal fragment. Table 18.6 summarizes the failure found by Messerer as reported by Nahum and Melvin.[23]

Diaphyseal fractures of the radius and ulna have been primarily classified by the anatomic and descriptive terms of the injury. Müeller et al.[17] have defined the injuries within their systematic classification. Figure 18.25 summarizes their classification. Two eponyms are

TABLE 18.6. Humerus strength.

	Male	Female
Torque (N = m)	70	55
Range	55–78	39–80
Bending (kN)	2.71	1.71
Range	2.35–2.94	1.18–2.35
Average maximum moment (N = m)	151	85
Long axis compression (kN)	4.98	3.61
Range	2.71–7.83	2.45–0.09

From Messerer, as reported in Naham and Melvin.[23]

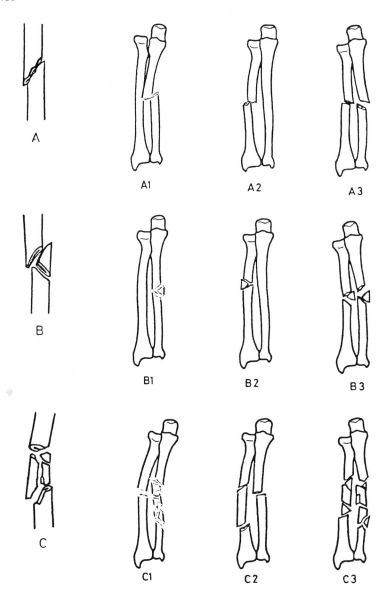

FIGURE 18.25. AO classification of radius and ulna fractures.

Radius/Ulna diaphysis: the groups

A1   Simple fracture, of the ulna, radius intact
A2   Simple fracture, of the radius, ulna intact
A3   Simple fracture, of both bones

B1   Wedge fracture, of the ulna, radius intact
B2   Wedge fracture, of the radius, ulna intact
B3   Wedge fracture, of the one bone, simple or wedge fracture of the other

C1   Complex fracture, of the ulna
C2   Complex fracture, of the radius
C3   Complex fracture, of both bones

TABLE 18.7. Radius strength.

	Male	Female
Torque (N = m)	22	17
Range	16–27	13–23
Bending (kN)	1.20	0.67
Range	0.98–1.77	0.54–0.88
Average maximum moment (N = m)	48	23
Long axis compression (kN)	3.28	2.16
Range	2.35–4.21	1.03–3.18

From Messerer, as reported in Naham and Melvin.[23]

TABLE 18.8. Ulna strength.

	Male	Female
Torque (N = m)	14	11
Range	8–21	9–13
Bending (kN)	1.23	0.81
Range	0.98–2.16	0.69–0.98
Average maximum moment (N = m)	49	28
Long axis compression (kN)	4.98	3.61
Range	2.15–7.83	2.45–5.09

From Messerer, as reported in Naham and Melvin.[23]

associated with forearm fractures: Monteggia and Galeazzi fractures. A Monteggia fracture is a fracture of the proximal ulna associated with a dislocation of the radial head. A Galeazzi fracture is a fracture of the distal radial diaphysis associated with a dislocation of the ulna at the wrist. Tables 18.7 and 18.8 list the reported strengths of the radius and ulna as determined by Messerer.

Lower Extremity

Hip dislocations are divided into five types. Type I is a dislocation without a fracture or with no more than a minor fracture of the acetabular rim. Types II, III, and IV are dislocations with increasingly severe fractures of the acetabulum. Type V is a dislocation with an associated fracture of the femoral head and can be with or without an acetabular fracture.

Epstein,[31] in discussing 559 hip dislocations seen from 1928–1970 at Los Angeles County University of Southern California Medical Center, indicated that most appeared from motor vehicle trauma, such as a posterior dislocation resulting from the knee striking the dash board. Epstein (referenced in Pietrafesa and Hoffmann[32]) noted that this is an injury that resulted from not using seat belts. Of the 800 dislocations he had evaluated, only five (0.6%) were restrained during the accident. In three of these five cases the seat broke from its mounting, and in the other two the victims had been wearing their seat belts extremely loosely.

In the classification of femur fractures, the bone is typically divided into three parts. Fractures involving the proximal femur are generally referred to as hip fractures. There are three basic type of hip fractures: (1) intracapsular, (2) intertrochanteric, and (3) subtrochanteric. The distal femur fractures would be in the supra- and intracondylar regions, and the rest would be diaphyseal fractures. Figure 18.26 illustrates the regions of a typical femur.

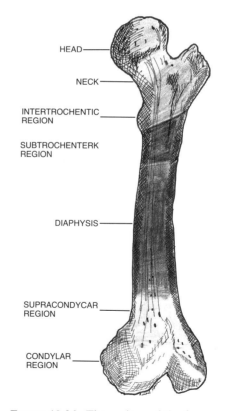

FIGURE 18.26. The regions of the femur.

Intracapsular hip fractures are those that involve the head and neck of the femur. They can be classified by the location along the neck. A subcapital fracture is just distal to the head, a transcervical is through the midportion of the neck, and a basilar neck fracture, which is actually extracapsular, is at the base just proximal to the intracondylar region of the femur. The Garden[33] classification is a straightforward system based on displacement. In this classification, which gives some prognosis of the injury, there are four types of fractures. A Garden I fracture is one in which the neck fracture is either incomplete or impacted. In a Garden II fracture, the fracture completely traverses the femoral neck, but there is no displacement of the fragments. A Garden III fracture has partial displacement of the two fragments. In a Garden IV fracture, there is complete displacement of the fragments.

A femoral neck fracture in geriatric patients tends to be a very low-energy injury.[34] There have been three mechanisms described for femoral neck fractures. Kocher,[35] at the turn of the century, described two possible mechanisms. The first was a direct blow on the greater trochanter resulting from a fall. The second was from lateral rotation of the extremity. The third mechanism, that of a fatigue failure of the neck, was proposed by Urovitz et al.[36] in 1977. In the nongeriatric patient, a femoral neck fracture usually results from major trauma.

Various systems of classification of fractures of the intertrochanteric region have been proposed. Boyd and Griffin[37] divided these fractures into four types. Evans[38] looked at the stability of the fractures and used this as his method of classification. Type I fractures started at the lesser trochanter and went proximal and lateral to the greater trochanter. They were stable if they were undisplaced or if medial bony apposition could be obtained during the reduction of the fracture at the time of internal fixation. If medial bone apposition could not be obtained, then the fracture was classified as unstable. Type II fractures have a reverse obliquity and start in the region of the lesser trochanter and go distal and lateral. These are also unstable because they tend to

displace after reduction because of the pull of the hip adductors. Stable fractures are relatively easy to treat because after anatomic reduction and fixation there is no tendency to lose the reduction, while unstable fractures are difficult to treat because it can be difficult to maintain reduction.

A subtrochanteric is a fracture within 5 cm of the lesser trochanter of the lesser trochanter. Fielding and Magliato[39] classified these proximal diaphyseal fractures according to the distance from the lesser trochanter. Type I fractures are at the level of the lesser trochanter. Type II fractures are within 2.5 cm of the lesser trochanter, and type III are from 2.5 cm to 5 cm below the inferior aspect of the lesser trochanter. DeLee[40] uses a clinically important concept and divides subtrochanteric fractures into stable and unstable fractures.

The ASOF classification of proximal femur fracture does not include subtrochanteric fractures, as these are considered diaphyseal fractures. The proximal femur is divided into three parts: part A is the intertrochanteric region, part B the neck, and part C the head. Figure 18.27 is the basis of the AO classification of proximal femur fractures.

The femur is not perfectly straight; it is slightly bowed anteriorly, that is, the convex side faces forward. This influences the fracture pattern when it is loaded indirectly through the knee, as would typically happen during a frontal accident when the knee strikes an object, such as the dashboard. Fractures of the femoral diaphysis may be classified by the descriptive terms for other shaft fractures. The Swiss method may also be used. Figure 18.28 summarizes the ASOF classification of femoral diaphyses fractures. The femur is one of the strongest bones in the human skeleton. Table 18.9 summarizes femur strengths.

The patella is the largest sesamoid in the body. It serves to give a mechanical advantage to the quadriceps. It can be injured by direct trauma, such as in striking a dashboard or indirectly from a strong contracture of the quadriceps on the partially flexed knee. Indirect injuries, which result from tension in the quadriceps, will cause either a tendon rupture, an avulsion fracture, or a transverse fracture of

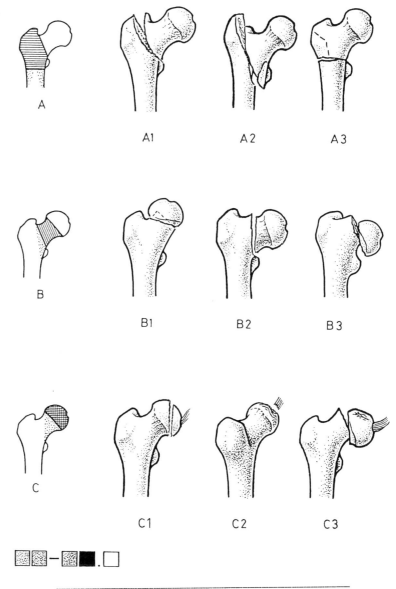

FIGURE 18.27. AO Classification of proximal femur fractures.

Femur proximal: the groups

A1 Trochanteric area fracture, pertrochanteric simple
A2 Trochanteric area fracture, pertrochanteric multifragmentary
A3 Trochanteric area fracture, intertrochanteric

B1 Neck fracture, subcapital, with slight displacement
B2 Neck fracture, transcervical
B3 Neck fracture, subcapital, with marked displacement

C1 Head fracture, split
C2 Head fracture, with depression
C3 Head fracture, with neck fracture

the patella. Direct injuries, which result from the patella being struck, will usually cause a comminuted and frequently stellate-appearing fracture.

Fractures of the tibia can be classified by the descriptive terms that describe the appearance of the fracture. Since the pattern of the fracture is a result of the forces that cause the

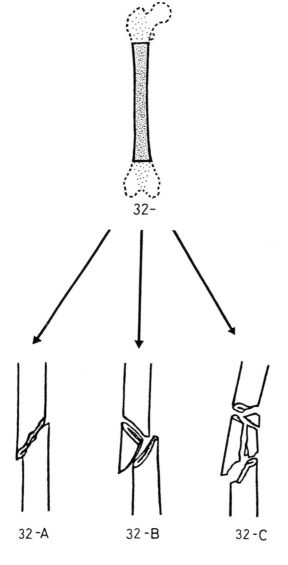

FIGURE 18.28. AO classification of femoral shaft fractures.

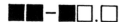

Femur diaphysis: the segment, the types

32-   Femur diaphysis
32-A Femur diaphysis, simple fracture
32-B Femur diaphysis, wedge fracture
32-C Femur diaphysis, complex fracture

fracture, these terms imply the mechanism of loading that caused the fracture. Most authors classify fractures of the tibia diaphysis without reference to the fibula. In fracture treatment, an unfractured fibula maintains length and general alignment of the leg (anatomically from the knee to the ankle, by definition). Injuries in which the tibia and fibula are fractured at the same level are more unstable than those in which the tibia and fibula are fractured at different levels. Müeller et al.,[17] in their classification of leg fracture, chose to evaluate

TABLE 18.9. Femur strength.

	Male	Female
Torque (N = m)	175	136
Range	141–222	78–207
Bending (kN)	3.92	2.58
Range	3.43–4.66	2.26–3.33
Average maximum moment (N = m)	310	180
Long axis compression (kN)	7.72	7.11
Range	6.85–8.56	5.63–8.56

From Messerer, as reported in Naham and Melvin.[23]

TABLE 18.10. Tibia strength.

	Male	Female
Torque (N = m)	89	56
Range	63–110	47–63
Bending (kN)	3.36	2.24
Range	2.30–4.90	1.86–2.65
Average maximum moment (N = m)	207	124
Long axis compression (kN)	10.36	7.49
Range	7.05–16.39	4.89–10.37

From Messerer, as reported in Naham and Melvin.[23]

TABLE 18.11. Fibula strength.

	Male	Female
Torque (N = m)	9	10
Range	6–12	8–16
Bending (kN)	0.44	0.30
Range	0.35–0.54	0.21–0.39
Average maximum moment (N = m)	27	17
Long axis compression (kN)	0.60	0.48
Range	0.24–0.88	0.20–0.83

From Messerer, as reported in Naham and Melvin.[23]

the tibia and fibula together. Since the status of the fibula affects treatment decisions, their classification is logical. It is also useful descriptively because the status of two bones are described with one code. The segment for the tibia and fibula is 42. Figure 18.29 is a drawing from Müeller et al. of the classification of tibia fractures. The letter and number are the two *'s in the five-digit classification, 42-**.x. For the simple fractures that are the "A" fractures and the wedge fractures that are the "B"

fractures, the subgroup that is indicated by the "x" after the decimal point in the five-digit code defines the condition of the fibula. For an unfractured fibula it is "1"; for a fibula fractured at a different level, it is "2"; and for the fibula fractured at the same level, it is "3." In "C" tibia fractures, this digit indicates the comminution and number of fragments in the tibia itself.

The tibia, since it supports most of the body weight, is the strongest long bone in our skeleton. Table 18.10 summarizes the strength of the tibia and Table 18.11 summarizes the strength of the fibula.

Ankle injuries can be classified by the mechanism causing them. However, to understand the classification, one has to understand the movement of the ankle. Unfortunately, more than one term is used to describe the same motion. One of the best descriptions of the complex motions of the ankle and hindfoot can be found in the chapter by VanderGriend, Savoie, and Hughes[41] in Rockwood et al.'s Fractures in Adults. There are six motions of the ankle and hindfoot. Plantarflexion and dorsiflexion are the up and down motions of the foot. In plantarflexion the foot moves downward and in dorsiflexion the foot moves upward. When one walks with a plantarflexed ankle, one is walking on the toes. If one walks with the ankle dorsiflexed, one is walking on the heel with the toes off of the ground. There can also be some internal rotation and external rotation. In internal rotation, one becomes more pigeon-toed, while with external rotation one's toes point outward. The final two motions are supination and pronation. In supination the ankle and hindfoot angulate to start to bring the medial aspect of the heel foot (great toe) off of the ground. In pronation, the motion is to bring the lateral aspect of the foot and heel from the ground. The fracture mechanism descriptions will usually often include two other terms, adduction and abduction. In adduction the hindfoot is moved toward the midline, that is, toward the other foot. In abduction, the hindfoot is moved laterally, that is, away from the other foot.

Pure vertical loading, such as one gets when jumping, falling, and landing in a standing

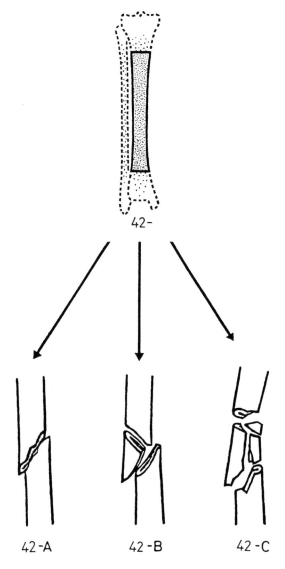

FIGURE 18.29. AO classification of tibia and fibula fractures.

Tibia/Fibula diaphysis: the segment, the types

42-   Tibia/Fibula diaphysis
42-A Tibia/Fibula diaphysis, simple fracture
42-B Tibia/Fibula diaphysis, wedge fracture
42-C Tibia/Fibula diaphysis, complex fracture

position will cause pillion fractures by the driving of the talus into the tibia. Reudi and Allgower[42] classified this fracture into three types. In type I, the fracture is essentially undisplaced. In type II, there is moderate com-

minution and displacement. And in type III, there is severe comminution and displacement. In the AO classification, these are the 43-xxx.x fractures: "43" indicates that it is the lower end of the tibia and "-xxx.x" is the type

FIGURE 18.30. AO classification of distal tibia fractures.

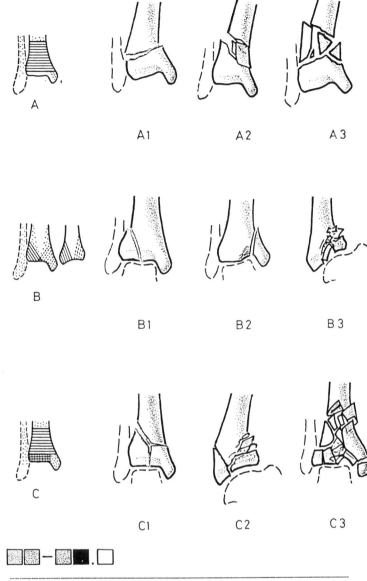

Tibia/Fibula distal: the groups

A1 Extra-articular fracture, metaphyseal simple
A2 Extra-articular fracture, metaphyseal wedge
A3 Extra-articular fracture, metaphyseal complex

B1 Partial articular fracture, pure split
B2 Partial articular fracture, split-depression
B3 Partial articular fracture, multifragmentary depression

C1 Complete articular fracture, articular simple, metaphyseal simple
C2 Complete articular fracture, articular simple, metaphyseal multifragmentary
C3 Complete articular fracture, multifragmentary

and severity of the injury. Figure 18.30 is the AO classification.

Supination and adduction of the ankle will cause a tear of the lateral ligament or fractures of the lateral malleolus distal to the syndesmosis between the tibia and fibula. In the most severe case there can also be a vertical fracture of the medial malleolus. Supination and external rota-

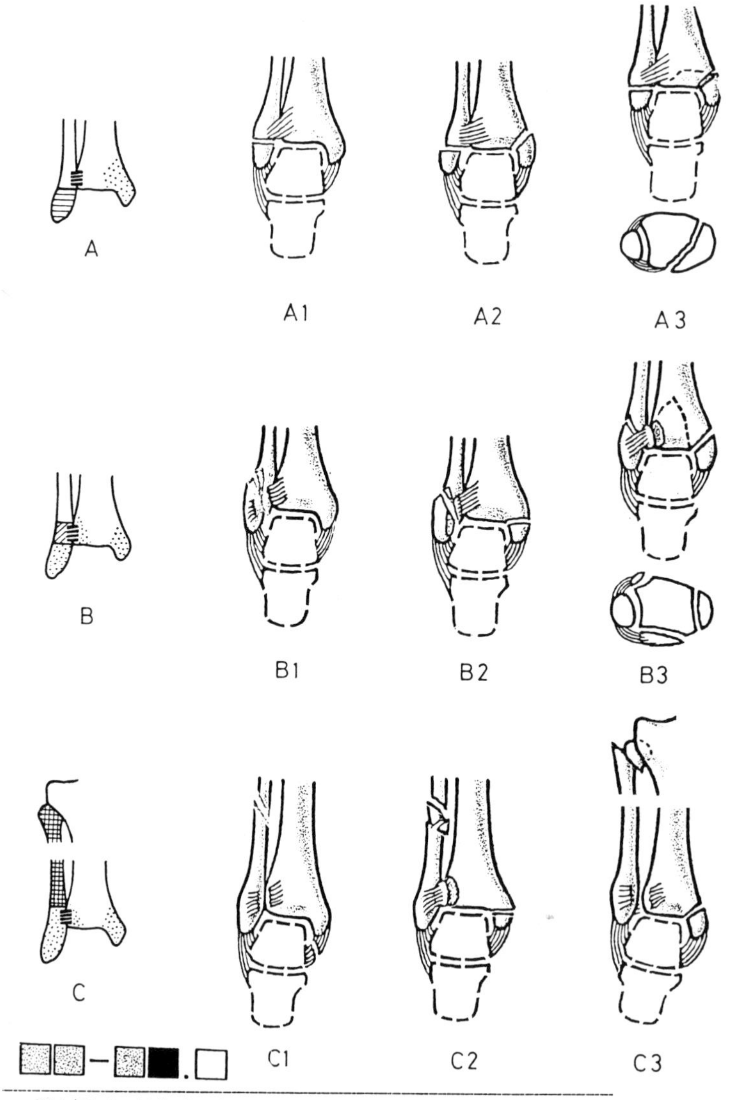

FIGURE 18.31. AO classification of ankle fractures.

Tibia/Fibula, Malleolar Segment: the groups

A1   Infrasyndesmotic lesion, isolated
A2   Infrasyndesmotic lesion, with a fracture of the medial malleolus
A3   Infrasyndesmotic lesion, with a postero-medial fracture

B1   Transsyndesmotic fibula fracture, isolated
B2   Transsyndesmotic fibula fracture, with a medial lesion
B3   Transsyndesmotic fibula fracture, with a medial lesion and Volkmann (fracture of the
     postero-lateral rim)

C1   Suprasyndesmotic lesion, diaphyseal fracture of the fibula, simple
C2   Suprasyndesmotic lesion, diaphyseal fracture of the fibula, multifragmentary
C3   Suprasyndesmotic lesion, proximal fibula

tion will lead to tears of the anterior tibiofibular ligament, or avulsion at the attachment on this ligament. If the force continued, one would also see a spiral fracture of the lateral malleolus and fractured medial malleolus or a tear of the deltoid ligament. In a pronation adduction injury, there is initially a fracture of the medial malleolus or a tear of the deltoid ligament, which is followed by tears of the anterior and posterior tibiofibular ligaments and an oblique fracture of the lateral malleolus. In a pronation external rotation injury the

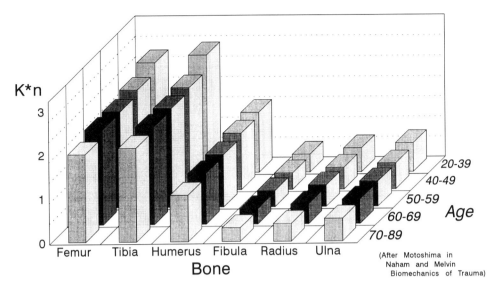

K*n

(After Motoshima in
Naham and Melvin
Biomechanics of Trauma)

FIGURE 18.32. A summary of the changes in bone strength with aging. (Modified from Motoshima.[43])

medial malleolus or deltoid ligament fails first, which is then followed by a spiral fracture of the lateral malleolus. In the AO classification, the malleoli are segment 44. Their general classification is summarized in Fig. 18.31.

Bones are not static; their strength varies. As one ages the strength of bones slowly lessens. Figure 18.32 summarizes the changes in bone strength with aging. Bones are strongest during the second and third decade and slowly weaken as one ages. Disease can affect strength. Early menopause can lead to severe osteoporosis in the female.

The big question biomechanically is not how do bones break, but why do bones not break more often? In many slips and falls there is enough energy to break a wrist or hip, yet most of the time there is no fracture. Why do more fractures not occur? Bone can be preloaded by muscle tension. The muscle tension and preloading can affect how bones fracture. But muscle pull can also be bad, for the forces of muscles pulling can also cause fractures. The classical model is fractures during electroconvulsive therapy (ECT), which not uncommonly occurred in patients who were not rendered temporarily paralyzed prior to receiving the ECT. The forces of the contraction of muscles can cause significant bony injury. Interesting fractures rarely occurred during

the initial ECT; rather, they occurred during subsequent treatment, indicating that fatigue is a factor in fractures.

As more is understood about fatigue, preloading, and the forces truly applied to bone, there will be a greater understanding of fractures, and it may become a bit easier to predict the force needed to cause a given bone to fail. The current data as reported in this chapter fail to account for these other factors.

References

1. Committee on Medical Aspects of Automotive Safety (1971) Rating the severity of tissue damage: I. The Abbreviated Injury Scale. JAMA 215:277–280.
2. Association for the Advancement of Automotive Medicine. *The Abbreviated Injury Scale: 1990 revision.* Association for the Advancement of Automotive Medicine, Des Plaine, IL, 1990.
3. Baker SP, O'Neill B, Haddon W, Long WB (1974) The Injury Severity Score: A method for describing patients with multiple injuries and evaluating emergency care. J Trauma 14: 187–196.
4. Champion HR, Sacco WJ, Carnazzo AJ, Copes W, Fouth WJ (1981) Trauma score. Crit Care Med 9:672–671.
5. Champion HR, Sacco WJ, Copes WS, Gann DS, Gennarelli TA, Flanagan ME (1989) A

revision of the trauma score. J Trauma 29: 623–629.

6. Boyd CR, Tolson MA, Copes WS (1987) Evaluating trauma care: the TRISS method. J Trauma 27:370–379.

7. Bondurant F, Cotler HB, Buckle R, et al (1988) The medical and economic impact of severely injured lower extremities. J Trauma 28: 1270–1273.

8. Johansen K, Daines M, Howey T, et al (1990) Objective criteria accurately predict amputation following lower extremity trauma. J Trauma 30:568–517.

9. Gregory JT, Gould RJ, Peclet M, et al (1985) The mangled extremity syndrome (M.E.S.): a severity grading system for multisystem injury of the lower extremity. J Trauma 25:1147–1150.

10. Müeller ME, Allgöwer, Schneider R, Willenegger. Manual of internal fixation: techniques recommended by the AO-ASIF group. Springer-Verlag, New York, 1990.

11. Gustilo RB, Mendoz RM, Williams DN (1984) Problems in the management of type III (severe) open fractures: a new classification of type III open fractures. J Trauma 24:742–746.

12. Winquest RA, Hansen ST Jr (1980) Comminuted fractures of the femoral shaft treated by intramedullary nailing. Orthop Clin North Am 11:633–648.

13. Salter RB, Harris WR (1963) Injuries involving the epiphyseal plate. J Bone Joint Surg [Am] 45A:587–622.

14. Rang M. The growth plate and its disorders. Williams and Wilkins, Baltimore, 1969.

15. Harkess JW, Ramsey WC, Harkess JW. Principles of fractures and dislocations. In Rockwood CA, Green DP, Bucholz RW (eds) Fractures in adults. JB Lippincott Company, New York, 1990.

16. Cotton FJ, Berg R (1929) "Fender fractures" of the tibia at the knee. N Engl J Med 201: 989–995.

17. Müeller ME, Nazarian S, Koch P, Schatzker J. Classification of fractures of long bones. Springer-Verlag, Berlin, 1990.

18. Seddon H (1942) A classification of nerve injuries. Br Med J 4260:237–239.

19. Post M (1989) Current concepts in the treatment of fractures of the clavicle. Clin Orthop Rel Res 245:89–101.

20. Allman FL (1967) Fractures and ligamentous injuries of the clavicle and its articulation. J Bone Joint Surg 49A:774–784.

21. Neer CS (1963) Fractures of the distal clavicle with detachment of the coracoacromial ligaments in adults. J Trauma 3:99–110.

22. Sankarankutty M, Turner BW (1975) Fracture of the clavicle. Injury 7:101–106.

23. Messerer O (1880) Uber Elasticitat und Festigcitat der Mnschlichen Knochen. Stuttgard J.G. Cotta. (Cited in Nahum AM, Melvin J. The biomechanics of trauma. Appleton-Century Crofts, Norwalk, CT, 1985.)

24. Klenermann L (1969) Experimental fractures of the adult humerus. Med Biol Eng 7:357–364.

25. Clemmons HM, Hammond G (1947) Spontaneous fracture of the humerus due to muscle violence. Guthrie Clin Bull 17:49–51.

26. Herzmark MH, Klune FR (1952) Ball-throwing fracture of the humerus. Med Ann Distric Columbia 21:196–199.

27. Peltokallio P, Peltokallio V, Vaalasti T (1968) Fracture of the humerus from muscular violence in sport. J Sports Med Phys Fitness 1:21–25.

28. Gregersen HN (1971) Fracture of the humerus from muscular violence. Acta Orthop Scand 42:506–512.

29. Chao SL, Miller M, Teng SW (1971) A mechanism of spiral fracture of the humerus: a report of 129 cases following the throwing of hand grenades. J Trauma 11:602–605.

30. Arfwidsson S (1957) Missle-throwing fracture of the shaft of the humerus. Acta Chir Scand 113:229–233.

31. Epstein HC (1974) Posterior fracture-dislocations of the hip. J Bone Joint Surg [Am] 56A:1103–1127.

32. Pietrafesa CA, Hoffmann JR (1983) Traumatic dislocation of the hip. JAMA 249:3342–3346.

33. Garden RS (1974) Reduction and fixation of subcapital fractures of the femur. Orthop Clin North Am 5:683–712.

34. Banks HH (1962) Factors influencing the results in fractures of the femoral neck. J Bone Joint Surg [Am] 44A:931–964.

35. Kocher T (1896) Beitrage zur Kentruss einiger praktisck wichtiger. Fractuformen, Basel Leipzig, Carl Sallman. (Cited in Rockwood CA, Green DP, Bucholz RW. Fractures in adults. Vol 2. JB Lippincott, Philadelphia, 1991.)

36. Urovitz EPM, Fornaiser VL, Risen MI, MacNab I (1977) Etiological factors in the pathogenesis of femoral trabecular fatigue fractures. Clin Orthop Rel Res 127:275–280.

37. Boyd HB, Griffin LL (1949) Classification and treatment of intertrochanteric fractures. Arch Surg 58:853–866.

38. Evans EM (1949) The treatment of trochanteric fractures of the femur. J Bone Joint Surg 31B: 190–203.

39. Fielding JW, Magliato HJ (1966) Subtrochanteric fractures. Surg Gynecol Obstet 122:555–560.

40. DeLee JC. Fractures and dislocations of the hip. In Rockwood CA, Green DP, Bucholz RW (eds) *Fractures in adults*. JB Lippincott, Philadelphia, 1991.

41. VanderGriend RA, Savoie FH, Hughes, JL. Fractures of the ankle. In Rockwood CA, Green DP, Bucholz RW. *Fractures in adults*. JB Lippincott, Philadelphia, 1991.

42. Reudi TP, Allgower M (1979) The operative treatment of intra-articular fractures of the distal tibia. Clin Orthop Rel Res 138:105–110.

43. Motoshima.

19
Child Passenger Protection

Kathleen Weber

Child restraint systems function in much the same way as occupant protection systems for adults, with a few important differences. For the average child restraint user, the primary difference is the wide variety of systems from which to choose. Children of different ages and sizes require different types of restraints, and, among each type, the way in which they are used can be critical for effective performance. This chapter describes the theory behind the design of restraint systems, relates these principles to the various types of child restraint systems available today, and indicates the circumstances in which children in these restraints may still be injured, particularly when the child restraints are misused. Finally, the issues of child injury potential and biomechanically based injury criteria are addressed, and research needs are identified.

Restraint System Theory

In a vehicle crash, there are actually a series of collisions. The primary impact is between the vehicle and another object, while the occupants continue to travel forward at the precrash speed. Unrestrained occupants then come to an abrupt stop against the decelerating vehicle interior or the ground outside the vehicle. Restrained occupants, however, "collide" with their belts, or other restraint system, very soon after the primary collision, with various benefits to the traveler. Finally, there are collisions between the body's internal organs and the bony structures enclosing them, which can be mitigated by the use of occupant restraint systems.

The front ends of vehicles are designed to crush during impact, thereby absorbing crash energy and allowing the passenger compartment to come to a stop over a greater distance (and longer time) than does the front bumper. By tightly coupling the occupants to the vehicle frame, through the use of snug-fitting belts, the occupants "ride down" the crash with the vehicle. For adults, there is usually only one link, such as a lap/shoulder belt, between the occupant and the vehicle. For children, however, there are usually two.

In the case of belts, which absorb little energy themselves, the tighter they are adjusted prior to the crash, the lower will be the body's initial deceleration into the belts. Other types of protection systems, such as padding or airbags, can themselves absorb impact energy between the occupant and the vehicle interior. Controlling the rate of the body's overall deceleration reduces not only the forces acting on the body's surface but also the differential motion between the skeleton and the internal organs. Hard surfaces or loose belts, on the other hand, stop the body abruptly when they are finally struck or pulled tight, applying more force to the body surface and giving its contents a harder jolt.

Tight coupling to the crushing vehicle addresses only part of the problem, however. To optimize the body's impact tolerance, the remaining loads must be distributed as widely as possible over the body's strongest parts. For adults, who prefer to face the front of the vehicle (or must do so to drive), this includes the shoulders, the pelvis, and secondarily the thorax. For children, especially infants, restraint over larger and sometimes different body areas is necessary.

Proper placement and good fit are important for effective occupant restraint. Serious restraint-induced injuries can occur when the belts are misplaced over body areas having no protective bony structure. Such misplacement of a lap belt can occur during a crash if the belt is loose or, with small children, is not held in place by a crotch strap or other positioning device. A lap belt that is worn or rides up above the hips can intrude into the soft abdomen and rupture or lacerate internal organs (King, 1985; Rutledge et al., 1991). Moreover, in the absence of a shoulder restraint, a high lap belt can act as a fulcrum around which the lumbar spine flexes, possibly causing separation of the lumbar vertebrae in a severe crash (Johnson and Falci, 1990; Nyquist and King, 1985).

The primary goal of any occupant protection system is to keep the central nervous system from being injured. Broken bones will mend and soft tissue will heal, but damage to the brain and spinal cord is currently irreversible. In the design of restraint systems, it may therefore be necessary to put the extremities, ribs, or even abdominal viscera at some risk in order to ensure that the head and spine will be protected.

Child Restraint Systems

There are several different types of restraint systems designed especially for children. These vary with the size of the child, the direction the child faces, and the placement of the vehicle seat belt. All types, however, work on the principle of coupling the child as tightly as possible to the vehicle frame, and many provide additional energy absorption through padding or structural deformation.

There is an important difference, however, between restraint systems for infants and young children and those for older children and adults. Child restraints are anchored to the vehicle with the seat belt provided, and the child is then secured to the child restraint with a separate harness and/or other restraining surface (shield). This results in two links between the vehicle and the occupant, rather than only one. It is therefore critical that both the seat belt and the harness be as tight as possible to allow the child to ride down the crash with the vehicle and thereby provide the child with the best crash injury protection. If properly used and secured, child restraints reduce the risk of death and serious injury to their occupants by approximately 70% (Kahane, 1986). By comparison, estimates of fatality reduction to adults in lap/shoulder belts average about 50% (Evans, 1986; Huelke et al., 1979; Partyka, 1988).

Infant Restraints

There are two types of restraint systems designed exclusively for infants. One places the infant facing the rear of the vehicle. The other allows the infant to lie flat, perpendicular to the direction of vehicle travel.

Rear-Facing Infant Restraints

In North America, the most common restraint system for infants under 20 lb (9 kg) is a semi-upright seat that faces the rear of the vehicle (Fig. 19.1). It is anchored in place with a seat belt, and internal harness straps secure the infant's shoulders. In an impact, the crash forces are transferred from the back of the restraint to the infant's back, which is its strongest body surface, while the restraint also supports the infant's head. Even in an oblique or lateral crash, the back of the rear-facing infant restraint swivels toward the direction of impact, still providing its occupant with effective protection. In rear-end and rollover crashes, which tend to be much less severe, the shoulder straps provide containment, and the restraint often rotates up against the vehicle seat back, completely enclosing the infant. For best protection and comfort, rear-facing restraints should be installed so that the back

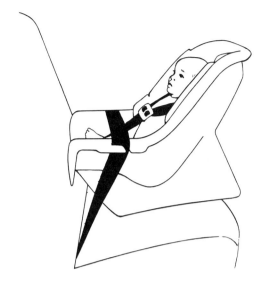

FIGURE 19.1. Rear-facing infant restraint.

surface is at approximately a 45° angle with respect to vertical. Although regulatory criteria allow the back angle to increase to 70° during a 30-mph impact test with a 6-month–size dummy, most infant restraints stay below 60°. Infants outgrow these restraints when they exceed 20 lb or the top of their head extends above the back of the restraint.

To work properly, the infant restraint must face rearward, and the harness straps must be over the shoulders and adjusted for a snug fit. If the infant's head or body needs lateral support, padding can be placed between the infant and the side of the restraint. Firm padding, such as a rolled towel, can also be placed between the infant and the crotch strap or buckle between its legs to keep the infant's pelvis from sliding forward. This is particularly helpful with premature infants (Bull and Stroup, 1985). Thick, soft padding should not, however, be placed under the infant or behind its back. Such padding will compress during an impact, leaving the harness straps loose on the infant's body.

Properly used, rear-facing restraints have proven to be extremely effective in actual crashes (Melvin, et al., 1980; National Transportation Safety Board, 1983). Unfortunately, parents and others who do not understand how

an infant restraint is designed to work will often install it facing forward (Cynecki and Goryl, 1984). A laboratory test of this type of incorrect use with an older but still widely used model of infant restraint indicates that there is a risk of serious neck injury from contact with the seat belt, which is designed to hold the restraint, not the infant, in place (Weber and Melvin, 1983). In this test, the shoulder straps were set properly over the infant dummy's shoulders, so the dummy slid under the seat belt until stopped at the neck by the belt (Fig. 19.2A). Current infant restraints have close-fitting crotch straps and do not allow the same sliding motion, but infants facing forward in these restraints are still subject to neck injury, to be discussed below. If the harness straps are not used, which is also a common misuse with either type of infant restraint, the dummy flexes at the waist around the lap belt (Fig. 19.2B). When the belt is fastened over the shell to anchor it in this incorrect manner, it is too high and too far away from the body to provide effective restraint. An infant in this situation would likely suffer spinal and internal abdominal injuries as its body is thrown into the seat belt.

It is therefore critical that infant restraints be used facing the rear of the vehicle. One reason parents face infants the wrong way is that they are told that the center of the rear seat is the safest seating position, but drivers would like to be able to see their babies in the rear seat. Infant visibility is especially an issue if the driver is the only adult in the car. Although the rear seat is a less hostile environment than the front, and the center-rear provides the most space between the child and the side of the vehicle, it is only "safest" if all other factors are equal. Facing an infant restraint forward in the back is much worse than restraining the infant rearward in the front. In fact, rear-facing infant restraints have performed very well in the front passenger seat, particularly when they rest against the instrument panel (Melvin et al., 1980). Many infant restraint models have a slot in the back for a vehicle shoulder belt, now available in both front and rear seats, so that it can help support the restraint in a crash (Fig. 19.3). (If the infant

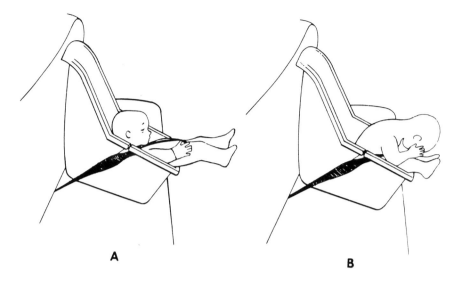

FIGURE 19.2. Infant restraints facing forward: (A) with, and (B) without harness in use.

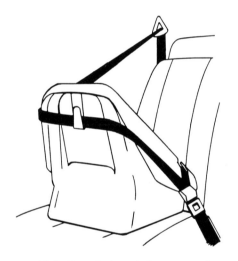

FIGURE 19.3. Rear-facing infant restraint with shoulder belt used for support.

cannot yet hold up its head, however, the belt may hold the restraint at an angle too upright for comfort and unrestricted breathing.)

Although the use of rear-facing restraints in the front seat has been recommended for some time, and the American Academy of Pediatrics (AAP) now specifically recommends that premature infants be placed in a seat location "that allows for observation by an adult during travel" (AAP, 1991), the recent appearance of passenger-side airbags has complicated this issue. Tests conducted at various facilities have indicated that certain types of child restraints, but particularly rear-facing ones, "could be struck by the airbag when it inflates in a crash. If this happens, a child in the restraint could be seriously injured" (SAE CRABI, 1991). Child restraint users are further cautioned to "always read the vehicle owner's manual and the child restraint instructions for directions on where and how to install a child restraint." For situations in which the driver is alone with a very young infant or there is no rear seat (two-passenger vehicles), it may not be possible to safely transport an infant.

Car-Bed Restraints

Another type of infant restraint is the car-bed or carry-cot (Fig. 19.4). This type is used more often in Europe and Australia but is generating interest in the United States because of concerns about premature infants with positional apnea (Willet et al., 1986). In a car-bed restraint, the infant lies flat, either prone or supine, and the bed is placed on the vehicle seat with its long axis perpendicular to the direction of travel and the baby's head toward the center of the seat (not next to the door). In a frontal crash, the forces are distributed along the entire side of the infant's body, while straps

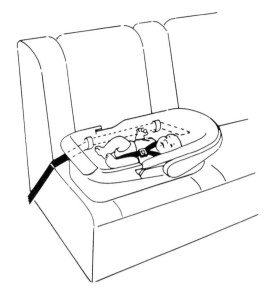

FIGURE 19.4. Car-bed infant restraint.

or a "baby bag," secured to the car-bed on each side with zippers, provides containment during rebound and rollover. In a side impact, however, the infant's head and neck are theoretically more vulnerable in a car-bed than in a rear-facing restraint, especially if the impact is on the side nearest the head and there is significant intrusion (Weber, 1990). Documented crash experience is too limited at this time to provide further insight into the actual injury risk.

Car-bed restraints are tested with the same dummy as rear-facing infant restraints, but the performance criteria merely relate to containment of the dummy. European regulations also limit the forward travel of the dummy and its chest acceleration (Glaeser et al., 1990). Such criteria would be useful additions to the United States standard. Canada does not at this time allow the sale of car-beds.

The potential effect of a deploying airbag interacting with a car-bed restraint is largely unknown, although preliminary testing indicates that its low profile may allow the car-bed to avoid significant interaction with some airbag designs. If future testing indicates no injurious effects under certain specified conditions, this may be a partial solution to the infant monitoring dilemma.

Convertible Restraints

Convertible child restraints are designed to be used rear-facing for an infant and forward-facing for a child over 1 year (Fig. 19.5). Most of the above information about rear-facing infant restraints also applies to rear-facing convertibles, including the caution about airbags. The important difference is that, because convertibles have a higher back-support surface, children can remain rear-facing in them longer than the same children can remain in infant-only restraints. In fact, most children seem to outgrow infant restraints within a few months and should then use a convertible restraint, still in the rear-facing position.

As required by regulation, manufacturers' instructions identify the transition to forward-facing in terms of body weight. This weight is usually 20 lb (9 kg) but ranges from 18 to 25 lb (8 to 11.5 kg). The lower end of the "turn-around" weight range is not based on any careful biomechanical evaluation of the tolerance of children to crash forces applied to the front of their bodies. Instead, the 6-month dummy used in United States and Canadian standard crash tests of infant restraints and rear-facing convertible restraints weighs 17.4 lb (8 kg). Most manufacturers, however, voluntarily test with a 20-lb, 9-month dummy, and some have tested with a 25-lb, 18-month dummy. The weight selected for the instructions may merely reflect the Federal standard, but most manufacturers have chosen to go beyond it. In reality, there is a considerable margin of safety built into convertible child restraints in the rear-facing position, and children would benefit from facing rearward as long as they, with their growing legs, can comfortably do so. The issue of how long a child should face rearward in order to avoid cervical and other serious injuries is currently a topic of international concern and will be discussed below.

While facing rearward, the shoulder straps should be left in slots below the child's shoulders, so that the straps can keep the child from ramping up the back of the restraint. When the child is eventually allowed to face

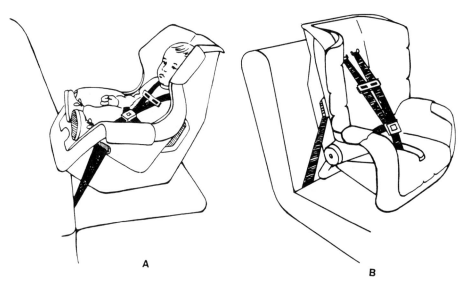

FIGURE 19.5. Convertible child restraint in (A) rear- and (B) forward-facing use.

forward, the shoulder straps must be raised to the highest slots, so that the strap forces press back against the shoulders and do not compress the shoulders and spine downward. More importantly, in convertible restraints with three pairs of strap slots, the uppermost are usually the only ones designed to withstand frontal crash loads.

Convertible restraints are tested in both rear-facing and forward-facing positions. Forward-facing tests use a dummy the size of a 3-year-old child weighing 33.3 lb (15 kg), and criteria assess body accelerations and forward travel or "excursion" of the head and knees. Most convertible child restraints, however, claim to be for children up to 40 or 45 lb (18 or 20 kg). In practice, the factors limiting use of a convertible restraint are usually the length of the harness straps or the width of the shell, and, before the weight limit is reached, the child no longer fits into the restraint.

Restraint Design Choices

There are many different convertible child restraint designs to choose from. Although all types of child restraints on the domestic market today perform very well in crash tests and have been very effective in protecting children in actual crashes (Kahane, 1986), differences

among the internal restraining systems should be noted.

The original strap arrangement in early child restraints was the 5-point harness, which was patterned after military and racing harnesses (Fig. 19.6A). There is a strap over each shoulder, one on each side of the pelvis, and one between the legs. All five come together at a common buckle. The function of the crotch strap is to hold the lap straps firmly down on top of the thighs, and thus it should be as short as possible. [Many child restraints in Europe and older ones in the United Kingdom do not have crotch straps, and their occupants are thus susceptible to submarining (Conry and Hall, 1987; Lowne et al., 1987.)] Because the crotch strap is merely a lap-strap positioning device, the primary lower torso restraint is still the combined lap straps. Although simple and effective, early five-point harness systems were difficult to adjust and buckle around a squirming child, and complaints about twisting and "roping" of the straps continue today. In recent years, however, easier means of adjusting five-point harnesses have been developed and are incorporated into newer models.

In the early 1980s, a creative designer replaced the lap portion of the harness with a padded tray-like shield (Fig. 19.6B). The

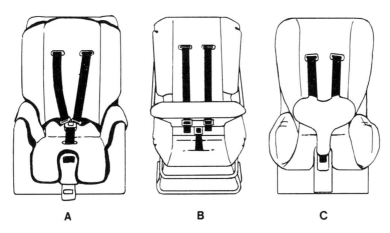

FIGURE 19.6. Restraining configurations: (A) 5-point harness, (B) harness/shield combination, (C) T-shield.

shoulder straps were attached to the shield, which kept them from twisting, and there was an easier means of adjusting those straps. The shield was still held in place by a crotch strap made of belt webbing. Other manufacturers quickly followed suit. Although these harness/shield combinations do not contact the body as low on the pelvis as the 5-point harness, they are much more convenient to use, and years of field experience have shown no performance problems.

At about the same time, a Japanese manufacturer developed another variation on the 5-point harness that incorporated a retractor on the shoulder straps (Fig. 19.6C). These straps were attached to a flat chest shield with a relatively rigid stalk, which in turn attached to the child restraint between the child's legs. The overall shape of the shield and stalk has been compared to an elephant's head or a bicycle seat and is now usually referred to as a T-shield. Eventually, similar designs began to appear in the American market, some with automatic retractors and some with manual strap adjusters.

Although ease of adjustment and one-handed operation of the T-shield provide a further level of convenience for parents, there are some theoretical problems with this restraint configuration. Because the length and angle of the stalk is fixed, it is not possible to adjust the shield to fit close to a small child's body or low across the pelvis. As discussed earlier, a loose-fitting restraining system does not couple the occupant tightly to the crushing vehicle, and higher forces on the body will result. The lower torso restraint of the lap belt is now replaced by a narrow vertical stalk that concentrates impact forces at the center of the pelvis rather than spreading the forces across the pelvic breadth, and lateral restraint provided by lap straps is also lost. Another concern is that the throat of a small child may be injured from contact with the top of the shield during a crash, especially in the forward-facing position. It is important to emphasize that these problems are, at the moment, only theoretical, because we are not aware of any injuries related to this type of restraining system used in actual crashes. In response to these criticisms, however, some T-shields have now been designed to make the stalk more flexible, to lower the height of the shield, and to provide two stalk attachment positions.

Misuse and Injury Potential

There are a variety of ways to misuse a convertible child restraint. Incorrect routing of the vehicle belt has been well documented among older models (Cynecki and Goryl, 1984; Shelness and Jewett, 1983). This could have anywhere from a minor to a disastrous effect on restraint performance, depending on the design and specific misrouting (Weber and Melvin, 1983). Other dangerous practices commonly observed include not using the harness straps at all, leaving the seat belt or harness straps very loose, having the crotch strap very long, or placing the shoulder straps under the child's arms. Loose belts or straps will not couple the child tightly to the crushing vehicle, and higher crash forces on the body will result. A long crotch strap will place the lap straps up around the waist, where they may intrude into the soft abdomen during impact. Shoulder straps routed under the arms may crush or intrude under the child's flexible rib cage and cause serious injury to thoracic and abdominal organs. When the crotch strap is too long and the shoulder straps are under the arms, or the shoulder straps merely connected by the plastic strap positioner, the child will flex around the straps at the waist, possibly causing fracture or dislocation of the lumbar spine and laceration of abdominal organs. These injuries would be similar to those produced by a lap belt misplaced around a child's waist.

The reasons for misuse of child protective devices are complex, as are the solutions. It is disturbing, for instance, that follow-up interviews with parents observed misusing a child restraint revealed that 70% to 90%, depending on the specific misuse, knew what they should have been doing but chose not to (Cynecki and Goryl, 1984). Only those with misrouted seat belts were largely unaware of their errors. As child restraint usage has increased and misuse identified as a serious problem (Petrucelli, 1989), designers and manufacturers have responded with design and labeling changes to discourage both intentional and unintentional errors. Newer child restraints have the seat belt routing paths labeled, and many have eliminated multiple openings through which the belt could be misplaced. One design has been verified to perform well with either of two seat belt paths. Crotch straps on most models are now of a short, fixed length, innovative means to easily adjust harness straps are proliferating, and diagrams are displacing text. To assist in identifying and prioritizing potential misuses in the product development process, analytical approaches using parent panels and a technique called Misuse Mode and Effects

Analysis (MMEA) have been proposed and are currently being evaluated (Bell, 1991; Czernakowski and Müller, 1991).

Although design changes and warnings have helped to reduce some misuses, in the end children are still dependent on parents or caregivers to take the time to fasten the harness, adjust it snugly, and secure the restraint in the right direction, tightly to the car.

Neck Injury in Forward-Facing Child Restraints

There has long been a concern that a child's cervical spine could be pulled apart from the weight of the head in a crash when the shoulders are held back (Burdi et al., 1969). In the United States, two documented cases of this type of injury have been identified that involve children at the traditional transition weight for changing from rear- to forward-facing. These children were 10 months old, weighing 8 kg, and 9 months old, weighing 9 kg, and received injuries to the cervical spine while restrained facing forward (Diekema and Allen, 1988; Fuchs et al., 1989). In both cases, the restraints were apparently properly installed and the harness straps used. One case resulted in separation of the odontoid process at C2, while the other resulted in a fatal atlanto-occipital dislocation. These injuries would have been avoided had the children been rear-facing rather than forward-facing in their convertible restraints at the time of the crash. There is also a documented case in which an 8-month-old child weighing "over 17 lb" escaped injury, because he was restrained rear-facing when involved in a very severe frontal crash in a two-passenger sports car (NTSB, 1983).

Media attention in Germany in 1989 sparked intensive study of the potential for cervical spine and spinal cord injury to children facing forward in conventional child restraints (Langwieder and Hummel, 1989; Morres and Appel, 1989), resulting in the identification of four cases involving children from 9 to 12 months restrained by four-point harnesses (no crotch strap). All resulted in tetraplegia, and one child died after 25 days.

These, the fatal American case, and other cases were presented at meetings of international experts in 1990 and 1991, and 11 cases of interest from Europe and North America were studied in detail (Tarriere et al., 1991). (Significantly, no cases could be found among accidents in Australia, where forward-facing child restraints for children over 6 months typically have 5- or 6-point harnesses and top anchor straps.) All crashes were frontal (10 to 2 o'clock), with velocity changes ranging between 24 and 60 km/h (15 to 37 mph). The European children were restrained by 4-point harnesses and the North American children by a 5-point or harness/shield system, with all apparently used as directed. None of the restraints were tethered at the top. The ages of the 11 children ranged from 6 to 23 months, and eight were female. Seven received injuries at the C1 or C2 level, and the other four were injured in the T1–T3 region. Two children, both 9 months, died, while the two girls of 23 months received only odontoid fractures with no permanent neurologic deficit. Only the oldest (18 months) of the remaining seven avoided para- or tetraplegia.

Fuchs et al. (1989) and Janssen et al. (1991) describe the differences between the material and geometric features of the child versus the adult spine and surrounding tissue that relate to the particular cervical, and particularly high cervical, injuries found among the former. These features result in considerable spinal mobility as well as spacing between the vertebrae and spinal cord that may mitigate the effects of this mobility. In spite of its fragile structure, injury to the cervical spine from all causes is rare in children (Janssen et al., 1991).

In trying to determine the actual mechanism of injury in a vehicle crash, it is important to determine whether there was head contact. Although it is apparently possible to stretch the ligaments and separate the vertebrae beyond the limits of the spinal cord, especially for infants under 1 year, head contact while the neck is in tension may be the more critical event when fractures and dislocations occur, especially among older children. This contact suddenly stops the free motion of the head, putting significant shear loads on the neck. Because there may be no external evidence on the head of such contact, it may take a detailed investigation of the crash dynamics and vehicle interior to come to a conclusion. Unfortunately, those who document injuries in the medical literature are not usually in a position to also investigate the vehicle, the restraint, and the actual circumstances of the crash, and thus this mechanism of injury may be overlooked.

Among the 11 cases cited above, experts determined that head contact was likely in at least six, with some cases more definite than others. If head contact is an important factor in the occurrence of neck injury, it follows that children in tethered child restraints would be much less likely to have head contact with the interior and therefore unlikely to suffer these injuries. In addition, preliminary tests comparing a tethered with a nontethered child restraint in frontal crashes, using a specially instrumented 3-year dummy, indicate that neck forces and moments are significantly lower in a tethered restraint (International Task Force on Child Restraining Systems, 1991; Tarriere et al., 1991). There is also some speculation that a 4-point harness and a reclined position (angled back for sleeping) are more strongly associated with neck injury than a 5-point harness and an upright position, but the reasons for this are not clear.

It must again be emphasized that these injuries are still very rare, considering the number of restrained children involved in crashes throughout the world and the number of infants who are improperly facing forward. A recent effort to find restraint-induced neck-injury cases in Great Britain resulted in only one possible case among 50 fatally injured children from 1972 to 1989 (UK Department of Transport, 1991). At the same time, many cases of severe frontal crashes in which fully restrained children have received no neck injury have been fully investigated and documented over the years (e.g., Dejeammes et al., 1984; Langwieder and Hummel, 1989; Melvin et al., 1980). Because of its potentially severe consequences, however, it will be important to continue to monitor this type of injury as more and more restrained children are involved in crashes.

Rear Facing versus Forward Facing

In Sweden, children are restrained in large rear-facing restraints until 3 or 4 years old (Fig. 19.7). These restraints sit away from the vehicle seat back to give the child more leg room, but, because of the need for an extra lower anchorage strap, they are not allowed by United States or Canadian regulations. These restraints, however, have extremely low injury and fatality rates (Carlsson et al., 1989; Turbell, 1989), and there are no reports of fatalities in Sweden among children in rear-facing restraints involved in frontal crashes. Laboratory tests have also shown that dummy acceleration and loading criteria are significantly lower with rearward- than with forward-facing systems (Janssen et al., 1991; Langwieder et al., 1990). Child restraint experts in Europe are discussing possible modification of child restraint weight classes to encourage the extension of rear-facing restraints to children up to 18 months. In the United States, child restraint advocates recommend transition at 1 year but are struggling to keep children rear-facing past 6 months and 17 lb.

What, then, are the factors that determine whether a child can safely use a forward-facing restraint? Weight is not the only indicator of

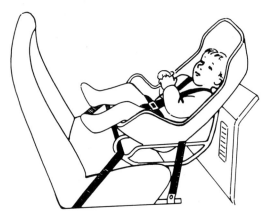

FIGURE 19.7. Large (Swedish) rear-facing child restraint.

skeletal and other physiological development. Other factors, such as age, height, and walking ability, need to be evaluated by anatomical and developmental experts, so that criteria can be established based on a combination of factors. Accident data, although sparse, need careful study to determine the types and mechanisms of injury seen in forward-facing infants and young children that do not occur with older children and adults, and at what thresholds these injuries cease to occur. Whatever the outcome of this research, however, it is clear that any extension of rear-facing restraint over current practice will be beneficial to children.

Child Boosters

When a child can no longer fit into a convertible child restraint, the next step is a booster. Most boosters are not themselves restraint systems, but rather they depend entirely on the vehicle belts to hold the child and the booster in place. Thus they facilitate the transition between a child restraint and seat belts. There are two different types of boosters: one is designed to be used with a lap belt only, and the other only with a lap/shoulder belt.

Shield Boosters

The most common type of booster in North America today is the low-shield booster (Fig. 19.8). It was designed to be used in seating positions with only a lap belt, which has been the rear seat environment in American cars until very recently. In most versions, the lap belt goes across the front of the shield, transferring the load against the belt to a wider, somewhat crushable surface on the child's abdomen. (One model is secured behind the child by the lap belt, and the shield is separately latched to provide restraint.) The low shield provides virtually no upper torso restraint. The primary value of this type of booster is that it raises the child up for better visibility and provides a buffer between the child and a lap belt that may try to ride up around the child's waist.

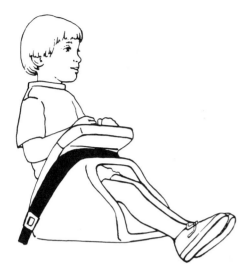

FIGURE 19.8. Low-shield booster.

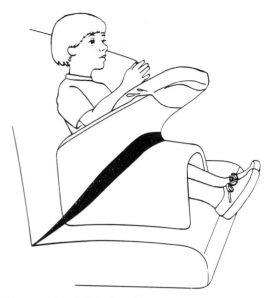

FIGURE 19.9. High-shield booster.

The original shield-booster (Fig. 19.9), which has a high shield rather than a low one, was developed in the mid-1960s (Heap and Grenier, 1968). The high shield acts much like an airbag, restraining the head and upper torso in a frontal crash while deforming to absorb energy. The only performance problem is that the shield sits at a fixed distance from the vehicle seat back and thus may not be snug against a slender child's body. The gap between the shield and the child results in extra head excursion. From a user's point of view, the restraint is considered easy to use if left buckled in place, but it is cumbersome to move from one vehicle to another. Some parents also perceive that the high shield blocks the child's view. By lowering the height of the shield, however, all the impact forces are concentrated on the upper abdomen, rather than being spread over the entire front of the child's trunk. There are indications from laboratory tests of low-shield boosters with a specially instrumented dummy that these abdominal forces may be excessive (Melvin and Weber, 1986), although field accident data has not confirmed this concern. Another advantage of the high shield is its ability to control head/neck motion and to protect the face during impact, which the low shield cannot do.

Shield boosters are subject to the same tests and criteria as forward-facing child restraints,

but the dummy kinematics are quite different (Melvin and Weber, 1986). Whereas the upper torso is held relatively upright in a five-point harness (Fig. 19.10A), the dummy folds around a typical low shield until the head contacts the legs (Fig. 19.10B). The motion around the high shield is somewhat in between (Fig. 19.10C), although the head excursion is greater because it starts out farther from the dummy. [It should be noted here for clarity that a shield restraint popular in Europe, which looks much like an American low shield, is sufficiently different in design and materials that it performs instead like a snug high shield (ITFCRS, 1991)].

Although some low-shield boosters have indicated in their instructions that a shoulder belt, if available, can be placed in front of the "taller child," this is now not recommended. The shield itself usually pushes the shoulder belt up and away from the child, making its angle worse with respect to the child's body. Moreover, routine impact tests have indicated that a shield restraint and a shoulder belt may not be compatible. When used with a lap belt alone, the dummy wraps around the low shield, pushing it more or less in equilibrium against the belt. When the upper torso is held back by the shoulder belt, the lower torso

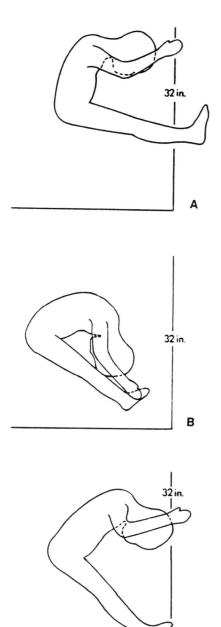

FIGURE 19.10. Dummy position at maximum torso bending: (A) 5-point harness, (B) low-shield booster, (C) high-shield booster.

the shoulder belt in front of the shield, or to place the shoulder belt behind the child.

At present, shield boosters are only required to be tested with the 3-year-old (33.3 lb, 15 kg) dummy, but most manufacturers voluntarily test them with a larger 6-year-old dummy (48 lb, 22 kg), and some also verify structural integrity with a 6-year dummy weighted to 60 lb (27 kg). However, the extra 3 inches (7.6 cm) of sitting height that goes along with the increase in weight from 48 to 60 lb in the average child (Weber et al., 1985) is not taken into account. It is not certain, therefore, whether the head and neck of a slender child weighing 60 lb can be adequately protected by a shield booster.

Belt-Positioning Boosters

A belt-positioning booster is designed to be used with a lap/shoulder belt (Fig. 19.11). It has small handles or guides under which the lap belt and the lower end of the shoulder belt are routed to position them better on a child's small body. The guides, functioning much like a crotch strap, hold the lap belt low and flat across the child's upper thighs. The inboard guide also pulls the shoulder belt toward the

moves forward and tends to slide under the shield, which in turn tends to rotate under the belt. The best approaches, in order of preference, are to limit use of shield boosters to a seat position with only a lap belt, to route

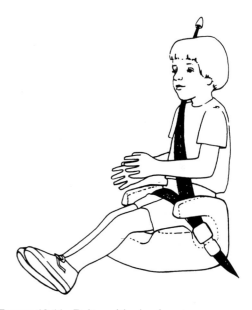

FIGURE 19.11. Belt-positioning booster.

child and makes its angle more vertical, so that it crosses the center of the child's chest. While low-shield boosters merely raise the child and transfer the lap belt load to a wide abdominal area, the belt-positioning boosters adapt vehicle belt systems to a child's body size, so that he or she can take advantage of the built-in upper and lower torso restraint.

The use of a belt-positioning booster with only a lap belt is not generally recommended, although Canadian regulations are not aimed at restricting such usage, as are those in the United States. The rationale is that, without upper torso restraint, the risk of head impact and consequent injury increases the more the child is raised off the vehicle seat. This is due primarily to the longer belt that is needed to go around both child and booster. As the belt is pulled tight during impact, the leading surface of the longer belt is higher and farther forward than the leading surface of a shorter belt that goes around only the child. The head of the child, whose body is rotating around this belt, will also travel farther forward than that of an unboosted child, allowing the head to hit interior surfaces that otherwise it would have missed (Weber and Melvin, 1983).

With respect to head/neck injury prevention, it is better for a child to sit directly on the vehicle seat when only a lap belt is available than to sit on a belt-positioning booster. If, however, the lap belt angle or seat contour is such that the belt will not stay low on the pelvis, it may be necessary to use the booster to prevent belt-induced spinal or abdominal injury, if a more satisfactory seat and restraint combination is not available.

Belt-positioning boosters originated in Australia and Sweden in the early 1970s, as a means of fitting lap/shoulder belts to children, and have been used there and elsewhere successfully ever since. Many come with high backs that not only give the child rear head support but also have belt guides to optimize the location of the shoulder belt. Although several models were manufactured in the United States in the early 1980s, they soon disappeared again because lap/shoulder belts were not generally available in rear seats where children sat, and parents were therefore required to install a special set of child shoulder straps. Now that rear-seat lap/shoulder belts are standard equipment, however, there is an urgent need for these boosters to help provide effective, comfortable, and convenient restraint for children in the 3-to-7 year age range who ride in outboard front- and rear-seat positions. Due to antiquated regulations, however, these boosters may not be sold in the United States unless they are labeled as being for children over 50 lb (23 kg).

To try to fill the gap, a new generation of booster has been developed that converts from a shield to a belt-positioning booster, depending on which type of belt system is available. These boosters have a low shield for use with a lap belt only, or the shield can be removed to leave belt-positioning guides for use with a lap/shoulder belt. Of the two restraint configurations, the lap/shoulder belt with the belt-positioning booster is the preferred system, because of its more effective upper-torso restraint and its better positioned lower-torso restraint. When used appropriately, however, both have performed well in actual crashes.

Because United States child restraint regulations, as of 1992, have not recognized the belt-positioning booster as a stand-alone device, there are no test requirements or performance criteria. (This situation is likely to change soon.) Canadian regulations do recognize this product but do not require a crash test to verify the performance of the belt-positioning function. Instead, Canadian regulations ensure that the seating surface is quite firm, so that the child will not compress the booster in a crash and possibly slide under the lap belt. Australian regulations include a weight limitation for boosters with backs, in order to avoid injurious loading of the child into the belt by the booster itself.

A child should use a booster only as long as it is needed to adapt the belts to the child's body size. As the child grows, his or her ears may rise above the top of low vehicle seat-backs, and the child will then not be protected from potential rear-impact neck injury. If a booster is still needed for belt fit, a model with a firm back should be selected.

Belt Compatibility, Integrated Systems, and ISOFIX

Thus far this chapter has primarily addressed the design of the child restraint itself and has only alluded to the seat belts that attach child restraints to vehicles. The original function of belts was to restrain only adult-size occupants, and some of their design parameters have been found to be in conflict with those that would best secure child restraints. These parameters include belt anchor location, buckle size, and type of retractor and latchplate. These and many other issues regarding child restraint compatibility with vehicle belts and seats have been the focus of a long-term effort by the Society of Automotive Engineers (SAE) Children's Restraint Systems Task Force. This effort has resulted in an SAE recommended practice (SAE J1819, 1990), which has already had a marked effect on domestic restraint design and has significantly improved vehicle/child-restraint compatibility for current North American products.

During this time, another approach for avoiding child-restraint installation difficulties was pursued in Sweden and is now being incorporated in American and French vehicle designs as well. This approach is a built-in or "integrated" child restraint (Karlbrink et al., 1989; Tingvall, 1987). The original concept included a rear-facing restraint for infants, but current production models are only for forward-facing children. The Swedish version is a fold-down booster seat to be used with a lap/shoulder belt, and which must be labeled in the United States as only for children over 50 lb (23 kg). The current American version includes both a booster seat and a special harness that meets FMVSS 213 requirements for children under 50 lb. In outboard positions, the integrated booster can also be used with the lap/shoulder belt. In addition to eliminating incompatibility problems, it is expected that integrated systems will be less subject to misuse and will provide improved frontal crash protection. The disadvantage, of course, is that integrated restraints cannot be moved to another vehicle.

Beyond the integrated child restraint is a concept called ISOFIX (Turbell, 1991). The proposal is for standard rigid interface hardware to be available in all vehicles and on all child restraints, so that child restraint installation would entirely bypass vehicle belts and the child restraint would not rely on the vehicle seat cushion for support. In addition to a likely reduction in misinstallation and an improvement in crash performance, the creators of the concept hope there can be an electrical interface to do such things as disable a passenger airbag.

Seat Belts for Children

There is no special age at which a child "can use a seat belt" by itself. Although vehicle seat belts are designed primarily with adult use in mind, they are not inherently unsuitable for children who can sit up unassisted. Seat belts are part of a continuum of restraint systems with varying levels of effectiveness for children. In general, more restraint is better than less, and good fit is important for effective restraint performance. Child restraints typically have more restraining surface area (e.g., five straps or a broad shield) than does a lap belt alone, and their restraining systems may be more easily positioned properly on a child's body. Good fit of a lap belt is as low as possible on the pelvis, touching or even flat across the thighs. A shoulder belt should cross the chest at midsternum and lie flat on the shoulder (Fig. 19.12).

Good fit for either a lap or lap/shoulder belt is dependent on the size of the occupant, and suitable occupant size varies considerably from one specific belt and seat combination to another. Children should be restrained whenever possible by systems designed for their small bodies or by seat belts adapted to their body size by a booster. However, if a child restraint or booster is not available, or if the child can no longer fit into one of these systems, then seat belts must be used.

To achieve the best fit, the child should be sitting fully upright with his or her pelvis as vertical and as far back into the seat as pos-

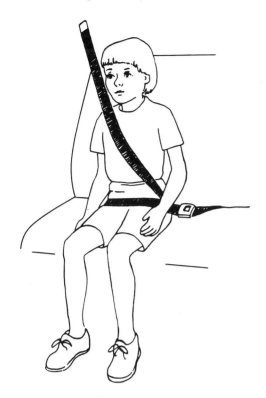

FIGURE 19.12. Child in lap/shoulder belt showing proper fit.

known to result in severe rib fracture and internal injuries (States et al., 1987).

If a lap/shoulder belt can be made to fit a sitting child, it can be a very effective restraint system and is certainly preferred over a lap belt alone. But the lap belt should definitely be used if no other restraint system is available. For infants, however, there is really no effective alternative to the rear-facing or car-bed restraint.

Child Injuries and Biomechanics

Accident experience has indicated that children are less prone to injury than adults under the same impact conditions, that the injuries they do receive are less severe, and that injuries of the same severity are less likely to result in permanent disabilities (Dejeammes et al., 1984; Gustafsson et al., 1987; Newman, 1979). There is evidence that the more flexible thorax of the child reduces the risk of internal injury, because the ribs bend rather than break, and bone fractures in general are less likely in children. The head is the site of most frequent injury for all occupants, but children receive relatively more head injuries than adults, because their head surface area is proportionally greater. At the same time, children are not suffering more severe head injuries than adults, despite the fragility of their skulls.

As the use of seat belts has been increasing, clinical literature has been focusing on injuries associated with their use (Anderson et al., 1991; Johnson and Falci, 1990), but age has not been found to be a predictor of abdominal injury associated with belts (Rutledge et al., 1991). Crash investigations also do not reveal that children are any more likely to submarine than adults, and serious neck injury is still rare among all restrained occupants. Finally, speculation that small children will eject over the top of a lap belt, because of a high center of gravity, and that they will submarine under the belt, are contradictory, and evidence of the former has not been documented.

Regarding the apparent ability of children to withstand impact better than their adult

sible. This will help place the lap belt in front of the pelvic bone below the anterior-superior iliac spines and will minimize the possibility of the belt sliding up and intruding into the soft upper abdomen. The lap belt must not be placed nor be allowed to ride up around the waist.

To place the shoulder belt away from the neck, the child should sit as close to the lower end as possible. Routing the shoulder belt behind the child is not recommended and should be done only if the belt would have to lie flat across the throat or face and no other seat position or restraint is available. Shoulder belts that touch the side of the neck will not cause injury as long as they are snug on the shoulder (Appleton, 1983; Corben and Herbert, 1981; NTSB, 1988). The shoulder belt should never be placed under the arm of a child or adult, because, in a crash, the resulting belt forces on the side of the rib cage are counterparts, one explanation for the case of the restrained occupant is fairly simple. The force on a body held by a seat belt is directly proportional to the weight of that body. For example, a man weighing 180 lb (82 kg) undergoing whole-body deceleration of 15 G will experience a total force on his belts of 2,700 lb (12 kN), while a 20-lb (9-kg) child in the same situation will experience only 300 lb (1.3 kN), spread over the restraint system. Even though the child's bony structure and connective tissue may be weaker than the adult's, the child's weight is so much less that the injury potential is less. An exception may be the weight of the head relative to the strength of the neck structures, and hence the concern about serious neck injury among restrained forward-facing children.

Stürtz (1980) and Dejeammes et al. (1984) have reviewed experimental data relating to the impact response and injury thresholds of children, addressed the problem of scaling adult and animal data to children, and performed laboratory tests correlating child dummy measurements with actual crash injuries (Stürtz) or with results of the few crash tests with child cadavers (Dejeammes). Both studies concluded that there were insufficient response and injury data in the literature to establish definitive tolerance limits, but more was known about the child thorax and extremities than other regions. The studies also agreed that data were virtually nonexistent for the child abdomen and pelvis, and neither study treated the neck in its review. (See neck injury discussion, above.) After incorporating new data from their dummy reconstructions, both studies concluded that thoracic acceleration tolerance of children is similar to that of adults, but the studies disagreed on the relative tolerance of the head/brain to injury. This difference of opinion may be due to the inclusion of noncontact acceleration by Dejeammes and consideration of only contact acceleration by Stürtz. Whereas Dejeammes et al. concluded that child head injury tolerance was higher than that of adults, Stürtz proposed contact Head Injury Criterion (HIC) values for use with a 6-year size dummy that are considerably below the adult dummy

threshold. This latter conclusion is supported by accepted techniques for scaling anthropometry data to predict injury. Although the smaller size alone would lead to an expected tolerance to higher accelerations, the lesser stiffness of the head structure more than offsets the size difference and leads to a significantly lower tolerance to contact accelerations, such as those generated by an airbag deployment close to a rear-facing infant restraint.

Because child response and injury data have historically been sparse and difficult to interpret, injury criteria for evaluating the performance of child restraint systems have been based on adult data and regulatory practice, and the dummies used to simulate children have lacked biofidelity. Preliminary efforts to scale adult injury criteria to children, with the little response data available, appears to be promising and may be used to evaluate restraint conditions for which there is no field experience (SAE CRABI, 1991). In addition, new design concepts can often be evaluated best by comparing their performance data with those of a system with known effectiveness.

At present, the most pressing need is for experts to evaluate anatomical, physiological, and accident data to determine a conservative but practical threshold at which a young child may be restrained facing forward without undue risk of neck injury, and for biomechanical and restraint design experts to determine the variables among forward-facing restraints that may lead to or reduce the likelihood of such injuries. For the future, a cooperative effort among several experts in biomechanics and impact trauma is needed to review and evaluate data from many sources to establish response corridors and injury thresholds for children. With this information, better dummies can be designed and better evaluations can be made of future child restraint systems.

Conclusion

The consistent and proper use of restraint systems for infants and children in automobiles can prevent hundreds of deaths and thousands of injuries each year. Infants require the most special treatment, with restraint systems designed to apply crash forces to their backs or the full length of their bodies. Children over 1 year also benefit from specially designed restraints that snugly conform to their small body shape, while providing elevation so that they can see the world around them. Seat belts, too, can provide good restraint, even for young children, provided that attention is paid to good belt location and fit. It is important to understand both the theory behind the design of restraint systems and how this theory has been applied to child restraints, in order to be able to evaluate their performance in a crash, to develop improved child restraint design, and to provide informed guidance concerning their selection and use.

Acknowledgment. The author would like to acknowledge the assistance of the illustrator, Kathleen Crockett Richards.

References

American Academy of Pediatrics, Committee on Injury and Poison Prevention and Committee on Fetus and Newborn. Safe transportation of premature infants. Pediatrics 87:120–122; 1991.

Anderson PA, Rivara, FP, Maier RV, Drake C (1991) The epidemiology of seatbelt-associated injuries. J Trauma 31:60–67.

Appleton I. *Young children and adult seat belts: Is it a good idea to put children in adults belts?* New Zealand Ministry of Transport, Road Transport Division, Wellington, August 1983.

Bell R. Misuse test panels, a technique for the identification and prevention of misuse of child restraints. *Association for the Advancement of Automotive Medicine, 35th annual conference,* 1991 October 7–9, Toronto. AAAM, Des Plaines, IL, pp 43–55, 1991.

Bowler M, Torpey S. *An evaluation of the Victorian baby safety bassinet loan scheme.* Victoria Road Traffic Authority, Hawthorn, July 1988.

Bull MJ, Stroup KB (1985) Premature infants in car seats. Pediatrics 75:336–339.

Burdi AR, Huelke DF, Snyder RG, Lowrey GH (1969) Infants and children in the adult world of automobile safety design: pediatric and ana-

tomical considerations for design of child restraints. J Biomech 2:267–280.

Carlsson G, Norin H, Ysander L. Rearward facing child seats. *Association for the Advancement of Automotive Medicine, 33rd conference,* 1989 October 2–4, Baltimore, MD. AAAM, Des Plaines, IL, pp 249–263, 1989.

Conry BG, Hall CM (1987) Cervical spine fracture and rear car seat restraints. Arch Dis Child 62:1267.

Corben CW, Herbert DC. *Children wearing approved restraints and adult's belts in crashes.* New South Wales, Traffic Accident Research Unit, Sydney, January 1981.

Cynecki MJ, Goryl ME. *The incidence and factors associated with child safety seat misuse.* DOT HS 806 676. Goodell-Grivas, Southfield, MI, December 1984.

Czernakowski W, Müller M. Misuse Mode and Effects Analysis (MMEA)—an approach to predict and quantify misuse of child restraint systems (CRS). *Association for the Advancement of Automotive Medicine, 35th annual conference,* 1991 October 7–9, Toronto. AAAM, Des Plaines, IL, pp 27–43, 1991.

Dejeammes M, Tarriere C, Thomas C, Kallieris D. Exploration of biomechanical data towards a better evaluation of tolerance for children involved in automotive accidents. SAE 840530. *Advances in belt restraint systems.* Society of Automotive Engineers, Warrendale, PA, pp 427–440, 1984.

Diekema DS, Allen DB (1988) Odontoid fracture in a child occupying a child restraint seat. Pediatrics 82:117–119.

Evans L (1986) The effectiveness of safety belts in preventing fatalities. Accid Anal Prev 18:229–241.

Fuchs S, Barthel MJ, Flannery AM, Christoffel KK (1989) Cervical spine fractures sustained by young children in forward-facing car seats. Pediatrics 84:348–354.

Glaeser KP, Langwieder K, Hummel T. Protection effects of child restraints—experience from accidents and sled tests with carry-cots. *Road Safety and Traffic Environment in Europe, proceedings,* 1990 September 26–28, Gothenburg, Sweden. Vol 1. VTI Report 362A. Swedish Road and Traffic Research Institute, Linkoping, pp 139–149, 1990.

Gustafsson H, Nygren A, Tingvall C (1987) Children in cars—an epidemiological study of injuries to children as car passengers in road traffic accidents. Acta Paediatr Scand Suppl 339:I1–25.

Heap SA, Grenier EP. *The design and development of a more effective child restraint concept.* SAE 680002. Society of Automotive Engineers, New York, 1968.

Huelke DF, Sherman HW, Murphy M, Kaplan RJ, Flora JD. *Effectiveness of current and future restraint systems in fatal and serious injury automobile crashes.* SAE 790323. Society of Automotive Engineers, Warrendale, PA, 1979.

International Task Force on Child Restraining Systems. Draft minutes of the meeting; 1990 April 30–May 4; Paris. Renault Automobiles Département des Sciences de l'Environnement, Nanterre, France, 1990.

International Task Force on Child Restraining Systems. Report of the 5th meeting; 1991 April 22–24; Paris. Renault Automobiles Département des Sciences de l'Environnement, Nanterre, France, 1991.

Janssen EG, Nieboer JJ, Verschut R, Huijskens CG. Cervical spine loads to retrained child dummies. SAE 912919. *35th Stapp Car Crash Conference, proceedings,* 1991 November 18–20, San Diego, CA. Society of Automotive Engineers, Warrendale, PA, 1991.

Johnson DL, Falci S (1990) The diagnosis and treatment of pediatric lumbar spine injuries caused by rear seat lap belts. Neurosurgery 26:434–441.

Kahane CJ. An evaluation of child passenger safety—the effectiveness and benefits of safety seats. DOT HS 806 890. National Highway Traffic Safety Administration, Washington, DC, February 1986.

Karlbrink L, Krafft M, Tingvall C. Integrated child restraints in cars for children aged 0–10. *12th International Technical Conference on Experimental Safety Vehicles,* 1989 May 29–June 1, Gothenburg, Sweden. Vol 1. National Highway Traffic Safety Administration, Washington, DC, pp 73–75, 1990.

King AI. Abdomen. In Melvin JW, Weber K (eds) *Review of biomechanical impact response and injury in the automotive environment.* DOT HS 807 042. University of Michigan Transportation Research Institute, Ann Arbor, pp 125–146, 1985.

Langwieder K, Hummel T. Children in cars—their injury risks and the influence of child protection systems. *12th International Technical Conference on Experimental Safety Vehicles,* 1989 May 29–June 1, Gothenburg, Sweden. Vol 1. National Highway Traffic Safety Administration, Washington, DC, pp 39–49, 1990.

Langwieder K, Hummel T, Felsch B, Klanner W. Injury risks of children in cars—epidemiology and effect of child restraint systems. XXIII FISITA Congress, 1990 May 7–11, Turin, Italy, Vol 1. Associazione Tecnica dell'Automobile, Turin, pp 905–919, 1990.

Langwieder K, Hummel T. Neck injuries to restrained children. IRCOBI Workshop on Future in Child Restraints, 1989 September 15, Stockholm. HUK-Verband, Munich, 1989.

Lowne R, Gloyns P, Roy P. Fatal injuries to restrained children aged 0–4 years in Great Britain 1972–86. *11th International Technical Conference on Experimental Safety Vehicles,* 1987 May 12–15, Washington, DC. National Highway Traffic Safety Administration, Washington, DC, pp 227–235, 1988.

Melvin JW, Weber K. Abdominal intrusion sensor for evaluating child restraint systems. SAE 860370. *Passenger comfort, convenience and safety.* Society of Automotive Engineers, Warrendale, PA, pp 249–256, 1986.

Melvin JW, Weber K, Lux P. Performance of child restraints in serious crashes. *American Association for Automotive Medicine, 24th conference,* 1980 October 7–9, Rochester, NY. AAAM, Morton Grove, IL, pp 117–131, 1980.

Morres H, Appel H. Paraplegia as result of unsafe child restraints. *IRCOBI Workshop on Future in Child Restraints,* 1989 September 15, Stockholm. Technical University, Berlin, 1989.

National Transportation Safety Board. Child passenger protection against death, disability, and disfigurement in motor vehicle accidents. NTSB SS-8301. NTSB, Washington, DC, September 1983.

National Transportation Safety Board. Children and lap/shoulder belt use. In *Performance of lap/shoulder belts in 167 motor vehicle crashes.* Vol 1. NTSB, Washington, DC, pp 63–71, March 1988.

Newman JA. *The restraint of school-age children in automobiles, a literature review.* Biokinetics, Ottawa, October 1979.

Nyquist GW, King AI. Spine. In Melvin JW, Weber K (eds) *Review of biomechanical impact response and injury in the automotive environment.* DOT HS 807 042. University of Michigan Transportation Research Institute, Ann Arbor, pp 45–92, 1985.

Partyka SC. Belt effectiveness in fatal accidents. In *Papers on adult seat belts—effectiveness and use.* DOT HS 807 285. National Highway Traffic Safety Administration, Washington, DC, June 1988.

Petrucelli E. Child restraint misuse in the USA: implications for crash protection. *IRCOBI Workshop on Future in Child Restraints,* 1989 September 15, Stockholm. Association for the

Advancement of Automotive Medicine, Des Plaines, IL, 1989.

Rutledge R, Thomason M, Oller D, Meredith W, Moylan J, Clancy T, Cummingham P, Baker C (1991) The spectrum of abdominal injuries associated with the use of seat belts. J Trauma 31:820–826.

Shelness A, Jewett J. Observed misuse of child restraints. SAE 831665. *Child Injury and Restraint Conference, proceedings*, 1983 October 17–18, San Diego, CA. Society of Automotive Engineers, Warrendale, PA, pp 207–215, 1983.

Society of Automotive Engineers. *Securing child restraint systems in motor vehicle rear seats*. SAE J1819. SAE, Warrendale, PA, 11 November 1990.

Society of Automotive Engineers, Child Restraint and Airbag Interaction Task Force. Unconfirmed minutes of the meeting, 1991 April 10, Romulus, MI.

States JD, Huelke DF, Dance M, Green RN (1987) Fatal injuries caused by underarm use of shoulder belts. J Trauma 27:740–745.

Stürtz G. Biomechanical data of children. SAE 801313. *24th Stapp Car Crash Conference, proceedings*, 1980 October 15–17, Troy, MI. Society of Automotive Engineers, Warrendale, PA, pp 513–559, 1980.

Tarriere C, Carlsson G, Trosseille X. Initial conclusions of an International Task Force on Child Restraining Systems. *13th International Technical Conference on Experimental Safety Vehicles*, 1991 November 4–7; Paris. Paper no. 91-S3-W-19. 18p. U.S. National Highway Traffic Safety Administration, 1993.

Tingvall C (1987) Children in cars–some aspects of the safety of children as car passengers in road traffic accidents. Acta Paediatr Scand Suppl 339:1–35.

Turbell T. ISOFIX status report. Swedish Road and Traffic Research Institute, Linkoping, May 1991. (Distributed as ISO/22/12/WG 1 N 220.)

Turbell T. Swedish programs for child protection in cars. IRCOBI Workshop on Future in Child Restraints, 1989 September 15, Stockholm. Swedish Road and Traffic Research Institute, Linkoping, 1989.

United Kingdom, Department of Transport. Occurrence of neck injuries to children in child restraints. April 1991. (Distributed as ISO/22/12/WG 1 N 219.)

Weber K. Comparison of car-bed and rear-facing infant restraint systems. *12th International Technical Conference on Experimental Safety Vehicles*, 1989 May 29–June 1, Gothenburg, Sweden. Vol 1. U.S. National Highway Traffic Safety Administration, pp 61–66, 1990.

Weber K, Lehman RJ, Schneider LW. *Child anthropometry for restraint system design*. UMTRI-85-23. University of Michigan Transportation Research Institute, Ann Arbor, June 1985.

Weber K, Melvin JW. Injury potential with misused child restraining systems. SAE 831604. *27th Stapp Car Crash Conference, proceedings*, 1983 October 17–19, San Diego, CA. Society of Automotive Engineers, Warrendale, PA, pp 53–59, 1983.

Willet LD, Leuschen MP, Nelson LS, Nelson RM (1986) Risk of hypoventilation in premature infants in car seats. J Pediatr 109:245–248.

Selected Child Restraint Regulations and References

Australia. *Child restraint systems for use in motor vehicles*. AS 1754–1989. Standards Australia, North Sydney, 1989.

Canada. *Child restraint systems*. CMVSS 213. Transport Canada, Ottawa, October 1989.

International Organization for Standardization. *Compilation of safety regulations and standards for children in cars*. ISO/22/12/WG 1 N 214. SIS/SMS, Stockholm, April 1991.

United Kingdom. *Rearward-facing infant restraint systems*. BS AU 202a. British Standards Institution, London, 1985.

Seat belt assemblies for motor vehicles, Part 2, Specification for restraining devices for children. BS 3254: Part 2. British Standards Institution, London, 1988.

Seat belt booster cushions. BS AU 185. British Standards Institution, London, 1983.

United Nations, Economic Commission for Europe. *Uniform provisions concerning the approval of restraining devices for child occupants of power-driven vehicles ("child restraint system")*. ECE Reg. 44, amended and supplemented as of November 1990. (Available: Swedish Road and Traffic Research Institute, Linkoping.)

United States. *Child restraint systems*. FMVSS 213. National Highway Traffic Safety Administration, Washington, DC, September 1992.

20
Isolated Tissue and Cellular Biomechanics

Lawrence E. Thibault

Introduction

The majority of our current concepts relating to the biomechanical aspects of human injury have come from research that may be described as macroscopic in nature. To this end human cadaver specimens, various animal models, anthropomorphic test devices, and both analytical and numerical simulations have served as the primary tools of investigation in our field to date. Collectively, the research findings from this endeavor have been responsible for the contemporary views of human injury tolerance criteria and they have led to numerous standards and regulations, and to the design of a safer mechanical environment.

The contributions of the biomechanics community in this regard have been enormous in the context of the overall national effort directed toward injury control and prevention. This volume should provide the reader with a sense of this achievement and an idea of how the macroscopic world of biomechanics has been the logical first step in estimating the effects of mechanical forces on the process of injury production and its sequelae.

This chapter focuses upon an or adjunct approach in the study of the biological effects of mechanical forces that are applied to living structures.

The approach utilizes isolated tissue and cell culture models and, therefore, may be considered more microscopic in contrast with the previously described research. It is simply another tool that the biomechanics community may employ to study this complex problem.

Investigations at the cellular and subcellular level have the following aims: (1) to understand the relationship between the macroscopic descriptors of the applied loads (contact force, impact velocity, and acceleration) and the associated deformation of the tissue; (2) to relate the tissue deformation to the field variables such as strain in order to describe the dynamic mechanical environment of the cell; and (3) to study the physiological or pathophysiological response of the cell to mechanical stimuli.

With the technology available today it is possible to measure with good precision the macroscopic loads that result from accident simulation. Further, using physical and mathematical models one can then estimate the deformations that occur at the organ or tissue level when an organism is subjected to these loads. It remains to develop the failure criteria for the elements that constitute the living structures. With the experimental methodologies available in recent years it is now possible to subject isolated tissue and cell cultures to controlled mechanical stimulation and to measure the physiological and biochemical events that are elicited by the stimuli and may relate to the functional or structural failure of these components.

In this regard one may think of mechanical stimulation as another physical factor along with the chemical, electrical, and thermal conditions that in concert constitute the environment of the cell. As in these other cases it is reasonable to assume that mechanical stimulation when "excessive" (operating out of the physiological range) will lead to injury or possibly cell death.

This chapter is not intended as an exhaustive review of the research associated with the biomechanics of injury at the tissue or cellular level since much of this work is relatively new and is not readily available in the literature as of this time. Rather, this report is intended to serve as a description of a process whereby one can move from the macroscopic to the more microscopic approach in the study of human injury. The examples cited herein are for illustrative purposes and for expediency

are taken from our work at the University of Pennsylvania. As such, they deal primarily with neural and vascular tissue studies and relate to our specific interest in central nervous system trauma.

Figure 20.1 depicts the process where the level of mechanical loading is first related to the tissue deformation through the use of physical or mathematical models. This deformation is then used as the stimulus to investigate the response of the living tissue or single cells. Studies such as these may then lead to an improved understanding of tissue failure criteria and new avenues to address the issues of theraputic intervention and rehabilitation.

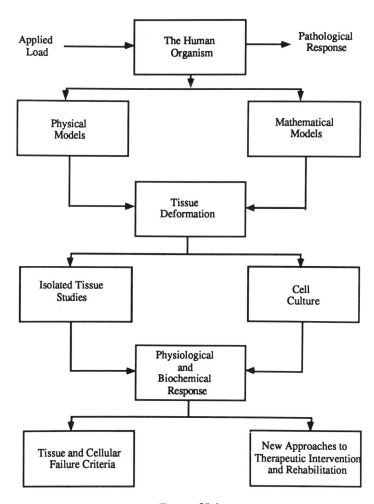

FIGURE 20.1

Transforming the Macroscopic Loads to Organ, Tissue, and Cellular Deformations

Central nervous system (CNS) trauma in general and brain injury in particular has been the subject of intensive biomechanics investigation for the past five decades. In this chapter CNS will be the example that is used to demonstrate the concepts of transition from the macroscopic to the microscopic level of biomechanics research. Some of the earliest studies[1-4] suggested that the translational and rotational accelerations of the head serve as a macroscopic descriptor and predictive index with regard to the incidence of brain injury. Subsequent investigations, ranging from human volunteer experiments to animal model studies,[5-8] confirmed that inertial loading and its magnitude, duration, and direction relative to the anatomy can produce a broad spectrum of neuropathological findings. These various forms of injury to the brain include the following: cerebral concussion, cortical contusion, focal intracerebral hematoma, subdural hematoma, and diffuse axonal injury with prolonged coma. Each of these pathologic entities is distinctive and represents the structural or functional failure of the discrete elements with the brain.

It is reasonable to imagine that the deformations of the neural and neuraovascular elements within the brain vary in magnitude and topographic distribution as some complex function of the loading conditions, geometry of the brain and skull, and the constitutive properties of the tissue. Attempts have been made to measure the in situ deformations[9-11] but the experimental difficulties have thus far prevented any detailed information from being obtained. Because these data are so important in providing insight into the mechanisms of injury other approaches have been employed. These methods enable one to estimate the field parameters under dynamic loading conditions and they fall into two categories: (1) physical models, which are designed as surrogates for the anatomic structures of interest and have been used extensively in experimental

mechanics to estimate local stress and strain; and (2) computational simulations, which are analytical and numerical methods employed to predict the detailed deformations of a structure under load.

Each of these methods has the limitation that it represents only an approximation of the actual anatomic structure. In the case of the skull and brain, for example, analytical models are constrained to use simple two- and three-dimensional approximations for the geometry such as circular cylindrical, spherical, or ellipsoidal structures. The constitutive properties of the tissue must by necessity be modeled in a manner that may oversimplify the problem. Finite element methods on the other hand are potentially capable of the more complex analysis. Numerical schemes have been developed that permit one to incorporate the nonlinear geometry of the structure and to accommodate a complete hierarchy of constitutive expressions for the material.

Physical models have been a critical component of mechanics research in that theoretical representations at the very least need experimental validation and experimental stress and strain analysis is a well-developed tool that has independently contributed to our knowledge of structural mechanics. The advantages of physical models relate to the fact that they are designed by the investigator. They are fabricated of synthetic materials that are selected by the designer to facilitate the measurements and they can be thoroughly instrumented as desired.

This section will discuss the use of these tools and their ability to provide insight into the relationship between the macroscopic loads and the detailed deformation of the tissue of interest.

Physical Models

To gain further insight into the biomechanics of head injury, it is important to clarify the response of the brain tissue to the range of mechanical loads believed to cause injury. Physical models can be used to relate the loading kinematics of controlled animal experiments to the resulting injury pathology by estimating the deformation field. In 1943, Holbourn quantified the strain distribution of a surrogate brain material during a controlled applied load.[12] Sagittal, coronal, and horizontal sections of wax skulls were filled with a 5% gelatin solution that closely represented the mechanical properties of brain tissue. While the skull was subjected to rotational loads, the photoelastic stresses within the material were mapped. Holbourn found that very high strain rates were produced in the superior margin of the brain in the sagittal model, the same region where an acute subdural hematoma occurs.

Holbourn used these results to postulate that a majority of the head injuries seen clinically were due solely to rotations of the head. Previously, many investigators had believed that a majority of injuries were produced primarily by the loose brain colliding against the rigid skull during impact loading. Holbourn suggested that injury resulted no from compression of the tissue components under such conditions, but rather from the shear strain induced in the brain tissue and neurovasculature under rotational loading conditions. This hypothesis was later confirmed by studies performed on a range of subprimates which showed that an array of head injuries (e.g., acute subdural hematoma, concussion, and diffuse axonal injury) could be produced using nonimpact, angular acceleration.[13–15] These animal experiments and the physical model studies by Holbourn established rotational loading as an important cause of head injury.

Despite the suggestion that rotational loads are an important cause of head injury, most of the subsequent physical models were subjected to nonrotational impact loading. More recently, however, Thibault et al. constructed physical models of the baboon brain, subjected them to sudden rotational loads, and compared the spatial distribution of measured strain in the surrogate brain to pathological data from primate head injury experiments.[16] Later, Margulies used physical models to investigate another type of head trauma (diffuse axonal injury) and to suggest a tolerance level for the onset of severe diffuse axonal injury in the baboon and adult human.[17,18] Physical models

can be used to measure how the strain response of the model is affected by changing the model geometry. The results from such an effort can be used to develop a scaling relationship that can be applied to a range of brain sizes. This scaling information can then be used to develop human injury tolerance levels.

Physical modeling can also be used to measure the changes that occur in brain deformation when brain tissue flows from the cranial vault during loading. During the course of dynamic loading, the regional rise in intracranial pressure causes brain material to flow through the foramen magnum at the base of the skull. Thus, the brain volume does not remain constant but decreases during the loading period thereby producing an "effective compressibility." However, the effect this exit of brain material has on the strain patterns in the brain remains unclear. Researchers have developed finite element models of the head that incorporate time-independent compressible material elements to simulate the exit of material, varying the value of the compressibility to fit physical model experimental data.[19,20] Without experimental validation of the effect of this material compressibility on the strain field, however, problems may arise when using these finite element models to extrapolate the response of the head under conditions for which no experimental results from physical models exist. Testing physical models with variable effective compressibility will determine the extent such changes have on the strain pattern.

A device that has been used to accelerate the physical models was also employed successfully in previous animal and physical modeling experiments in our laboratory. The system consists of a six-inch Bendix HYGE actuator and linkage assembly that delivers a distributed inertial load to the primate head or physical model (Fig. 20.2). Amplitude of the peak acceleration and pulse duration can be controlled by adjusting the set pressure applied to the cylinder, while acceleration waveshape can be changed by altering the geometry of the metering pin. A more detailed description of the HYGE device can be found elsewhere.[16,17] An accelerometer (Endevco Instruments, San

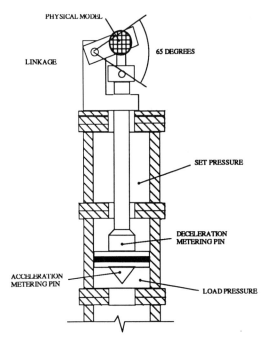

FIGURE 20.2

Juan Capistrano, CA) is mounted on the mechanical linkage arm and provides the loading data under these controlled kinematical conditions.

The physical models used in previous investigations by Thibault et al. and Margulies[16,17] are described elsewhere. Various idealized geometries (including cylinders and hemicylinders), baboon skulls, and three types of human skulls (neonatal, pediatric, and adult) (Carolina Biological Supply) have been subjected to controlled inertial loading. These skull models are prepared as hemisections and an example of a sagittal plane model is shown in Fig. 20.3. In this particular example the skull was cut 1.0 to 1.5 cm lateral to the sagittal midline and was manufactured to facilitate the insertion of a surrogate spinal column. The intended use of this particular model was to investigate the superior margin strains as they may serve to estimate the degre to which the parasagittal bridging veins are stretched. The distal end of the spinal column was fitted with a removable plate, permitting one to vary the membrane across the distal end, thereby changing the effective compressibility of the material.[21]

Cylindrical aluminum cans are constructed to contain the prepared skulls. Six threaded holes ($1/4'' \times 20''$) located on the face of the can provide a method to fasten a plexiglas cover plate to the can. This cover plate is equipped with an O-ring to ensure a water-tight seal between the aluminum can and the cover plate. The interior of the skull and spinal column is coated with flat while enamel to enhance photographic resolution during high-speed filming. The skull/spinal column assembly is potted in position using a polymer/resin mix (Castolite, Buehler Corp., Evanston IL). The interior of the skull/spinal column will then be cleaned in preparation for the initial layer of surrogate brain tissue. A polymer gel (Sylgard Medical gel, Dow Corning, Midland, MI) with mechanical properties similar to brain tissue will be poured into the model to a level 1.0 cm from the sagittal midline. After the gel cures, an orthogonal black enamel grid (7 mm spacing) is painted on the gel surface and allowed to dry thoroughly to permit any paint solvents to evaporate. At this time, a second layer of gel can be poured to the level of the sagittal midline and a second grid is painted in the spinal column region. After full drying of the enamel, the final layer of gel is then poured and allowed to cure.

The motion of the physical model is filmed using a HYCAM high speed camera at a rate of 6600 frames per second. A sequence of photographs ($8'' \times 10''$) can be developed from selected frames of the high-speed film and a digitizer is used to record the location of the grid intersections in the photographs.

The locations of these intersections are then stored on an IBM compatible computer (Dell Computer Corp., Austin TX), and subsequently analyzed to calculate strain and strain rate in the desired regions of interest. Examples of the still frame computer reconstructed images are shown in the undeformed and deformed condition in Fig. 20.4. The deformed grid corresponds to that point in time when the deceleration was a maximum. One can see that it is possible to compute the strains within the model as a function of the loading conditions and investigate both the temporal and spatial variations within the field.

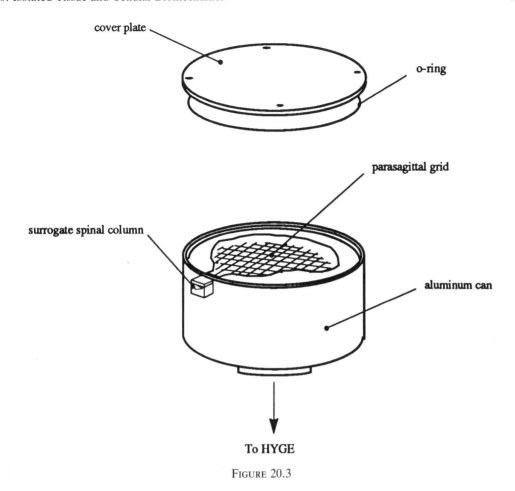

To HYGE

FIGURE 20.3

Presented in Fig. 20.5 is an example of such a computation for a grid element located in the central region of the superior margin. This type of data will be used later to develop experiment parameters for stimulating isolated tissue and cell culture models. However, the data can be used independently to validate analytical and numerical simulations or to develop empirical scaling relationships that may be important in and of themselves for the purpose of scaling animal model studies to man.

Computational Simulations

Mathematical models of head injury facilitate the study of the spatial and temporal responses of the brain structure across a broad range of inputs, whereas physical models are confined to discrete load levels dictated by the limits of the equipment. Bycroft, and Lee and Advani developed the first analytical model for head injury caused by rotational loads.[22,23] They applied a symmetric torsional acceleration to an elastic sphere, and transformed the solution to a viscoelastic solution using the correspondence principle. The analytical solution showed that large shear strains could be generated in the region of the brain stem.

Liu and Chandran modeled the brain as an elastic sphere encased in a rigid spherical shell.[24] Subjecting the model to rotational acceleration produced high stresses in the cortical and subcortical regions, indicating that rotational loads could produce injuries such as gliding contusions and subdural hematomas. Subsequent models of the same geometry,

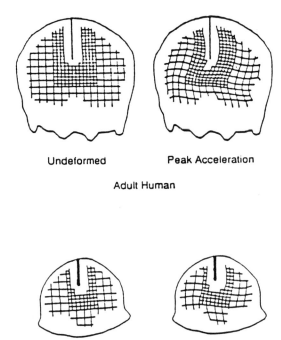

Undeformed   Peak Acceleration

Adult Human

Undeformed   Peak Acceleration

Nonhuman Primate

FIGURE 20.4

levels on the mechanical properties of brain tissue.

Ljung developed viscoelastic models of different geometries (infinitely long cylinder, cylinder with one closed end, and a sphere) and placed a special emphasis on deformation in the superior sagittal sinus.[25] Misra extended the geometric analysis by studying a prolate spheroid filled with a Kelvin material and subjected it to an angular acceleration pulse.[26] Misra concluded that geometry may well have an important effect on the spatial and temporal distribution of strain, especially in the cortical and subcortical areas. Margulies investigated the strains deep within the white matter of a viscoelastic cylindrical model and compared here results with physical model simulations and the pathology of subhuman primate studies where the rotational accelerations in the coronal plane resulted in diffuse axonal injury with prolonged coma.[27] Meaney conducted a similar injury-specific analysis of a viscoelastic structure designed to simulate the sagittal plane of the brain and focused on the superior margin strains. His model was used in concert with physical model studies and isolated tissue experiments to determine the threshold levels of inertial loading that are responsible for acute subdural hematoma.[21] His numerical computations are depicted in Fig. 20.6.

subjected to other loading conditions, displayed the ability of the models to predict a threshold for concussion. In the process it drew attention to the dependency of these injury

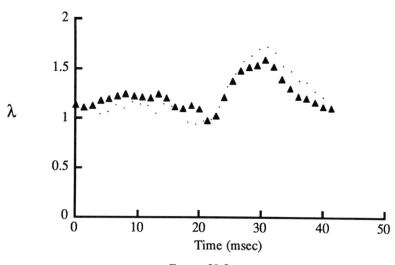

FIGURE 20.5

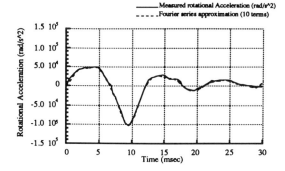

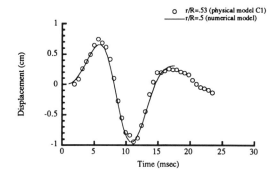

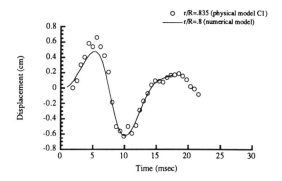

FIGURE 20.6

Shown in this figure is a Fourier series approximation of the inertial load compared with the actual forcing function of the experiment. This series approximation was used to drive the mode. Subsequently one can see the comparison of the numerical estimation of the deformation at various locations within the simulation and the actual experimental data obtained from the physical model study. This interplay between the computational

simulations and experimental data from physical model studies is important if we are to have reasonable confidence in this research endeavor.

In recent years the use of finite element methods to investigate the structural response of the brain to inertial loading has become a potentially important adjunct to experimental and analytical methods. In this past decade finite element programs have been used to investigate the structural response of the brain to inertial loading. Khalil and Viano reviewed the early use of such computational methods and their review is recommended by this author as supplemental reading. Linear analysis approaches have been used by investigators in order to estimate the deformations that occur within the brain under dynamic loading conditions. These estimates are restricted in that the deformations and rotations of the structure are assumed to be small. More recently, software has become available that permits the investigator to analyze large deformation problems with a comprehensive hierarchy of constitutive expressions for the materials. Programs such as DYNA have been used by a number of researchers. Their simulations require a detailed knowledge of the geometry of the structure and the constitutive properties of the brain material, but they are not restricted to the small deformation assumptions of previous numerical schemes. Most recently a simulation using this approach was conducted and compared to the results of the physical model studies that were discussed earlier, with favorable agreement. Again, it is our belief that this interaction between the experimental and computational approaches in biomechanics is prudent.

Experimental Methodologies to Investigate the Response of Isolated Tissue and Cell Culture Models to Controlled Mechanical Stimulation

Based upon the previous discussion, the neural and neurovascular elements of the CNS experience deformations that can result in a continuum of injury response in the sense that there are levels of strain that produce no response, spontaneously reversible forms of trauma, and irreversible injury and cell death. If the physical and mathematical models can help us to estimate the deformations experienced by the components of the CNS then it is reasonable to explore methods of subjecting isolated tissue elements or single cells to controlled mechanical stimulation. This section is an attempt to answer the following questions in this regard:

1. Can we develop the experimental methods that enable us to deform tissue or cells in culture in a controlled and reproducible manner?
2. Can we measure the load deformation characteristics of the living material?
3. Is it possible to examine the physiological response at the tissue and cellular level to dynamic mechanical stimulation in a way that may shed light upon tolerance criteria and detailed mechanisms of injury?

Researchers in our lab and others have examined the role of mechanical forces in the etiology of head injury by observing the response of an isolated unmyelinated axon to rapid elongation.[28,29] A graded depolarization in response to increasing levels of strain and strain rate in the squid giant axon has been observed. This graded response suggests a spectrum of injury severity for individual axons, ranging from mild, reversible injury for stretch ratios less than or equal to 1.10 to permanent deficit at 1.20 and structural failure at 1.25 which will be discussed later. Diffuse axonal injury (DAI) observed in a subhuman primate model appears morphologically as microscopic abnormalities distributed throughout the while matter, independent of any focal injury.[14,30,31] It would be of great interest to understand this abnormality and it may be possible to conduct such studies on the isolated axon. One feature of the axonal damage observed is abnormally shaped nodes of Ranvier, structures unique to myelinated nerves. In addition, the variation in the mechanical structure between the node and

internode suggests that strains may not be distributed uniformly along the myelinated fiber, as is assumed for the unmyelinated axon. Thibault et al. dynamically stretched frog sciatic nerve bundles, a myelinated nerve preparation, and measured the compound action potential as an indicator of functional viability.[32] Response to injury varied from a transient alteration in the signal with small stretch to an irreversible change in the compound action potential following a large stretch. Gennarelli et al. demonstrated that dynamic elongation of guinea pig optic nerves resulted in axonal damage similar to that seen morphologically in cases of human DAI.[33] While these studies suggest functional and structural changes of myelinated nerves as a result of dynamic stretch, mechanically loading a nerve bundle does not result in a reproducible, quantifiable load on each axon. The responses of many axons are measured, leading to a final correlation between some "average" response and the overall or "average" load. Using a single myelinated nerve fiber, on the other hand, allows for the measurement of an individual axon response to a known loading condition. Gray and Ritchie demonstrated functional changes, including reversible conduction block and altered action current, in a single myelinated frog axon due to static stretch.[34] However, when the axon was stretched 5% in less than one millisecond, no consistent change in potential was measured. The lack of single fiber response to dynamic injury in Gray and Ritchie's experiment is likely due to two factors. First, applying a 5% stretch to the portions of the bundle nearest the dissected single fiber does not translate directly to a 5% fiber stretch because the single fiber may slip within the bundle. More importantly, a 5% stretch may be too small to elicit an injury response. Data from Galbraith's dynamic elongation experiments on squid axons indicate only a small transient depolarization in response to a 5% stretch.[29] Therefore, the response of a single myelinated nerve fiber to larger dynamic strains still needs to be studied before conclusions can be drawn concerning the consequences of dynamic stretch injury.

In addition to investigating the response of the neural tissue we have been studying the effects of mechanical stimulation on blood vessel specimens. Our animal model data suggest that a myogenic response to mechanical stimulation can result in a vasospasm with the associated alterations in blood flow and metabolism. Because of the cylindrical nature and the relatively small sizes of the axons and vessels miniature material testing machines have been developed and are integrated onto a microscope stage. This approach is shown schematically in Fig. 20.7.

The device consists of a solenoid driver, an isometric force transducer, a linear variable displacement transducer, as well as a fluid perfusion system. Further details are given in Figure 20.8. This device has been designed to produce high strain rate deformations in the biological specimens to simulate the deformations approximated by phusical and mathematical simulations. The materials testing platform is centered upon a Nikon Diaphot inverted microscope. The microscope serves as a platform for micromanipulators, measurement systems, and the mechanical driver for producing loads on the specimens. The microscope itself was modified to allow a Wild dissecting microscope to be attached in such a way that the vessel or the myelinated or

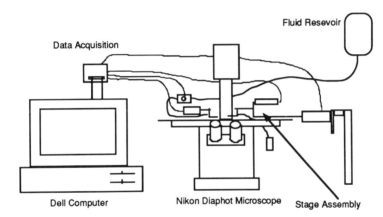

FIGURE 20.7

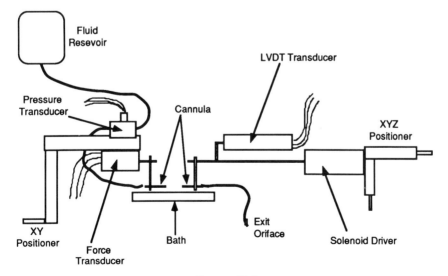

FIGURE 20.8

unmyelinated axon may be easily mounted. In addition to normal optical studies a Cohu CCD video camera and recorder can be attached directly to the microscope to visually record the experimental event for qualitative and quantitative analysis of the deformations. The entire platform is incorporated on a saddle that was originally designed by Galbraith for use in deformation experiments on the squid giant axon. The saddle is mounted on the microscope's normal stage. The micro-manipulators are incorporated into the saddle for orienting and positioning of the specimen and the chamber for maintaining viable specimens. The driver (as a subassembly) as well as all of the major measurement systems are also attached to the saddle.

Both single axons and isolated blood vessels have been used in these systems to measure the mechanical stimuli and the biological response. In the case of the axons measurements of membrane potential, voltage clamp current, and cytosolic free calcium concentration have been made. In the case of the isolated blood vessels we have recorded on video tape a spontaneous contraction of the vessel in response to high strain rate uniaxial loading. A brief discussion of these methods and the techniques associated with the preparations will follow.

A single myelinated nerve fiber is isolated for use from the sciatic nerve of a frog. Medium size frogs (*Rana pipiens*, 3″–3.5″) are obtained from West Jersey Biological through University Laboratory Animal Resources. The frogs are housed for a short period and then euthanized prior to the dissection procedure according to an approved experimental protocol (IACUC No. E-890214). In brief, the sciatic nerve–gastrocnemius muscle complex is dissected from the leg of a frog. Under a dissecting microscope, one of the branches of the nerve into the muscle is isolated and the connective tissue sheath of this nerve bundle is split open and cut away. A single nerve fiber is isolated from the group by cutting through all other fibers. In this manner, several milli-meters of a single myelinated fiber, approxi-mately 15 μm in diameter, can be exposed. For the dynamic stretch experiments, the fiber is

mounted into custom made glass micropipets. The pipets, shown with a mounted fiber in Figure 20.9, are made by drawing glass capillary tubing (2 mm OD, 1.6 mm ID) to a 15 to 20 mm inner diameter tip using a pipet puller. An internal constriction is made in the tapered region by applying heat locally as the pipet hangs vertically. This method is described in detail by Chonko et al.[45] To mount the fiber into the pipet tips one end of the single axon is cut free of the nerve bundle as the pre-paration lays in the experimental chamber immersed in Ringer's solution. Using an xyz-micromanipulator (Narishige, model ML-8), a micropipet is positioned very close to the free end of the fiber. A vacuum is applied through flexible tubing attached to the end of the micropipet which draws the fiber inside the pipet until it reaches the constriction. A con-tinuous vacuum holds the fiber in place against the constriction during experimentation. The mounting procedure is completed by cutting the opposite end of the fiber free of the nerve bundle and drawing it into a second micropipet, as described above.

Mechanical loading of the blood vessels was accomplished by a solenoid directly attached to a chuck assembly that in turn was coupled to a cannula. This solenoid is a Ledux model 189711-025 and has been positioned parellel to the axis of loading. The solenoid chosen has been rated at producing a force of 2.6 pounds in 10 msec for a stroke of 0.2 inches. This solenoid is rigidly attached to the mounting chucks in direct line.

The solenoid can be triggered either manu-ally via a function generator with a step up amplifier or via a computer-controlled system. These systems provide for varied and easily controllable loading conditions. Also in-corporated into this system is a Trans-Tek 0217-000 linear variable displacement trans-ducer which is mounted parallel to the drive shaft of the main pulley for measurement of the displacement of the shaft. The blood vessel is attached over a blunted 30-gauge needle which has had its surface roughened. The blood vessel is then tied on with size 6-0 suture. This cannula is then attached to a mounting arm to allow access into the inner portion of

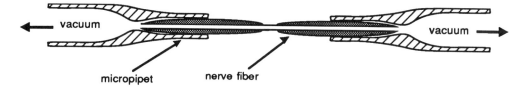

FIGURE 20.9

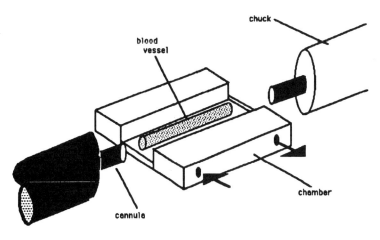

FIGURE 20.10

the blood vessel for electrodes or other probes. This entire chuck assembly attaches directly to the solenoid driver which is mounted on a XYZ micropositioner. A micromanipulator can be used for introduction of electrodes or probes into the blood vessel interior. The other side of the vessel is also cannulated and then attached to the force transducer lever arm to allow the vessel to have fluid perfused through the cannula.

In order to maintain vessel viability, the specimens need to be immersed in an oxygenated Krebs solution. The solution is circulated and the temperature controlled. The chamber (Fig. 20.10) is made of plexiglass with the bottom milled out and replaced by a glass coverslip. The chamber trough is 3 cm wide and allows for the most accurate preparation of solution and environmental control.

Two external reservoirs of 500-ml containers use a simple gravity feeding system to maintain a constant pressure head. A third resevior is used to remove excess fluid from the chamber.

The solution is oxygenated by means of a gas bubbler connected to a gas cylinder (95% O_2/5% CO_2) which allows oxygen to be bubbled through these containers before the solution leaves the feed system. The pressure head was chosen to deliver 4 ml/min for perfusion to maintain vessel viability. In addition, a pressure transducer is incorporated into the feed system to measure the pressure drop over the vessel and thus provide a quantitative determination of response of the vessel with regard to the pressure drop flow relations.

In addition to the methods described, which were designed to subject isolated axons and blood vessels to controlled mechanical stimulation, we have developed techniques to apply loads to cells in culture. This cell culture system permits one to investigate the effects of mechanical deformation on neural and vascular tissue physiology, morphology, and biochemistry. Cells are grown on a transparent, circularly clamped, elastomeric substrate which is deflected into a spherical cap by a uniform pressure applied to the underside of the substrate. The resulting biaxial tension in the substrate creates a state of biaxial strain in the attached monolayer of cells. Control features permit the magnitude, rate, duty cycle, and frequency of the applied strain to be varied. Figure 20.11 depicts the deformation of the substrate.

The chamber, designed for use on a microscope stage, serves as a modified cell culture dish and is comprised of a cap, a cylindrical well, and a ported, sealed reservoir. A transparent, segmented polyetherurethane urea sheet, Mitrathane (Matrix Medica, Denver), is clamped by an O-ring to the bottom of the well and serves as the compliant base for the well and the substrate on which the cells are grown. The base of the well is attached to a reservoir into which air is cyclically injected and exhausted. The pressure generated within the reservoir deforms the compliant base into a spherical cap with an associated biaxial strain of the attached cells. The top of the well is joined to a removable cap, allowing for conventional biochemical and physiologic assays as well as cell culture maintenance to be performed under sterile conditions. An optical path through the apparatus is present as a result of glass windows in the cap and reservoir and permits direct microscopic visualization of the deforming cells grown on the transparent compliant base. The chamber fits easily into conventional incubators and can be sterilized by gas or steam in the preassembled state.

The pressure source is a regulated tank of compressed air whose inlet and exhaust to the reservoir are controlled by a solenoid valve. A solid state timing circuit controls cycling of this valve. In this setup, the duty cycle was set at 50% and the frequency ranged from 0 to 5 Hz. The magnitude of strain as well as the strain rate can be varied. Peak strain is varied by controlling the gas pressure in the reservoir. Strain rates are varied by restricting the flow of gas into the reservoir, thereby controlling the filling time and, hence, the rate of deformation of the substrate.

Ideally, the circularly clamped, flat substrate inflates into a hollow spherical cap. When cut in cross-section through the peak deflection, this cap would appear as an arc (see Fig. 20.12A).

The average substrate stretch ratio, as shown in Fig. 20.12A, is defined as follows:

$$\lambda_{sub} = \frac{s}{2a} = \frac{\theta R}{a} \qquad (1)$$

where

λ_{sub} = the calculated substrate strain
s, a, θ, and R are defined in Fig. 20.12A.

The substrate strain is a biaxial elongation and can be related to the substrate stretch ratio:

$$\varepsilon_{sub} = \lambda_{sub} - 1 \qquad (2)$$

where ε_{sub} = the calculated substrate strain, and q and R can be defined in terms of w_0 and a, which are readily measurable.

$$\theta = 2\alpha = \arctan\left(\frac{w_0}{a}\right) \qquad (3)$$

$$R = \frac{a^2 + w_0^2}{2w_0} \qquad (4)$$

where a is defined in Fig. 20.12A.

Substituting Eqs. (1), (3), and (4) into Eq. (2) and expanding utilizing the trigonometric series expansion for arctan gives Eq. (5):

$$\varepsilon_{sub} = \frac{2}{3}\left(\frac{w_0}{a}\right)^2 - \frac{2}{15}\left(\frac{w_0}{a}\right)^4$$
$$+ \frac{2}{35}\left(\frac{w_0}{a}\right)^6 \cdots \qquad (5)$$

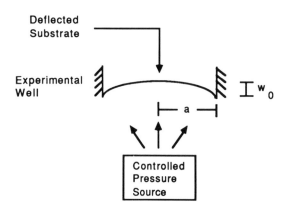

FIGURE 20.11

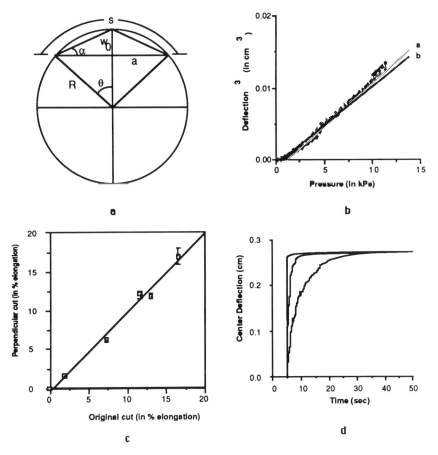

FIGURE 20.12

In these experiments in which $w_0/a < 0.5$, terms of order higher than 2 can be neglected without significant loss of precision, giving the following:

$$\varepsilon^{sub} = \frac{2}{3}\left(\frac{W_0}{a}\right)^2 \qquad (6)$$

Thus, the average elongating strain can be related directly to the center deflection and the radius of the well. Figure 20.12B represents a load-deflection curve for the substrate. The lines a and b represent the loading and unloading phase of the substrate deformation. As can be seen, the behavior is that of a classical membrane with little hysteresis. Figure 20.12C demonstrates the isotropic behavior of the substrate over the range of strains from zero to approximately 20%. These data were obtained

by making silicone rubber molds of the deformed membrane and measuring arc length from orthogonal cuts in the mold. Dynamic deformation is controlled by a variable restriction at the inlet to the reservoir beneath the membrane. Strains can be imparted to the cultured cells over a broad range of strain rates. Figure 20.12D shows three such conditions. The rise time in an approximation of the step response is approximately 25 msec.

Experiments were conducted to determine the actual strain on cells produced by graded deformation of the substrate. Fluorescent beads (0.6 μm diameter) were attached to cultured endothelial cells, and the culture was centered on a microscope stage. A distinct cell with at least two beads attached to its surface was chosen for study. Photomicrographs were taken of the beads prior to and after graded deformation of the substrate. The separation between beads on the surface of the cell was then measured and plotted against deformation of the substrate. The results of one experiment are shown in Fig. 20.13.

These experiments demonstrated that the measured deformation of endothelial cells was linear with the deformation of the substrate, but cell strain varied from 40% to 80% of the substrate. Presumably, the deformation response of a cell to substrate extension depends upon its attachments and its structure; consequently, it is important to determine cell strain in each preparation studied.

Nevertheless, it is possible to subject a population of cells to dynamic biaxial extension and to measure the biological response to such stimulation.

Thus far, we have described the mechanical methodologies to stimulate the tissue or cells in culture. It remains to describe the techniques that are currently being used to assess the biochemical and physiological consequences of mechanical stimulation.

It is important to first note that my colleagues and I have placed particular emphasis upon the role of calcium in mediating the physiological response of cells in the injury process. Therefore, we have gained most of our experience in this area of cellular bio-

mechanics and the injury process by evaluating changes in intracellular calcium in response to mechanical trauma.

Functional Response of Tissue and Cell Culture Models to Mechanical Injury

Calcium is a likely candidate to play a role in the cell's injury response as the importance of calcium in normal cell function is well established and abnormal levels of intracellular calcium are known to be damaging to cellular components. Calcium is essential in maintaining the structural integrity and the normal function of nervous tissue.[35-36] Cell injury can occur when an external stimulus damages the cell membrane, thereby impairing its ability to act as a barrier to extracellular calcium. The resulting increased calcium influx can overwhelm the cellular mechanisms that normally maintain a low, relatively constant intracellular calcium concentration.[37,38] If the cell is unable to sequester or expel sufficient calcium, the cytosolic free calcium level may surpass a critical threshold, triggering a series of pathological events. For instance, the disassembly of microtubules begins at calcium concentrations above $10\,\mu M$ and is greatly accelerated at millimolar concentrations.[36] Neurofilament degradation by calcium-activated neutral proteases begins when calcium concentrations reach 50 to $100\,\mu M$.[39,40] These disrupted cytoskeletal elements, unable to diffuse across the membrane, may lead to an osmotic pressure gradient and subsequent swelling. In a nerve fiber, the accumulation of intracellular debris may occur at or near the nodes of Ranvier where the axon diameter changes significantly. Jones and Cavanagh demonstrated that, for neurofilament degradation induced chemically over a period of weeks, paranodal or nodal swelling occurred due to the accumulation of filamentous masses in myelinated peripheral nerves.[41] Increased calcium influx following membrane damage has other consequences. Variations in intracellular calcium can disrupt normal axon functions, such as axoplasmic

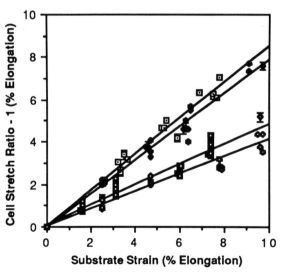

FIGURE 20.13

transport. Ochs et al. found that exposing a desheathed nerve to 25 to 100 mM extracellular calcium resulted in blocked axoplasmic transport after about two hours, probably due to microtubule depolymerization.[35] In addition, efforts to maintain low intracellular calcium by sequestration or extrusion may lead to diminished mitochondrial function and metabolic depletion of the cell.[37-39] This sequence of events leading to cell injury or death— altered membrane permeability or membrane damage, calcium influx, structural disruption— has been hypothesized for cells in general that are exposed to biochemical agents that alter the cell membrane. Balentine observed that the sequelae of spinal cord impact injury, disruption of the myelin and granular dissolution of the axoplasm, were likely a result of increased intracellular calcium. The mechanism by which the impact injury caused an elevated calcium concentration, however, was not addressed.

In our work, it has been hypothesized that dynamic mechanical elongation of a nerve fiber creates transient membrane defects or "pores" which effectively increase membrane permeability and allow a damaging influx of calcium. Intracellular calcium transients resulting from the rapid mechanical deformation of cells have been demonstrated by other researchers in this lab. Using the fluorescent calcium indicator dye, Quin2, Winston recorded elevated calcium levels in endothelial cells attached to a biaxially strained substrate and demonstrated the cells' ability to recover to resting calcium concentration.[42] Using a similar technique, cytosolic free calcium transients were measured in vascular smooth muscle cells.[43] In the unmyelinated squid giant axon, an increased intracellular calcium concentration in response to a dynamic uniaxial elongation was measured with an ion-selective internal microelectrode.[44] The calcium transients for several levels of stretch will be discussed later in the chapter. For a stretch ratio less than or equal to 1.1, the giant axon spontaneously recovered to its resting calcium concentration. Above this level of stretch, however, the intracellular calcium concentration remained abnormally high or increased to

the calcium concentration in the external bath.

Measurements of intracellular free calcium transients following stretch injury are made using the fluorescent calcium indicator dye, fura-2 (Molecular Probes, Inc.). The lipid-soluble form of the dye, fura-2/AM, diffuses across the axolemma. Once in the axoplasm, the acetoxy-methyl ester is cleaved from the dye molecule by endogenous esterases, leaving fura-2 free acid which binds ionic calcium. Upon binding calcium, the excitation spectrum for the fluorescent dye shifts.[46] The maximum fluorescence of unbound fura-2 occurs at about 360 nm wavelength excitation while the peak for Ca^{2+}-bound dye is close to 340 nm.[46,47] Therefore, the intensity of the emitted fluorescence at two wavelengths yields a relative measure of the amount of bound and unbound dye in the cell. A ratio of these measurements is used to calculate the intracellular free calcium concentration.

The shift in the fluorescence maximum upon binding Ca^{2+} can be exploited by using two excitation wavelengths, one near the Ca^{2+}-saturated maximum and the other near the Ca^{2+}-free maximum. If the concentrations of free and bound dye are sufficiently dilute that the fluorescence of each species is proportional to its concentration, then the fluorescence intensity at the two excitation wavelengths is given by:

$$F_1 = S_{f1}C_f + S_{b1}C_b$$
$$F_2 = S_{f2}C_f + S_{b2}C_b \qquad (1)$$

where C_f is the concentration of free fura-2, C_b is the concentration of Ca^{2+}-bound fura-2, and the S values are proportionality constants. Since Ca^{2+} and fura-2 form a 1:1 complex, C_f and C_b are related by

$$C_b = \frac{C_f[Ca^{2+}]}{K_d} \qquad (2)$$

where K_d is the dissociation constant. Substituting (2) into (1) and taking the ratio $R = F_1/F_2$ yields an equation for the calcium ion concentration:

$$[Ca^{2+}] = K_d \frac{R - R_{min}}{R_{max} - R} \left(\frac{S_{f2}}{S_{b2}}\right) \qquad (3)$$

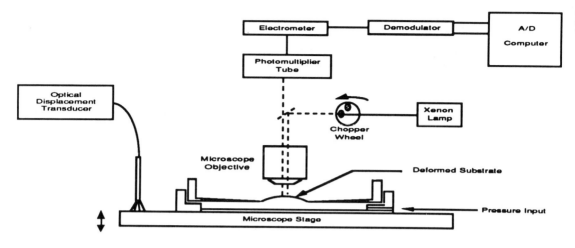

FIGURE 20.14

where R_{min} is the fluorescence ratio with zero calcium (S_{f1}/S_{f2}) and R_{max} is the ratio at calcium saturation (S_{b1}/S_{b2}). It is important to note that the calculated calcium concentration is independent of the dye concentration. This will make the calcium measurement insensitive to variations in the amount of dye loaded between different experiments and variations of absolute fluorescence due to photobleaching during the course of one experiment. However, any autofluorescence must be subtracted before the ratio is taken. Both isolated sinle axons and neural and vascular cells in culture using this intracellular indicator with a system depicted in Fig. 20.14.

Single myelinated nerve fibers have been successfully loaded with the fluorescent indicator dye, fura-2, according to the protocol specified in the methods section. The fibers remained viable after dye loading, as demonstrated by stimulating the nerve while still attached to the muscle, and observing a muscle twitch.

A change in the intracellular free calcium concentration in the single fiber has been demonstrated in response to ionophore treatment. An alternate fluorescence measurement system was used. Exciting the dye-loaded fiber with alternating 340 nm and 360 nm wavelength light and detecting the emitted fluorescence using a silicon intensifier target tube (SIT) camera (Hamamatsu Photonics), images of the

fiber displaying the spatial distribution of intracellular calcium were obtained every 4 sec. Averaging the calcium concentration over a region of the image including most of the node, the resting level of intracellular calcium was calculated for images taken over a 2-min period and found to be approximately 100 nM. The data in Fig. 20.15 shows that several minutes after the addition of ionomycin (Molecular Probes, Inc.) to the Ringer's solution bathing the nerve, the averaged nodal calcium concentration had risen from this resting level to about 900 nM.

A similar ionophore experiment was performed on a single fiber using the experimental

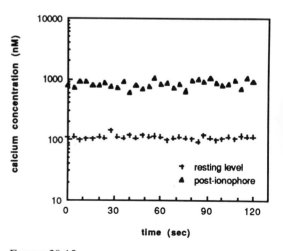

FIGURE 20.15

system described in this proposal. Again, a rise in the intracellular calcium concentration was measured in response to treatment of the nerve with an ionophore (4-bromo A-23187, Molecular Probes, Inc.). However, because this system is capable of much greater sampling rates, up to 500 Hz, the transient increase as well as the steady state change in calcium concentration can be detected. The results of this experiment are shown in Figure 20.16.

Figure 20.17 depicts three experiments using the calcium sensitive fluorescant indicator dye, Quin 2. Figure 20.17A shows the response of endothelials cells to a stretch of approximately 8% at a strain rate of $10 \sec^{-1}$. Current from the photomultiplier tube is proportional to calcium concentration in the cytosol. Figure 20.17B shows a series of six identical stimuli which were delivered to cell following exposure to a 0.1% gluteraldehyde solution. Each stimulus was delivered at 1-min intervals and the figures are plotted on the same graph for convenience. One can follow the accumulation of calcium and the ultimate death of the cell. Trypan blue stain was used to confirm the observation. Figure 20.17C demonstrates the spontaneous accumulation of calcium following a traumatic level of cell deformation.

Vascular smooth muscle and neural cells in culture have exhibited a similar response to mechanical stimulation. Isolated tissue elements such as the squid giant axon and the single myelinated fiber from the frog sciatic nerve have demonstrated functional changes as measured by the resting membrane potential as can be seen in Fig. 20.18. This series of studies was conducted using the squid giant axon. For increasing levels of stretch at high strain rates the axon depolarizes to levels that are exponentially dependent upon the mechanical stimulus. Using ion-selective microelectrodes the intracellular calcium concentrations were also measured and have been shown to increase as a function of the uniaxial elongation, again at high strain rates. Examples of these results are shown in Figure 20.19.

Clearly it is possible to controllably deform isolated tissue elements and cells in culture, and to measure the electrical and chemical changes that may be elicited by the mechanical stimulus. These tools extend our capabilities in the context of injury biomechanics by providing opportunities to investigate the effects of mechanical deformation on the living elements that constitute the organs and organisms when these structures are subjected to forces from the external environment.

Analysis of the Mechanisms of Cell Injury

It is this topic area that may serve to bring together the molecular biology and the bio-

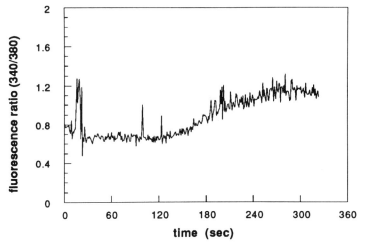

FIGURE 20.16

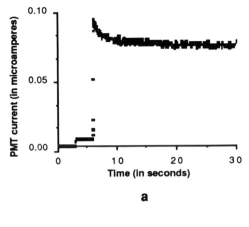

a

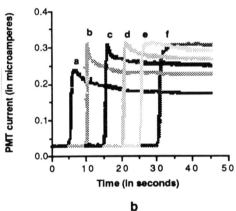

b

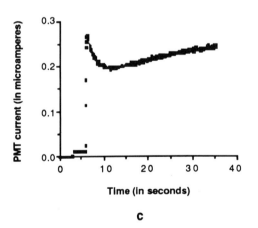

c

FIGURE 20.17

mechanics communities that have a common interest in understanding the mechanisms of injury to the cell. At this level the biomechanician is challenged by the structural complexity of the cell, its transport mech-

anisms, and the myriad of biochemical processes that are potentially influenced by the state of stress or strain that the cell structure may endure.

The mechanism by which dynamic elongation initiates the injury sequence is hypothesized to be a stretch-induced transient change in membrane permeability. In 1981, Ganot et al. reported increased membrane conductance in the *Myxicola* giant axon in response to a rapid transverse mechanical stimulus.[48] The reversal potential of the mechanically altered conductance for small stimuli was very close to that of the leak conductance, suggesting a similarity between these two pathways. A mechanically induced conductance increase in a biological membrane was also described by Terakawa and Watanabe.[49] Slow injection of a small fluid volume into a squid giant axon produced a hyperpolarization and increased membrane conductance, perhaps as a result of increased potassium or leak conductance.

Using a model cell membrane consisting of lipid bilayer and gramicidin channels, Hunter measured membrane conductance in response to biaxial strain at various strain rates.[50] Although gramicidin channel conductance was not strain dependent, increased membrane conductance with strain was measured for bilayers containing no gramicidin that had an initial, unstressed conductance of greater than $3 \times 10^6 \, pS/cm^2$. Hunter hypothesized that these bilayers contained microscopic defects that allowed increased conductance with dynamic membrane strain.

The above studies have demonstrated changes in biological membrane conductance as a function of mechanical deformation. These conductance changes need to be related to the physiologic consequences of stretch injury to form a coherent injury hypothesis. In our research, strain-dependent membrane conductance and accompanying changes in ion transport have been modeled in order to develop an analytical expression describing the experimental stretch-induced calcium transients.

An analytical model is being developed to describe the change in calcium permeability of

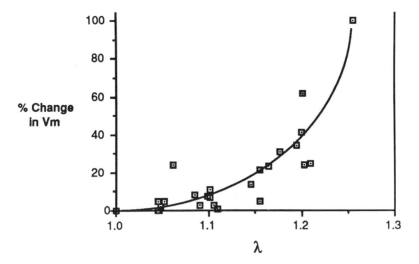

FIGURE 20.18

FIGURE 20.19

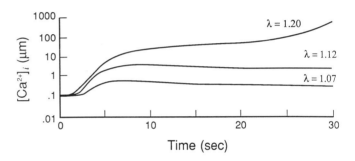

strain. In this model, the membrane is treated as a viscoelastic matrix material containing cylindrical elastic inclusions representing membrane proteins. Applying a dynamic tensile strain to the nerve fiber deforms the nodal membrane where local stress concentrations develop at the inclusion–matrix interface, leading to the formation of transient defects or "pores." These defects in the membrane cause an increase in nonspecific leak conductance, allowing calcium to diffuse down its concentration gradient into the axoplasm. From measurements of nodal displacement during dynamic stretch of a single myelinated axon, as described previously, a transfer function for nodal strain resulting from fiber strain will be established.

Calculation of the inclusion–matrix interface stress concentration due to an applied strain is based on Hashin's formulation of the inclusion problem.[51] Hashin solves the problem of an isotropic elastic spherical inclusion imbedded in an infinite three-dimensional isotropic elastic matrix. Using the correspondence principle and geometrical modifications, Hashin's analysis will be applied to the case of an isotropic linearly elastic cylindrical inclusion in an isotropic viscoelastic matrix.

An expression for the diffusivity of calcium ions in the membrane, taking into account the hindered diffusion through membrane pores, will be developed using pore theory. As a first approximation, the membrane defects will be considered right cylindrical pores of length l,

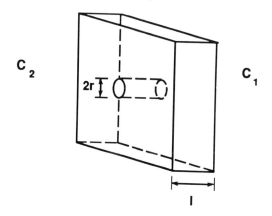

FIGURE 20.20

equal to the thickness of the membrane, and radius $r(t)$, as shown in Fig. 20.20. The time varying function for the pore radius will be chosen considering the stress concentration calculations described above and data in the literature on lipidprotein interactions. To simplify the analysis, electrical interactions between solute molecules and between solute molecules and the pore walls are neglected. Calcium ions are assumed to be rigid spheres of radius a, calculated from the Stokes–Einstein relation:

$$a = \frac{R\,T}{6\pi\eta\,D\,N}$$

where R = gas constant, T = absolute temperature, η = solution viscosity, D = free diffusion coefficient of molecule, and N = Avogadro's number.[45]

The diffusivity of calcium ions in the membrane is decreased from that in free solution by two factors: steric hindrance at the entrance to the pore, and friction between the pore wall and diffusing molecule. In order to enter the pore, the center of a diffusing molecule of radius a must pass through the central region of the pore swept out by a radius of $r(t) - a$ so as not to collide with the pore edge.[52] Therefore, the relative area for diffusion can be expressed as a ratio of this area available to the molecule to the actual pore area. That is,

$$\frac{A(t)}{A_o(t)} = \frac{\pi[r(t) - a]^2}{\pi r^2(t)} = \left(1 - \frac{a}{r(t)}\right)^2,$$

where if $a \ll r$, A/A_o approaches one, corresponding to free diffusion.[53] If $a = r$, A/A_o will equal zero, and the molecule will be sterically excluded from the pore.

The fractional decrease in diffusivity due to friction between the molecule and the pore wall can be calculated using:

$$\frac{f_o}{f(t)} = 1 - 2.104\,\frac{a}{r(t)} + 2.09\left[\frac{a}{r(t)}\right]^3 - 0.95\left[\frac{a}{r(t)}\right]^5,$$

where f_o corresponds to the frictional drag on the freely diffusing molecule (i.e., $a \ll r$).

Combining these two effects to obtain an expression for the hindred diffusivity of the molecule in the membrane results in creates transient membrane pores, the pore radius is proportional to the stretch ratio for a uniaxial elongation such as that applied to the squid axon. This assumes that increasing the level of strain does not solely increase the number of pores in the membrane. Furthermore, assuming the permeability of the axolemma to calcium is determined by the hindered diffusivity of calcium in the membrane (see below), the flux of calcium into the axoplasm, and thus the peak intracellular calcium concentration, is proportional to the strain-dependent calcium diffusivity. This proportionality is, of course, complicated by the sequestration of calcium into intracellular stores. However, that the data in Fig. 20.21 exhibits a trend similar to the relative diffusivity curve of Fig. 20.22 suggests that pore theory is an appropriate choice for the analysis of stretch-induced calcium transients.

$$D_m(t) = D_{free}\left(1 - \frac{a}{r(t)}\right)^2\left(1 - 2.104\,\frac{a}{r(t)} + 2.09\left[\frac{a}{r(t)}\right]^3 - 0.95\left[\frac{a}{r(t)}\right]^5\right).$$

The relative diffusivity, or $D_m(t)/D_{free}$, is plotted in Fig. 20.22.

Considering the membrane a barrier of thickness l separating two solutions of constant calcium concentrations C_1 and C_2, as in Fig. 20.12, the calcium flux can be written as

FIGURE 20.21

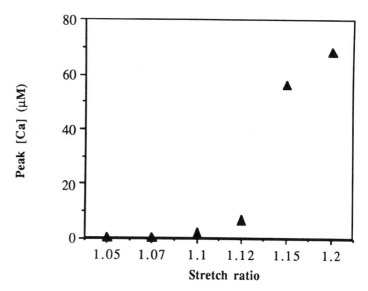

FIGURE 20.22

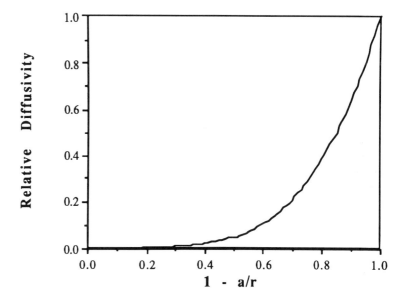

$$J(t) = P(t)[C_2 - C_1],$$

where $J(t)$ is the diffusion flux across the membrane and $P(t)$ is the permeability of the membrane to calcium. Assuming that diffusion of calcium through membrane pores is the primary determinant of membrane permeability to calcium,

$$P(t) = \frac{a(t)D(t)}{l},$$

where $a(t)$ is the area fraction of pores in the membrane, and $D(t)$ is the hindered calcium diffusivity calculated earlier. In this analysis, interaction between pores and end effects of the pores are neglected.

Flux experiments are being carried out in this lab to characterize the size of the strain-induced pores using radiolabeled ions of various radii. This data may provide a method to separate the effects of pore size and the number of pores, which together determine the flux.

It is hypothesized that the deformation of the cell's membranes causes an increase in permeability to ions due to the formation of defects or pores. This theory of mechanically induced poration is supported by the observation that osmotically swelled red cells become permeable to the relatively large hemaglobin molecule.[54] Furthermore, upon removal of the osmotic gradient, the membrane's integrity is restored. The red cell membrane is capable of only a 2 to 4% increase in area before lysis occurs.[54] Regions of high strain can recruit lipid from adjacent regions to relieve the strain. Therefore, the rate at which the strain is applied will determine the extent of the induced poration. Further, it is assumed that within limits, the pore formation is transient and reversible just as the red cell reseals when the distending pressure is removed.

Closure

With the exception of crush injury, the mechanical forces that lead to the CNS trauma are applied dynamically with a characteristic time course of 50 msec or less. Little is known, however, regarding the time course of the pathophysiological response of the tissue. The models developed in our laboratory are designed to investigate the underlying mechanisms of injury, determine the threshold of mechanical stimuli that produces injury, and explore the time course of the pathophysiological events in order to define windows of opportunity and strategies for therapeutic intervention. The macroscopic analysis of CNS injury is complicated by the fact that the tissue or organ response is dictated by the cellular response. We are attempting to move biomechanics and injury research toward the areas of membrane mechanics, cytomechanics, and transport process analysis at the cellular level.

In the past, we had used a primate model to replicate specific forms of injury. We focused our attention on Diffuse Axonal Injury (DAI) and Acute Subdural Hematoma (ASDH) because epidemiological data indicated that these forms of injury were responsible for approximately 70% of the mortality and morbidity associated with brain injury. By subjecting physical models or surrogates of the skull-brain structure to loading conditions which produced these discrete forms of brain injury in the primate model, we were able to estimate the magnitude and temporal nature of the deformations that were experienced by the various neural and neurovascular elements in association with these injuries. With this information, we developed a strategy to investigate the biomechanics of injury at the isolated tissue and cellular levels in order to begin to simplify this complex analysis. Accordingly, we designed instrumentation that permits the study of isolated axons, blood vessels, and cells in culture under conditions of controlled mechanical deformation. Utilizing these technologies, we demonstrated that high strain rate deformation of the axolemma led to an elevated level of intracellular calcium.

Cell membrane ionic permeability is directly affected by high strain rate deformation which leads to an immediate elevation in cytosolic free calcium ion concentration. This traumatic rise in cytosolic free calcium in neurons has been implicated in cytoskeletal disruption, functional impairment, cell swelling, and ultimately cell death, while in smooth muscle cells the event can lead to spontaneous contraction. Neural tissue can respond by sequestering calcium or pumping it from the cytoplasm. However, the pumping mechanisms are dependent on oxidative metabolism and may be compromised if blood flow to the tissue is reduced by vessel reactivity or structural failure.

Our current findings suggest that the cerebrovasculature responds to mechanical deformation under conditions of high strain rate loading. This response, in the form of a transient spasm, could result in regional reduction of cerebral blood flow. to investigate the mechanism of this mechanically induced vasospasm, we return again to the cellular level and now focus on the smooth muscle element of the vessel wall. We have preliminary data demonstrating elevated levels of intracellular calcium in smooth muscle cells in culture.

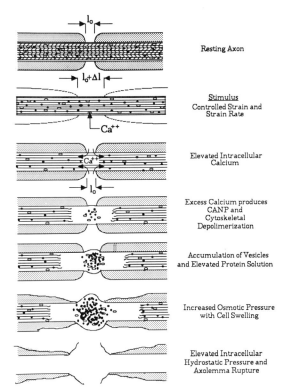

Resting Axon

$l_0 + \Delta l$

Stimulus
Controlled Strain and
Strain Rate

Ca^{++}

Elevated Intracellular
Calcium

l_0

Excess Calcium produces
CANP and
Cytoskeletal
Depolimerization

Accumulation of Vesicles
and Elevated Protein Solution

Increased Osmotic Pressure
with Cell Swelling

Elevated Intracellular
Hydrostatic Pressure and
Axolemma Rupture

FIGURE 20.23

Transient changes in cytosolic free calcium can produce a spontaneous contraction and, on a more macroscopic level, can lead to vasospasm. We hypothesize that, in situ, these events occur in concert with the neural tissue insult as previously described.

Figure 20.23 demonstrates our current thinking with regard to the injury cascade that can occur as a direct result of dynamic elongation of the axon for example. This process will be exacerbated if there is an interruption in local blood flow accompanying the direct mechanical insult since the cell requires energy to actively pump calcium from the cytosol.

This chapter is intended to demonstrate that this line of research can lead to new views of how we can apply the rigorous tools of experimental and theoretical biomechanics to the analysis of tissue, cellular, and subcellular structures.

Acknowledgments

I would like to take this opportunity to thank my former students Drs. Susan Margulies, James Galbraith, Flaura Winston, Catherine Hunter, David Meaney, Kenneth Barbee, and Robert Boock for it has been their hard work that has enabled us to move in this direction. My current students Katherine Saatman, Adam Landsman, Robert Cargill, Lynn Bilston, Daniel Goldstein, Kristen Belliar, and Kirk Thibault are continuing this work.

I would also like to thank the National Institutes of Health, the National Highway Traffic Safety Administration, and the Centers for Disease Control for their support over these last 10 years.

References

1. Gurdjian ES, Lissner HR, Patrick LM (1962) Protection of the head and neck in sports. JAMA 182:509–512.
2. Denny-Brown D, Russell WR (1941) Experimental cerebral concussion. Brain 64:93–164.
3. Holbourn AHS (1945) Mechanics of brain injuries. Br Med Bul 3:147–149.
4. Ommaya AK, Hirsch AE, Flamm ES, Mahone RH (1966) Cerebral concussion in the monkey: an experimental model. Science 153:211–212.
6. Ommaya A, Gennarelli TA (1974) Cerebral concussion and traumatic unconsciousness. Brain 97:633–654.
7. Gennarelli TA, Thibault LE (1972) Pathophysiologic responses of rotational and translational accelerations of the head. In Proceedings of the 16th Stapp Car Crash Conference, SAE, pp 296–308.
8. Gennarelli TA, Thibault LE (1982) Biomechanics of acute subdural hematoma. J Trauma 22:680–696.
9. Ommaya AK, Hirsch AE, Martinez JL (1966) The role of whiplash in cerebral concussion. In Proceedings of the 10th Stapp Car Crash Conference, November.
10. Shatsky S, Alter WA, Evans DE (1974) Traumatic distortions of the primate head and chest: correlation of biomechanical, radiological, and pathological data. In Proceedings of the 18th Stapp Car Crash Conference, SAE, pp 351–381.
11. Prudenz R, Sheldon C (1946) The lucite calvarium—a method for direct observation of the brain. II. Cranial trauma and brain movement. J Neurosurg 3:487.
12. Holbourn AH (1943) Mechanics of head injuries. Lancet 2:438–441.

13. Abel J, Gennarelli T, Segawa H (1978) Incidence and severity of cerebral concussion in the rhesus monkey following sagittal plane acceleration. In: Proceedings of the 22nd Stapp Car Crash Conf. SAE, pp 33–53.

14. Gennarelli T, Thibault L, Adams J, Graham D, Thompson C, Marcinin R (1982) Diffuse axonal injury and prolonged coma in the primate. Ann Neurol 12:564–574.

15. Gennarelli TA, Ommaya AK, Thibault LE (1971) Comparison of translational and rotational head motions in experimental cerebral concussion. In Proceedings of the 15th Stapp Car Crash Conference, November.

16. Thibault L, Bianchi A, Galbraith J, Gennarelli T (1982) Analysis of the strains induced in physical models of the baboon brain undergoing inertial loading. In Proceedings of the 35th ACEMB 8.

17. Margulies S, Thibault L. A proposed human tolerance criteria for diffuse axonal injury. J Biomechanics (in press).

18. Margulies SS, Thibault LE (1989) An analytical model of traumatic diffuse brain injury. J Biomech Eng 111:241–249.

19. Ward CC, Thompson RB (1975) The development of a detailed finite element brain model. In Proceedings of the 19th Stapp Car Crash Conf, pp 641–674.

20. Lee MC, Melvin JW, Ueno K (1987) Finite element analysis of traumatic acute subdural hematoma. In Proceedings of the 31st Stapp Car Crash Conf, pp 67–77.

20a. Khalil TB, Viano DC Critical issues in finite element modeling of head impact. In Proceedings of the 26th Stapp Car Crash Conf, pp 87–102.

20b. Cheng LY, Rifai S, Khatua T, Pziali RL (1989) Finite element analysis of diffuse axonal injury. In Proceedings of the 33rd Stapp Car Crash Conf.

20c. Tong P, DiMasi F, Carr G, Galbraith C, Eppinger R, Marcus J, Finite element modeling of head injury response to inertial loading. In Proceedings of the 12th Int Tech Conf of Exp. Safety Vehicles, Gothenburg, Sweden.

21. Meaney DF (1991) Biomechanics of acute subdural hematoma in the subhuman primate and man. University of Pennsylvania PhD dissertation.

22. Lee YC, Advani SH (1970) Transient response of a sphere to torsional loading—a head injury model. Math Biosci 6:473–486.

23. Bycroft GN (1973) Mathematical model of head subjected to an angular acceleration. J Biomech 6:487–495.

24. Liu YK, Chandran KB, von Rosenburg DV (1975) Angular acceleration of viscoelastic (Kelvin) material in a rigid speherical shell—a rotational head injury model. J Biomechan 8:285–292.

25. Ljung C (1975) A model for brain deformation due to rotation of the skull. J Biomech 8:263–274.

26. Misra JC, Chakravarty S (1984) A study on rotational brain injury. J Biomech 17:459–466.

27. Margulies S (1987) Biomechanics of traumatic coma in the primate. University of Pennsylvania, PhD Dissertation.

28. Goldman DE, Wells JB (1983) Longitudinal stretch of squid giant axon. Biophys J 41:52a.

29. Galbraith JA (1988) The effects of mechanical loading on the electrophysiology of the squid giant axon. PhD dissertation, University of Pennsylvania.

30. Gennarelli TA, Thibault LE, Tipperman R, et al. Axonal injury in the optic nerve: a model of diffuse axonal injury in the brain. J Neurosurg 71:244–253.

31. Graham DI, Adams JH, Legan S, Gennarelli TA, Thibault CE (1985) The distribution, nature and time course of diffuse axonal injury. Neuropathol Appl Neurobiol 11:319.

32. Thibault LE, Gennarelli TA, Tipton HW, Carpenter DO (1974) The physiologic response of isolated nerve tissue to dynamic mechanical loads. ACEMB 16:176.

34. Gray JAB, Ritchie JM (1954) Effects of stretch on single myelinated nerve fibres. J Physiol 124:84–99.

35. Ochs S, Worth RM, Chan S-Y (1977) Calcium requirement for axoplasmic transport in mammalian nerve. Nature 270:748–750.

36. Schliwa M, Euteneuer U, Bulinski JC, Izant JG (1981) Calcium lability of cytoplasmic microtubules and its modulation by microtubule-associated proteins. Cell Biol 78:1037–1041.

37. Morgan BP, Luzio JP, Campbell AK (1986) Intracellular Ca^{2+} and cell injury: a paradoxical role of Ca^{2+} in complement membrane Attack. 7:399–411.

38. Schanne FAX, Kane AB, Young EE, Farber JL (1979) Calcium dependence of toxic cell death: a final common pathway. Science 206:700–702.

39. Balentine JD (1988) Spinal cord trauma: in search of the meaning of granular axoplasm and

vesicular myelin. J Neuropathol Exp Neurol 47:77–92.

40. Kamakura K, Ishiura S, Suzuki K, Sugita H, Toyokura Y (1985) Calcium-activated neutral protease in the peripheral nerve, which requires μM order Ca^{2+}, and its effect on the neurofilament triplet. J Neurosci Res 13:391–403.

41. Jones HB, Cavanagh JB (1983) Distortions of the nodes of Ranvier from axonal distension by filamentous masses in hexacarbon intoxication. J Neurocytol 12:439–458.

42. Winston FK (1989) The modulation of intracellular free calcium concentration by biaxial extensional strains of bovine pulmonary artery endothelial cells. PhD dissertation, University of Pennsylvania.

43. Barbee KA (1991) Cellular response of vascular smooth muscle to mechanical stimuli. PhD dissertation, University of Pennsylvania.

44. Thibault LE, Gennarelli TA, Margulies SS, Marcus J, Eppinger R (1990) The strain dependent pathophysiological consequences of inertial loading on central nervous system tissue. In Proceedings of the 1990 International IRCOBI Conf, Lyon, France.

45. Chonko AM, Irish III JM, Welling DJ (1978) Microperfusion of isolated tubules. In Methods in Pharmacology. Martinez-Maldonado, ed. Plenum, New York.

46. Grynkiewicz G, Poenie M, Tsien RY (1985) A new generation of Ca^{2+} indicators with greatly improved fluorescence properties. J Biol Chem 260:3440–3450.

47. Tsien RY, Poenie M (1986) Fluorescence ratio imaging: a new window into intracellular ionic signaling. Trends Biochem Sci 11:450–455.

48. Ganot G, Wong BS, Binstock L, Ehrenstein G (1981) Reversal potentials corresponding to mechanical stimulation and leakage current in *myxicola* giant axons. Biochim Biophys Acta 649:487–491.

49. Terakawa S, Watanabe A (1982) Electrical responses to mechanical stimulation of the membrane of squid giant axons. Pflügers Arch 395:59–64.

50. Hunter CM (1988) Effects of mechanical loading on ion transport through lipid bilayer membranes.

51. Hashin Z (1969) The inelastic inclusion problem. Int J Engng Sci 7:11–36.

52. Renkin EM (1955) Filtration, diffusion, and molecular sieving through porous cellulose membranes. J Gen Physiol 38:225–243.

53. Pappenheimer JR, Renkin EM, Borrero LM (1951) Filtration, diffusion and molecular sieving through peripheral capillary membranes. Am J Physiol 167:13–46.

54. Evans E, Waugh R, Melnik L (1976) Elastic area compressibility modulus of red cell membrane. Biophys J 16:585–595.

21
Vehicle Interactions with Pedestrians

Thomas F. MacLaughlin, David S. Zuby, Jeffrey C. Elias, and C. Brian Tanner

Introduction

Each year in the United States motor vehicles kill nearly 7,000 pedestrians, accounting for 15% of the nation's motor vehicle traffic fatalities.[1] Nonfatally injured pedestrians number over 110,000,[2] and many suffer serious, disabling injuries. Developing vehicle-based countermeasures to reduce the severity of this trauma has often been considered an intractable problem, consequently limiting efforts in this area. In recent years, however, accident data analyses have provided a more thorough understanding of the pedestrian accident environment. The most frequently and seriously injured body regions, as well as sources for those injuries have been identified. Based on this knowledge, research to reduce pedestrian trauma has begun to yield encouraging results.

Pedestrian accidents are largely an urban problem.[3,4] About 80%, including more than half of the fatalities, occur on urban and residential roads. Preimpact braking is present in 70% of these, reducing impact speeds an average of nearly 20 km/h.* As a result, pedestrians are struck at relatively low impact speeds; 90% are at speeds of 48 km/h or less, as shown in Fig. 21.1. This accounts for half of all harm suffered by pedestrians. Harm[5] is a measure of the importance of trauma and is computed by weighting injuries according to their severity, as well as by frequency of occur-

rence. The relatively low-speed nature of pedestrian accidents is encouraging, because the chances of reducing pedestrian trauma through vehicle modifications are much greater at these lower speeds. This information has provided research incentive to focus on impacts in the 0 to 48 km/h speed range.

Young people appear to be overrepresented as pedestrian accident victims. Figure 21.2 shows that pedestrians through age 15 sustain 40% of all pedestrian injuries and account for 30% of the total pedestrian harm at collision speeds of 48 km/h and below. Although the Fatal Accident Reporting System (FARS) reports that child fatalities have declined nearly 35% over the last decade,[1] child trauma is still a significant part of the pedestrian problem, and continues to deserve serious attention.

Areas of the body most seriously injured are the head and thorax. Leg injuries, though generally much less serious, are more frequent. Use of the harm concept permits an accounting of the relative importance of trauma to the different parts of the body. Figures 21.3 and 21.4 show the distribution of harm by body region and source for impact speeds not exceeding 48 km/h. The contributions of the different injury severity levels are also shown. Head and thorax[†] injuries account for three-quarters of the harm. Severe injuries, those

---

*Metric units are used throughout this chapter. Note that 1 km/h is equivalent to 0.62 mph.

[†] Thorax injury includes "hard" abdomen injury; i.e., injury to body regions protected by the lower thoracic cage (73% of all abdomen injuries).

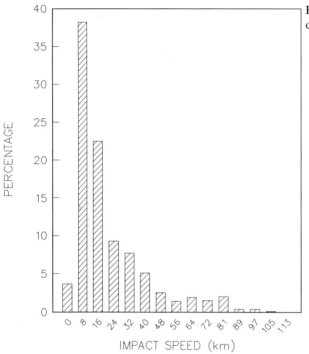

FIGURE 21.1. Impact speed–based distribution of pedestrian victims. (From MacLaughlin.[3])

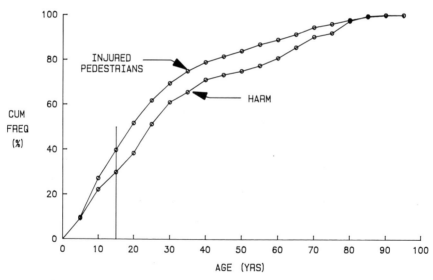

FIGURE 21.2. Cumulative frequency and harm of injured pedestrians by age. (From MacLaughlin.[3])

with Abbreviated Injury Scale (AIS) ratings of 4 and 5,[6] are major contributors. The information in the previous two figures is combined in Table 21.1 to show the most harmful injury source/body region contacts. All contacts resulting in at least 2% of the harm are listed. Head, thorax, and leg impacts against hoods, fenders, vehicle faces, and bumpers are highlighted. They produce over 50% of pedestrian harm in the less than 48 km/h speed range.

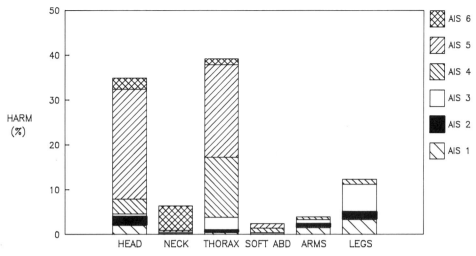

FIGURE 21.3. Distribution of pedestrian harm by body region and injury severity. (From MacLanghlin.[3])

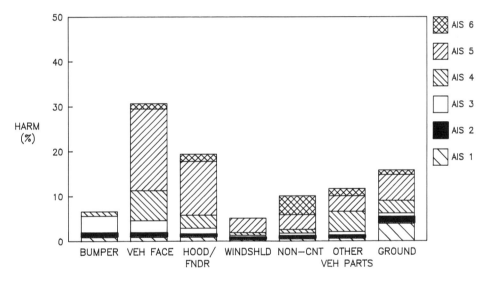

FIGURE 21.4. Distribution of pedestrian harm by injury source and injury severity. (From MacLaughlin.[3])

Early efforts to include long-term impairment measurements[4] suggested an increase of approximately 25% in the relative importance of both head and leg trauma, and about a 25% reduction in thorax trauma importance. Much more work is required to establish quantitatively the significance of injury impairment and disability in the motor vehicle crash environment.[7]

Most of the information in Figs. 21.3 and 21.4 was based on accident data collected in the 1970s and early 1980s. The design and distribution of motor vehicles in the United States have changed in recent years, undoubtedly changing these harm distributions. Passenger cars today have lower front profiles and shorter hoods, which would tend to shift thorax and child head impacts from the vehicle face to the hood/fender surface and move a number of head-to-hood impacts into the cowl and windshield. Offsetting this trend is the increasing proportion of light trucks and vans

TABLE 21.1. Most harmful *injury source/body region* combinations in pedestrian accidents ≤48 km/h.

	Injury source/body region	Harm %
*	Vehicle face/thorax	17%
*	Hood-fender/head	11%
	Ground/head	10%
	Other vehicle parts/thorax	9%
*	Vehicle face/head	8%
*	Hood-fender/thorax	7%
*	Bumper/legs	7%
	Noncontact/neck	5%
	Windshield/head	5%
	Noncontact/thorax	4%
*	Vehicle face/legs	3%
	Ground/thorax	2%
	Total harm	88%

* Head, thorax, and leg injuries caused by hoods, fenders, vehicle faces, and bumpers.

(LTV) being used as personal vehicles and therefore being involved in pedestrian collisions. Collecting new pedestrian accident data is vital to continued understanding of the accident environment. Nonetheless, the currently available data are adequate and appropriate for defining research to effectively reduce injury severity.

From the accident information described above, the National Highway Traffic Safety Administration (NHTSA) established a research and development program with the goal of reducing the injury consequences of motor vehicle/pedestrian collisions. Contacts being addressed are head impacts against hoods, fenders, and cowls; thorax impacts against vehicle faces, hoods, and fenders; and leg impacts against bumpers and vehicle faces. The strategy is similar for the three body regions. First, an experiment to simulate the impact is developed. This involves building a component test device and developing or confirming associated injury criteria. Next, the component test equipment is used to assess impact performance of representative production vehicles, and to identify particular design configurations that exhibit lower potential for injury. Finally, if required, structural modifications are made to an exemplar vehicle to improve performance and demonstrate

possible benefits. Care is taken to assure that design changes are simple, low in cost, and within current production technology. The following sections describe the status of this research for head, thorax, and leg protection, and present the authors' views of future research needs.

Head Injury Research

Pedestrian Kinematics

Understanding the kinematics of vehicle/pedestrian interactions is important when examining head injuries because of their influence on the severity of the impact. Simulations of pedestrian accidents have been attempted with human cadaveric specimens, anthropometric dummies, and computer simulations, each with varying degrees of success.

Cadavers represent the most human-like surrogates for the study of pedestrian impact kinematics. Experiments using cadavers indicate that the motion of a pedestrian is very "fluid" when struck by a vehicle. The body wraps around the front of the vehicle, closely following the contours of the fascia and hood. Disadvantages of cadavers are their limited availability and repeatability, coupled with difficult instrumentation and handling procedures.

Several pedestrian cadaver experiments, however, are referenced in the body of pedestrian injury research literature. Pritz[8] compared the dynamic responses of cadaveric specimens with those of anthropomorphic dummies. King et al.[9] reported numerous measurements of body segment accelerations for both cadavers and dummies. Similar experiments in Europe include a comparative analysis of the responses of cadavers and various dummies.[10]

Anthropomorphic test dummies also have been used to study pedestrian kinematics. Dummies used for pedestrian examinations are generally modified versions of the devices used to assess the safety of vehicle occupants. The durability and availability of dummies allows for more extensive testing than is possible with

FIGURE 21.5. MADYMO pedestrian models. (From Hoyt and Chu.[12])

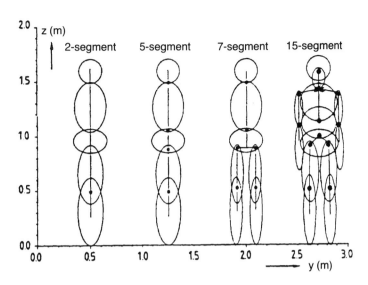

cadaveric specimens. However, high-speed films of pedestrian impacts using dummies show that their body segments generally appear to be too inflexible to accurately duplicate the complex pedestrian collision event. After initial contact with the bumper of the striking vehicle, a dummy tends to rotate about its center of gravity, as the lower limbs rebound from the bumper. Dummy kinematics notably differ from observed cadaver kinematics. Despite these shortcomings, successful dummy experiments have been conducted.

Finally, mathematical computer models based on rigid body dynamics have been used to predict pedestrian impact kinematics. Analyses using generalized commercial software as well as specific models are reported in the literature. Van Wijk et al.[11] examined the efficacy of two-dimensional models with varying degrees of complexity. The commercial program, MADYMO, was used to create two-dimensional models of a pedestrian consisting of two, five, and seven rigid body segments as well as a three-dimensional model with 15 body segments (Fig. 21.5). The results of impact simulations were compared with pedestrian dummy tests.

Unfortunately, most pedestrian models are based largely on dummy characteristics, and produce simulations that have many of the limitations observed in dummy impact tests.

An exception is the work of Hoyt and Chu,[12] who used the two-dimensional version of MADYMO to develop a nine-segment adult pedestrian model to simulate the kinematics from two cadaver tests.

Head Impact Simulation

Component test methods appear to be a practical way to evaluate the potential for injury resulting from specific body region to vehicle surface impacts. Realistic component tests, simulating the impact of the pedestrian's head onto the hood, can be performed if the head's impact velocity is known. Typical head trajectories and resulting velocities at impact with the vehicle surface have been determined from studies of pedestrian kinematics described earlier.

A typical pedestrian head trajectory in cadaver tests reported by Pritz[8] is shown in Fig. 21.6. Head-to-hood impact velocities relative to the vehicle, reported as ratios of the initial vehicle/pedestrian impact speeds, ranged between 0.7 and 0.9.[13] Interestingly, maximum head velocities were reported to occur before impact with the hood. In cadaver studies conducted by European researchers, average head impact velocity ratios ranged from 1.0 to 1.37.[10,14] The higher velocity ratios in the European studies probably resulted

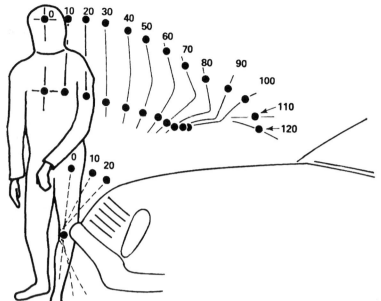

FIGURE 21.6. Pedestrian head trajectory from cadaver tests. (From King et al.[9] Reprinted with permission © 1976, Society of Automotive Engineers, Inc.)

because smaller vehicles were used than in the United States study.[13] Consequently, the cadavers' heads did not strike the hoods, but rather most impacted the windshields. Pedestrian dummies were reported to experience head impact velocities similar to those measured for cadavers.[8,10]

The computer models reported by Van Wijk et al.[11] predicted head impact locations within the range measured from the dummy experiments. However, head impact velocities from the two-dimensional models were higher than observed in the dummy experiments. The three-dimensional model produced more realistic head impact velocities, which suggested that rotation of the pedestrian's body about an imaginary spinal axis and arm/hood interaction affected head impact velocity in ways that could not be analyzed with the two-dimensional models. Hoyt and Chu's[12] "cadaver" model, and an eight-segment version representing children, produced impact kinematics that were reasonable and generally agreed with accident report descriptions. The average ratio of head impact velocity to initial vehicle contact velocity from these reconstructions was 0.9.

A rigid head form impact test device, capable of producing the head impact speeds experienced by pedestrians, was developed by Pritz et al.[15] and Brooks et al.[16] It contains instrumentation for measuring acceleration and location of the head form, providing data for calculation of various head injury criteria.[17–19] The test device was used to reconstruct vehicle damage patterns observed in specific pedestrian accidents involving head impacts to confirm the feasibility of predicting injuries in the laboratory. Fourteen adult pedestrian accidents were reconstructed to develop relationships between the measurable injury criteria and the severity of "real world" injuries.[20] Figures 21.7 and 21.8 show the relationships between injury severity, expressed as maximum AIS and probability of death (POD) and the Head Injury Criterion (HIC). These verify that a HIC value of 1,000 is an accurate indicator of the threshold of serious head injury (AIS 3, POD approximately 7%), and HIC 1,500 appeared to be a threshold of severe/critical injury (AIS 4–5, POD approximately 26%).

Evaluation of Pedestrian Head Injury Potential of Vehicles

The component impact test method was employed to evaluate the potential for injury

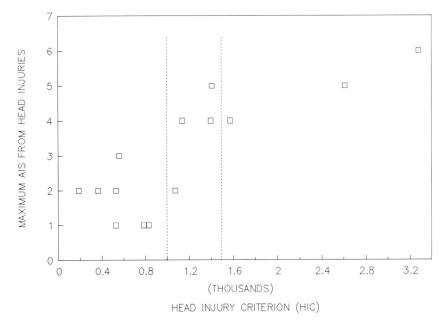

FIGURE 21.7. Maximum Head Injury AIS versus Head Injury Criteria (HIC). (From MacLaughlin and Kessler.[21] Reprinted with permission © 1990, Society of Automotive Engineers, Inc.)

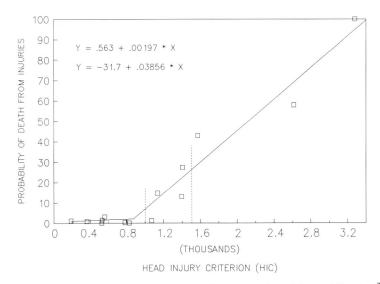

FIGURE 21.8. Probability of Death (POD) versus HIC. (From MacLaughlin and Kessler.[21] Reprinted with permission © 1990, Society of Automotive Engineers, Inc.)

resulting from impacts to various vehicle features. Typically, component impact tests have been conducted at the upper range of likely impact velocities. Because the vehicle/pedestrian impact velocity for more than 90% of pedestrian accidents is less than 48 km/h,[3] and because the ratio of head impact speed to vehicle/pedestrian impact speed is approximately 0.9 for vehicles in the United States,[12,13] most component tests have been conducted at impact velocities of less than 43 km/h. The potential injury severity of experimental impacts have been evaluated principally with the HIC. Good performance is indicated by simulated pedestrian impacts, which produce HIC values of less than 1,000.

The results of component impact testing suggest that the front surface of the vehicle can be characterized by three sections with different injury potential. The central hood is defined by the area of the hood that lies more than 150 mm from any hood edge. The hood/ fender area includes the hood surface within 150 mm of the side edges as well as the tops of the fender panels. The rear hood area lies between the front edge of the windscreen and a line 150 mm forward of the rear hood edge. Accident data indicate that pedestrian head impacts are distributed fairly uniformly within these regions.[21]

Impacts to central hoods produced a wider range of HIC and resulting POD values than the other two areas.[22] Some of the hoods appeared to offer good head protection. As a consequence, a detailed central hood test procedure was developed, and the hoods of several passenger cars, light trucks, and vans

were thoroughly evaluated.[21] Considerable reduction of injury severity could be realized if all vehicles' central hood surfaces were similar to those that produced the lowest HIC values. The rear hood area, however, exhibited more severe impacts than the central hood area. Figure 21.9 illustrates that impacts within 150 mm of the rear hood edge typically produced higher HIC values than impacts more than 150 mm forward of the rear hood edge.[21] Impacts to the hood/fender area produced the highest HIC values of the three vehicle areas that have been described.[13,22]

Attributes of vehicle front end design that affect the severity of simulated pedestrian head impacts include the clearance between the hood surface and engine compartment components, the hood material, and the hood reinforcement structure. Consideration of these and other elements of vehicle front end design could reduce head impact injury severity.

The experimental results suggest that for impact velocities between 37 and 44 km/h, the head form must be allowed between 58 and

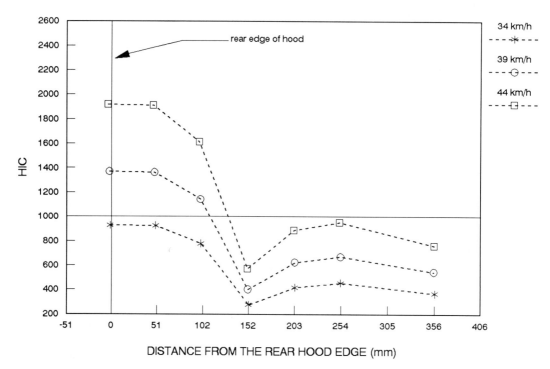

FIGURE 21.9. Effect of impact location on impact severity (HIC). (From Kessler et al.[22])

76 mm dynamic displacement beyond the hood surface to maintain HIC below 1,000.[13,21,22] Dynamic displacement may exceed the available under-hood clearance if the engine compartment components are not rigidly mounted. In most cases, however, engine compartment components are rigid and massive by comparison to the head form and hood sheet metal. These observation suggest that pedestrian head impacts to exterior body panels with more than 58 mm clearance to the nearest engine compartment component can potentially produce only minor injuries.

Hood material also influences injury severity. Test results demonstrate that conventional sheet steel body panels absorb the energy of the head's impact, producing relatively low forces and consequently low HIC values. One aluminum hood was tested, exhibiting desirable energy-absorbing characteristics. The greater dynamic displacement observed in this test suggested a need for more clearance. Impacts to several hoods manufactured from plastic fiber composites indicate that such hoods exhibit poor energy-absorbing characteristics and are considerably stiffer than most steel hoods. Consequently, the threat of severe head injury is considerably greater from impacts to these contemporary plastic composite hoods than from conventional steel hood impacts.[22]

The structure of the underside reinforcement of the hood also affects the severity of simulated pedestrian head impacts.[22,23] Tests on two vehicles with nearly identical exterior geometry and different reinforcement structures illustrated that the vehicle with heavier reinforcements (Fig. 21.10) produced more severe impacts than the more lightly reinforced vehicle (Fig. 21.11). Although under-hood clearances differ in the two vehicles, the performance difference was attributed primarily to the variation in hood reinforcement.

Pedestrian Head Injury Countermeasures

Modifying the front ends of vehicles to reduce the severity of pedestrian injuries has been

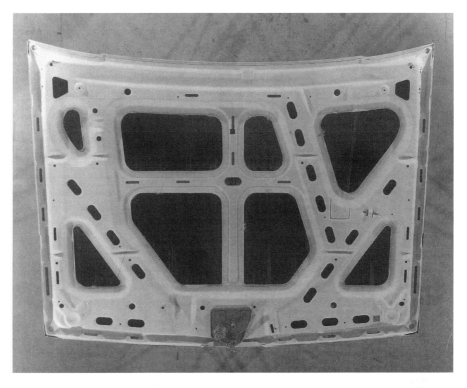

FIGURE 21.10. Hood with heavy reinforcement structure. (From Kessler.[23])

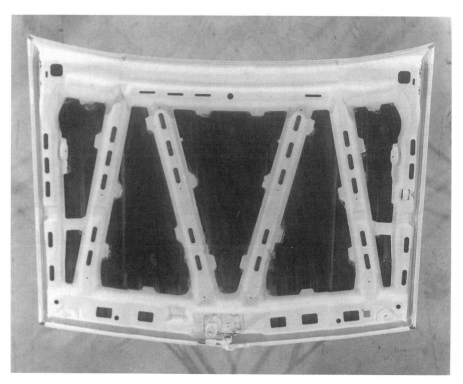

FIGURE 21.11. Hood with light reinforcement structure. (From Kessler.[23])

considered impractical by many. Observations from component impact tests, however, have suggested several practical modifications that may have significant effects. These injury countermeasures do not depart from conventional design and manufacturing practice, and appear to be cost-effective.

The hood/fender region produced the most severe indication of injury in component impact tests. Recent demonstrations of pedestrian injury countermeasures have shown that this area can be softened and made more energy absorbent by reducing the local stiffness of the fender and providing clearance between the fender surface and apron structure. Such modifications to the fender of a Mercedes-Benz 124 series vehicle reduced maximum impact forces to 30% below those measured in similar impacts to 123 series vehicles.[24] The stiffness of the fender was decreased with a combination of perforating an inner fender surface and using a Z-profile as shown in Fig. 21.12. Similar results, which include a 40% reduction of HIC, are observed for

comparable modifications of a Ford Taurus by Zuby et al.[25] (Fig. 21.13). Clearance below the fender surface was achieved by removing the flanges from the hood edge (to simulate a commonly used hemmed joint) and from the top of the upper apron. The inner fender surface was perforated to soften it, similar to the Mercedes-Benz 124. Figure 21.14 shows the Taurus modifications. While the removal of a flange from a structural member may not seem practical, Fig. 21.15 illustrates that the upper aprons of other production vehicles are manufactured without a clearance-reducing flange below the fender surface. Additional reduction of injury potential, and quite possibly HIC below 1,000 at a 37 km/h head impact velocity, could be achieved by improving the perforation pattern and slightly lowering the upper apron.

The 124 series Mercedes-Benz also included injury-reducing countermeasures in the rear hood region. A 20% reduction of impact force was realized by styling the rear hood sheet steel to provide about 10 mm more clearance

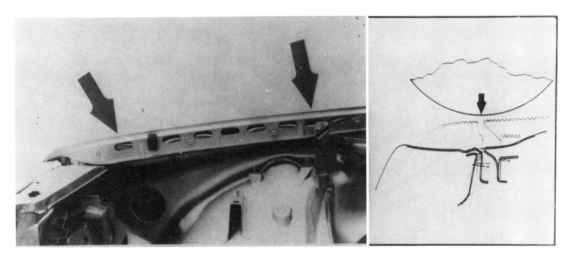

FIGURE 21.12. Hood/fender structure of Mercedes 124 series vehicle. (From Zuby et al.[25])

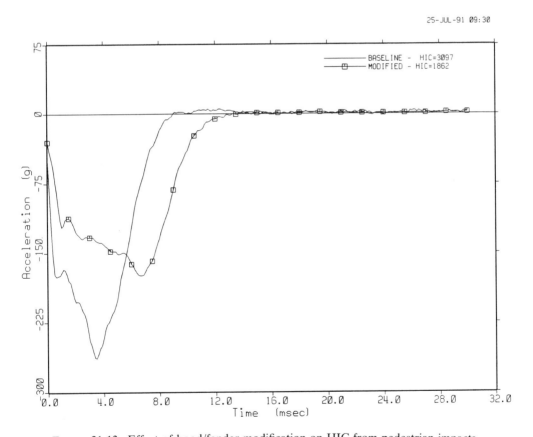

FIGURE 21.13. Effect of hood/fender modification on HIC from pedestrian impacts.

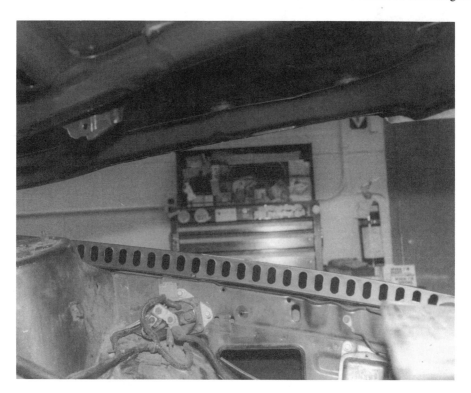

FIGURE 21.14. Ford Taurus hood/fender modifications.

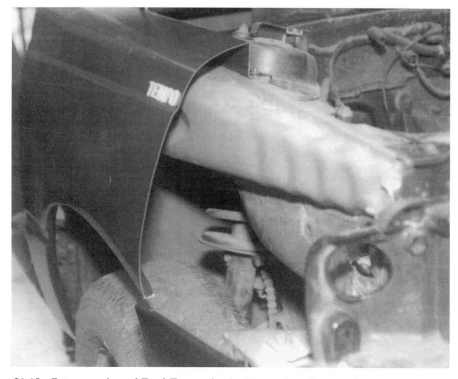

FIGURE 21.15. Cut-away view of Ford Tempo fender illustrating absence of up-standing apron flange.

between wiper hub and reinforcement cross member than was available in the 123 series vehicles.[24] NHTSA researchers have considered replacing the upper portion of the heavy sheet steel fire wall of the Taurus with a frangible seal. Figure 21.16 shows the head form acceleration and HIC for rear hood impacts with an intact upper fire wall compared to the results from impacts without the upper fire wall. These results suggest that HIC values below 1,000 at 37 km/h impact velocity, are quite possible in the rear hood regions of typical production vehicles.

Thorax Injury Research

Thorax Impact Simulation

Component testing is also an effective way to simulate pedestrian thorax impacts against vehicle surfaces. Developing the test technology is more difficult than for the head. Thoracic surrogates suitable for injury assessment must have human-like force-deflection responses, whereas the head can be treated as essentially rigid. Also, thorax responses and injury criteria are not well defined for children, despite their frequency as accident victims.

The NHTSA developed a family of thoracic surrogates to simulate pedestrian impacts in the laboratory.[26,27] Configurations representing 3-, 6-, 9-, and 12-year-old children and the 50th percentile adult male have been constructed. Because pedestrians generally travel a path perpendicular to that of the striking vehicle,[28] the surrogates were developed to simulate the most representative accident condition, a lateral impact to the chest. The component test devices are designed to represent a distributed loading condition with full thoracic involvement for each age group. The

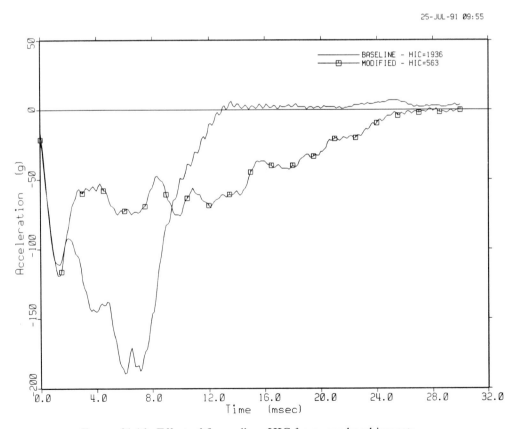

FIGURE 21.16. Effect of fire wall on HIC from rear hood impacts.

design is based on a lumped mass analytical model of the human thorax.

Figure 21.17 shows the adult thoracic surrogate. A round metal plate and guide rods represent the effective rib mass. The carriage with its accompanying weights represents the spine and remaining effective thoracic mass. A closed cell polyethylene foam is used to simulate both the stiffness and damping characteristics of the ribs and the thoracic viscera. A smaller and less dense piece of foam is covered by "dummy skin" to simulate the skin and muscles exterior to the ribs.

The biofidelity of a dummy or component test device rests in its ability to accurately reproduce human-like responses. The parameters used to evaluate the impact biofidelity of these thoracic surrogates include the acceleration and relative displacement of the rib and spine masses and the reaction force. Because of the variability of test results with cadavers or other biological specimens, ranges are used to create a standard for evaluating the accuracy of impact test devices.

The Association Peugeot-Renault (APR) measured reaction forces and the physical displacement of the chest wall in a series of cadaver drop tests; the International Standards Organization (ISO) developed thoracic surrogate response recommendations from this data.[29] Figure 21.18 illustrates that the force response of the adult pedestrian thoracic surrogate lies near the ISO corridor for a 22.5-km/h, 2-m drop. Figure 21.19 shows the response of the pedestrian surrogate compared to an ISO corridor developed from 27 km/h side impact simulation sled tests. The NHTSA developed another set of recommended responses from similar side impact simulations with cadavers.[30,31] The reaction forces and accelerations of the ribs and spine were measured. Figures 21.20 and 21.21 compare the upper rib and spine acceleration responses of the pedestrian thoracic surrogate with the recommended response developed by NHTSA.

A comparable body of data for evaluating biofidelity of the child thoracic surrogates does not exist. Little or no information exists for child impact response characteristics. Hamilton et al.[32] used a scaling technique with the force and deflection data of the ISO drop tests to develop impact responses for 3-, 6-, 9-, and 12-year-old children. His technique accounted for differences in physiology between children and adults as well as age and

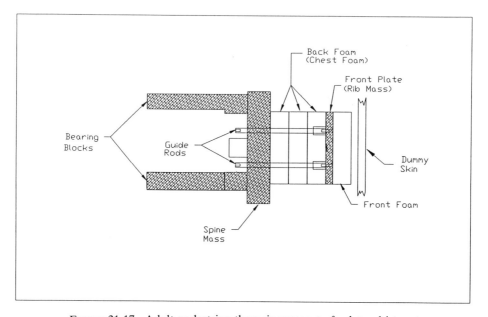

FIGURE 21.17. Adult pedestrian thoracic surrogate for lateral impact.

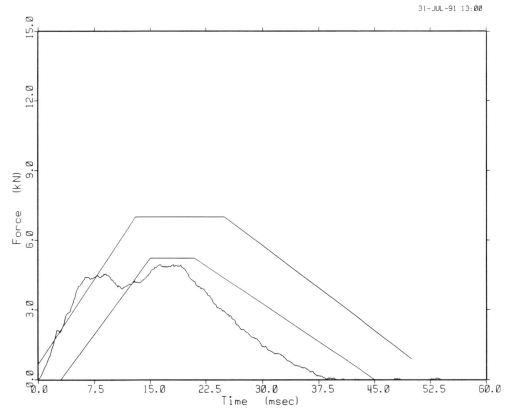

31-JUL-91 13:00

FIGURE 21.18. Adult pedestrian surrogate response and ISO force corridor for 22.5 km/h, drop test condition.

weight differences. The scaled responses were used to design the child thoracic surrogates. Figures 21.22 and 21.23 compare the cadaveric force and deflection from a 23-km/h, 2-m drop scaled to represent thoracic response of the 3-year-old. The responses of the 3-year-old pedestrian thoracic surrogate are included for comparison.

The thoracic surrogates are laboratory test devices that are capable of consistent, repeatable, and reproducible human-like impact responses. They simulate impact conditions with distributed loading. Injury criteria are used to relate measured forces, displacements, and accelerations to probable injury severity levels. The injury criteria used in assessing thoracic injury for pedestrians are the same criteria used for vehicle occupants in side collisions: the Thoracic Trauma Index (TTI), Viscous Injury Criterion (V*C), and crush.

The TTI is an acceleration based criterion with modifying factors to account for age and size.[30,31] The kernel value [TTI(d)][33] currently used to evaluate occupant protection in side collisions is the average of the maximum filtered spine and rib accelerations. A TTI value of less than 85g has been proposed as the maximum exposure for adult crash test dummies.

Crush is a deflection-based criterion that measures chest compression.[34] It is usually expressed as a percentage of the test subject's chest dimension. The criterion is based on correlation between chest deflection and the occurrence of rib fractures that are associated with other thoracic injuries. Chest deflections in the range of 28% to 35% generally represent AIS-3 level injuries in adults.

The Viscous Injury Criterion (V*C) is a deflection-based criterion that includes the

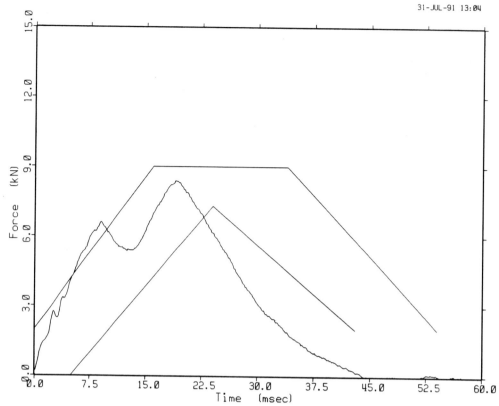

FIGURE 21.19. Adult pedestrian surrogate response and ISO force corridor for 27 km/h, sled test condition.

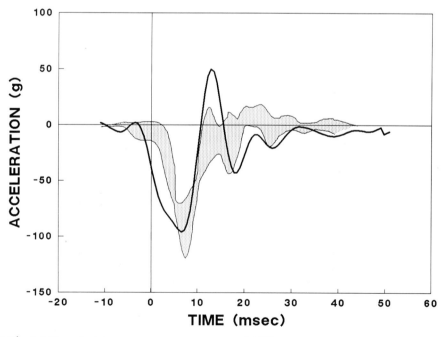

FIGURE 21.20. Adult pedestrian surrogate response and NHTSA upper rib acceleration corridor for 27 km/h, sled test condition.

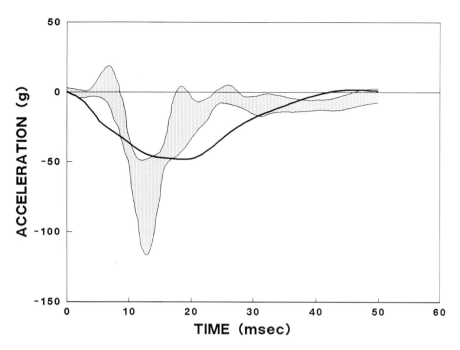

FIGURE 21.21. Adult pedestrian surrogate response and NHTSA spine acceleration corridor for 27 km/h, sled test condition.

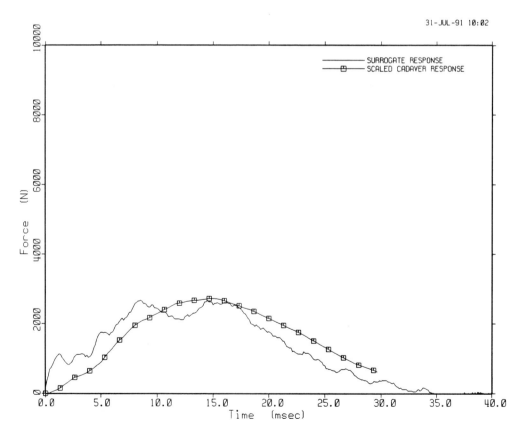

FIGURE 21.22. A 3-year-old pedestrian surrogate response and scaled cadaver thoracic force for 22.4-km/h, 2-m drop test condition.

31-JUL-91 15:00

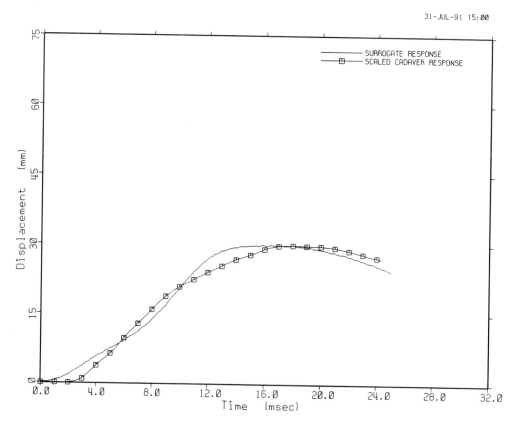

FIGURE 21.23. A 3-year-old pedestrian surrogate response and scaled cadaver thoracic displacement for 22.4-km/h, 2-m drop test condition.

contributing factor of velocity to injury.[35,36] The amount of crush, expressed as a percentage of the half chest breadth, and the crush rate are multiplied to calculate V*C. A value of 1 m/sec is believed to represent the onset of serious injury.

Accident reconstructions were performed by the NHTSA to develop a relationship between measurable criteria and injury severity for children. Pedestrian accidents in which the impact conditions and resulting vehicle damage were well documented were selected for reconstruction. Because the vehicles were only moderately damaged by the child pedestrians, it was difficult to evaluate the accuracy of the reconstructions. The injury data from the laboratory tests were quite scattered and the results were limited to approximate threshold values for serious injury. The onset of serious injury for children seemed to occur at

lower levels than for adults. The threshold values were 60g for TTI, 25% for crush, and 0.38 m/sec for V*C.[37]

Production Vehicle Testing

After developing the equipment and procedures to simulate pedestrian thorax impact, a representative sample of the current production vehicle fleet was tested to establish a general performance level and determine what vehicle design features may affect injury severity levels. Early problem identification studies indicated that thoracic injuries caused by impact with the vehicle face region comprised a significant segment of the total pedestrian injuries. To address this issue, the initial series of testing simulated small children being struck by the vehicle face with full thoracic involvement and no wraparound to the upper hood surface. The chest height of small children is at or below the height of the leading edge of the hood, and little or no rotation of the upper body is observed at impact. Therefore, the thorax impact speed is assumed to be essentially the same as the vehicle speed. Twenty-four cars and five LTVs were tested over a range of impact speeds.[38]

The results of the fascia tests demonstrated the relative aggressiveness of rigid structures common to the front-end design of most passenger vehicles. Such features as soft fascias, frangible headlight covers, and non-rigid headlight housings were less hostile, but even the best-performing vehicles produced injury levels that exceeded threshold values for impacts over 29 km/h. The three injury criteria showed similar results. Figure 21.24 shows the range of values for chest deflection expressed as a percentage of half the chest breadth plotted against test speed. This illustrates the potential injury reduction that could be realized if all vehicles performed as well as the best-performing vehicle. Despite this possibility for significant injury reduction, vehicle faces still present a high potential of severe thorax injury for small children impacted at speeds over 29 km/h.

The front profiles of passenger cars have changed significantly in recent years. Today's hoods are lower and leading hood edges are much less prominent. As a result, a smaller portion of the child pedestrian population will encounter full thoracic impact with the fascia of the car. The increased slopes of many current hood designs raise the probability that the child's thorax will contact the relatively flat hood surface of the car. This type of impact is typically seen with an adult victim.

Impact onto the upper hood surfaces of a vehicle offers several potential benefits. The hood structure is less rigid than the vehicle face, allowing more dynamic deflection. The upper surfaces are relatively flat and smooth, and tend to distribute the impact loading more uniformly. Finally, the velocity of the thorax impact should be significantly reduced from the initial vehicle/pedestrian impact velocity as the upper body rotates onto the hood of the vehicle.

Current testing being conducted by the NHTSA simulates 6-year-old, 12-year-old, and adult pedestrian impacts into the upper hood and fender surfaces of contemporary vehicles. Full lateral thoracic involvement normal to the hood surface is assumed with lower hood

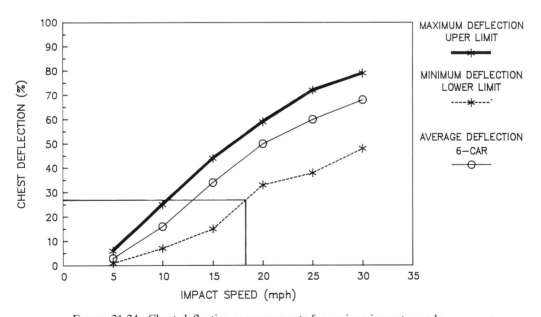

FIGURE 21.24. Chest deflection measurements for various impact speeds.

profiles of current production vehicles. Most of the 6-year-old child impacts occur on the upper surfaces of the front fascia or the forwardmost surfaces of the hood and fender. The target areas for 12-year-old child and adult thoracic impact simulations are the hood and fender surface. This overlaps the regions addressed by the head impact studies. An important consideration of future testing will be determining what effects head injury countermeasure designs have on thorax injury severity levels.

The initial impact speed for these upper surface tests is 32 km/h. Preliminary results indicate that this speed will produce a range of thorax injury levels about the threshold values.

Lower Limb Injury Research

Injuries to the pedestrian lower limb rarely pose as serious a threat to life as injuries to the head and thorax. However, the leg is the body region most often severely injured. Generally, these injuries do not exceed an AIS 3; thus, the resulting harm is less than the harm associated with life-threatening head and thorax injuries. But, severe injury to the lower limb often results in long and difficult periods of rehabilitation for the victim. In many cases, pedestrian leg injuries result in some degree of disability or lead to future development of degenerative joint disease. This makes it difficult to accurately describe the societal costs of pedestrian lower limb injuries, but many researchers believe their importance may be underestimated. The costs of this disability and disease are not well known, but research is continuing on the development of new injury cost scales with the work of Yates et al.,[39] Zeidler et al.,[40] and States and Viano.[7]

Lower Limb Injury Tolerances

The success of research to prevent pedestrian lower limb injuries depends upon understanding the injury mechanisms and tolerances for the different structures of the leg. Two types of loads are considered significant causes of pedestrian leg injuries. First, lateral impact causes shear to occur when the bumper and

hood edge of the vehicle strike the leg. Both the femur and tibia might be affected, depending on the position of the pedestrian relative to the car. Lateral impact tolerances of the femur have been reported in the range of 3,500 to 7,500 Newtons (N) by Gibson et al.[41] Many sources agree that the average tolerance is about 4,000 N.

There seems to be some controversy about the tibia's tolerance to lateral impact. Cesari et al.[42] measured impact forces of 3,300 N in cadaver tests resulting in tibia fracture. Kajzer[43] suggested that 4,000 N would be a reasonable impact tolerance for the lower leg and tibia and others have concurred. These findings contrast with reports by Snider et al.,[44] who reported impact tolerance between 1,500 and 3,000 N for dynamic impact to the tibia. This difference may arise from differences in test procedure; Kajzer tested complete lower legs while Snider tested the tibia alone.

The second important mechanism causing lower limb injury is lateral bending. Bending not only contributes to long bone fractures, but also is considered the most important cause of injury to the knee and ankle joints. According to the parameters of a mathematical model developed by Fowler and Harris,[45] the bending tolerance is 212 N-m for the femur and 214 N-m for the tibia/fibula combination. Nyquist et al.[46] also tested the bending strength of the tibia during impact. They found tolerance levels somewhat higher than those used by Fowler and Harris, and they differentiated between tibias from males and females. The male bending strength was 320 N-m, while the female bending strength was only 280 N-m. Examples of serious knee injuries include intra-articular fracture and ligament tears. The strengths of several ligaments have been measured by Aldman et al.[47] Unfortunately, these data cannot be used to predict the injury tolerances without an accurate kinematic model of the knee structure, which has not been developed.

The bending response and tolerance of the ankle and knee joints are not well known. While ankle injuries occur very rarely to pedestrians, knee injuries are quite common; therefore, understanding the knee response is critical. The load mechanism being studied is a lateral bending of the extended knee, which can cause damage for small deformations. The most commonly reported value for the onset of serious injury from lateral bending is 200 N-m. This load corresponds to about 6° of angular deflection.

Leg Impact Simulations

The pedestrian lower limb impact can be simulated through mathematical modeling, cadaver experiments, full-scale dummy tests, or component testing. The benefits and short-comings of these approaches, as applied to head impact simulation, generally apply to the leg impact problem as well. Additional efforts have been made, however, with regard to using full-scale dummies in simulating the bumper/leg impact.

Cadaver legs bend significantly in pedestrian impact simulations because the bones fracture or the knee joint fails. Standard test dummies cannot reproduce these effects because they lack lateral knee compliance. Several modifications for dummy knees have been proposed to deal with this problem.

One modification was described by Pritz.[48] A short length of half inch diameter threaded rod was added just below the standard knee. Under sufficient lateral loads, this modified knee deformed plastically. The length of rod was determined by force-rotation measurements taken from cadaver tests and further verified by quasi-static tests of intact cadaver legs.

Another effort by Fowler and Harris[45] added an additional joint near knee level that would allow lateral rotation. The torque required to initiate rotation was controlled by adjustable clutch plates, which were normally set to allow rotation for torques greater than 200 N-m. An advantage of this modification was that the plates retained their maximum amount of rotation.

Even with the modified knees described above, full dummies only roughly approximated the response of cadavers in full-scale pedestrian tests. Therefore, researchers have concentrated their efforts on developing component test devices, each of which would simulate only a part of the pedestrian impact. The head and thorax impactors described earlier in this chapter are examples of component devices.

The modified knee joint of Bunketorp et al.[49] consisted of a central ball and socket joint constrained on either side by simulated collateral ligaments made of copper (Fig. 21.25). The joint was designed to simulate the structure of the knee. This research tool was used to determine the effects of various loads on different parts of the knee joint. Bunketorp et al. also used cadaveric lower limbs with a weight added through a ball joint at the top of the leg to simulate the body mass. The cadaveric legs were used to study injuries that occurred due to various pedestrian impact loading patterns.

Pritz and Pereira[50] developed a device to simulate the upper leg impact into the hood edge. It was a single segment device that could be launched into the hood edge of a vehicle to measure the load imparted to a pedestrian in an impact. Cadaver tests provided data for determining the effective mass and surface material stiffness of the projectile. A drawing of this impactor is shown in Fig. 21.26.

A newer model of the lower limb was developed by Aldman et al.[51] This model incorporated the knee joint modification made by Pritz with some of the simplifications of the earlier cadaver leg tests. As in the cadaver leg tests, the upper body was represented only by a lumped mass connected to the lower limb through a ball joint. The segments of the lower leg had masses and centers of gravity similar to those of the average human, but with a simplified construction. They were rotationally symmetric and used steel tubes as bones that were covered with a layer of foam to give appropriate impact response. The knee was instrumented with strain gauges to measure loads (see Fig. 21.27).

Cesari et al.[52] incorporated the above model into a device called the Rotationally Symmetric Pedestrian Dummy (RSPD). New aspects of the model include the addition of a plastically deforming ankle joint and a wooden foot. The ankle joint will deform plastically under a

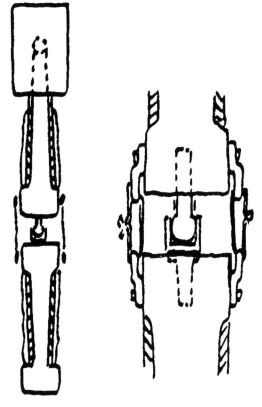

FIGURE 21.25. Aldman and Bunketorp's early component lower leg test device. (From Pritz and Pereira.[50])

moment of 40 N-m, while the knee joint deforms when the moment reaches 70 N-m. In addition, the masses of the RSPD leg have been increased by a factor of 1.5 because the RSPD is actually a simplified full pedestrian dummy, which simulates both legs of the pedestrian with a single structure.

Currently, the designs of the upper and lower leg impactors are being updated. Early testing of a lower limb impactor is under way at Institute National de Recherche sur les Transports et lur Securite (INRETS).[53] This work, led by Cesari, has resulted in a lower limb model consisting of two segments joined by a plastically deforming knee joint. The segment masses are based on the Hybrid III 50th percentile dummy, with the lower segment containing the mass of the foot. The knee now consists of two separate bending

elements, and deforms plastically under a load of 200 N-m. The dynamic rotation of each of the segments can be measured during the test. In addition, static shear deformation is measured and impact forces are determined based on the segment accelerations and masses. Finally, the impactor requires less space and energy, because it is a free-flying device.

A new upper leg impactor based on Pritz's design, currently under development by Harris and Lawrence, will attempt to deal with two problems. Its effective mass will not simply be a function of the pedestrian size, but also a function of the vehicle geometry. Furthermore, the geometry will also be used to determine the direction and location of impact.

Impact Simulation Results and Findings

The component test devices described above were used to study vehicle parameters to determine their influence on the loads transferred to the bones and joints of the leg during an impact. These parameters can be divided into two broad categories: vehicle front end geometry, and front end compliance.

Early researchers identified several vehicle geometric parameters thought to be important in determining pedestrian lower limb injuries. Two critical vehicle parameters for lower leg and knee injuries are the bumper height and lead. Definitions of these measurements are shown in Fig. 21.28.

The likelihood of knee injury is greatest when the bumper impact occurs directly to the knee. When this happens, several severe failures of the joint may occur. The force of high-speed impacts will cause the joint surfaces themselves to fracture. If the impact speed is lower, the forced bending of the knee leads to severe ligament damage. In some cases, both types of injury occur. These severe injuries are also associated with damage to important nerves and blood vessels that pass through the knee region. Many of these injuries can lead to long-term and sometimes permanent disability or degenerative joint disease. Most require surgical reduction. The effects of such an

FIGURE 21.26. Pritz/upper leg component test device. (From Cesari et al.[52])

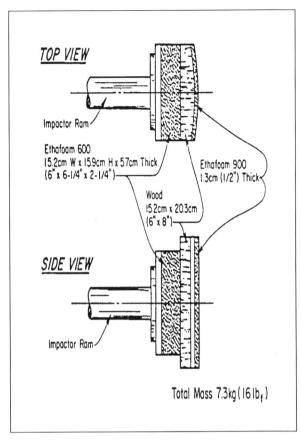

impact are generally worse when the bumper lead is large.

Studies by Aldman et al.[47,51] and Bunketorp et al.[49] have shown that the load transferred to the knee is lowest when the center of the bumper impact occurs below the knee, just above the center of gravity of the lower leg. Unfortunately, currently regulated bumper heights are about the same height as the knee of the 50th percentile male. Other researchers have shown that a softer secondary bumper or substructure mounted just below and about 5 to 15 mm ahead of standard bumpers could reduce the severity of pedestrian lower leg injuries. The secondary bumper may be more beneficial than a lower primary bumper.

Even with lower bumpers, violent impacts are likely to cause fractures of the lower leg. Impacts with rigid surfaces at high speeds produce fragmented fractures, which are associated with serious soft tissue injury. Broader impact surfaces might be employed to avoid such severe injuries. This idea is compatible with the secondary bumper modification previously described.

Hood edge height and contour are the most important parameters to consider for injuries to the upper leg and pelvis. It has been observed that the most severe pelvis and thigh injuries suffered by adult pedestrians are caused by vehicles with square profiled hood edges that are 85 to 100 cm high. In addition, such vehicles generally are worse for the child thorax. Hip and thigh injuries can be reduced by lowering and rounding the profile of the hood edge. However, such changes are also important in determining the severity of head and thorax injuries. Thus, hood edge designs

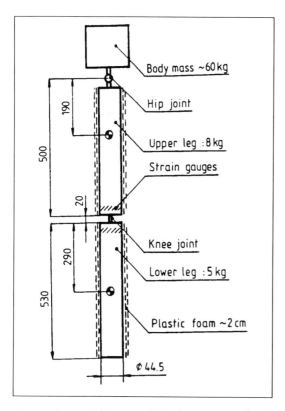

FIGURE 21.27. Aldman and Bunketorp's rotationally symmetric lower leg component test device. (From Cesari et al.[52])

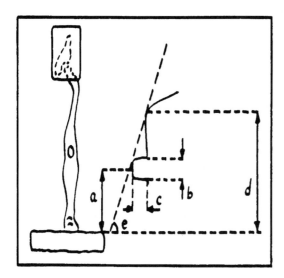

FIGURE 21.28. Important vehicle front parameters in pedestrian lower limb testing. (From Cesari et al.[52]) a = bumper level; b = bumper width; c = bumper lead distance; d = bonnet edge height; e = bumper lead angle (front inclination angle).

for pedestrian injury mitigation must consider the entire pedestrian problem.

Early pedestrian researchers thought that the primary vehicle parameter that influenced pedestrian injury was the compliance of the vehicle. However, significant changes in compliance are difficult to achieve because bumpers are required to protect the car in low-speed collisions. It was found that even vehicles with the softest allowable front designs cause severe injuries in pedestrian tests. Nonetheless, some improvements to vehicle compliance in conjunction with geometric modifications could be helpful in reducing pedestrian lower limb injury. Softer front structures would be less likely to cause compound fractures and soft tissue injuries, thus reducing overall healing time and disability.

As stated earlier, current bumper heights are about the same as that of the 50th percentile adult knee. Lowering bumpers, however, could benefit pedestrians and vehicle occupants as well. In particular, the occupants of the struck vehicles in side impacts would be less likely to suffer injuries if bumper heights more closely matched vehicle sill heights. Studies from the National Accident Sampling System (NASS) have shown that the rate of serious injuries in vehicles struck in the side by the fronts of cars with minimum bumper heights (203 to 302 mm) is less than one-third that for cars struck in the side by the fronts of cars with maximum bumper heights (406 to 531 mm). Similarly, the cars with high bumpers cause severe injury more than twice as often as cars with bumper heights of 305 to 404 mm in similar side impacts.

Future Research Needs

Although significant progress has been made in addressing the pedestrian injury problem, much remains to be done. In this section, the authors describe the research and development activities that are most needed.

New in-depth pedestrian accident investigations should be conducted. Information from accident studies has been valuable in formulating effective research to reduce pedestrian trauma. Some aspects of the problem, however, are changing. Vehicle designs and materials are different than those of 10 to 20 years ago. Front profiles of cars are much lower and smoother; hoods are generally shorter; "soft" plastics are used extensively in fascia designs; and plastic body panels are becoming more prevalent every year. Vehicle distribution and use are also shifting. LTVs appear in greater numbers and are primarily used as personal and family vehicles, rather than commercial vehicles. These changes emphasize the importance of continuing efforts to collect updated pedestrian accident data, so that research efforts can be refined to increase their effectiveness.

An injury impairment scale is needed. The NHTSA essentially was limited to using harm to determine research priorities for addressing various pedestrian body regions, because the initial work to establish levels of injury impairment was not refined. Consideration of impairment is especially important for the pedestrian trauma problem. Head and thorax injuries produce approximately equivalent harm, but recent work indicates that moderate (AIS 2) brain injury can have long-term impairment consequences,[7] an outcome unlikely for moderate thorax trauma. Lower extremity injuries greatly outnumber head and thorax injuries, but result in much less harm, because of significantly lower injury severity levels. Leg injuries involving joints (e.g., the knee), however, can lead to permanent impairment and resulting disability, even though injury severity may be moderate. Thus, an injury impairment scale would be valuable for obtaining improved comparisons of the consequences of trauma to different body regions, and, therefore, establishing more accurate pedestrian research priorities.

Improved computer simulations of the vehicle/pedestrian collision should be developed. These models typically are used to determine head and thorax impact velocities, which are affected by vehicle/pedestrian collision speed, vehicle geometry, fascia stiffness, and other parameters. The accuracy of these predictions has been limited by the difficulty in formulating models that closely simulate the complex collision event. Large kinematic differences occur between cadaver and dummy experiments from differences in stiffness, energy absorption, and flexibility of body segments of dummies and humans. Efforts are under way to create models that duplicate the kinematics resulting from vehicle/cadaver impact tests, rather than dummy tests, and to determine the value of three-dimensional, rather than two-dimensional, representations.

Cowls, fender tops, and the rear and side edges of hoods tend to be very stiff and need to be "softened" to reduce the threat of head injury to pedestrians. Recent tests with modified hood/fenders suggest that significant improvement is feasible. Impact tests suggest that plastic hoods and fenders, especially, need to be designed with greater attention given to pedestrian head protection.

As an understanding of pedestrian thorax injury threat from impact on hood and fender surfaces is developed, structural modifications will be studied. Thorax injury countermeasures will have to be compatible with changes made to improve head protection. If the two requirements conflict, some compromises based on the relative societal consequences may be necessary.

Although prototype component test devices are being developed, more work is needed before they can be used to test and evaluate vehicles for their potential in causing leg injury. The knee in particular is considered the most vulnerable leg region; accurately simulating knee injury is complex, and requires properly duplicating joint articulation. Furthermore, the injury tolerance of the knee joint is not well defined. Once completed, leg impactors should be used to develop and evaluate vehicle concepts for reducing pedestrian lower extremity trauma. Countermeasures to protect pedestrians need to be examined for their potential compatibility with side impact occupant protection. Lowered vehicle profiles and reduced bumper heights, for example, have been cited in the literature as potentially beneficial to both pedestrians and vehicle occupants in side collisions.

Conclusion

Pedestrian trauma inflicted by motor vehicles is a serious national problem. The resulting human suffering affects tens of thousands of lives every year in the United States alone, and is especially tragic when children are the victims.

Recent research indicates that injury severity is strongly influenced by vehicle design, and can be greatly reduced by altering designs in ways that are technically feasible and cost-effective. Results of this research should dispel the commonly held notion that the only viable solution to the pedestrian injury problem is preventing the accidents.

Greater awareness of the role of vehicle design is an essential first step in seeking solutions. By considering pedestrian protection in the early stages of new vehicle development, manufacturers can incorporate safer structures with little or no increased cost. This process can begin now. As research progresses and new understanding is gained, even safer designs will evolve.

Everyone in the motor vehicle research community plays an important role. Continued efforts by researchers in government, the motor vehicle industry, and the private sector are essential to developing effective vehicle-based injury countermeasures to reduce pedestrian trauma.

References

1. Fatal Accident Reporting System 1989. A decade of progress. National Highway Traffic Safety Administration, DOT HS 807 693, March 1991.
2. Office of Regulatory Analysis, Plans and Policy, National Highway Traffic Safety Administration. Analysis of target population—injuries received by contacting the hood, upper fender and cowl of passenger cars and light trucks. January 1990 (unpublished).
3. MacLaughlin TF, Hoyt TA, Chu S-M. NHTSA's Advanced Pedestrian Protection Program. Eleventh International Technical Conference on Experimental Safety Vehicles, National Technical Information Service, Springfield, VA, 1987.
4. Hoyt TA, T01 report—problem determination—vehicle/pedestrian collisions. National Highway Traffic Safety Administration, March 1985 (unpublished).
5. Malliaris AG, Hitchcock RJ, Hedlund JH. A search for priorities in crash protection. SAE 820242. Crash Protection SP-513. Society of Automotive Engineers, Warredale, PA, 1982.
6. Genarelli TA, et al. The Abbreviated Injury Scale, 1985 revision. The American Association of Automotive Medicine, Arlington Heights, IL, 1985.
7. States JD, Viano DC. Injury impairment and disability scales to assess the permanent consequences of trauma. Accident analysis and prevention. Vol 22, No. 2. Pergamon Press, Great Britain, pp 151–160, 1990.
8. Pritz HB. Comparison of the dynamic responses of anthropometric test devices and human anatomic specimens in experimental pedestrian impacts. Twenty-Second Stapp Car Crash Conference P-77. Society of Automotive Engineers, Inc., Warrendale, PA, SAE 780894, 1978.
9. King AI, Krieger KW, Padgaonker AJ. Full-scale experimental simulation of pedestrian-vehicle impacts. Twentieth Stapp Car Crash Conference P-66. Society of Automotive Engineers, Inc., Warrendale, PA, SAE 760813, 1976.
10. Brun-Cassan F, et al. Comparison of experimental collisions performed with various modified side impact dummies and cadavers. Twenty-Eighth Stapp Car Crash Conference Proceedings P-152. Society of Automotive Engineers, Inc., Warrendale, PA, SAE 841664, 1984.
11. Van Wijk J, Wismans J, Wittebrood L. MADYMO pedestrian simulations. Pedestrian Impact Injury and Assessment P-121. Society of Automotive Engineers, Inc., Warrendale, PA, SAE 830060, 1983.
12. Hoyt TA, Chu S-M. Analytical pedestrian accident reconstruction using computer simulation. (Report# DOT HS 806 970.) National Technical Information Service, Springfield, VA, 1986.
13. Pritz HB. Effects of hood and fender design on pedestrian head protection. (Report# DOT HS 806 537.) National Technical Information Service, Springfield, VA, 1984.
14. Cavallero C, et al. Improvement of pedestrian safety: influence of shape of passenger car-front structures upon pedestrian kinematics and injuries: evaluation based on 50 cadaver tests.

Pedestrian Impact Injury and Assessment P-121, Society of Automotive Engineers, Inc., Warrendale, PA, SAE 830624, 1983.

15. Pritz HB. Experimental investigation of pedestrian head impacts on hoods and fenders of production vehicles. Society of Automotive Engineers, Warrendale, PA, SAE 830055, 1983.

16. Brooks DL, Collins JA, Guenther DA. Experimental reconstructions of real world pedestrian head impacts. (DOT/NHTSA Basic Agreement #DTNH22-83-A-072779, VRTC Task Order #OSU-84-4059.) The Ohio State University, Columbus, OH, 1985.

17. Gadd CW. Use of a weighted impulse criterion for estimating injury hazard. *Proceedings of the Tenth Stapp Car Crash Conference* P-12. Society of Automotive Engineers, New York, NY, SAE 660793, 1966.

18. Stalnaker RL, McElahney JH, Roberts VL. MSC tolerance curve for head impacts. ASME paper ul-WA/BHF-10. American Society of Mechanical Engineers, New York, NY, 1971.

19. Saul RA. An overview of the mean strain criterion development. National Highway Traffic Safety Administration, October 1991 (unpublished).

20. Hoyt TA, MacLaughlin TF, Kessler JW. Experimental pedestrian accident reconstructions—head impacts. (Report# DOT HS 807 288.) National Technical Information Service, Springfield, VA, 1988.

21. MacLaughlin TF, Kessler JW. Pedestrian head impact against the central hood of motor vehicles—test procedure and results. *Thirty-Fourth Stapp Car Crash Conference Proceedings* P-236. Society of Automotive Engineers, Inc., Warrendale, PA, SAE 902315, 1990.

22. Kessler JW, Hoyt TA, Monk MW. Pedestrian head injury reduction concepts. (#DOT HS 807 432.) National Technical Information Service, Springfield, VA, 1988.

23. Kessler JW. Development of countermeasures to reduce pedestrian head injury. *Eleventh International Technical Conference on Experimental Safety Vehicles—Proceedings.* National Technical Information Service, Springfield, VA, 1987.

24. Sturtz G. Experimental simulation of the pedestrian impact. Tenth International Technical Conference on Experimental Safety Vehicles (DOT HS 806 916). National Technical Information Service, Springfield, VA, 1986.

25. Zuby DS, Elias JC, Tanner CB, MacLaughlin TF. NHTSA pedestrian protection programs—status report. National Highway Traffic Safety Administration, September 1991 (unpublished).

26. Hamilton MN. Experimental study of thoracic injury in child pedestrians. *Eleventh International Conference on Experimental Safety Vehicles—Proceedings.* National Technical Information Service, Springfield, VA, 1987.

27. Hamilton MN, Wiechel JF, Guenther DA. Development of a child lateral thoracic impactor. *Passenger comfort, convenience and safety: test tools and procedures* P-174. Society of Automotive Engineers, Warrendale, PA, SAE 860368, 1986.

28. Brooks D, Wiechel J, Sens M, Guenther D. A comprehensive review of pedestrian impact reconstruction. *Accident reconstruction: automobiles, tractor-semitrailers, motorcycles, and pedestrians* P-193. Society of Automotive Engineers, Inc., Warrendale, PA, SAE 870605, 1987.

29. ISO recommendations for body segment response in lateral impacts. ISO/TC22/SC12/WG5, Document N139, February, 1987.

30. Eppinger RH, Morgan RM, Marcus JH. Development of dummy and injury index for NHTSA's thoracic side impact protection research program. *SAE transactions.* Vol 93. Society of Automotive Engineers, Warrendale, PA, SAE 840885, 1984.

31. Morgan RM, Marcus JH, Eppinger RH. Side impact—the biofidelity of NHTSA's proposed ATD and efficacy of TTI. *Proceedings of the Thirtieth Stapp Car Crash Conference* P-189. Society of Automotive Engineers, Warrendale, PA, SAE 861877, 1986.

32. Hamilton MN, Chew H, Guenther DA. Adult to child scaling and normalization of lateral thoracic impact data. *Proceedings of the Thirtieth Stapp Car Crash Conference* P-189. Society of Automotive Engineers, Warrendale, PA, 1986.

33. Federal Register Part II Department of Transportation, National Highway Traffic Safety Administration. 49 CFR Parts 571, et al., Federal Motor Vehicle Safety Standards; Side Impact Protection; Rules, Vol 55. No. 210, Oct 30, 1990 Rules and Regulations pp 45722–45780.

34. Melvin JW, Webber K. Review of biomechanical response and injury in the automotive environment. *The engineering design, development, testing and evaluation of an advanced anthropomorphic test device, phase 1: concept*

definition (DOT HS 807 224). National Technical Information Service, Springfield, VA, 1988.

35. Viano DC, Lau IV. Thoracic impact: a viscous tolerance criterion. Tenth International Technical Conference on Experimental Safety Vehicles (DOT HS 806 916). National Technical Information Service, Springfield, VA, 1986.

36. Lau IV, Viano DC. The viscous criterion—basis and applications of an injury severity index for soft tissues. *Proceedings of the Thirtieth Stapp Car Crash Conference* P-189. Society of Automotive Engineers, Warrendale, PA, 1986.

37. Elias JC, Monk MW, Hamilton MN. Experimental child pedestrian accident reconstruction—thoracic impact (Report #DOT HS 807 420). National Technical Information Service, Springfield, VA, 1988.

38. Elias JC, Monk MW. NHTSA pedestrian thoracic injury mitigation program—status report. Proceedings of the Twelfth International Conference on Experimental Safety Vehicles, 1989.

39. Yates DW, et al. A system for measuring the severity of temporary and permanent disability after injury. *Proceedings of the 33rd Annual Meeting of the Association for the Advancement of Automotive Medicine.* Association for the Advancement of Automotive Medicine, Arlington Heights, IL, 1989.

40. Zeidler F, et al. Development of a new injury cost scale. *Proceedings of the 33rd Annual Meeting of the Association for the Advancement of Automotive Medicine.* Association for the Advancement of Automotive Medicine, Arlington Heights, IL, 1989.

41. Gibson TJ, Hinrichs RW, McLean AJ. Pedestrian head impacts: development and validation of a mathematical model. *Proceedings of the 1986 IRCOBI Conference—Zurich, Switzerland.* IRCOBI Secretariat, BRON, France, 1986.

42. Cesari D, Cavallero H, Roche H. Mechanisms producing lower extremity injuries in pedestrian accident situations. *Proceedings of the 33rd Annual Meeting of the Association for the Advancement of Automotive Medicine.* Association for the Advancement of Automotive Medicine, Arlington Heights, IL, 1989.

43. Kajzer J. Bumper system evaluation using an experimental pedestrian dummy. *Proceedings, Twelfth International Technical Conference on Experimental Safety Vehicles* (U.S. G.P.O. 1990-268-345:20365). National Technical

Information Service, Springfield, VA, 1989.

44. Snider JN, Fuller PM, Wasserman JF. The response of the human lower leg to impact loading. *Proceedings, 1988 IRCOBI Conference—Bergisch Gledbach, W. Germany.* IRCOBI Secretariat, BRON, France, 1988.

45. Fowler JE, Harris J. Practical vehicle design for pedestrian protection. *Proceedings, Ninth International Technical Conference on Experimental Safety Vehicles.* National Technical Information Service, Springfield, VA, 1982.

46. Nyquist GW, et al. Tibia bending and response. *Proceedings, 29th Stapp Car Crash Conference* P-167. Society of Automotive Engineers, Warrendale, PA, SAE 851728, 1985.

47. Aldman B, Thorngren L, Bunketorp O, Romanus B. An experimental model system for the study of lower leg and knee injuries in car pedestrian accidents. *Proceedings, 1980 IRCOBI Conference—Oxford, England.* IRCOBI Secretariat, BRON, France, 1980.

48. Pritz HB. Comparison of the dynamic responses of anthropomorphic test devices and human anatomic specimens in experimental pedestrian impacts. *Proceedings of the 22nd Stapp Car Crash Conference* P-77. Society of Automotive Engineers, Warrendale, PA, SAE 781024, 1978.

49. Bunketorp O, Aldman B, Thorngren L, Romanus B. *Clinical and experimental studies on leg injuries in car-pedestrian accidents.* Society of Automotive Engineers, Warrendale, PA, SAE 826049, 1982.

50. Pritz HB, Pereira JM. Pedestrian hip impact simulator development and hood edge location consideration on injury severity. *Proceedings, 27th Stapp Car Crash Conference* P-134. Society of Automotive Engineers, Warrendale, PA, SAE 831627, 1983.

51. Aldman B, et al. Load transfer from the striking vehicle in side and pedestrian impacts. *Proceedings, Tenth International Technical Conference on Experimental Safety Vehicles* (DOT HS 806 916). National Technical Information Service, Springfield, VA, 1986.

52. Cesari D, Cavallero C, Roche H. Evaluation of the round symmetrical pedestrian dummy leg behavior. *Proceedings, Twelfth International Technical Conference on Experimental Safety Vehicles* (U.S. G.P.O. 1990-268-345:20365). National Technical Information Service, Springfield, VA, 1989.

53. Cesari D. Presentation at the 6th meeting of ISO/TC22/SC10/WG2, Columbus, Ohio, November 9, 1990.

Index